Essentials of Computers for Nurses

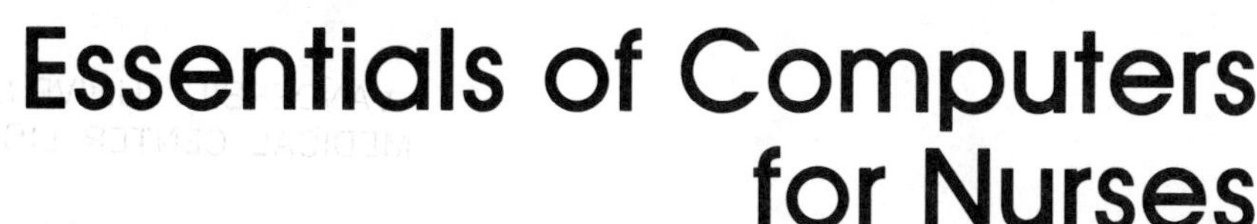

Essentials of Computers for Nurses

Virginia K. Saba, R.N., Ed.D.
Graduate Faculty
Georgetown University School of Nursing
Washington, DC

Kathleen Ann McCormick, R.N., Ph.D., F.A.A.N.
National Institutes of Health
National Institute on Aging
Gerontology Research Center
Baltimore, Maryland

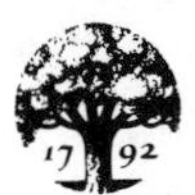

J. B. LIPPINCOTT COMPANY Philadelphia
London Mexico City New York St. Louis São Paulo Sydney

Sponsoring Editor: Diana Intenzo
Manuscript Editor: Elizabeth P. Lowe
Indexer: Carol M. Kosik
Design Director: Tracy Baldwin
Designer: Anne O'Donnell
Production Supervisor: J. Corey Gray
Production Coordinator: Barney Fernandes
Compositor: Progressive Typographers
Printer/Binder: R.R. Donnelley & Sons Company
Cover Printer: Philips Offset

The authors and publisher have exerted every effort to ensure that drug selection and dosage set forth in this text are in accord with current recommendations and practice at the time of publication. However, in view of ongoing research, changes in government regulations, and the constant flow of information relating to drug therapy and drug reactions, the reader is urged to check the package insert for each drug for any change in indications and dosage and for added warnings and precautions. This is particularly important when the recommended agent is a new or infrequently employed drug.

6 5 4 3 2 1

Library of Congress Cataloging in Publication Data

Saba, Virginia K.
Essentials of computers for nurses.

Includes bibliographies and index.
1. Nursing—Data processing. 2. Information storage and retrieval systems—Nursing. I. McCormick, Kathleen A. II. Title. [DNLM: 1. Computers—nurses' instruction. 2. Nursing. WY 26.5 S113e]
RT50.5.S23 1986 001.64'024613 85-10218
ISBN 0-397-54457-X

This book was written by Virginia K. Saba and Kathleen A. McCormick in their private capacity. No official support or endorsement by the U.S. Public Health Service or the National Institute on Aging is intended or should be inferred.

Foreword

There are no more timely topics than computers and the applications of computer technology to nursing. Once in a decade one is privileged to encounter a book that provides knowledge of new technology combined with its applications to a long-established profession. Such is *Essentials of Computers for Nurses,* authored by Dr. Virginia K. Saba and Dr. Kathleen A. McCormick, who are pioneers and authorities on computer technology in nursing. Both have been career nurses in the U.S. Public Health Service Commissioned Corps; Dr. Saba, formerly of the Division of Nursing, Health Resources and Services Administration, is now on the graduate faculty of Georgetown University School of Nursing while Dr. McCormick continues to serve in the Public Health Service at the National Institutes of Health. Their combined talents in computer technology, with Dr. Saba's additional education and experience in the area of scientific and technical information systems and Dr. McCormick's additional preparation as a nurse physiologist, give meaning to the phrase "high tech—high touch."

Through the efforts of these distinguished nurses and the innovative programs they have introduced in conjunction with other government officials, nurses both here and abroad are learning to become computer literate through national and international conferences, developmental research, and educational courses on the basic concepts and applications of computer technology to nursing. Dr. Saba spearheaded the nursing sessions at the Symposium on Computer Applications in Medical Care (SCAMC). She also was instrumental in the development of the first newsletter and journal in this field, *Computers in Nursing.* Drs. Saba and McCormick were both instrumental in establishing and leading the first national professional effort focused on computer applications in nursing: The American Nurses' Association Council on Computer Applications in Nursing.

The book provides comprehensive coverage of the information essential to understanding computers as well as state-of-the-art computer applications to nursing. The reader will find particularly helpful the historical perspective of the computer and its introduction into the field of nursing.

The authors describe computer elements and how they function and define and describe such terms as hardware, software, data processing, and systems theory. They also present details of computer systems currently in use in nursing. In addition, they explain how to develop computerized nursing information systems for all types of patient care facilities.

And now, while innovative technology is being developed rapidly, this book is fundamental in that it identifies and justifies a new direction in the nursing profession: it is responsive to technology while maintaining a level of care for the patient that is both compassionate and of high quality. With examples, illustrations, and tables, the authors show how computerized nursing information systems help nurses monitor the quality of care provided, evaluate the nursing process, and manage nursing services.

The authors accept computers as being capable of providing an important technology for health care. They have articulated the concepts of computer technology concretely and explicitly and specified what steps are necessary to develop nursing information systems and to make full use of emerging technologies. Most important, the reader can learn to deal with technological change and thus become an informed specialist or, in popular parlance, *computer literate.*

Another important aspect of this book is its implication of how federal health policies can influence the ways in which computer programs will develop. Such federal policies shape various strategies for ensuring the delivery of optimal care in the most cost-effective way. The federal government has financed the assessment, implementation, and evaluation of computer technology in hospitals, communities, schools of nursing, and research centers.

Each of these programs has demanded manpower and resources. If we analyzed the megatrends of computer-related policy, we would uncover new laws, new programs, and new resources being targeted for computer technology in the future. Thus, public policy objectives identify the issues that are raised on the public agenda, the process by which laws are passed committing resources to programs that affect people, the development or withdrawal of rules and regulations that interpret laws, the process of program implementation, and the evaluation of the usefulness of a program. Those knowledgeable in computer technology will have greater opportunities for input into public policy formulation. This textbook describes how computers will influence public policy and characterizes several current federally funded programs that use computer technology.

The impact of computers on health care delivery cannot be separated from the costs of health care. Economic considerations have become dominant in public policy formulation in health. Computers can be used in the implementation of the diagnosis related groups (DRGs) as cost-saving technology to provide information on the magnitude of health expenditures; to identify inflationary budgets; and to provide cost-effective, timely information needed to evaluate actual expenditures for nursing services.

There are potential limitations to a full commitment by the nursing profession to computer technology, but by highlighting them, as the authors have, nurses and health policy officials can plan strategies to accomplish professional goals by using the technologies appropriately. For example, nurses may overestimate the capacity of the federal government to affect nursing practice through the increased support of technology. There is, however, a major emphasis today on diminishing the federal role and expanding health programs at the state and local levels. In addition to the role of states, the importance of private industry in health care has also increased. One nursing strategy identified in this book shows how to work more closely with the private sector—the computer industry—in the development of nursing information systems for patient care. Many policy decisions made by industry have had an important impact on the applications of computers in nursing. Many of those decisions have also had an impact on the policy decisions and resources committed by the federal government.

This is an appropriate time to assess recent developments related to computers in health care to determine the direction in which we will be, or ought to be, headed during the next decade. As we approach the year 2000, any changes that might occur in nursing education, practice, research, and administration will be occurring simultaneously as changes occur in the attitude of the American people toward computer technology. Some will favor the changes and others will not.

Furthermore, the book deals with the ripple effect of the computerized nursing information systems. These systems have increasingly moved into hospitals and also into community health care agencies, nursing schools, and research centers. As their use expands from hospitals — where they have been most in vogue — we find them in home care programs, in health maintenance organizations (HMOs), day care centers for the young and the elderly, and even in birthing centers. Hence, the authors review the use of computers in hospitals and in the community to determine how this technology can improve the continuity of care from home to hospital and back home again.

With each expansion come new questions about personnel, resources, public policy, accessibility, and economics. Thus, we find new regulations, new laws, and new evaluations are developing that impact nursing. The authors therefore explore such questions as how computers will change the nursing process, help identify inflationary budgets, provide cost-effective information, and influence public policy.

This textbook provides nurses with fundamental information so that they can develop strategies to help shape public policies and the use of computers in health care. The authors raise the question of what strategies would be appropriate for optimizing the use of computers without sacrificing the direct patient care that nurses value. Then, addressing this question, the authors suggest that nurses might consider the following strategies: ensuring more even distribution of computers in all health care settings, providing more support for further computer-use development, developing nurse organizations and network efforts, performing studies using reliable databases, and encouraging financial incentives to motivate nurses to become involved with computer applications.

Overall, the book seeks to provide all of the information nurses need to understand the changing face of a technologically oriented nursing profession and to prepare nurses better for the nursing profession — both for today and for tomorrow.

In summary, nurses have an important and unique contribution in helping shape computer use in health policy. The challenge will be for nurses to use computers to demonstrate explicitly the outcomes of nursing practice, to formulate realistic strategies for allocating resources, and to finance expanded uses of computers that enhance health care delivery and nursing education. This is the challenge that nurses face. This textbook provides the foundation for information needed to prepare the informed user of computers to utilize computers in the nursing profession, both now and in the future.

Faye G. Abdellah, R.N., Ed. D., Sc. D., F.A.A.N.
Deputy Surgeon General and Chief Nurse Officer
Public Health Service
U.S. Department of Health and Human Services
Washington, D.C.

Preface

Essentials of Computers for Nurses was written for students preparing for a nursing career and for practicing nurses who need basic information about using computers in the health field. The book begins with a discussion of nursing history, starting with Florence Nightingale's era, and then presents the parallel historical development of the computer, explaining in lay language the meanings of computer terms such as hardware, software, data processing, systems theory, and nursing information systems. The book describes early computer systems before moving on to a description of the complex, multifaceted systems in use today. It suggests ways of determining whether or not certain information systems are feasible and cost effective for specific agencies. In addition, it discusses how the need for information can be best handled—it considers smaller and larger units and time sharing, and how these factors fit an agency's objectives.

This book emphasizes specific uses of nursing information systems. Chapter 8 explains how to plan, design, and develop a nursing information system; how to maintain it; and how to evaluate its functional and technical performance in terms of improvement in nursing practices. This chapter gives nurses the tools and methods for developing a nursing information system.

The last section, Part D, provides possible applications of computer systems in nursing administration, nursing practice, nursing research, and nursing education. Part D also helps prepare nurses for aspects of care, which, as the book explains, are enhanced through the conscientious and skillful application of computers to nursing. Such ability gives nurses a new and creative approach to patient care.

This part of the book provides examples of available systems rather than evaluating them. Here, too, gleaned from various computer–nursing conferences, are descriptions of computer applications that nurses have discovered. Many of these experiences with computers have not yet been publicized.

This book is based on a course we taught, which was effective in developing student competencies in the essentials of computer technology in nursing. It is sequenced in a format that leads the reader from a complete understanding of computers to an overview of present applications. We, the authors, each focusing on a different area of computer technology in nursing, have signed our own chapters in the Contents, but we each contributed suggestions and revisions throughout the entire book.

Each chapter provides a set of learning objectives, a general overview of the facts, and questions and answers that can be used as a simple classroom guide. In addition, Part D includes examples of applications and discussion issues. Suggestions for hands-on experiences are also listed to provide a link between the content of the book and actual exercises.

In the foreword, Dr. Faye Abdellah, Deputy Surgeon General and Chief Nurse Officer of the U.S. Public Health Service, looks toward the future use of computer technology in nursing practice. She explores how computer use will affect health policy in both government and private industry.

Our approach should motivate readers to become knowledgeable about computer use in nursing. We believe that this volume will teach nursing administrators, clinical practitioners, researchers, educators, and students to be computer literate.

Virginia K. Saba, R.N., Ed.D.
Kathleen Ann McCormick, R.N., Ph.D., F.A.A.N.

Acknowledgments

The authors wish to acknowledge their gratitude to all those whose belief in and support of this volume enabled it to come into being. We thank especially Ann Bradford, Helen Foerst, Helen Hudson, Evelyn Lazzari, William Losaw, and Elliot Shefrin for reviewing the manuscript. Also of importance were the contributions of Patricia Barnett, Jack Benson, Shirley Casey, Morris Krowitz, Lillie Simmons, and Rita Wolferman.

We can do little more than bow down in gratitude before the persons to whom we dedicate this book: Dr. Alfred T. Joseph, Francis Michael McCormick, and Franick McCormick.

Contents

PART A
Historical Perspectives of the Computer and Nursing *1*

1 Historical Perspectives of Nursing *2*
Virginia K. Saba
Historical Perspectives of Computers in Nursing 3
Development of Computer Applications in Nursing 8
Landmark Events of Computers and Nursing 13
2 Historical Perspectives of the Computer *26*
Virginia K. Saba
Early Computer Developments 26
Recent Computer Developments 31
Computer Generations 34
Computer Industry Growth 41

PART B
The Computer *45*

3 Computer Hardware *46*
Virginia K. Saba
Definition of a Computer 46
Computer Classes 47
Computer Characteristics 47
Computer Types 48
Computer Functional Components 50
4 Computer Software *73*
Virginia K. Saba
Computer Programs 73
Programming Languages 76
Programming 79
5 Data Processing *87*
Virginia K. Saba
Data Processing 87
Data Processing Operations 88
Data Storage Organization and Structure 88
Data Processing Methods 93
Data Processing Types 93

Data Security 94
Privacy 95

PART C
Computer Systems *99*

6 Systems Theory and Systems *100*
Virginia K. Saba
Systems Theory 100
Systems 101
Computer Systems 105
Information Systems 105
Management Information Systems 107
Hospital Information Systems 110
7 Nursing Information Systems *116*
Virginia K. Saba
Background 116
Overview of Applications 120
8 Developing a Nursing Information System *125*
Virginia K. Saba
Committee and Project Staff 125
Planning Phase 127
Analysis Phase 131
Design Phase 136
Development Phase 147
Implementation and Evaluation Phase 150

PART D
Nursing Applications *163*

9 Administrative Applications *164*
Kathleen Ann McCormick
Nursing Administrative Information: An Overview 164
Essential Components of Nursing Services Information 165
Essential Components of Nursing Unit Management Information 176
Selected Administrative Applications 180
Issues 197
Suggestions for Hands-on Experiences 198
10 Prospective Payment Applications *203*
Kathleen Ann McCormick and Maureen Rothermich Miller
Prospective Payment: An Overview 203
Computer Systems: Facilitating Nursing Information Management Under Cost Containment Efforts 206
Available Computerized Systems 207
Impact of Computerized Prospective Payment Systems on Nursing Administrators 219
Issues 220

11 Community Health Applications *224*
Virginia K. Saba
Community Health Nursing 224
Community Health Management Information Systems 229
Ambulatory Care Systems 245
Special-Purpose Applications 249
Issues 254
Suggestions for Hands-on Experiences 254

12 Nursing Practice Applications *260*
Kathleen Ann McCormick
Manual to Computer Nursing Documentation: Historical Perspective 260
Standards Governing Computerized Documentation 261
Automated Nursing Notes 261
Documenting Practice with Mainframes and Minicomputers 263
A Computerized Nursing Record from Admission to Discharge—A Composite View 282
Microcomputers in Nursing Documentation 283
Issues 294
Suggestions for Hands-on Experiences 295

13 Intensive Care Unit, Emergency Room, and Operating Room Applications *300*
Kathleen Ann McCormick
Background 300
Computers' Capabilities in Intensive Care Environments 301
Computer Applications in the Intensive Care Unit 301
Computer Applications in the Emergency Room 324
Computer Applications in the Operating Room 325
Issues 326

14 Research Applications *330*
Kathleen Ann McCormick
Computers in the Nursing Research Process 330
Computers in Clinical Nursing Research 351
Issues 358
Suggestions for Hands-on Experiences 359

15 Educational Applications *362*
Kathleen Ann McCormick
Computer-Based Education 362
Computer-Assisted Instruction 363
Computer-Managed Instruction 395
Computer-Assisted Video Instruction 397
Other Educational Applications 398
Potentials for Home Computers 401
Issues 402
Suggestions for Hands-on Experiences 403

Glossary *409*
Answers to Study Questions *416*
Index *435*

Essentials of Computers for Nurses

PART A

Historical Perspectives of the Computer and Nursing

1 Historical Perspectives of Nursing

Objectives

- Describe what needs in the nursing profession influenced the introduction of the computer into nursing.
- List the legislation that influenced computer usage.
- Describe the early computer applications in hospitals and public and community health agencies and in education and research.
- List the significant landmark events in the developing relationship between computers and nursing.

The computer, a powerful tool in the broad field of technology, is modernizing the nursing profession. Computers are now essential equipment in many hospitals, community health agencies, academic and research centers, and other nursing settings. Computers are thus part of the nurse's everyday life, and nursing, long recognized as a caring profession, is now entering a technological era.

Computer technology can enable nurses to become more accountable and to handle society's health care needs more efficiently. However, as in all fields, efficiency and accountability depend largely on how well computers are used and understood.

Nursing departments in health care facilities are concerned not only with quality of care but with cost-effective management. Computerized nursing information systems (NISs) help nurses monitor the quality of care, manage nursing services, and evaluate the nursing process. Computers are used for planning, budgeting, policymaking, and administrative activities. With a computerized NIS, nursing staffs can allocate resources, classify patients, and plan nurse staffing and scheduling. Moreover, NISs help with nursing education and research programs, which continue to test new computer methods and models in order to focus on the changing role of nursing in the health care arena.

Computer systems enable nurses to do the following:

- Document, organize, store, and process large volumes of data
- Communicate and retrieve information for timely decision making
- Generate aggregated information for quality, cost control, evaluation, and research
- Educate and instruct students about nursing knowledge and skills
- Conduct research to help improve the profession

In order to understand what these technological advances mean, this textbook will describe nursing before the application of computer technology, what the computer can do, and what effect computer systems will have on the nursing profession.

This chapter discusses the needs of the nursing profession that brought the computer into nursing—namely, nursing practice, nursing standards, nurse supply, nursing services, nursing education, nursing research, and legislation. Further, it includes information on the development of computer applications in nursing, primarily in hospitals, community health agencies, educational institutions, and research programs. Finally, it encompasses the continuing education efforts, including national and international conferences and workshops on computers and nursing, that have resulted in a better understanding of the value of computers in the nursing profession. The chapter is divided into the following major categories:

- Historical perspectives of computers in nursing
- Development of computer applications in nursing
- Landmark events of computers and nursing

HISTORICAL PERSPECTIVES OF COMPUTERS IN NURSING

Computer technology was introduced into the nursing profession in response to needs in the following segments of the profession plus nursing-oriented legislation:

- Nursing practice
- Nursing standards
- Nurse supply
- Nursing services
- Nursing education
- Nursing research
- Legislation

Nursing Practice

The need for computers in nursing has arisen because nursing practice has become more complex in the past 100 years. Historically, nursing theory began with Florence Nightingale, whose *Notes on Nursing: What It Is, and What It Is Not,* alluded to the need for a computing device. Nightingale described the need for nurses to record manually "the proper use of fresh air, light, warmth, cleanliness, and the proper selection and administration of diet" (Nightingale, 1859, p. 6). The purpose of documenting such observations, she implied, was to collect, store, and retrieve data to manage patient care intelligently (Seymer, 1954).

Until the 1930s, nursing notes on patient care generally included discussions of the medical record. In 1937, Henderson recommended that nurses write nursing care plans as a tool for planning, providing, and communicating patient care. This recommendation was reinforced in a textbook chapter devoted to writing care plans (Harmer and Henderson, 1939).

By 1960, 100 years after Florence Nightingale wrote on the six canons of nursing, assessment of nursing practice had become part of the patient's record. Various assessment tools had been developed. Abdellah and associates (1960) used 21 nursing problems to describe nursing practice. Henderson (1964) and Henderson and Nite (1978) categorized nursing care into 14 major activities. In 1975, the National Conference Group on the Classification of Nursing Diagnoses proposed a list of 37 nursing diagnoses, which nurses began to use in assessing patients' health problems (Gordon, 1981; Roy, 1975; Gebbie, 1976). Nurses began to list their methods and develop frameworks to assess patients' needs, thus documenting their own practice. In 1982, the North American Nursing Diagnoses Association

TABLE 1-1 *Changing Criteria for Nursing Practice Assessment*

TYPE OF ASSESSMENT CRITERIA	NUMBER OF ASSESSMENT CRITERIA	INITIATOR	YEAR
Canon (rule)	6	Nightingale	1859
Nursing problem	21	Abdellah and associates	1960
Activities and conditions	14	Henderson	1964
Nursing diagnosis	37	National conference group on the classification on nursing diagnoses	1975
Nursing diagnosis	50	North American Nursing Diagnoses Association	1982

(NANDA) approved 50 nursing diagnoses as a basis for assessing health problems that required intervention (Kim and colleagues, 1984). Table 1-1 lists these changing criteria for assessment.

Nursing Standards

The standards of nursing practice imposed by hospital organizations were formalized in 1951 when the Joint Commission on Accreditation of Hospitals (JCAH) was established. The JCAH stressed the need for adequate records on patients in hospitals and set standards for nursing documentation in the medical record (Namdi and Hutelmyer, 1970).

The JCAH, which considered nursing notes to be a legal document, in the 1970s expanded the scope of nursing practice in hospitals. It wanted the nursing process documented in the following areas: assessment, planning, implementation, and evaluation (JCAH, 1970). In 1981, the group advocated that hospitals classify patient requirements in order to determine nursing resources and to allocate nurse staffing more effectively (Alward, 1983; JCAH, 1981).

As these improvements were discussed and implemented during the past two decades, some hospitals began to use data-processing methods to update their medical and nursing record systems. Computer systems in health care settings began to provide an information processing capability that could collect, store, and retrieve information needed to assess, document, and communicate patient care.

Nurse Supply

In addition to the need to document nursing practice and increasing requirements for nursing records, the need to assess the supply of nurses also prompted the introduction of computers into nursing.

The number of hospitals increased in the early 1900s, and hospitals sought to keep pace with scientific and medical advances and new surgical procedures. Therefore, more nurses were needed to meet the updated needs for patient care.

During World War II (1941–1946), federal legislation was passed to recruit and educate a large number of nurses to meet the emergency war effort. As a result of federal funding for the Cadet Nurse Corps (PL 74), schools of nursing graduated some 117,000 nurses for the wartime emergency (FSA, 1950). However, this increase in supply still could not meet the demand for more nurses, and continuing concern about nurse supply and the corresponding need for nursing education made an inventory of nurses essential.

In 1949, the American Nurses' Association (ANA) took the first inventory of all registered nurses (ANA, 1949). The ANA periodically conducted inventories until 1978 in order to describe the population of currently licensed registered nurses. In 1977, the National Sample Survey was initiated by the U.S. Public Health Service and now periodically estimates and describes the registered nurse population.

Still another group began to count nurses. In 1937 the Division of Nursing, U.S. Public Health Service, Department of Health, Education and Welfare, in cooperation with state and territorial directors of public health nursing, took its first annual census of nurses employed in public health agencies (DN, 1975). This census was conducted periodically through 1979 and also served to describe the agencies providing public and community health nursing services.

These counts were initially tabulated either manually or with the use of IBM cards and early data-processing equipment. Beginning with the 1966 ANA inventory and the 1970 public health nursing census, data were stored on magnetic tapes and processed by computer.

Nursing Services

The need for complex calculations within nursing services also prompted the introduction of the computer. Studies conducted in the early 1920s had shown that the ratio of staff nurses to patients varied greatly among hospitals (Roberts, 1954). Most of the descriptive information on nurse staffing from 1930 through the 1960s featured the ratio of patients to personnel and the number of nursing care hours per patient per day. These figures were determined by staffing studies using time and functional study methods (Aydelotte, 1973).

However, in the 1960s, most studies used standard engineering methods; that is, they dealt primarily with four major techniques centering on time and task frequency, work sampling, observation, and self-reporting of nursing activities. Such studies produced patient classification schemes as a means of determining staffing requirements; generally they characterized the patient in terms of acuity of illness or ability for self-care. Many other studies attempted to measure the quality of care, but they were essentially questionnaires used as tools to measure the quality of patient satisfaction. The need for the computer became evident as the requirements for nursing resources became more complex and the volume of data increased.

Nursing Education

Like other segments of the nursing profession, nursing education began to use computers as educational programs developed and grew. Formal education for nurses was suggested by Florence Nightingale, and her concepts have influenced nursing education over the years. She advocated that "ladies" have a sound education to be prepared for "nursing work"—caring for the sick and preventing disease in homes and in public or private institutions. She distinguished the educated nurse, who would be prepared for superior positions, from the "ordinary" practitioners of care (Nightingale, 1859).

In the early 1900s, as the number of hospitals increased, schools of nursing were established in the hospitals. Training nursing students in these hospital schools was viewed as an economical way of staffing the hospitals. The students, in turn, cared for the sick under physicians' supervision (Gortner and Nahm, 1977).

Over a 50-year period, several studies have focused on nursing education. Goldmark (1923), Brown (1948), Bridgman (1953), and Lysaught (1973) conducted studies that made the same recommendation: the minimum professional nursing education should be at the baccalaureate level. Brown (1948) said, for example, that an effective educational system was critical, since nurses must be prepared to handle increased medical knowledge and adapt to expanding health care programs.

The education of nurses was also a concern of the ANA, and in 1926 the association formed a committee on the grading of nursing schools whose main objective was to examine the quality of nursing education. The committee's report, known as the Burgess Report, recommended that nursing standards be raised and stressed the need for "quality" nursing education (Gortner and Nahm, 1977).

During World War II, the number and size of nursing schools increased to accommodate the war effort. Beginning in the 1950s, the 2-year community and junior college programs were introduced, replacing many hospital schools of nursing (Montag, 1954). Also, graduate education began, making it possible for nurses to specialize in education, research, administration, supervision, and advanced clinical practice.

The expansion of nursing schools and programs and the increased numbers of nursing students indicated an urgent need for a device such as the computer to manage school and student records. In addition, students needed assistance in learning more as the core of nursing knowledge expanded. In addition to the classroom aids, students needed access to learning materials outside class time.

Nursing Research

Nursing research began with statistical analyses performed by Florence Nightingale, who was involved not only in nursing education and practice, but also in nursing statistics and nursing research (Werley, 1981). She manually collected and analyzed pertinent information because she realized the need for solid nursing data in order to improve the health care delivery system of her day.

Since those days, the emphasis on nursing research has been sporadic. Although several studies were conducted to investigate specific problems (*e.g.,* determining the direction of nursing education, improving nursing practice, determining nurse supply and requirements, developing educational standards, and highlighting nurse staffing needs), not until 1955 did nursing research advance. This was primarily due to the federal funding that came from the Public Health Service Act of 1944. Funds were provided for nursing research through grants to educational and health care institutions and individuals (Vreeland, 1964; Gortner and Nahm, 1977). This federal support facilitated the development of nursing research. Thus, nursing began to use the computer as a research tool. This new tool enhanced both theoretical and clinical nursing research.

Legislation

Several federal legislative acts that were passed during the past 25 years required computer assistance for implementation. These acts also emphasized documentation for reimbursement of patient care services (Table 1-2).

The Nurse Training Act of 1964 (PL 88-581) and subsequent nurse training legislation, including the more recent Omnibus Budget Reconciliation Act of 1981 (PL 97-35), provided extensive financial support to both institutions and students for nursing education. It mandated various activities for determining requirements and projecting the supply of nurses. The Division of Nursing, U.S. Public Health

TABLE 1-2 *Selected Legislation That Influenced Documentation of Patient Care*

LEGISLATION AND YEAR	PUBLIC LAW
Nursing Training Act of 1964	88-581
Social Security Amendments of 1965 (Medicare and Medicaid)	89-97
Quality Assurance Program; Professional Standards Review Organizations (PSROs) — 1972	92-603
Health Services Research, Health Statistics, and Medical Libraries Act of 1974	93-353
National Health Planning and Resources Development Act of 1974	93-641
Omnibus Budget Reconciliation Act of 1981	97-35
Social Security Amendments of 1983; Prospective Payment System (DRGs)	98-21

Service, Department of Health and Human Services, was responsible for administering the legislation. These new laws initiated information systems, which helped implement them.

The Social Security Amendments of 1965, that is, Medicare and Medicaid (PL 89-97), which were enacted to improve and increase health services to the aged and medically indigent, also affected nursing documentation. These amendments provided reimbursement of costs of health care services for eligible persons over age 65 and for certain low-income persons. This legislation also promoted the development of patient care information systems to document care received and provide information needed for reimbursement.

Other legislation included the Quality Assurance Program of 1972 (PL 92-603), which established Professional Standards Review Organizations (PSROs) to evaluate and monitor health care. The first step for implementing this legislation was to collect and analyze data on quality of care.

Then, in 1974 the Health Services Research, Health Statistics, and Medical Libraries Act (PL 93-353) was passed. This act mandated that the National Center for Health Services Research (NCHSR) undertake research activities covering all aspects of health services in the country. NCHSR supported numerous grants and contracts that focused on the technological solutions to health care problems facing the nation. Its program initiated projects using computer technology to develop innovations in the health care system. These projects focused on computer applications to support not only the needs of health care administrators, but also the providers of care.

The National Health Planning and Resources Development Act of 1974 (PL 93-641) established health planning agencies throughout the nation. This authorization also established the need for planning methods and criteria, which required extensive information from hospitals, professional organizations, and other community health agencies. Further, it mandated the creation of the National Health Planning Information Center (NHPIC), which contained a nursing component. This nursing component provided information to the nursing community on health planning including nurse personnel planning (Saba and Skapik, 1979). NHPIC housed a reference collection as well as a computerized database with literature on health planning methodologies including health resources personnel, facilities, and finance studies. The NPHIC database is now part of the MEDLARS' (*MED*ical *L*iterature and *A*nalysis *R*etrieval *S*ystem) as the Health Planning & Admin (Health Planning and Administration) on-line database at the National Library of Medicine.

Then, Title VI of the Social Security Amendments of 1983 (PL 98-21), commonly known as diagnosis related groups (DRGs), was passed, providing a prospective payment system to replace the retrospective cost-based reimbursement system in use. Payment for in-hospital Medicare and Medicaid patient services was to be based on 467 DRGs. This new system has caused hospitals to monitor and analyze patient care costs even more closely. It requires that the patients' diagnoses and charges for services be integrated with data from billing, general ledger, and medical records. Such integration is extremely difficult without a computerized information system.

Many other legislative acts, extensions, and amendments have been passed by Congress to improve health care and services, all of which require accurate record keeping. The computer was and is essential.

• • •

These historical perspectives highlight some of the changes in the nursing profession since Florence Nightingale's time. These changes deal primarily with redefining nursing practice, advancing nursing education, managing nursing services, and planning nursing research. Expansion in all fields has clearly made it necessary for nurses and nursing to study and use the technological advances that affect the delivery of care. The computer is the mechanism needed to manage the complex and voluminous data being collected to implement these changes.

DEVELOPMENT OF COMPUTER APPLICATIONS IN NURSING

Beginning in the 1950s, as the computer industry grew, computer use in the health care industry also developed. During this early period, hospitals and community health agencies started to use the computer primarily for business office functions. However, by the mid-1960s, hospitals began to include some patient care applications in their computer systems. Projects for designing and developing these patient care activities could be found in a variety of hospitals, community health agencies, and other health care facilities. Vendors were even marketing software "packages" to automate many hospital functions. However, because of the limitations of technology, their progress was slow.

During the late 1960s and early 1970s, as computers were improved and technological advancements were devised, computer applications and information systems in health care facilities grew. The introduction of on-line data communication, teletypewriter, and cathode ray tube (CRT) terminals added another essential dimension to the computer. Such innovations made computer systems more accessible and usable. In addition, several hospital information systems (HISs) were designed and developed. These systems became the forerunners of those that exist today. Some were developed under contracts or grants from various Department of Health, Education and Welfare agencies, such as the National Center for Health Services Research (NCHSR, 1980).

During this period, nurses began to recognize the computer's potential for improving documentation of nursing practice and the quality of care. They, too, began pioneering the use of the computer for repetitive activities inherent in managing hospital patient care. They assisted in designing and developing nursing components for information systems affecting patient care in hospitals, public and community health agencies, and ambulatory care settings. Further, they were instrumental in designing systems for education and research.

Some of the early HISs, which may still exist, are described in this section. Each in its own way incorporated nursing care activities and sought to improve documentation and management of patient care.

Hospital Applications

Burroughs/Medi-Data HIS

Probably one of the earliest hospital information systems was the Burroughs/Medi-Data HIS, developed at Charlotte Memorial Hospital in Charlotte, North Carolina. The system was designed to provide far more accurate information, faster communication, and standardized patient care documentation.

The initial system contained the patient diagnosis and other pertinent information on the patient and a care plan containing physicians' and nurses' orders. The nursing portion of the system consisted of a database of 200 symptoms or conditions requiring nursing action; called "initiators of care." The nurses used the computer system by entering an "initiator of care" for each patient through a cathode ray tube (CRT) terminal. As a result, they were able to devise a standardized care plan used to document care given. The computer system generated summary reports and the care plans for each shift (Somers, 1971; Smith, 1974).

Texas Institute for Rehabilitation and Research

The Texas Institute for Rehabilitation and Research in Houston also developed one of the first HISs. This hospital data management system focused on the individual patient care process and used CRTs connected to the hospital's own computer (Cornell and Carrick, 1973; Giebnik and Hurst, 1975; Valbona and Spencer, 1974). Nurses were some of the most frequent users of this system, which processed a significant portion of the patient record. The system also included standardized nursing care plans for documenting nursing notes, patients' levels of independence, and activities of daily living (Cornell and Bush, 1971). The system generated patients' care treatment plans and their daily schedules. This organization of care needed and care given helped the nursing staff allocate its resources more efficiently.

Institute of Living

The Institute of Living, Hartford, Connecticut, developed the first real-time computerized psychiatric information system designd to facilitate patient care (Lindberg, 1977). The system provided an integrated patient record that included nurses' progress notes as well as other pertinent patient care information. The nursing component consisted of a checklist of 215 nursing observations of patient behaviors arranged into 18 descriptive groups. These were originally presented on machine-readable forms and later graphically displayed on CRTs for the nursing staff to check. Through the selection of the various nursing observations, the computer provided a list of patient behaviors. The computer also provided the scores of patients' personality assessments; these were tabulated daily and became a significant part of the nurses' progress notes (Rosenberg and Carriker, 1966).

PROMIS

Another system in the forefront of data handling was PROMIS (Problem-Oriented Medical Information System), developed at the Medical Center Hospital of Vermont in Burlington. PROMIS incorporated the content of the Problem-Oriented Medical Record (POMR) (Weed, 1969). The major purpose of PROMIS was to establish a system that collected, stored, and processed all relevant medical information on a patient in order to provide "feedback" to providers of care as a means of evaluating the care given. PROMIS incorporated the four phases of medical care: collection of information (database), development of a problem list, development of a plan of action, and follow up for each problem (progress notes) (Lindberg, 1977; Giebnik and Hurst, 1975).

PROMIS also incorporated nursing video displays called "frames," which consisted of nursing care protocols for patients' specific diseases. Frames helped nurses formulate SOAP plans for patients' care (*i.e.*, *S*ubjective symptoms, *O*bjective signs, *A*ssessment, and *P*lans) (Hanchett, 1981). CRTs, which were activated with a light pen (marker), were used to enter data into this and other systems of this time (Gane, 1972; McNeill, 1979).

PROMIS was used for nearly 4 years on a gynecology ward and for 6 months on a medical ward. It was then redeveloped and used on a medical ward for approximately three years. When federal funds were halted in 1981–1982, research and development of the PROMIS system ceased, and it was removed from the hospital.

Technicon MIS

Still another system that incorporated nursing care plans was the Technicon Medical Information System (TMIS) developed at El Camino Hospital, Mountain View, California. This hospital-wide computer system managed all patient information during a given hospital stay. The nursing component consisted of nursing care protocols generated from the patient's medical diagnosis. The system predicted outcome measures that were used as guides to record patients' problems and care plans. Literally thousands of nursing care protocols were developed for this system. It also used CRTs that were activated with a lightpen (Mayers, 1974; Cook and McDowell, 1975; Cook and Mayers, 1981).

• • •

These are just some of the early efforts in the development of hospital information systems with nursing as an integral part. However, as vendors began to develop and market computer systems in the late 1970s and early 1980s, few offered nursing care applications for documenting patient care. Billing and accounting systems were primarily being marketed, plus systems that documented and processed medical orders.

Public and Community Health Applications

During the late 1960s and early 1970s, several public and community health agencies also began to systematize the collection of data on patients in ways that might make use of the computer feasible. Thus, several agencies attempted, and others began, to process nursing activities and other statistical data using the computer. This occurred primarily because of the complex reporting and reimbursement requirements of federal legislation such as Medicare and Medicaid. Several contracts and grants were awarded, primarily by the Division of Nursing, U.S. Public Health Service, Department of Health, Education and Welfare, to assist such agencies in developing computerized information systems.

Rockland County Project

Conducted by the Rockland County Health Department, New York, this was one of the earliest projects in public health (1971). Its purpose was to computerize the patient progress methodology, a methodology used to trace patients' progress in public health nursing settings. It attempted to determine patient care requirements so that a detailed patient classification and nurse staffing system for local public health nursing agencies could be established. However, because of limitations in funding as well as in the technological developments of the computer at that time, the system was never completely developed.

Buffalo Project

Another attempt to computerize patient care needs was the Buffalo project, conducted by the State of New York at Buffalo. The project, "Systematic Nursing Assessment," attempted to develop a standardized patient assessment form that could be computerized. It was designed to assist nurses in assessing patients' needs and in making patient care decisions (Taylor and Johnson, 1974). Although the tool was developed for the hospitalized patient, it was also adapted for community health nursing patients. Again, the computer technology did not lend itself to processing the numerous variables, and the tool was not computerized.

Philadelphia Project

Also in the early 1970s, the Philadelphia project was conducted by the Community Nursing Services of Philadelphia (1976), a local visiting nurse association. The project's goal was to develop a system that could be used to evaluate community health nursing services and to plan services efficiently. The system, which was designed to evaluate the process of patient care in order to establish criteria needed to predict care requirements, was completed but never implemented.

New Jersey System

In 1969 a contract was awarded to the New Jersey Department of Health to develop a statewide public health nursing system. The New Jersey system developed a home visiting management information system whose focus was to provide information on home visiting services statewide. The Home Health Care System was developed and implemented virtually across the state in the early 1970s. It was a batch system, whereby nurses in agencies used precoded forms to collect patient information. The forms were then sent to the state's computer facility for processing. Reports were generated and returned to assist nursing directors in managing their agencies. Since processing the forms was slow and tedious, the agency directors, in many instances, received information that was outdated. Finally, in the late 1970s, the system was abandoned (Saba and Levine, 1981).

COSTAR

Another early computerized information system was COSTAR (*CO*mputer *ST*ored *A*mbulatory *R*ecord system), an ambulatory care system. It was developed in the late 1960s at Massachusetts General Hospital's Laboratory of Computer Science for the ambulatory patients served by the prepaid Harvard Community Health Plan (Barnett, 1976). Its purpose was to computerize medical records so that patient care encounter data could be integrated to meet providers' medical, financial, and administrative needs. The initial system used precoded encounter forms that all health care providers, including nurses, completed. A standardized dictionary provided uniform documentation. The forms were manually completed and then keyed into the computer in batches. The system provided selected portions of the patient's medical record, producing various quality controls essential for patient management. Later, a CRT was used for on-line interaction between the users (*i.e.,* nurses) and the computer located at the laboratory. The on-line system also allowed for retrieval of patient information using the CRT.

Indian Health Service HIS

Another pioneering system, designed by Bell Aerospace Company for the Papagoe Indian Reservation, Tuscon, Arizona, was the Indian Health Service Health Information System (HIS). This health care system was designed to provide a centralized lifelong surveillance and to document and communicate the health care services, status, and conditions of all the Papagoe reservation residents who had received health care services. It provided a centralized database that contained medical summaries and information on patients including all health care services received (inpatient, outpatient, and public health nursing) (Brown and colleagues, 1971; Giebnik and Hurst, 1975). All health care providers who had use of a computer terminal had access to the patient files, including nurses. For example, the public health nurse could obtain, through the use of a CRT in her office, the latest health care information before visiting a patient in the home.

• • •

Also, in the late 1960s and early 1970s, several state and large local health departments and nonofficial agencies, including visiting nurse associations, developed or contracted with vendors for computerized information systems to administer public health and community health nursing services. Generally, the health departments' systems provided statistical reports required by local, state, and federal agencies. The voluntary agency systems provided billing and other financial data, primarily focusing on providing the reports and financial information needed for reimbursement of patient services.

Educational Applications

During the 1960s, special computerized information systems were also being developed in educational institutions. Computer-based education (CBE), which encompassed computer-assisted instruction (CAI) and computer-managed instruction (CMI), became visible on college campuses. Systems were designed to provide automated means of individualizing student instruction while serving a large number of students simultaneously.

PLATO

PLATO (*P*rogrammed *L*ogic for *A*utomatic *T*eaching *O*peration), the first CBE system to be developed, was designed for students using a CRT to interact with the computer in the classroom. Many nursing courses were adapted using PLATO, and it became an excellent tool for drill and practice courses. This new educational tool individualized the learning process and provided instant feedback of student progress (Bitzer and Boudreaux, 1968). The system tracked student progress and was also considered a CMI management tool.

Research Applications

One major research application of the computer to nursing was the development of computerized document retrieval systems. These systems are invaluable to researchers, who must index and search for literature as a first step in designing and developing research projects.

MEDLARS

In the late 1950s and early 1960s, the National Library of Medicine (NLM) developed MEDLARS (*MED*ical *L*iterature and *A*nalysis *R*etrieval *S*ystem). The NLM was established in 1936 as the library for the Surgeon General and the medical community and to contain the national collection of published literature for the medical sciences, including nursing. It also houses the world's largest collection of documents related to biomedical literature (MEDLARS, 1983).

MEDLARS used the computer not only to index the medical literature but also to produce the *Index Medicus*. In 1965 the "Special List Nursing," a special file in the MEDLARS database, was established as part of MEDLARS. This special file not only indexed the nursing periodical literature, but it prepared the *International Nursing Index* for publication by the American Journal of Nursing Company (Saba, 1981; INI, 1975).

In 1972 MEDLARS became an on-line system and was renamed MEDLINE (or MEDLARS on-line). MEDLINE became the first of several MEDLARS databases available nationwide. As a result, computerized searches of the medical and nursing literature became possible.

• • •

As computer usage continues to proliferate in the health care field, so are computer applications in nursing expanding in all areas of service—hospitals, community health agencies, and other health care facilities. The computer has proved valuable in the development of information systems. It improves nursing practice documentation to help provide high-quality patient care, and it improves the management and staffing of nursing units. It automates patient care plans and schedules, and it manages classification systems. Computerized information systems assist students in educational institutions and nursing researchers in document retrieval.

LANDMARK EVENTS OF COMPUTERS AND NURSING

The introduction of computers into the nursing profession has been relatively slow, although several landmark events have occurred over the past dozen years. These have included various types of continuing education programs, national and international conferences, and other events highlighting progress in the use of computers in nursing (Table 1-3.) All have promoted computer literacy (understanding of computers) among nurses.

NLN Invitational Conference

In 1973, the first invitational conference on management information systems for public and community health agencies was funded by the Division of Nursing, U.S. Public Health Service, Department of Health, Education and Welfare under the auspices of the National League for Nursing (NLN) (NLN, 1974). This national conference was followed by five workshops, held around the country, and a state-of-the-art national conference on the topic 3 years later (Fig. 1-1). The workshops and conferences were designed to teach public and community health nurses how to investigate, initiate, and implement computerized management information systems for their respective agencies. They offered guidelines and demonstrated how systems could be used for statistical reporting, cost analysis, and agency administration (NLN, 1976). The work of the participants resulted in several publications (see the bibliography).

Research Conference

In 1977 an invitational research conference entitled "Research Conference on Nursing Information Systems" was sponsored by the University of Illinois, College of Nursing, in Chicago. This conference, which recognized nursing's involvement in the design and development of nursing information systems, focused on the

TABLE 1-3 *Landmark Events of Computers and Nursing*

YEAR	TITLE	SPONSOR	SITE
1973	Invitational Conference on Management Information Systems for Public and Community Health Agencies	NLN, Division of Nursing, U.S. Public Health Service	Fairfax, VA
1974–1975	Five Workshops on Management Information systems for public and community health agencies	NLN, Division of Nursing, U.S. Public Health Service	Nationwide
1976	State of the Art Conference in Management for Public and Community Health Nursing Agencies	NLN, Division of Nursing, U.S. Public Health Service	Washington, DC
1977	Research Conference on Nursing Information Systems	University of Illinois College of Nursing	Chicago
1979	TRIMIS Conference on Computers in Nursing: A User's Perspective	TRIMIS Army nurse consultant team, Walter Reed Hospital	Washington, DC
1980	Early workshop on computer usage in health care: A National Survey	University of Akron School of Nursing, Continuing Education Department	Akron, OH
1981	First National Conference on Computer Technology and Nursing	NIH Clinical Center, TRIMIS Army nurse consultant team, and Division of Nursing, U.S. Public Health Service	Bethesda, MD
1981	Fifth Annual Symposium on Computer Applications in Medical Care (SCAMC-5)	SCAMC, Inc.*	Washington, DC
1982	Study Group on Nursing Information Systems	University Hospitals of Cleveland, Frances Payne Bolton School of Nursing, Case Western Reserve University, and National Center for Health Services Research, U.S. Public Health Service	Cleveland, OH
1982	International meeting: Working Conference on the Impact of Computers on Nursing	Working group, International Medical Informatics Association, and other British organizations	London and Harrogate, Yorkshire, England

1982	Second National Conference on Computer Technology and Nursing	NIH Clinical Center, TRIMIS Army nurse consultant team, and Division of Nursing, U.S. Public Health Service	Bethesda, MD
1982	Sixth Annual Symposium on Computer Applications in Medical Care (SCAMC-6)	SCAMC, Inc.*	Washington, DC
1982	First newsletter — *Computers in Nursing*	School of Nursing, University of Texas at Austin	Austin, TX
1983	MEDINFO-83: Fourth World Congress on Medical Informatics	International Medical Informatics Association	Amsterdam
1983	Third National Conference on Computer Technology and Nursing	NIH Clinical Center, TRIMIS Army nurse consultant team, and Division of Nursing, U.S. Public Health Service	Bethesda, MD
1983	Seventh Annual Symposium on Computer Applications in Medical Care (SCAMC-7)	SCAMC, Inc.*	Baltimore
1983	Second Annual Joint Congress and Conference	American Association for Medical Informatics	San Francisco and Baltimore
1983	Newsletter — *Computers in Nursing*	JB Lippincott	Philadelphia
1984	Fourth National Conference on Computer Technology and Nursing	NIH Clinical Center, TRIMIS Army nurse consultant team, and Division of Nursing, U.S. Public Health Service	Bethesda, MD
1984	Eighth Annual Symposium on Computer Applications in Medical Care (SCAMC-8)	SCAMC, Inc.*	Washington, DC
1984	Third Joint National Congress and Conference	American Association of Medical Informatics	San Francisco and Washington, DC
1984	First journal — *Computers in Nursing*	JB Lippincott	Philadelphia
1984	Council on Computer Applications in Nursing (CCAN)	ANA	Kansas City, MO
1984	National Forum on Computers in Health Care and Nursing	NLN	New York

*SCAMC, Inc. sponsored the symposium in cooperation with numerous professional societies, governmental organizations, universities, and health care organizations, including the Division of Nursing, HRSA, PHS, DHHS.

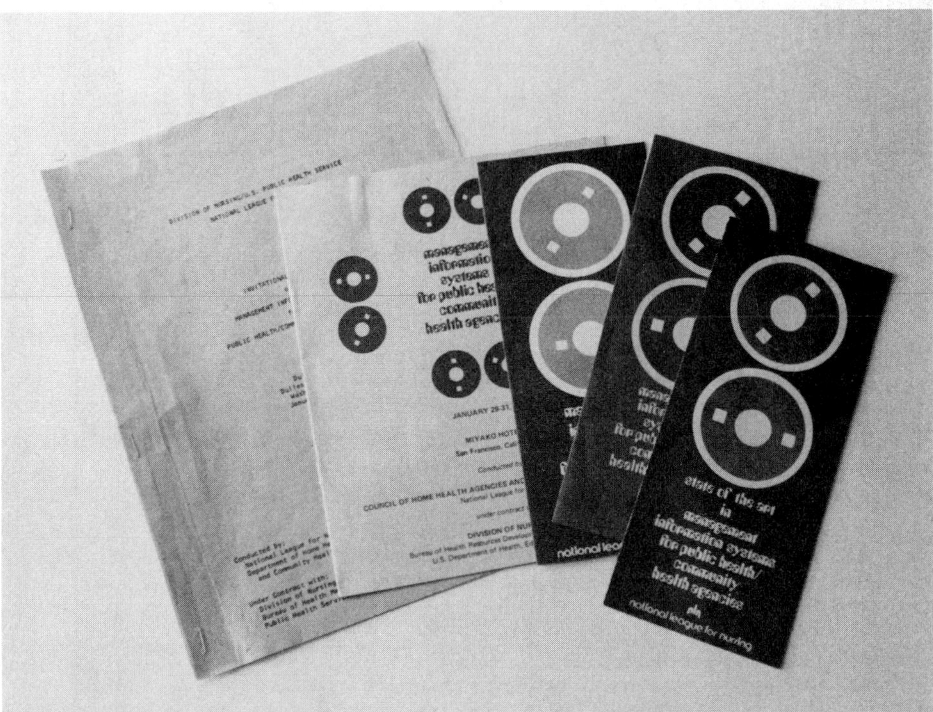

FIG. 1-1. National League for Nursing conferences and workshops.

state-of-the-art of nursing information systems and on the use of computer technology in the delivery of patient care. The meeting highlighted computer applications in documenting all aspects of nursing care, including nursing care plans, elements of the nursing process, and nursing notes. Several discussions on nursing applications in other health, patient, hospital, and medical information systems took place at this conference, which also provided new information on a number of special purpose applications, such as patient monitoring systems, patient classification and outcome measures, and information systems for public health and community nursing (Werley and Grier, 1981).

TRIMIS Conference

In 1979, the Tri-Service Medical Information Systems (TRIMIS) Army Nurse Consultant Team at Walter Reed Hospital held a conference entitled "Computers in Nursing: A User's Perspective." Its purpose was to expose nurses to the emerging role of computers in health care, particularly in nursing. Speakers emphasized the new partnership developing between nursing and the computer.

Early Workshop

In 1980 a workshop on computer usage in health care was conducted by the University of Akron School of Nursing. This 1-week credit workshop was held to orient nurses to all aspects of computer applications in nursing. Several nurses with expertise in computer technology presented various computer applications.

First National Conference

During 1981, other events affected nurses' computer literacy. The Clinical Center Nursing Department, National Institutes of Health (NIH), in collaboration with the Division of Nursing, U.S. Public Health Service, Department of Health and Human Services, and the Army Nurse Consultant Team (TRIMIS) at Walter Reed Hospital held their first national conference, at the NIH Clinical Center (Fig. 1-2). It focused on state-of-the-art computers and nursing. More than 700 nurse administrators, practitioners and clinicians, researchers, and educators attended (NIH, 1983).

Fifth Annual Symposium

Also in 1981, the Fifth Annual Symposium on Computer Applications in Medical Care (SCAMC) expanded its program to include nursing sessions. At four nursing sessions, papers dealt with nursing information systems and nursing aspects of computer technology. The symposium offered technical sessions, demonstrations, workshops, tutorials, hands-on experience, poster sessions, and exhibits of existing systems for the health care industry. It provided nurses a unique oppportunity to learn how computer applications could affect nursing care (Heffernan, 1981) (Fig. 1-3).

Study Group

In 1982 a study group on nursing information systems, sponsored by the University Hospitals of Cleveland, the Frances Payne Bolton School of Nursing, Case Western Reserve University, in cooperation with the National Center for Health Services Research, Office of the Assistant Secretary of Health, U.S. Public Health Service, was convened. This group discussed issues and described the categories of data needed for a nursing information system. The group identified the functions, structures,

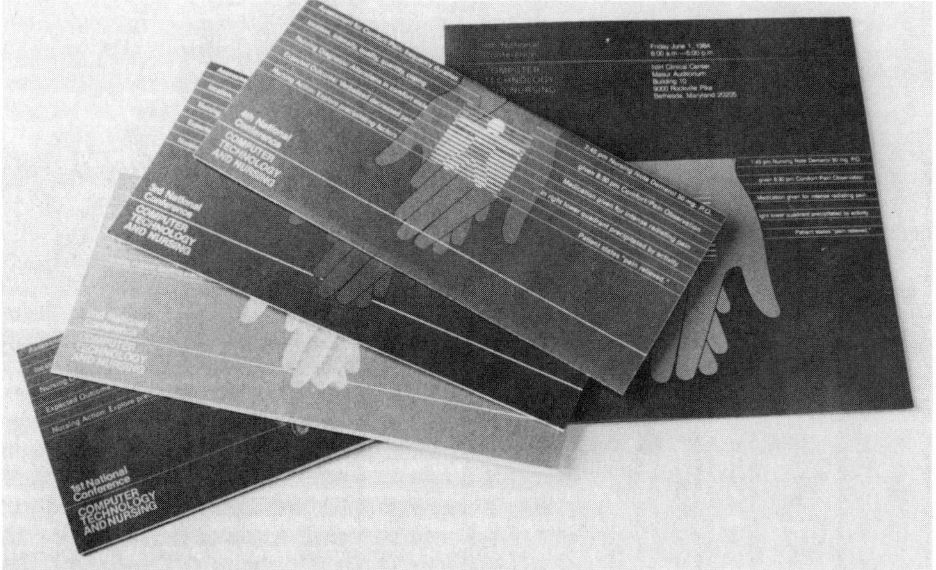

FIG. 1-2. National conferences, National Institutes of Health.

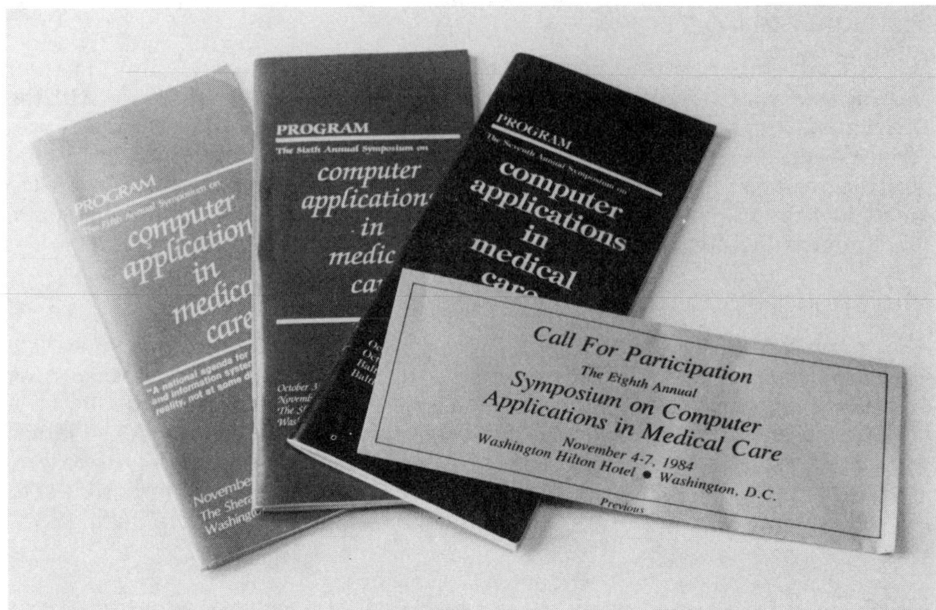

FIG. 1-3. Annual Symposiums on Computer Applications in Medical Care.

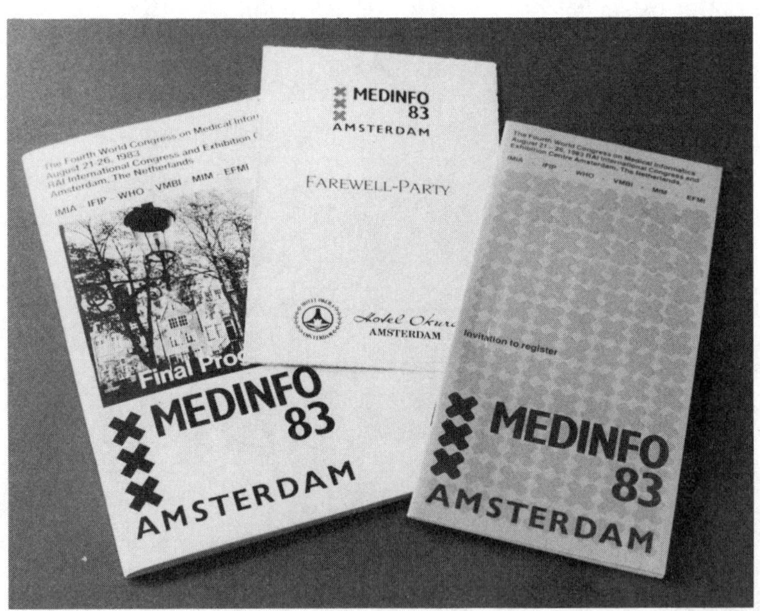

FIG. 1-4. MEDINFO 83.

and areas needed to computerize nursing information (Kiley and colleagues, 1983; Study Group, 1983).

International Meeting

In 1982 one of the first major international meeting for nurses and professionals interested in nursing and computers, the International Medical Informatics Association's (IMIA) "Working Conference on The Impact of Computers on Nursing," was held in the United Kingdom. This conference consisted of an open forum in London, followed by a closed workshop in Harrogate, Yorkshire (Scholes and colleagues, 1983).

MEDINFO 1983

For the first time, at the fourth World Congress on Medical Informatics, MEDINFO 1983, held in Amsterdam, a large international group of nurses participated in two one-day nursing sessions. On one day scientific papers on computer applications in nursing were presented; the second day consisted of seminars focusing on nursing systems (Van Bemmel and colleagues, 1983; Fokkens and colleagues, 1983) (Fig. 1-4).

Second Annual Congress and Conference

Also in 1983, the American Association for Medical Systems and Informatics (AAMSI), a newly formed organization, began holding nursing sessions at its second annual congress and conference. AAMSI began holding two meetings a year — one on the East Coast in the fall and one on the West Coast in the spring.

• • •

NIH and SCAMC held meetings in 1982 and 1983; the fourth National Conference on Computers and Nursing was held in 1984 at NIH. The Eighth Annual Symposium on Computer Applications in Medical Care (SCAMC-8) offered nurses six clinical nursing sessions, four panels, and four tutorials.

First Journal

Also in 1984, *Computers in Nursing,* the first nursing journal to focus on computer applications in nursing, was published by JB Lippincott Co. The journal, which originated in 1982 at the School of Nursing, University of Texas at Austin as a newsletter, now has an editorial staff of eight in the field of computers and nursing (Fig. 1-5).

• • •

These were the most significant of the many national and international meetings and developments on the topic of computer applications in nursing. The success of these conferences and the appearance of a journal demonstrated the intense interest nurses had in learning more about computers and their uses. In the early 1980s, many programs were sponsored by continuing education departments in colleges and universities nationwide. Such programs offered special courses, workshops, and meetings to introduce nurses to computers and computing (Fig. 1-6).

• • •

Today, nurses are learning to use computers in their work. This is commonly referred to as being "computer literate." Nurses are designing, developing, and

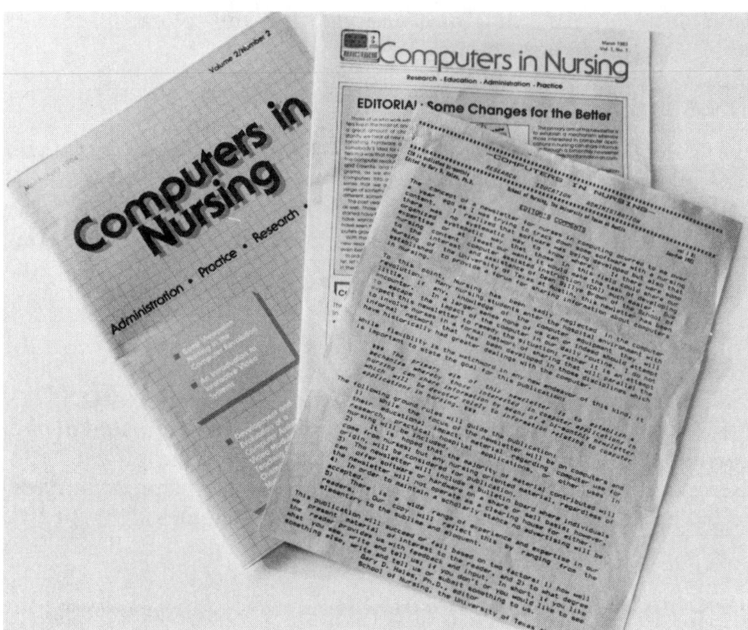

FIG. 1-5. Newsletter and journal on computers in nursing.

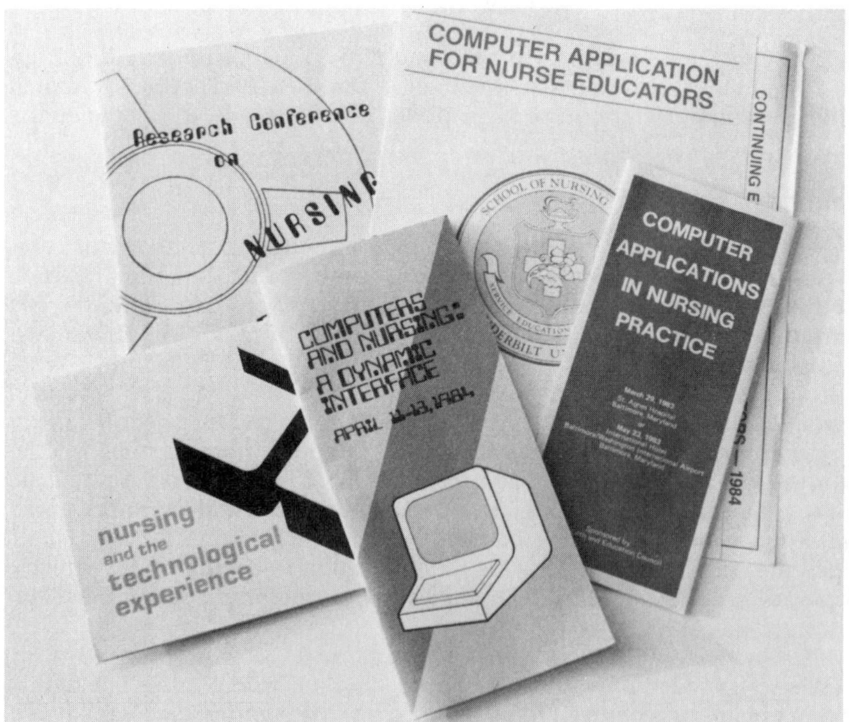

FIG. 1-6. Examples of computers and nursing workshops and meetings.

implementing nursing information systems. They are using computers to provide documentation needed for their timely reports and to assist them in providing safe quality care at a reasonable cost.

SUMMARY

In summary, this chapter highlights the historical perspectives of nursing and the computer, the developments of computer applications in nursing, and the developmental landmarks.

The chapter describes how advances in nursing practice, nursing standards, nurse supply, nursing services, nursing education, nursing research, and legislation promoted the need for computers in nursing.

Computer applications in nursing and several computerized information systems are described. They include Burroughs/Medi-Data HIS, Texas Institute for Rehabilitation and Research, Institute of Living, PROMIS, and Technicon MIS. These systems are considered to be the forerunners of many systems that are used today in hospitals. In public and community health, several applications were described. They include Rockland County, Buffalo, and Philadelphia projects; the New Jersey system; COSTAR; and Indian Health Services HIS. Finally, PLATO, the educational system, and MEDLARS, the research system, were described. Landmark events of computers and nursing include the following: the NLN Invitational, Research, and TRIMIS conferences; an early workshop; the four NIH conferences; the annual Symposiums on Computer Applications in Medical Care; the Study Group; the international meetings, MEDINFO 1983; the AAMSI Annual Congress and Conference; and the first journal on computers in nursing. These national and international conferences, symposiums, and workshops contributed to the development of nurses' computer literacy.

STUDY QUESTIONS

1. List the needs of the nursing profession that influenced the introduction of the computer into nursing.
2. Name the nurse who greatly influenced nursing practice, education, and research.
3. Who sets the standards for nursing practice in hospitals?
4. Who conducted the first inventory of all registered nurses and when was it conducted?
5. List the four key people who conducted studies in nursing education.
6. In what year did nursing research begin to receive federal support?
7. Name at least three legislative acts that influenced the introduction of the computer into nursing.
8. Name three of the five early hospital computer applications.
9. What is COSTAR and what does the acronym stand for?
10. Name the first computer-based education system.
11. What is MEDLINE and what does the acronym stand for?
12. Who sponsored the first national conference on management information system for public and community health agencies in 1973?
13. When and where was the first international computer meeting involving nurses held?
14. Name an organization that annually sponsors a symposium on computer application in medical care that offers nursing sessions.

15. What is the name of the first nursing journal on computers and when was it first published?

REFERENCES

Abdellah F, Beland I, Martin A, Matheney R: Patient-Centered Approaches to Nursing. New York, Macmillan, 1960

Alward RR: Patient classification systems: The ideal vs. reality. J Nurs Admin 13(2):14–19, 1983

American Journal of Nursing: International Nursing Index. New York, American Journal of Nursing Company, 1975

American Nurses' Association: Inventory of Professional Registered Nurses. New York, American Nurses' Association, 1949

Aydelotte M: Nursing Staffing Methodology: A Review and Critique of Selected Literature (DHEW Dec–NU [NIH] 73-433). Washington DC, U.S. Government Printing Office, 1973

Barnett OG: Computer-Stored Ambulatory Record (COSTAR) (DHEW pub. no. HRA 76-3145). Rockville, MD, National Center for Health Services Research, 1976

Bitzer MD, Boudreaux MC: Using a computer to teach nursing. Nurs Forum 8(3):234–254, 1969

Bridgman M: Collegiate Education for Nursing. New York, Russell Sage Foundation, 1953

Brown EL: Nursing for the Future. New York, Russell Sage Foundation, 1948

Brown VB, Mason WB, Kaczmarski M: A computerized health information service. Nurs Outlook 19(3):158–161, 1971

Community Nursing Services of Philadelphia: Development of a Computerized Record System to Store and Summarize Information Relevant to Administration. Evaluation and Planning of Nursing Services (contract no. 1-NU-241271). Washington, DC, Division of Nursing, Health Resources Administration, Department of Health, Education and Welfare, 1976

Cook M, Mayers M: Computer-assisted data base for nursing research. In Werley H, Grier K (eds): Nursing Information Systems, pp 149–156. New York, Springer, 1981

Cook M, McDowell W: Changing to an automated information system. Am J Nurs 75(1):46–51, 1975

Cornell S, Bush F: Systems approach to nursing care plans. Am J Nurs 71(7):1376–1378, 1971

Cornell SA, Carrick AG: Computerized schedules and care plans. Nurs Outlook 21(12):781–789, 1973

Division of Nursing: Surveys of Public Health Nursing: 1968–1972 (DHEW pub. no. HRA-76-8). Washington, DC, U.S. Government Printing Office, 1975

Federal Security Agency: The United States Cadet Nurse Corps. Washington, DC, U.S. Government Printing Office, 1950

Fokkens O, Haro AS, Van Derwerff A, et al (eds): MEDINFO 83 Seminars. Amsterdam, North-Holland, 1983

Gane D: The computer in nursing. In Hurst J, Walker H (eds): The Problem-Oriented System, pp 251–257. New York, Medcom Press, 1972

Gebbie KM (ed): Summary of the Second National Conference: Classification of Nursing Diagnoses. St. Louis, Clearinghouse – National Group for Classification of Nursing Diagnoses, 1976

Giebnik GA, Hurst LL: Computer Projects in Health Care. Ann Arbor, Health Administration Press, 1975

Goldmark J: Nursing and Nursing Education in the United States. New York, Macmillan, 1923

Gordon M: Identifying data through the nursing diagnosis approach. In Werley H, Grier M (eds): Nursing Information Systems, pp 32–35 New York, Springer, 1981

Gortner SR, Nahm MH: An overview of nursing research in the United States. Nurs Res 26(1):10–33, 1977
Hanchett ES: Appropriateness of nursing care. In Werley H, Grier M (eds): Nursing Information Systems, pp 235–242. New York, Springer, 1981
Hannah KJ: The computer and nursing practice. Nurs Outlook 24(9):555–558, 1976
Harmer B, Henderson V: Textbook of the Principles and Practice of Nursing, 4th ed. New York, Macmillan, 1939
Heffernan S (ed): Proceedings: The Fifth Annual Symposium on Computer Application on Medical Care. New York, IEEE Computer Society Press, 1981
Henderson V: The nature of nursing. Am J Nurs 64(8):62–68, 1964
Henderson V, Nite G: Principles and Practice of Nursing, 6th ed. New York, Macmillan, 1978
Joint Commission on Accreditation of Hospitals: Accreditation Manual for Hospitals: Chicago, Joint Commission on Accreditation of Hospitals, 1981
Kiley M, Holleran EJ, Weston JL, et al: Computerized nursing information systems (NIS). Nurs Manage 14(7):26–29, 1983
Kim MJ, McFarland GK, McLane AM (eds): Classification and Nursing Diagnoses. Proceedings of the Fifth National Conference. St Louis, CV Mosby, 1984
Lindberg D: The Growth of Medical Information Systems in the United States. Lexington, MA, The Lexington Books, 1977
Lysaught JP: From Abstract Into Action. New York, McGraw-Hill, 1973
Mayers M: Standard Nursing Care Plans. Palo Alto, K. P. Co. Medical Systems, 1974
McNeill DG: Developing the complete computer-based information system. J Nurs Admin 9(12):34–46, 1979
Montag M: Experimental programs in nursing education. Nurs Outlook 2(12):620–621, 1954
Namdi MF, Hutelmyer CM: A study of the effectiveness of an assessment tool in the identification of nursing care problems. Nurs Res 19(4):354–358, 1970
National Center for Health Services Research: Computer Applications in Health Care (NCHSR research report series, DHHS pub. no. [(PHS)] 80-3251). Hyattsville, MD, National Center for Health Services Research, 1980
National Institutes of Health: First National Conference: Computer Technology and Nursing. Bethesda, MD, National Institutes of Health, 1983
National Institutes of Health: MEDLARS: The computerized literature retrieval services of the National Library of Medicine. (NIH Brochure pub. no. 83-1286). Bethesda, MD, National Library of Medicine, 1981
National League for Nursing: State of the Art in Management Information Systems for Public Health/Community Health Agencies: Report of a Conference. New York, National League for Nursing, 1976
National League for Nursing: Management Information Systems for Public Health/Community Health Agencies: Report of the Conference. New York, National League for Nursing, 1974
New Jersey State Department of Health: Study of Home Health Agencies in New Jersey (contract no. 1-NU-04147). Washington, DC, Division of Nursing, Health Resources Administration, Department of Health, Education and Welfare, 1969
Nightingale F: Notes on Nursing: What It Is and What It Is Not (facsimile of 1859 edition). Philadelphia, JB Lippincott, 1946
Roberts M: American Nursing: History and Interpretation. New York, Macmillan, 1954
Rockland County Health Department: Rockland County Pilot Study: Nursing Care of the Sick (contract no. H 108-67-35). Washington, DC, Division of Nursing, Health Resources Administration, Department of Health, Education and Welfare, 1971
Rosenberg M, Carriker D: Automating nurses' notes. Am J Nurs 66(5):1021–1023, 1966
Roy C: A diagnostic classification system for nursing. Nurs Outlook 23(2):90–94, 1975
Saba VK: A comparative study of document retrieval system of nursing interest, Dissertation No 8124656. Diss Abstr Internat 42(5):1837A, 1981

Saba VK, Levine E: Patient care module in community health nursing. In Werley H, Grier M (eds): Nursing Information Systems, pp 243–262. New York, Springer, 1981
Saba V, Skapik K: Nursing information center. Am J Nurs 79(1):86–87, 1979
Scholes M, Bryant Y, Barber B (eds): The Impact of Computers on Nursing: An International Review. Amsterdam, North-Holland, 1983
Seymer LR: Selected Writings of Florence Nightingale. New York, Macmillan, 1954
Smith EJ: The computers and nursing practice. Supervisor Nurse 5(9):55–62, 1974
Somers J: A computerized nursing care system. Hospitals 45(8):93–100, 1971
Study Group Nursing Information Systems: Special report: Computerized nursing information systems: An urgent need. Res Nurs Health 6(3):101–105, 1983
Taylor DB, Johnson OH: Systematic nursing assessment: A step toward automation (DHEW pub. no. 7417). Washington, DC, U.S. Government Printing Office, 1974
Valbona C, Spencer WA: Texas Institute for Research and Rehabilitation Hospital computer system (Houston). In Collen M (ed): Hospital Computer Systems, pp 662–700. New York, John Wiley & Sons, 1974
Van Bemmel JH, Ball MS, Wigertz O (eds): Medinfo 83 (2 vols). Amsterdam, North-Holland, 1983
Vreeland EM: Trends in nursing education reflected in the federal medical services. Mil Med 129(5):415–422, 1964
Weed L: Medical Records, Medical Education and Patient Care. Cleveland, Case Western Reserve University Press, 1969
Werley H: Nursing data accumulation: Historical perspective. In Werley H, Grier M (eds): Nursing Information Systems, pp 1–10. New York, Springer, 1981
Werley H, Grier M (eds): Nursing Information Systems. New York, Springer, 1981

BIBLIOGRAPHY

Austin CJ: Information Systems for Hospital Administration. Ann Arbor, Health Administration Press, 1979
Ball M: Fifteen hospital information systems available. In Ball M (ed): How to Select a Computerized Hospital Information System, pp 10–27. Basel, Switzerland, S. Karger, 1973
Ball M: Medical data processing in the United States. Hosp Finan Manage 28(1):10–30, 1974
Ball MJ, Hannah KJ: Using Computers in Nursing. Reston, VA, Reston Publishing, 1984
Blum BI (ed): Computers and Medicine: Information Systems for Patient Care. New York, Springer-Verlag, 1982
Blum B: Proceedings: The Sixth Annual Symposium on Computer Applications in Medical Care. New York, IEEE Computer Society Press, 1982
Bronzino JD: Computer Applications for Patient Care. Reading, MA, Addison-Wesley, 1982
Bullough B, Bullough V: Issues in Nursing. New York, Springer, 1966
Cohen G (ed): Proceedings: The Eighth Annual Symposium on Computer Application in Medical Care. New York, IEEE Computer Society Press, 1984
Coleen MF (ed): Hospital Computer Systems. New York, John Wiley & Sons, 1974
Dayhoff RE (ed): Proceedings: The Seventh Annual Symposium on Computer Applications in Medical Care. New York, IEEE Computer Society Press, 1983
Fedorowicz J: Will your computer meet your case-mix information needs? Nurs Health Care 4(9):493–497, 1983
Fiddleman RH, Kerlin BD: Preliminary Assessment of COSTAR V at the North (San Diego) County Health Services Project (grant no. CS-D-000001-03-0). McLean, VA, The MITRE Corporation, 1980
Fordyce E: Theorists in nursing. In Flynn J, Heffron PB (eds): Nursing from Concept to Practice, pp 237–258. Bowie, MD, Brady, 1984
HCFA Legislative Summary: Prospective Payment Revision: Title VI of the Social Security Amendment (PL 98-21, no. 381-858:343). Washington, DC, U.S. Government Printing Office, 1983

Henderson V: On nursing care plans and their history. Nurs Outlook 21(6):378–379, 1973

Henderson V: The Nature of Nursing. New York, Macmillan, 1966

Hope GS: Delivery system and nursing in the 21st century. In Virgo JM (ed): Health Care: An International Perspective, pp 215–224. Edwardsville, IL, International Health Economics and Management

Kalish PA, Kalish BJ: Federal Influence and Impact on Nursing (NTIS pub. no. HRP-0900636). Annandale, VA, National Technical Information Service, 1977

Kemeny JG: Man and the Computer. New York, Charles Scribner, 1972

Kerlin B, Greene P: COSTAR: An Overview and Annotated Bibliography (contract no. 233-79-3201). McLean, VA, The MITRE Corporation, 1981

McCloskey J: Nursing care plans and problem-oriented health records. In Werley H, Grier M (eds): Nursing Information Systems, pp 119–126. New York, Springer, 1981

Naisbitt J: Megatrends: Ten New Directions Transforming our Lives. New York, Warner Books, 1982

National Center for Health Services Research: Automation of the Problem-Oriented Medical Record (NCHSR Research Summary Series, DHEW pub. no. HRA 77-31770). Rockville, MD, National Center for Health Services Research, 1979

National Center for Health Services Research: The Program in Health Services Research (DHEW pub. no. [HRA] 78-3136). Hyattsville, MD, National Center for Health Services Research, 1976

National League for Nursing: Selected Management Information Systems for Public Health/Community Health Agencies. New York, National League for Nursing, 1978

National League for Nursing: Management Information Systems for Public Health/Community Health Agencies: Workshop Papers. New York, National League for Nursing, 1975

National League of Nursing Education: A Study of Nursing Services in Fifty Selected Hospitals. New York, National League of Nursing Education, 1937

Office of Technology Assessment: Diagnoses Related Groups (DRGs) and the Medical Program: The Implications for Medical Technology. (Technical memorandum OTA-TM-H-17). Washington, DC, U.S. Congress, Office of Technology Assessment, 1983

Randall AM: Surviving the '80's and beyond: Strategic planning for health care data processing. In Virgo JM (ed): Health Care: An International Perspective, pp 115–132. Edwardsville, IL, International Health Economics and Management Institute, 1984

Saba VK: The computer in public health: Today and tomorrow. Nurs Outlook 30(9):510–514, 1982

Stewart IM: The Education of Nurses: Historical Foundations and Modern Trends. New York, Macmillan, 1943

Stratman WC: A Demonstration of PROMIS (NCHSR Research Summary Series, DHEW pub. no. [PHS] 79-3247). Hyattsville, MD, National Center for Health Services, 1979

Veazie S, Dankmyer T: HISs, MISs & DBMSs: Sorting out the letters. Hospitals 51(20):80–84, 1977

Virgo JM (ed): In Health Care: An International Perspective. Edwardsville, IL, International Health Economics and Management Institute, 1984

Vreeland EM: Nursing research programs in the public health service: Highlights and trends. Nurs Res 13(2):148–158, 1964

Wesseling E: Automating the nursing history and care plan. J Nurs Admin 2(3):34–38, 1972

2 Historical Perspectives of the Computer

Objectives

- Describe the developments that led to the modern computer.
- Describe major contributions in the development of the modern computer.
- Identify the five computer generations.
- Discuss the growth of the computer industry.

The computer, like the nursing profession, has a history that spans several centuries. People have used devices for counting as far back as recorded history shows. Many people, most working independently, helped to translate the computer concept into reality. It took a long time for the first computer to emerge; however, since its appearance, computer development and use have grown with extraordinary speed and revoluntionary effects.

This chapter covers the earliest known computing devices to the latest computers. The history of the computer can be described by two major series of events. The first highlights the early developments of a number of computer devices, and the second highlights the recent technological developments that influenced today's computers. These major computer developments are listed in Tables 2-1 and 2-2. A brief description of computer generations and a discussion of the phenomenal growth of the computer industry are also included.

This chapter discusses the following major topics:

- Early computer developments
- Recent computer developments
- Computer generations
- Computer industry growth

EARLY COMPUTER DEVELOPMENTS

Early significant computer developments include the following:

- Abacus
- Calculators
    - Napier's bones
    - Pascal's calculator
    - Leibniz's calculator
- Jacquard's loom
- Babbage's analytical engine
- Hollerith's tabulator

TABLE 2-1 *Early Computer Developments*

INVENTION	EVENT	YEAR
Abacus	First computing device	600 BC
Napier's bones	Early computing device for multiplication and division	1617
Pascal's calculator	First mechanical calculator to add and subtract	1642
Leibniz's calculator	First mechanical calculator to multiply and divide	1694
Jacquard's loom	First automatic weaving machine	1804
Babbage's analytical engine	First design of the modern computer	1833
Hollerith's tabulator	First electric tabulator and sorter	1889

Abacus

People have used some device for counting and computing as far back as recorded history shows. The abacus, which is derived from the Greek *abox,* meaning a "board," is one of the earliest. Used for centuries in Egypt and appearing in the Near East and China approximately 2000 years ago, it was a primitive device in which numbers were represented by beads fixed on a frame with a crossbar (Fig. 2-1).

Calculators

It was not until the 1600s, just before the Industrial Revolution, that a number of other computing devices appeared. The first, Napier's bones, invented by John Napier in 1617, was an ingenious multiplication system using numbered white rods that, when arranged side by side, could easily be manipulated to multiply numbers (Fig. 2-2).

In 1642, the first mechanical calculator, the forerunner of today's adding machine, was invented by Blaise Pascal (1623–1662). His ingenious device was used for addition and substraction (Fig. 2-3). Gottfried von Leibniz's calculator, invented in 1694, was an advance over Pascal's machine because it could multiply, divide, and take square roots as well as add and subtract (Randall, 1983; Capron and Williams, 1982).

Jacquard's Loom

In 1804, an automatic weaving loom designed for the textile industry by Joseph M. Jacquard was the first machine to use paper cards, which were prepunched with coded information to program and automatically control the weaving process (Fig. 2-4). These coded cards were the forerunner of the punched card.

TABLE 2-2 *Recent Computer Developments*

INVENTION	EVENT	YEAR
Aiken's Mark I	First large-scale digital calculator	1944
Echert and Mauchley's ENIAC	First electronic digital computer	1946
Von Newmann's stored program	Concept of the stored computer program	1946
EDSAC, EDVAC, WHIRLWIND I	Experimental computers	1949, 1951, 1951
UNIVAC I	First commercial computer	1951

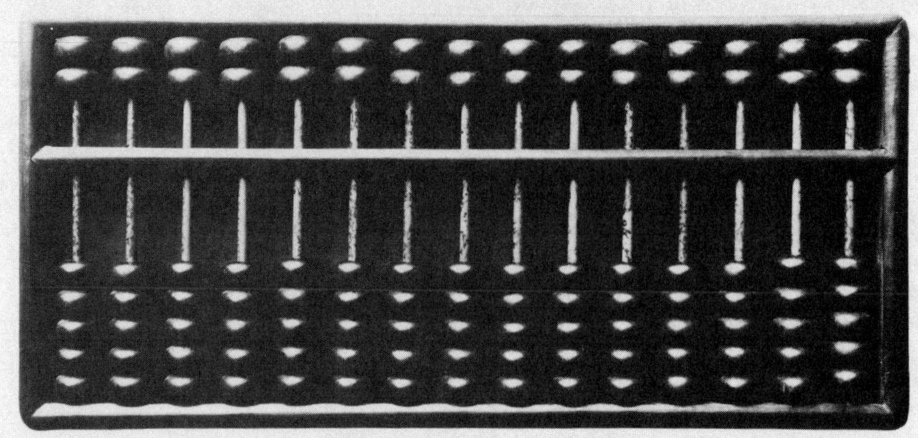

FIG. 2-1. The abacus. (Smithsonian Institution photo no. 19876)

Babbage's Analytical Engine

Charles Babbage (1791 – 1871), considered to be the father of the computer, made significant advances in the history of computing (Fig. 2-5) and in 1812 conceived and later built the "difference engine" to mechanize algebraic functions (Fig. 2-6). In 1833, he designed his "analytical engine," which was supposed to carry

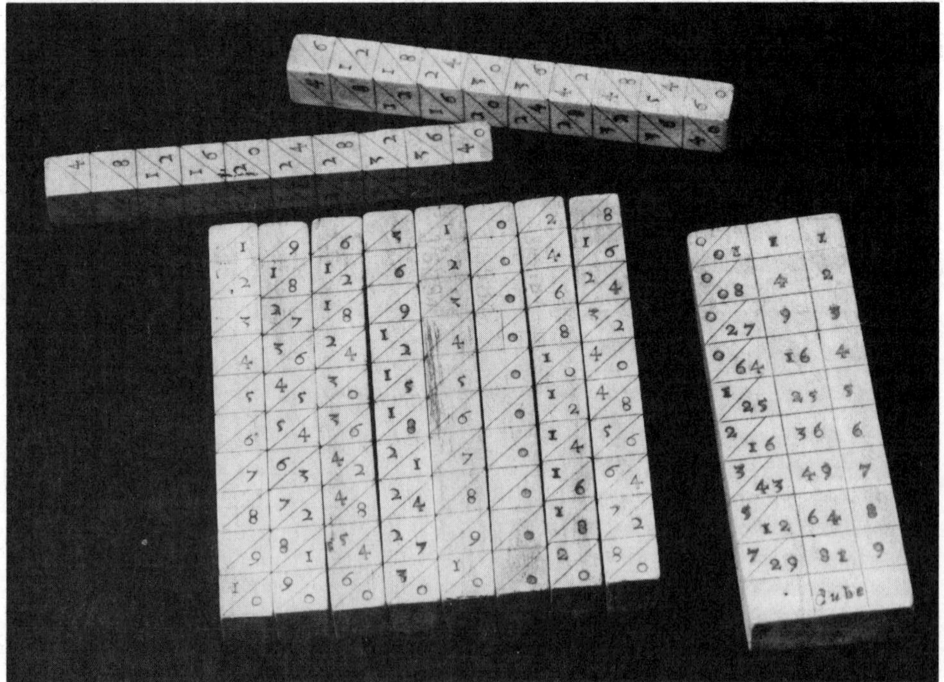

FIG. 2-2. Napier's rods. (Smithsonian Institution photo no. 58996-C)

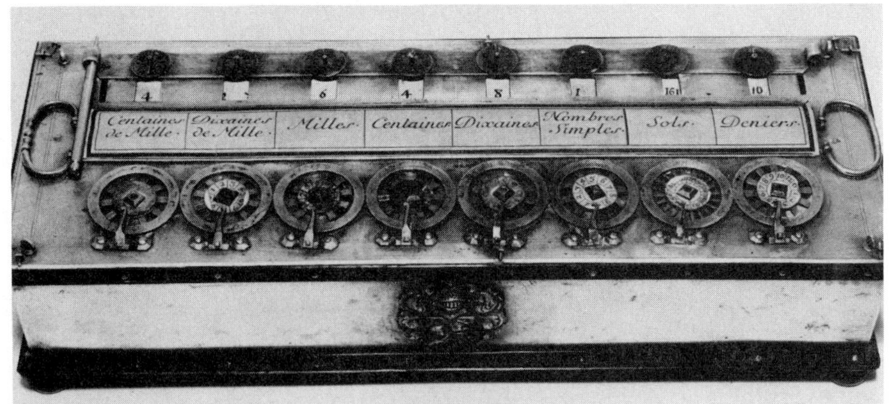

FIG. 2-3. Pascal's calculator. (Courtesy IBM archives)

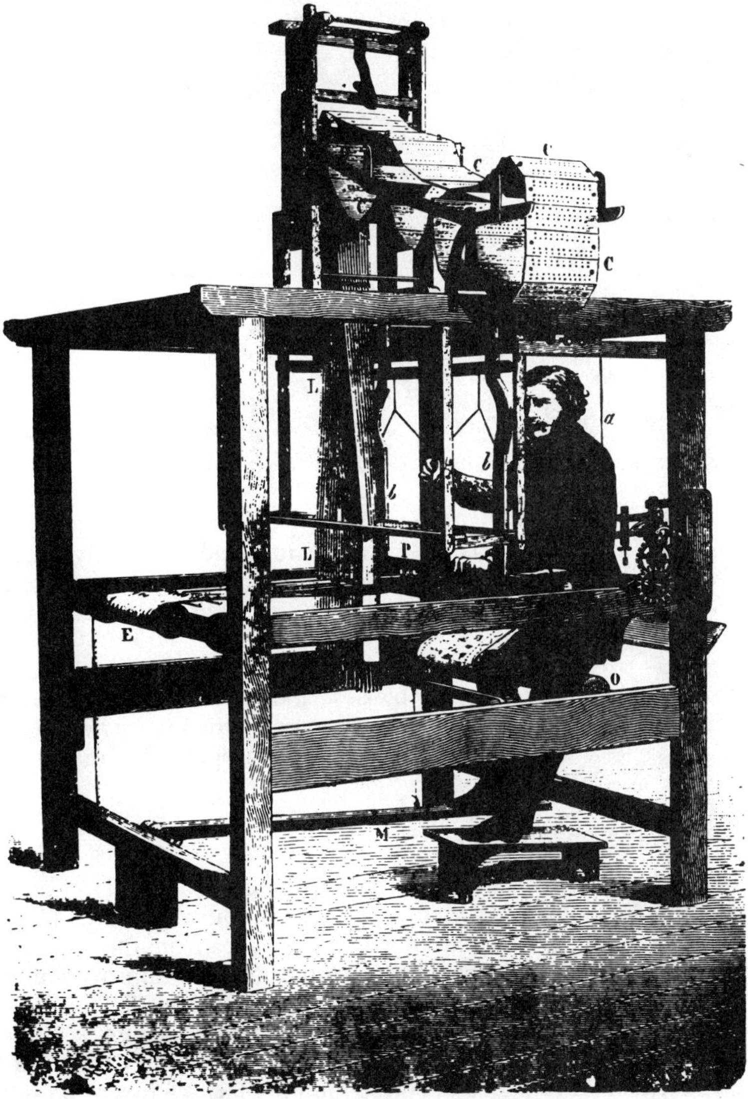

FIG. 2-4. Jacquard's loom. (Courtesy IBM archives)

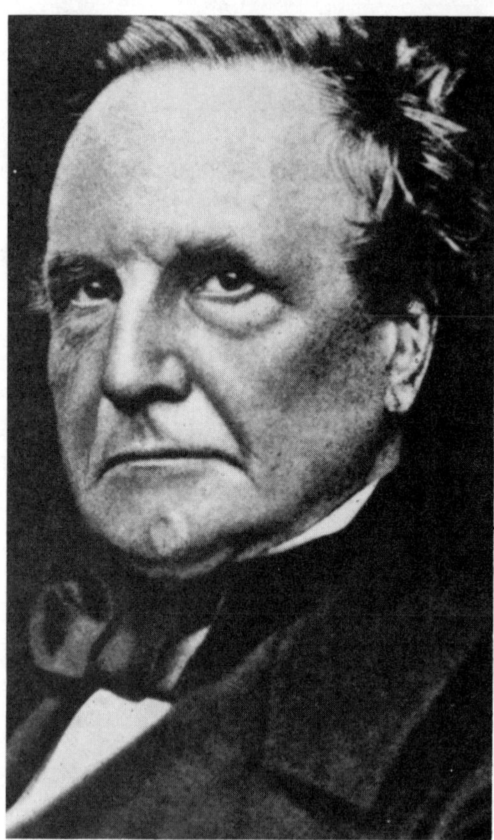

FIG. 2-5. Charles Babbage. (Courtesy IBM archives)

out all kinds of mathematical computations and essentially contained all the basic components found in today's computer (IBM, 1974; Wilkes, 1983; Randell, 1983). Known as "Babbage's folly," it was never built. Babbage was just 100 years ahead of his time.

It is of interest that Ada, the Countess of Lovelace and Babbage's friend, enriched "Babbage's folly" by describing in her translation of a paper on his analytical engine a computer program using the binary numbering system. In this regard, she is considered to be the first programmer (Shaw, 1983; Heller and Martin, 1982).

Hollerith's Tabulator

In 1889, Herman Hollerith invented an electrical tabulator and sorter that could read the holes that recorded coded data on punched cards (IBM, 1974; Randell, 1983) (Fig. 2-7). Hollerith borrowed the idea from the coded cards used to program Jacquard's automatic weaving loom and later improved his punched card and designed the 80-column punched card that is still used today. He left his position at the Census Bureau to establish his own company, which in 1924 became the firm known as the International Business Machines (IBM) Corporation.

Little of significance occurred after Hollerith's invention until World War II.

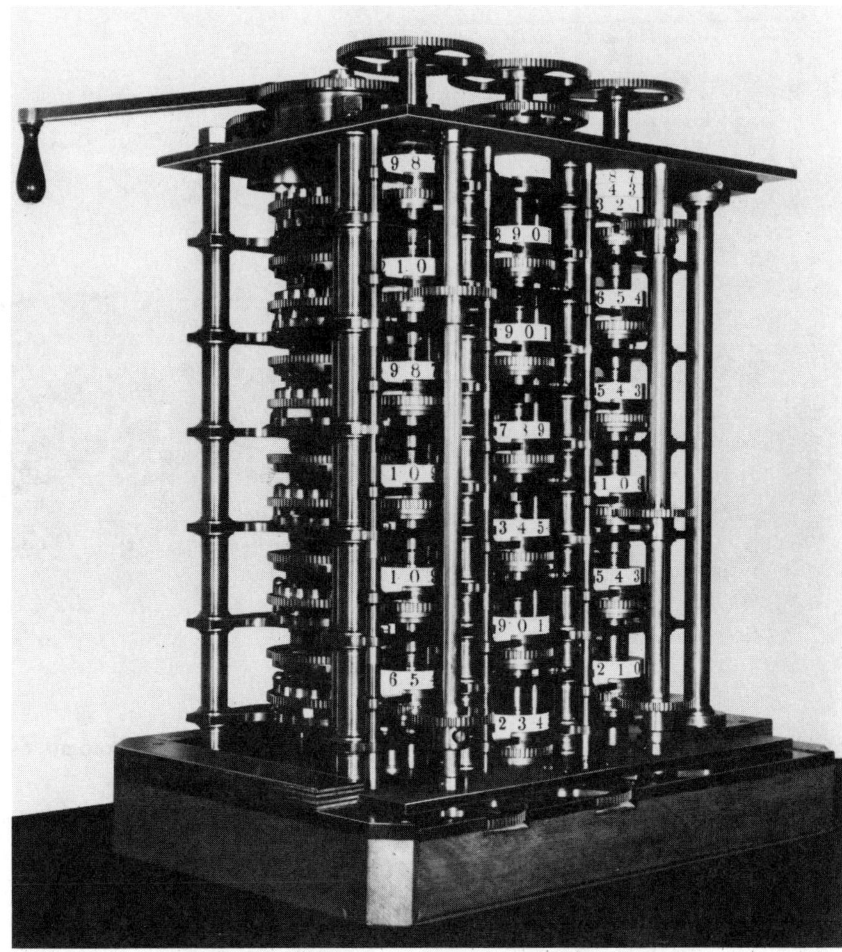

FIG. 2-6. Babbage's difference machine. (Courtesy IBM archives)

RECENT COMPUTER DEVELOPMENTS

The development of today's computer spans a very short period, compared to the centuries that led up to its creation. World War II probably had the most impact because it speeded up research and development (Heller and Martin, 1982; Randell, 1983). Many scientists in the United States, Great Britain, and Germany made technological advancements that influenced computer design and ushered in more reliance on the computer—a period sometimes called the "second Industrial Revolution."

In the United States the first large-scale computers were conceived and built in university projects sponsored by the military. The military needed a way to produce rapid calculations for ballistics and other requirements (Reid, 1982; RM Davis, 1977). The major developmental designs that represent recent computer history are shown in Table 2-2 and described in this chapter.

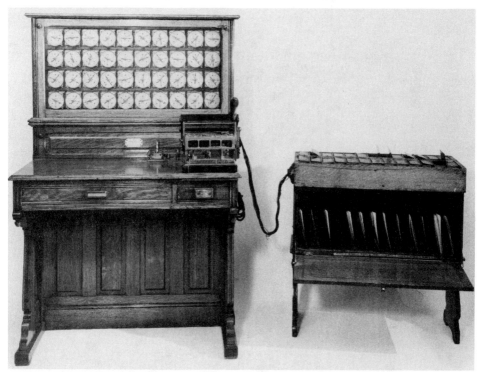

FIG. 2-7. Hollerith's tabulator and sorter. (Smithsonian Institution photo no. 64563)

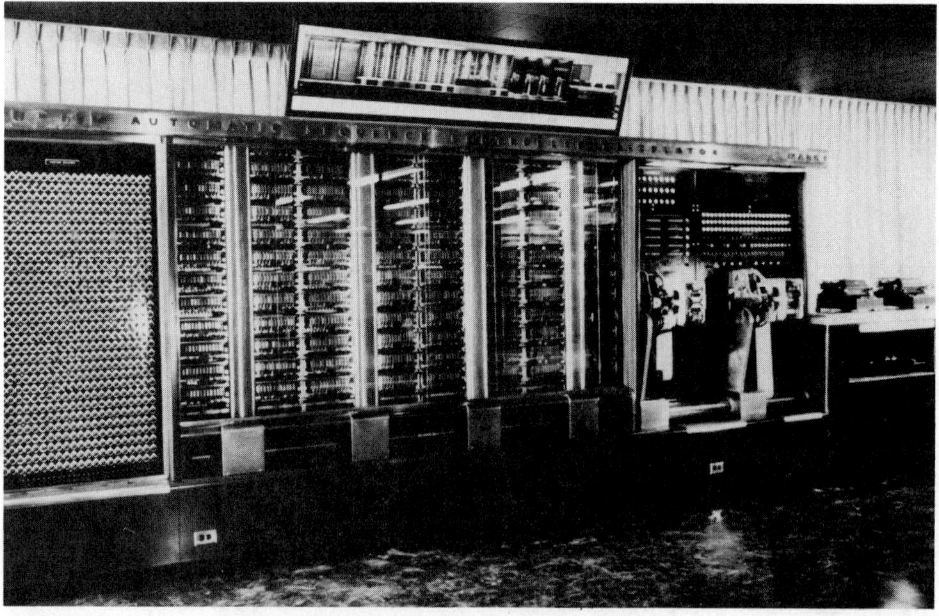

FIG. 2-8. Mark I. (Smithsonian Institution photo no. 55749)

Developments that affected the design of the modern computer primarily include the following:

- Mark I
- ENIAC
- Stored program concept
- EDSAC, EDVAC, WHIRLWIND I
- UNIVAC I

Mark I

In 1944, Professor Howard Aiken, a Harvard University engineer, with the aid of IBM, built the first large-scale, automatic electric computer, the Mark I (Fig. 2-8). It was the largest machine ever built to incorporate the ideas of Charles Babbage, who had lived a century earlier. At Harvard, it was used for several years to calculate tables for the military (IBM, 1984; Randell, 1983).

ENIAC

The Mark I was followed by the first electronic digital computer, the ENIAC (*E*lectronic *N*umerical *I*ntegrator *A*nd *C*alculator) (Fig. 2-9), completed in 1946 at the University of Pennsylvania by J. Presper Eckert Jr. and Dr. John Mauchly. The ENIAC, which weighed 30 tons and contained 19,000 vacuum tubes, was also built to assist the military. It did not use any stored programs.

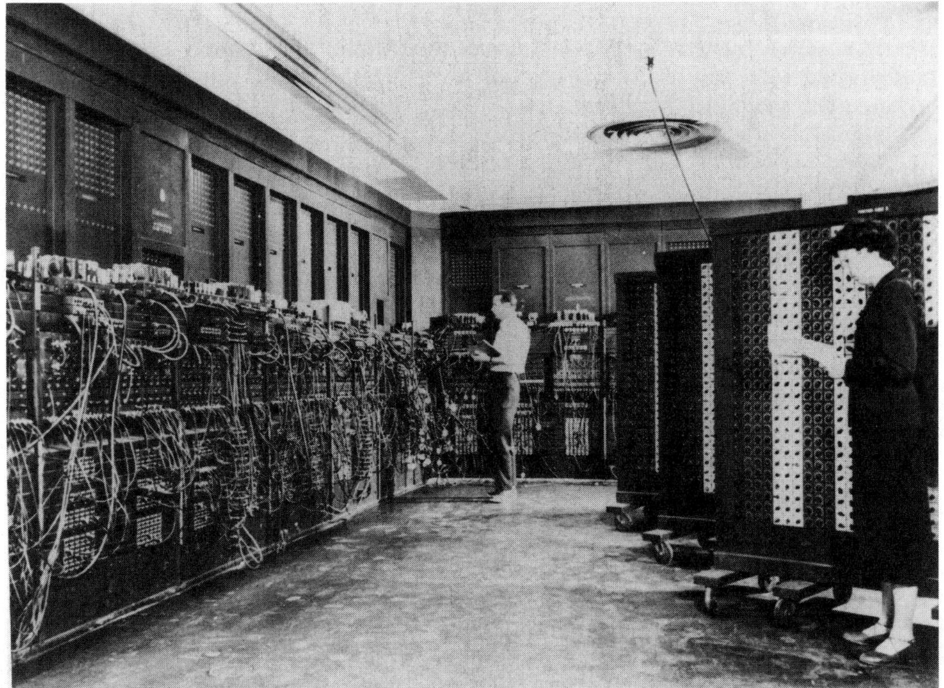

FIG. 2-9. ENIAC. (Smithsonian Institution photo no. 53192)

Stored Program Concept

It was not until later in 1946 that Dr. John Von Newmann originated the stored program by suggesting that the computer could store both numbers (data) and a program of operating instructions that could be automatically processed. He also recommended using the binary (two numbers) instead of the decimal (ten numbers) system to process data. Dr. Von Newmann also recommended several other features that are found in today's digital computers.

EDSAC, EDVAC, WHIRLWIND I

As a result of Von Newmann's recommendations, three computers were built incorporating his concepts. These computers were experimental and established the basic architecture for today's computer (Capron and Williams, 1984).

EDSAC

The EDSAC (*E*lectronic *D*elay *S*torage *A*utomatic *C*alculator), developed by Maurice Wilkes of Cambridge University in Great Britain, is famous for performing the very first computations using the stored program concept and binary numbers.

EDVAC

The EDVAC (*E*lectronic *D*iscrete *V*ariable *A*utomatic *C*omputer), developed by Echert and Mauchley for the U.S. Army at the Aberdeen Proving Grounds in Aberdeen, Maryland, also used Von Newmann's stored program concept and binary numbers.

WHIRLWIND I

WHIRLWIND I, built at the Massachusetts Institute of Technology in Cambridge, contributed to many hardware and software developments. Its most important advance was magnetic core memory.

UNIVAC I

In 1951, the UNIVAC I (*UNIV*ersal *A*utomatic *C*omputer) (Fig. 2-10), produced by Eckert and Mauchly, now of the Remington Rand Corporation, became the first commercially available electronic computer (IBM, 1974; Maynard, 1983). Incorporating Von Newmann's stored program and using the binary numbering system, the UNIVAC I consisted of 5000 vacuum tubes that, because of their size, were expensive to manufacture. The vaccum tubes required a great deal of electrical power and generated a great deal of heat, thus necessitating air conditioning. Thus, the UNIVAC I initiated the Computer Age and the four Computer Generations.

COMPUTER GENERATIONS

The history of the computer is incomplete without a description of computer generations. Each generation of computers represents advancements in the electronic components. Generally, these components (or logic circuits) were replaced with devices that improved the computer's processing power. An overview depicts the rapid changes that have occurred in recent computer history. There are many opinions regarding the number and dates of the computer generations. However, many authorities agree that four computer generations have occurred, and a fifth is expected (Table 2-3). The five computer generations, which are generally defined

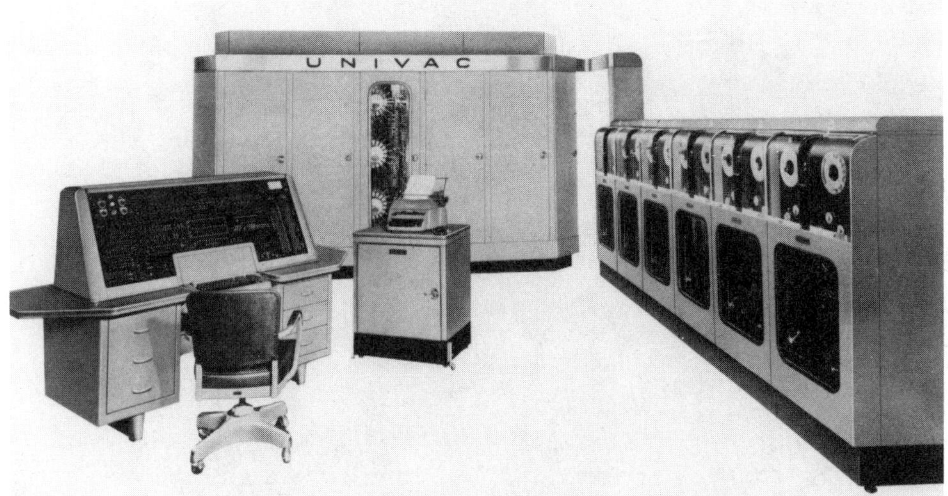

FIG. 2-10. UNIVAC I. (Smithsonian Institution photo no. 72-2616)

according to their electronic components, include the following: (Hopper and Mandell, 1984; Rosen, 1983):

- First generation: vacuum tubes
- Second generation: transistors
- Third generation: integrated circuits
- Fourth generation: large-scale integrated circuits
- Fifth generation: new hardware architecture and software

First Generation

Vacuum Tubes

The first-generation computers had logic devices consisting of vacuum tubes that resembled electric light bulbs (Figs. 2-11 and 2-12). They were used to build the first commercial computers from 1951 to 1958 (Hopper and Mandell, 1984). These computers had limited storage capacity and primarily used punched cards or magnetic tapes for their input, output, and secondary storage.

During this generation Sperry Rand Corporation produced the first commercial computer—UNIVAC I. Several other computer companies (IBM, RCA, Burroughs Corporation, National Cash Register Corporation, and Honeywell Corporation) also entered the field, developing alternate versions of these first-generation computers (Rosen, 1983).

TABLE 2-3 *Computer Generations*

GENERATIONS	ELECTRONIC COMPONENT	YEAR
First generation	Vacuum tubes	1951–1958
Second generation	Transistors	1958–1964
Third generation	Integrated circuits	1964–1974
Fourth generation	Large-scale integrated circuits	1975–present
Fifth generation	New hardware architecture and software	1990

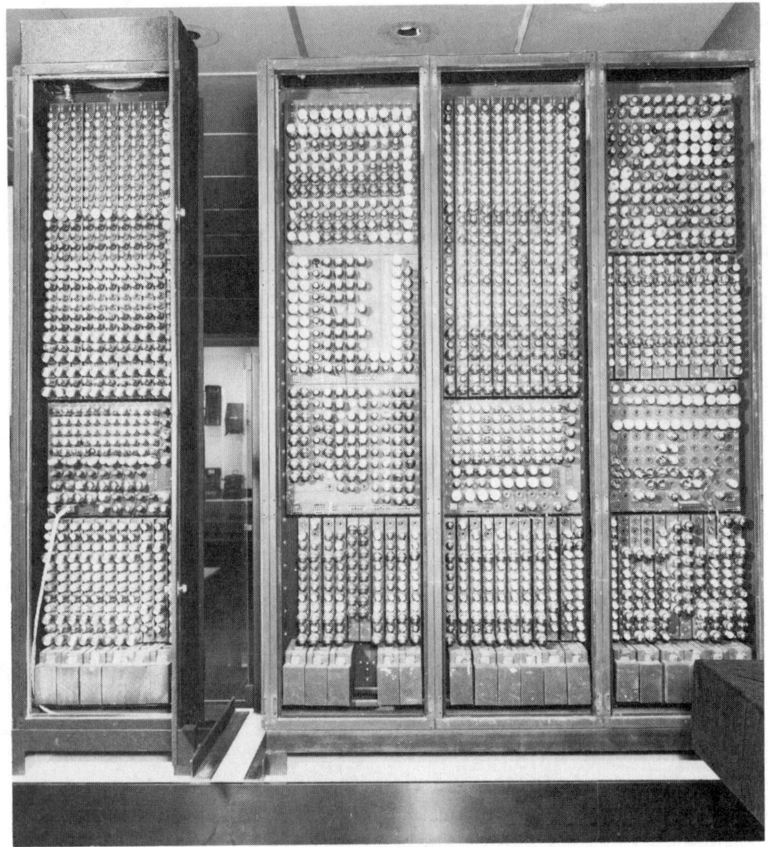

FIG. 2-11. ENIAC's vacuum tubes. (Smithsonian Institution photo no. 61797 A)

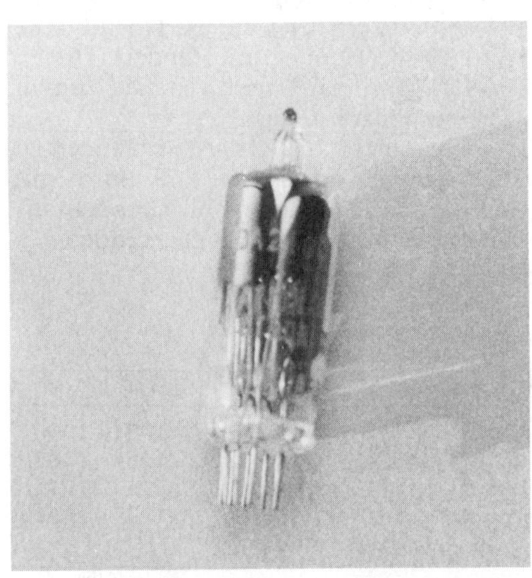

FIG. 2-12. Vacuum tube.

Second Generation

Transistors

The second-generation computers prevailed from approximately 1958 until 1964 and were characterized by the use of transistors, which replaced the vacuum tubes. The transistor, introduced by Bell Laboratories, was smaller, faster, and more flexible and reliable than the vacuum tubes. Furthermore, it required less electrical power, generated less heat, and was cheaper to produce (Fig. 2-13).

The transistor increased the speed and storage capacity of the second-generation computers, which used magnetic tapes for input, output, and secondary storage and began to use the early high-level programming languages. They were faster, more flexible, and more reliable than their predecessors and had a larger memory.

Third Generation

Integrated Circuits

The third-generation computers, introduced about 1964, were characterized by integrated circuits (IC), which replaced the transistor. The ICs were transistors imprinted on a silicon wafer. They were more reliable than the transistors, since they were made of semiconductor material; they lasted longer; they were more compact and therefore faster; they were also cheaper to produce, and, because of their size, they required less electrical power and generated less heat (Yau and Brasch, 1983). They led to the production of faster, more reliable, and more efficient computers, which again increased their storage capacity and processing speed.

The third-generation computers began to use the magnetic disk for input, output, and secondary storage and many new high-level programming languages. In addition, they began to use an operating system that made it possible to process more than one computer program at a time. Finally, they began to use on-line terminals. Such terminals allowed many users at different locations access to the computer at one time.

Minicomputer

During this generation the most spectacular growth was also seen in minicomputers, which began to be developed around 1959. The Digital Equipment Corporation (DEC), one of the largest companies in this field, introduced its PDP series.

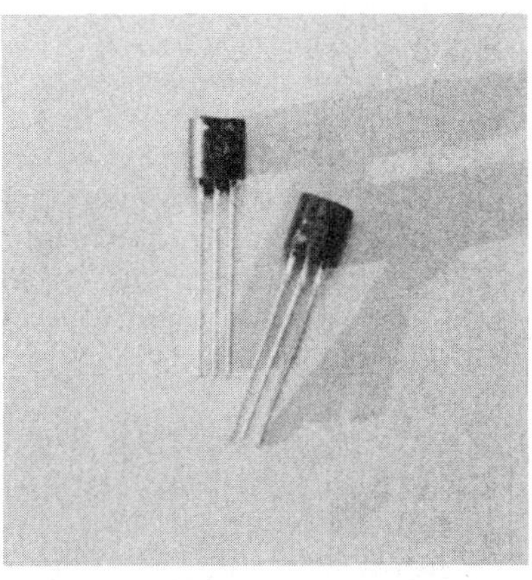

FIG. 2-13. Transistor.

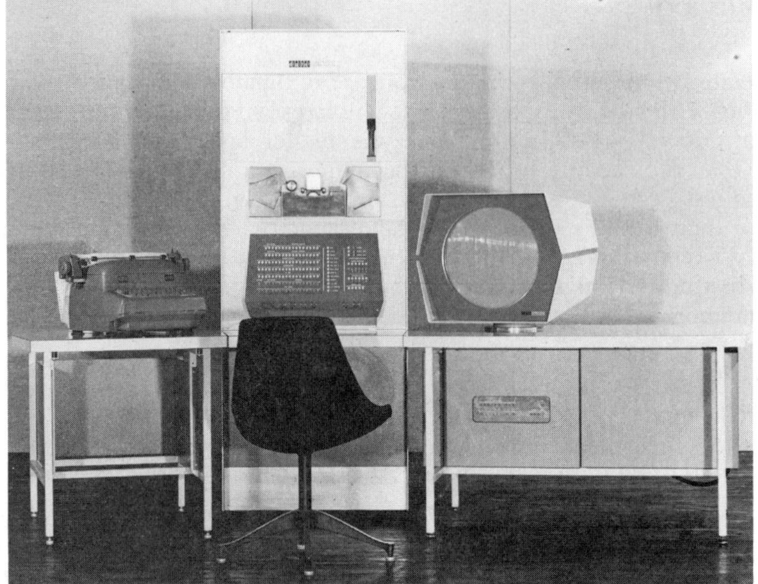

FIG. 2-14. Early minicomputer—DEC PDPI. (Courtesy Digital Equipment Corp.)

The minicomputer was small, yet functioned like a larger computer and cost less. The PDP-8, one of the most popular of the minicomputer series, was the same size as a medium-sized file cabinet (Fig. 2-14).

Computer experts differ on when the third generation of computers ended. Hopper and Mandell (1984) consider 1971 the end of this generation, when large-scale integrated (LSI) circuits called microprocessors were introduced. Rosen (1983) cites 1975 as their end, the year when the microprocessor on a chip and microcomputer were introduced.

Fourth Generation

Large-Scale Integrated Circuits

The fourth-generation computers emerged with the introduction of the LSIs, which were microminiaturized circuits chemically etched on silicon chips. They were called microprocessors and are commonly known as chips.

The chip called Intel 4004 was introduced in 1971 by Ted Hoff and Robert Noyce, both of Intel Corporation. This single silicon chip, approximately $\frac{1}{6}$-inch long and $\frac{1}{8}$-inch wide, contained the computer's microminiaturized circuits (2250 transistors) (Bylinsky, 1975; Science, 1978; Boraiko, 1982) (Figs. 2-15 to 2-17).

The fourth-generation computers contain advanced circuitry and are extremely sophisticated. They again have increased storage capacity, reliability, durability, and processing speed of the mainframe and minicomputers.

Microprocessor on a chip and Microcomputer

The chip was further refined and tested until 1975, when the microprocessor on a chip was produced, chemically joining all the components on the central processing unit on one chip. This chip, when connected with a memory chip and other

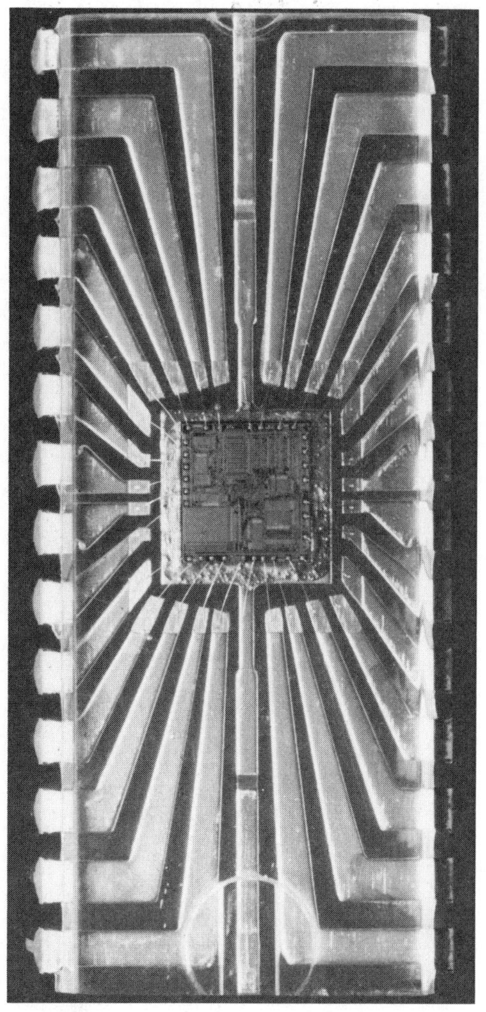

FIG. 2-15. Chip configuration. (Smithsonian Institution photo no. 77-6966)

chips, formed the first microcomputer. It was introduced in a January 1975 *Popular Electronics* magazine advertisement, under the name Altair-8800, as a computer kit for hobbyists and is considered the first commercially available microcomputer (Libes, 1983; Vacroux, 1975). Microcomputers thus entered the computer field and joined mainframes and minicomputers. Microcomputers led to the creation of many new input, output, and storage media and devices.

Fifth Generation

Much discussion exists on what fifth-generation computers will look like and when they will appear. According to the Institute of New Generation Computer Technology (1983), the fifth-generation computer's hardware architecture and software will make a quantum leap from those in use today. Fifth-generation computers not only will process large amounts of data faster than today's machines, but they will also solve complex problems and make inferences, similar to human reasoning.

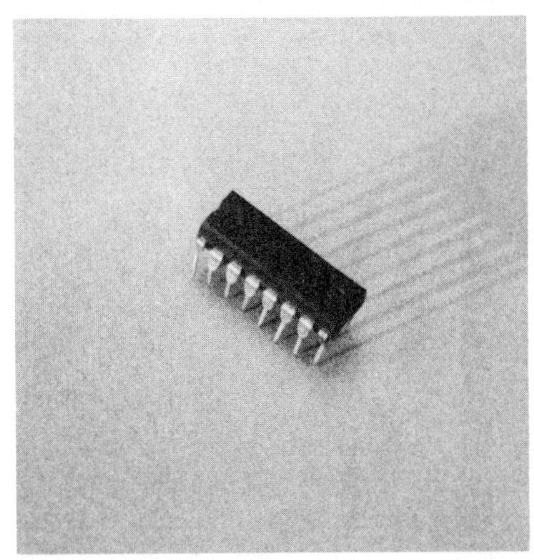

FIG. 2-16. Chip.

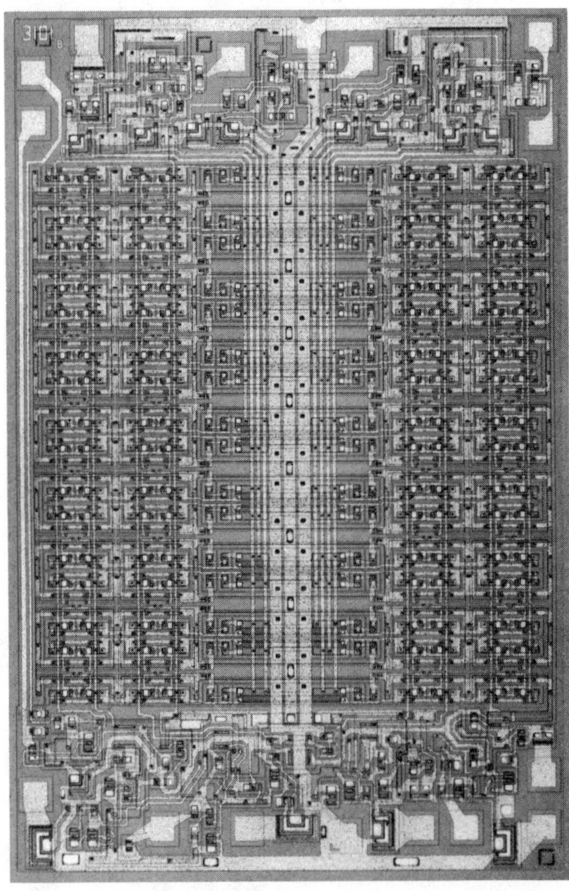

FIG. 2-17. Earliest chip made. (Courtesy Intel Corp.)

Further, they will be able to interpret and process the English language. The Americans and the Japanese are competing to achieve these goals by 1990 (Roth, 1983; Elmer-Dewitt, 1983). A replacement for the silicon chip is also a possibility. In any event, both the Japanese and Americans are researching new types of computer hardware architecture and software for tomorrow's computers.

COMPUTER INDUSTRY GROWTH

The growth of the computer industry has been tremendous. In the early 1950s, when computers were first commercially introduced, only a few large-scale models existed. However, by the mid-1950s, almost 1000 computers, primarily owned by the federal government, were in existence in the United States (RM Davis, 1977). By the mid-1960s, an estimated 30,000 large general-purpose computers were functioning.

By 1976, more than 20 years after the first production of computers, the number had increased to some 220,000 (RM Davis, 1977), and by 1980, an estimated 500,000 microcomputers existed (Shelly and Cashman, 1980). By 1983, several million computers were estimated to exist. If the use of the microprocessor in all the various games, automobiles, and appliances were considered, then the total would be about 100 million (M Davis, 1983).

SUMMARY

This chapter provides an overview of the historical developments of the computer. It describes the many people and inventions that led to the creation of the modern computer — mainframe, minicomputer and microcomputer.

Early computer developments began with the first computing device — the abacus — and then Napier's bones, Pascal's and Leibniz's calculators, Jacquard's loom, and Babbage's analytical engine, ending with Hollerith's tabulator. Recent computer developments began during World War II and are still emerging. They started with the first computer, Mark I, which led to the ENIAC, stored program, EDSAC, EDVAC, and WHIRLWIND I, and finally the production of the first commercial computer, UNIVAC I.

Next, the chapter discusses the five generations in the Computer Age — that is, the development of vacuum tubes, transistors, integrated circuits, large-scale integrated circuits, and the new hardware and software. One major development was the introduction of the chip, which revolutionized the computer age. The chapter concludes by describing the development of the computer industry from the early 1950s to the 1980s.

STUDY QUESTIONS

1. What five inventions or people influenced the early development of the computer?
2. Who is considered the father of the computer?
3. Who built MARK I, the first large-scale computer, and where was it built?
4. What is the name of the first electronic computer?
5. Who was responsible for the stored-program concept?
6. Name the three experimental computers used to develop the modern computer.
7. What is the name of the first commercially available computer?

8. How many generations of computers are there to date?
9. List the type of electronic component for each of the computer generations.
10. In what form was the first microcomputer introduced in 1975?

REFERENCES

Boraiko A: The chip: Electronic minimarvel that is changing your life. National Geographic 162(4):421–458, 1982
Bylinsky G: Here comes the second computer revolution. Fortune 92:134–138, 182, 184, November 1975
Capron HL, Williams BK: Computers and Data Processing, 2nd ed. Menlo Park, CA, Benjamin/Cummings, 1984
Davis M: The chip at 35. Personal Computing 8(7):127–131, 1983
Davis RM: Evolution of computers and computing. Science 195(4283):1096–1102, 1977
Elmer-Dewitt P: Finishing first with the fifth. Time 122(5):57, August 1, 1983
Heller RS, Martin CD: Bits 'n Bytes about Computing: A Computer Literacy Primer. Rockville, MD, Computer Science Press, 1982
Hopper GM, Mandell SL: Understanding Computers. New York, West Publishing, 1984
Institute of New Generation Computer Technology: Outline of research and development plans for fifth-generation computer systems. Byte 5(46):396–401, 1983
International Business Machines Corporation: More about Computers. Armonk, NY, International Business Machines Corporation, 1974
Libes S: Editor's page. Microsystems 4(5):8–9, 1983
Maynard MM: UNIVAC I. In Ralston A, Reilly ED Jr (eds): Encyclopedia of Computer Science and Engineering, 2nd ed, pp 1546–1547. New York, Van Nostrand Reinhold, 1983
McLeod R Jr, Forkner I: Computerized Business Information System: An Introduction to Data Processing. New York, John Wiley & Sons, 1982
Randell B: Digital computers: History: Origins. In Ralston A, Reilly ED Jr (eds): Encyclopedia of Computer Science and Engineering, 2nd ed, pp 532–535. New York, Van Nostrand Reinhold, 1983
Reid TR: Birth of a new idea. The Washington Post, July 25, 1982, pp B1, B5
Rosen S: Digital Computers: History: Contemporary and future. In Ralston A, Reilly ED Jr (eds): Encyclopedia of Computer Science and Engineering, 2nd ed, pp 540–554. New York, Van Nostrand Reinhold, 1983
Roth AD: Japanese fifth generation initiative: How will it impact the U.S. Gov Comput News 2(6):1, 14–15, 1983
Science: The numbers game. Time 111(7):54–58, February 20, 1978
Shaw M: Ada. In Ralston A, Reilly ED Jr (eds): Encyclopedia of Computer Science and Engineering, 2nd ed, pp 8–11, New York, Van Nostrand Reinhold, 1983
Shelly GB, Cashman TJ: Introduction to Computers and Data Processing. Brea, CA, Anaheim, 1980
Stern RA, Stern N: An Introduction to Computers and Information Processing. New York, John Wiley & Sons, 1982
Vacroux AG: Microcomputers. Sci Amer 232(5):32–40, 1975
Wilkes MV: Babbage, Charles. In Ralston A, Reilly ED Jr (eds): Encyclopedia of Computer Science and Engineering, 2nd ed, pp 157–158. New York, Van Nostrand Reinhold, 1983
Yau SS, Brasch FM: Computer circuiting. In Ralston A, Reilly ED Jr (eds): Encyclopedia of Computer Science and Engineering, 2nd ed, pp 306–317. New York, Van Nostrand Reinhold, 1983

BIBLIOGRAPHY

Abelson P, Hammond A: The electronics revolution. Science 195(4283):1087–1091, March 18, 1977
The age of miracle chips. Time, pp 44–45, February 20, 1978

Bernstein J: When the computer procreates. The New York Times Magazine, pp 9; 34–88, February 15, 1976
Covert C: Chip shots: A brief history of the indispensible silicon chip. TWA Ambassador 16(1):102–106, 1983
Denning PJ: Third generation computer systems. Comput Surv 3(4):176–213, December, 1971
Enlander D: Computers in Medicine: An Introduction. St Louis, C.V. Mosby, 1980
Frederick O: The computer moves in. Time, pp 14–24, January 3, 1983
Golden F: Big dimwits and little geniuses. Time, pp 30–32, January 3, 1983
Machine of the year: The computer moves in. Time, 121(1):13–40, January 3, 1983
Pylyshyn ZW (ed): Perspectives on the Computer Revolution. Englewood Cliffs, NJ, Prentice-Hall, 1970
Ralston A, Reilly ED Jr (eds): Encyclopedia of Computer Science and Engineering, 2nd ed. New York, Van Nostrand Reinhold, 1983
Rosen S: Electronic computers: A historical survey. Comput Surv 1(1):7–36, 1969
Rowan H: High industry productivity. The Washington Post, pp G1–G2, March 16, 1980
Sanders DH: Computers and Management. New York, McGraw-Hill, 1970
Schrage M: Xerox scientist to head supercomputer effort. The Washington Post, p C7, January 1, 1983
Shelly GB, Cashman TJ: Computer fundamentals for an information age. Brea, CA, Anaheim Publishing, 1984
Wilkes MV: Digital computers: History: Early. In Ralston A, Reilly ED Jr (eds): Encyclopedia of Computer Science and Engineering, 2nd ed, pp 535–540. New York, Van Nostrand Reinhold, 1983

PART B

The Computer

3 Computer Hardware

Objectives

- Understand how a computer works.
- Define and describe a computer.
- Describe the various computer types, classes, and characteristics.
- Describe the five functional components of the computer.
- List the various devices and media used by the computer.

The computer has a specific purpose and functions according to a logical design. In the health care industry and especially in the nursing profession, computers are used to aid in processing data for patient care. Computers also serve as tools for other nursing activities.

The term *computer hardware* refers to the computer's physical components —the machine itself. The computer consists of many different components, including the outside or peripheral devices. The machine components and devices enable the computer to process data. To understand how a computer processes data, it is necessary to examine the components and devices that compromise computer hardware.

This chapter covers various aspects of computer hardware including classification, characteristics, and types. In addition, it highlights the various functional components of the computer and describes the various devices and media used to communicate, store, and process data. It includes the following major categories:

- Definition of a computer
- Computer classes
- Computer characteristics
- Computer types
- Computer functional components

DEFINITION OF A COMPUTER

The computer is an electronic information-processing machine that processes data as directed by a stored sequence of instructions. It uses various input and output devices to communicate with the user. In essence, it is a machine that accepts and stores data in a required form and processes the data by doing arithmetic and performing logical operations. For example, the computer can determine if one number is greater than another and then supply the results in readable form (Morris, 1983).

COMPUTER CLASSES

Three broad classes of computers exist:

Analog
Digital
Hybrid

The analog computer operates on continuous data, measuring continuous analogous quantities such as voltage, current, temperature, and pressure. The digital computer operates on discrete numerical digits; it solves problems by performing arithmetic calculations and logical comparisons using numbers or digits (0 or 1)in machine-readable binary form to represent data. Because most of the computers used in the health care industry, other than the various monitors, are digital, this book focuses on them unless otherwise specified. The hybrid computer, as its name implies, contains features of both the analog and the digital and is used for specific applications such as complex signal processing.

COMPUTER CHARACTERISTICS

The computer is generally described in terms of the following four major characteristics:

- Automatic
- Electronic
- General purpose
- Digital

Automatic

The computer is automatic because it is self-moving; that is, it automatically processes data using computer programs called *software*. Computer programs are sets of instructions organized in a logical series of steps that specify how the computer is to "run" or process a "job," allowing the computer to perform the instructions without any human assistance.

Electronic

The computer is electronic because it uses microelectronic components etched on silicon chips for its circuitry. This means that its basic building blocks are extremely small. Electronic impulses that pass through the microminiaturized circuits named "logic gates" permit the computer to perform high-speed operations (Morris, 1983).

General Purpose

The computer is general purpose because the user can program it to process all types of problems. It can solve any problem that can be broken down into a set of understandable sequential instructions. The computer program (software), written in what is called a programming language or software, consists of English-like words used to code the computer program. (Chapter 4 includes an explanation of software.)

Digital

The computer is digital because it works with discrete "numbers" or numerical digits, using the logic of the binary numbering system. The values for all data and instructions—numbers, letters, and symbols—are represented by combinations of binary digits, 0s or 1s, that signify on and off impulses.

COMPUTER TYPES

Three distinct types of computers exist:

- Mainframe
- Minicomputer
- Microcomputer

Each type of computer was developed as the computer industry evolved, and each was developed for a different purpose. The three types differ in size, composition, storage capacity, processing time, and cost. They generally have different applications and are found in many different places in the health care industry.

Mainframe

The mainframe is the fastest and largest type of computer. Mainframes are composed of many pieces of hardware; at the minimum, a mainframe includes a console, cathode ray tube (CRT) terminals as input/output devices, a central processing unit (CPU) with a main memory, an auxiliary memory, and printers as output devices.

The console is used by an operator to communicate with the CPU. CRTs are used to key type and display input. The printers print the information the computer produces. These input/output devices can be close to (local) or far from (remote) the computer. Both are connected to the computer through some type of communication device. Auxiliary memory, on the other hand, uses storage devices that must be directly accessible to the main memory. Thus, the CPU and auxiliary memory storage devices are usually housed together, separate from the terminals (peripheral devices), in a specially designed room equipped with temperature and humidity control (Fig. 3-1).

The mainframe has the largest storage capacity (memory) and the fastest operating and processing time of all current computers. Generally, these machines are so expensive that they are leased or rented instead of purchased.

Mainframes are primarily found in large health care facilities such as hospitals, state health departments, or other community health agencies. Used to collect, store, and process extensive amounts of data from many sources to provide timely information for decision making, mainframes also process the large integrated hospital information systems (HISs) currently being implemented in health care institutions.

Minicomputer

The minicomputer is a miniature version of the mainframe. The first minicomputer, produced by the Digital Equipment Corporation (DEC) in 1959, has, like the mainframe, gone through several generations of development (Rosen, 1983). It was developed during the same period as the mainframes to satisfy the processing needs of smaller institutions and organizations.

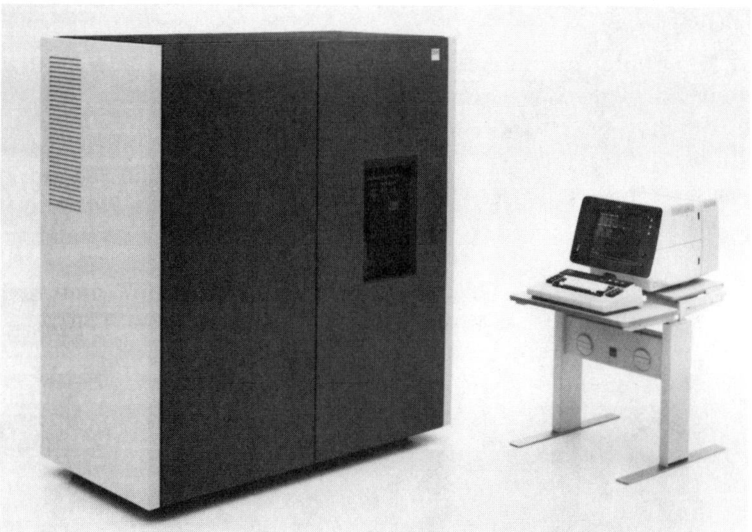

FIG. 3-1. Mainframe computer and console. (Courtesy IBM)

A minicomputer is composed of essentially the same hardware as a mainframe but is smaller and weighs much less. In fact, it may even be placed on a desk or located in the corner of a room. Unlike the mainframe, it may not require special air-conditioned facilities (Fig. 3-2). The minicomputer has a smaller storage capacity (memory), and its operating and processing time is usually slower than the mainframe. It costs less than a mainframe; therefore, a large number of users can afford to purchase it outright.

Minicomputers are found in many medium-sized hospitals and community health agencies. Used for similar applications as the mainframes but on a smaller scale, minicomputers are also used as single-purpose systems in specialty departments such as the laboratory, pharmacy, or nursing department. They are also used in medium-sized community health agencies to process financial and statistical data.

Microcomputer

The microcomputer, the newest and smallest of the three types of computers, is sometimes called a personal computer, desktop computer, or home computer. With the introduction of the microprocessor "chip,," the microcomputer became a reality in 1975 (Libes, 1983). It has made the computer accessible to most providers in the health care industry.

The microcomputer functions like the mainframe and minicomputer; however, its hardware components differ. Instead of having many pieces of hardware, a microcomputer is assembled as a complete desktop or portable unit that contains a keyboard, CRT or video display terminal (VDT) screen, disk drive(s), and CPU. The keyboard, which resembles a typewriter, serves to handle input data. The CRT/VDT or televisionlike screen dislays data for review. The CRT or VDT also can select input data by a lightpen, "mouse," or other type of pointer. In addition, it allows a user to view the output, which is generated by an attached printer (optional). Disk drives are input/output devices, allowing for data to be transferred

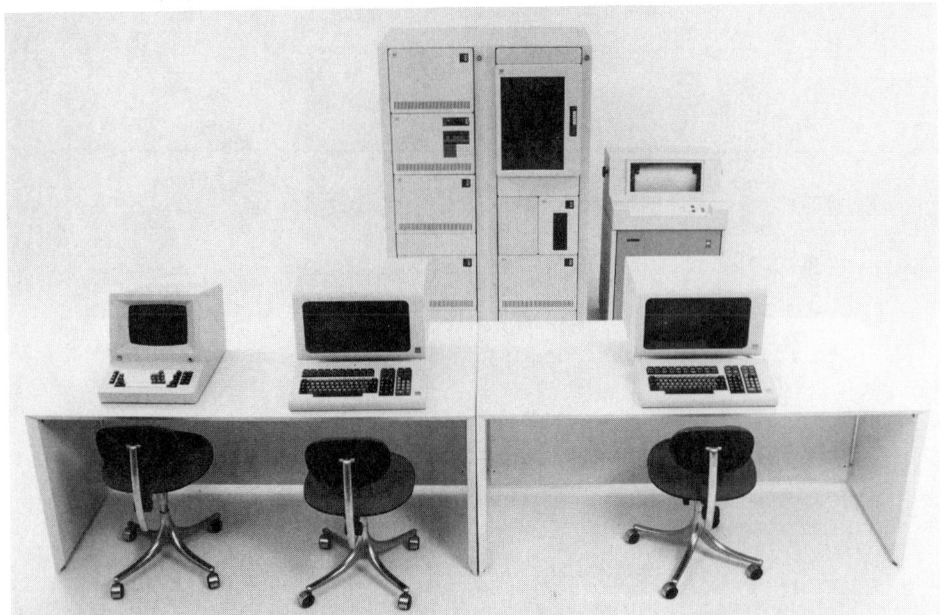

FIG. 3-2. Minicomputer with printer and CRT terminals. (Courtesy IBM)

from disk (diskettes) to and from the CPU. The CPU, the internal component of the microcomputer, consists of a microprocessor on a chip (Fig. 3-3).

The microcomputer usually processes one program "job" at a time and generally can accommodate only one user at a time. However, technology is changing so fast that some microcomputers are beginning to look and perform like small minicomputer systems. The microcomputer has the slowest operating and processing time and is the least expensive of the three types of computers. It stands alone or, if properly connected, can become a terminal to another computer.

Microcomputers are used in all areas of the health care industry. Hospital nursing departments use them to process patient classification, nurse staffing, nurse scheduling, and personnel management. Microcomputers are much in evidence in educational settings for computer-assisted instruction (CAI) and computer-managed instruction (CMI) and in research settings for various applications.

COMPUTER FUNCTIONAL COMPONENTS

The computer has five functional components that compromise computer hardware, the physical equipment of a computer system. They represent the visible parts of the computer. These components, listed in Figure 3-4, are basic to all computer systems and are not limited to any one specific computer manufacturer. They include the input and output units, the CPU (consisting of the control unit, the arithmetic and logic unit, and the main memory unit), and the auxillary memory unit, which is an extension of main memory (Morris, 1983; Hopper and Mandell, 1984).

This section presents a brief overview of these functional components. Also described are the various computer hardware devices and media that implement

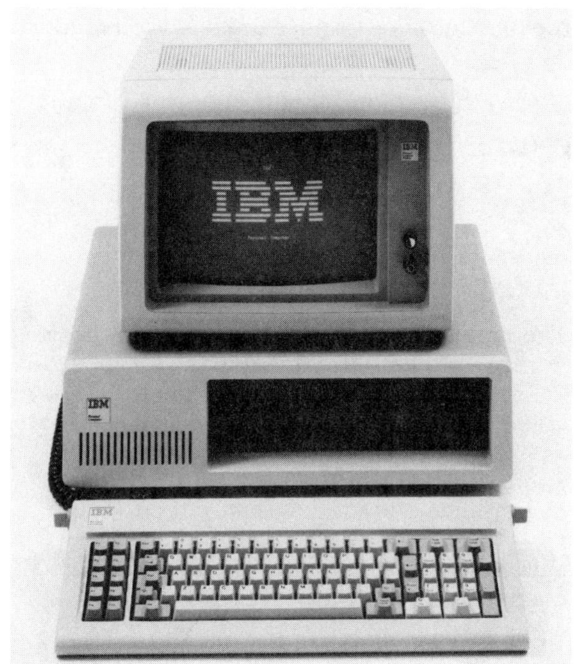

FIG. 3-3. Microcomputer—IBM Personal Computer. (Courtesy IBM)

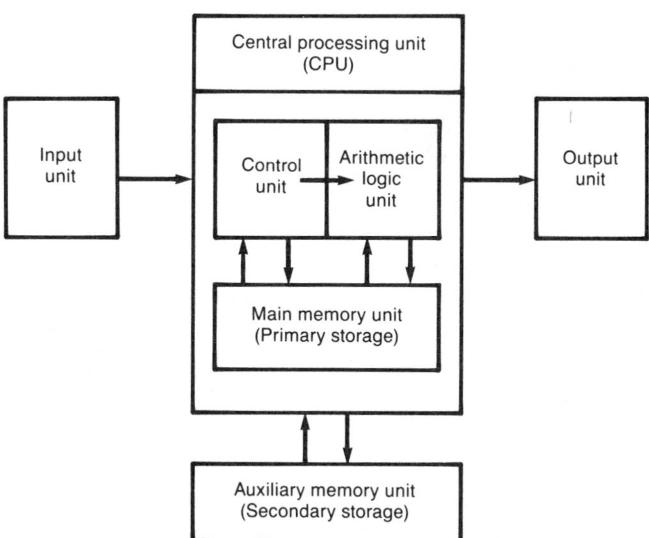

FIG. 3-4. Five functional components of the computer. (After Morris GJ: Digital computers: General principles. In Ralston A, Reilly ED Jr (eds): Encyclopedia of Computer Science and Engineering, 2d ed. New York, Van Nostrand Rheinhold, 1983, and Hopper GM, Mandell SL: Understanding Computers. New York, West Publishing, 1984)

the functions of these five units. They include the following:

- Input unit
- CPU — Control unit
- CPU — Arithmetic/logic unit
- CPU — Main memory unit
    - Auxiliary memory
- Output unit

Input Unit

The input unit acts as a "reception desk," accepting data and instructions and translating them into binary digits for input into the computer's memory in the CPU. Several different types of input devices, sometimes called peripheral devices, communicate with the computer system and are described below.

Input Devices and Media

Most available input devices are used for direct computer input and include devices to key type (using a method to display what is being keyed), read, or sense data. Many of the input devices and media are also used for output or storage. The common ones include the following:

- Terminal
    - Keyboard
- CRT terminal
- Other terminals
    - Hard copy terminal/teletypewriter
    - Portable terminal
    - Hand-held terminal
- Punched card
- Paper tape
- Optical character recognition (OCR)
- Magnetic-ink character recognition (MICR)
- Magnetic media
- Voice/Image

Terminal

A terminal, an input/output device primarily used to communicate with the computer, converts input data and instructions into binary codes and transmits them into computer memory. A terminal connected to a mainframe or a minicomputer is generally located far away from the main computer but convenient for computer users. However, it remains an integral part of a microcomputer.

Terminals generally are directly connected or use a modem, an interface device, to communicate with the computer through telephone lines (Fig. 3-5). Communication media such as cable, microwave, or even satellite are sometimes used. The modem (modulating and demodulating device) translates digital data into waves (analog) for transmission over the communication lines to the computer system and converts the waves back to their original digital form for input into the computer (Garfield, 1984).

There are primarily two different types of terminals—dumb and smart. The dumb terminals simply transmit keyed data to and from the computer without processing in any way; they merely enter and display data (input and output). The

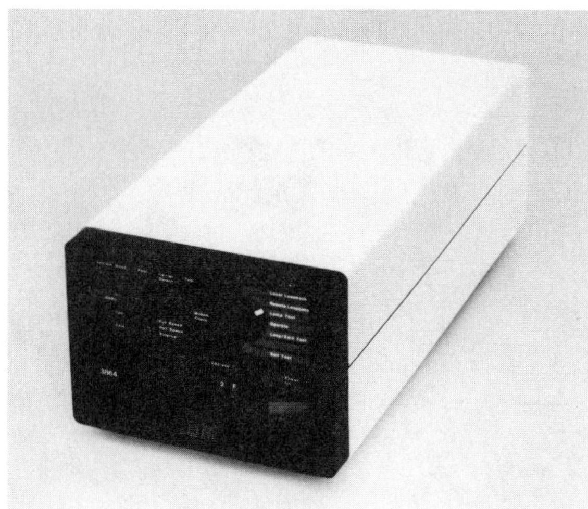

FIG. 3-5. Modem. (Courtesy of IBM)

smart terminals store, edit, and minimally process data before transmitting the data to the computer, thus enabling a user to edit data entered according to predefined rules. Also used to receive and display output data, some of the smart terminals can be programmed to perform computer processing tasks. These are sometimes called ***intelligent terminals.***

Terminals are also used in teleprocessing, which means using a computer through one or more communication links. In teleprocessing, terminals are located in many different places without having a computer in each; they are connected to a computer by a communication network. The computer is shared by several different users, which is called ***timesharing.***

Teleprocessing is found in small hospitals or community health agencies that cannot afford a mainframe or minicomputer system. These agencies generally contract with a vendor or service bureau and time-share computer services.

Terminals also allow for message switching, which means that messages are transmitted between terminals in the computer system. Message switching is sometimes found in HISs, where messages are sent to and from various departments.

Keyboard. The keyboard, an input device, is an integral part of any terminal. It is generally the part of the terminal that communicates with the computer. A device resembling a typewriter, it also contains numeric and several functional keys that vary in number and position. Generally a keyboard is found with a CRT or VDT screen, hard copy/teletypewriter, portable terminal, or hand-held terminal. A keyboard must be operated by a computer user.

Cathode Ray Tube Terminal

A CRT terminal is the most common input/output device, consisting of a keyboard and display screen. It is also called a video display terminal (VDT). Data are input primarily through the typewriterlike keyboard, but depending on the model, data may be selected and input with a lightpen, a finger, or a pointer/cursor (Fig. 3-6).

Other Terminals

A variety of other terminals communicate with the computer. Some more common ones are the hard copy/teletypewriter and portable and hand-held terminals.

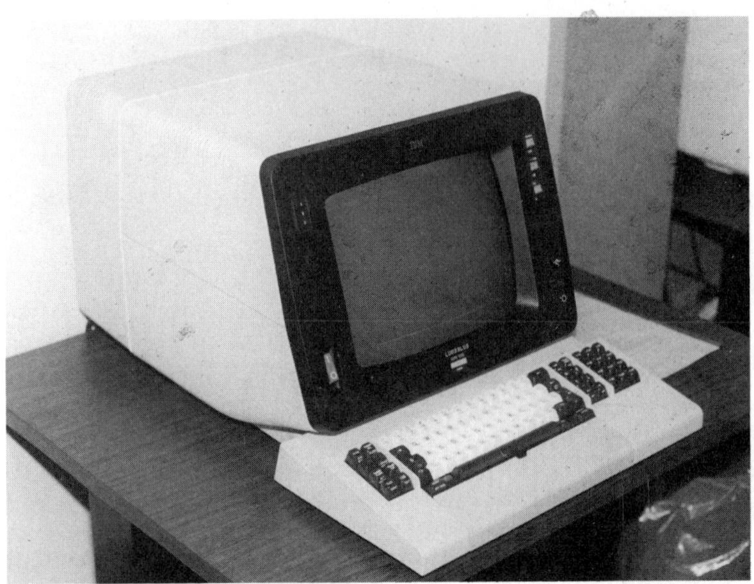

FIG. 3-6. CRT terminal, showing keyboard and video display/screen.

Hard Copy Terminal/Teletypewriter. The hard copy terminal, also called a teletypewriter, is an input/output device resembling a typewriter. It uses hard copy (paper) to record data being keyed in as input and prints output onto paper.

Portable Terminals. A portable terminal, generally a battery-run terminal consisting of a keyboard and a small VDT screen that displays three or four lines of typing, can be carried in a briefcase. This type of terminal can store and process limited amounts of data, which can be communicated to a central computer using a modem or other standard interfaces.

Hand-Held Terminal. The hand-held terminal, sometimes called a key pad, generally contains a limited set of numbers, letters, and symbols. It resembles an electronic calculator and is used to enter numbers or coded data and display limited data. It can store limited data in the battery-run unit or interface directly with a computer system. Nurses use these terminals in different ways; for example, they can record and store a patient's vital signs and then transmit the information directly into a hospital computer system. This type of terminal has many uses in data collection in all types of health care settings (Fig. 3-7).

Punched Card

The punched card was the most commonly used input and output medium for both mainframes and minicomputers until the CRT emerged. Invented by Herman Hollerith in 1889, the punched card was used as input for all early computers (Finkelstein, 1983). It is a paper card that stores data through punched holes arranged in predefined locations. The most common punched card contains 80 columns, each with 12 locations for punching (Fig. 3-8). It contains enough locations to represent the essential numbers, letters, and special symbols needed to code data.

Keypunched holes represent data. Once keyed, data are verified for accuracy and then batched together for computer input into a card reader. A punched card reader is the input device that mechanically or optically senses the holes in the

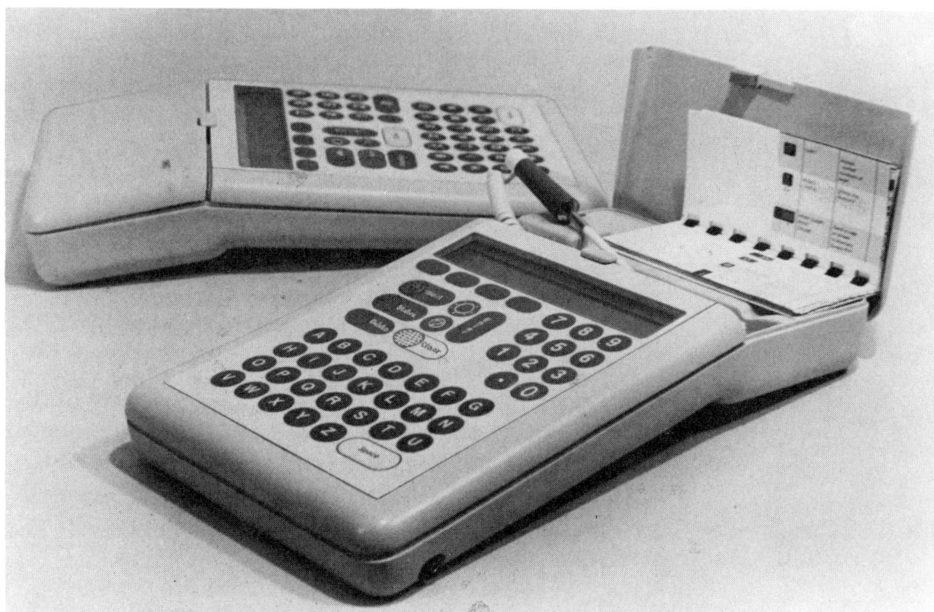

FIG. 3-7. Portable nursing unit terminal. (Courtesy NCR Corp.)

punched cards and automatically converts them into electronic impulses for the computer to read (Fig. 3-9).

Paper Tape

Paper tape serves the same purpose as punched cards. Data are recorded by a special arrangement of punched holes along the length of the paper tape. Paper tape is rarely used today.

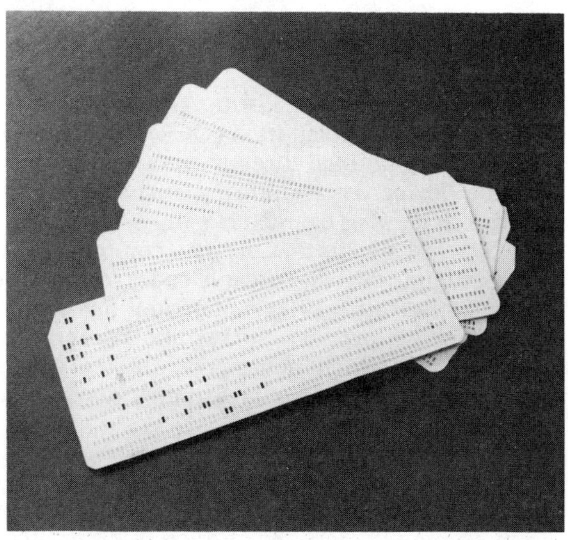

FIG. 3-8. Punched cards.

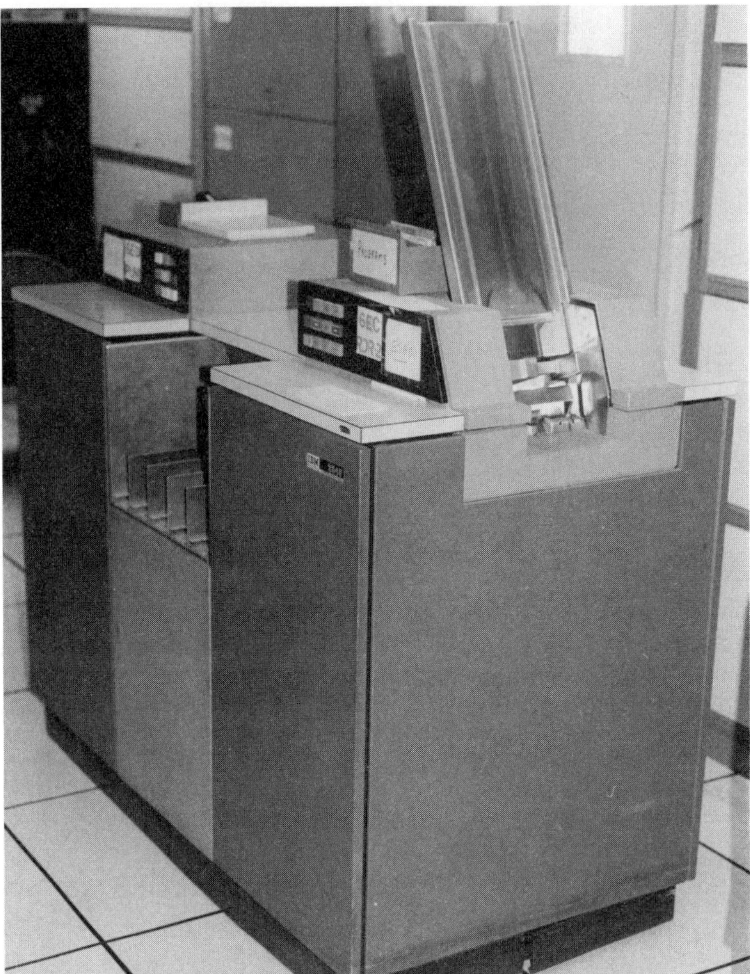

FIG. 3-9. Punched card reader.

Optical Character Recognition

Optical character recognition (OCR) is a specialized computer input medium that allows data to be read directly from a form or document. An electronic optical scanning device or an optical character reader reads special marks, bar codes, numbers, letters, or characters (Fig. 3-10). Such a device converts the characters into electrical signals that become computer input.

An example of OCR-readable codes are those outlined areas on the answer sheet of the nursing state board examinations that are filled in with pencil. The bar codes called universal product code symbols (zebra-striped bars) are another example. Ten bars, about 1 inch long, signify different numbers to code groceries or medical items. If read with a special scanning device, they can become input into some hospital inventory systems (Fig. 3-11).

Magnetic-Ink Character Recognition

Magnetic-ink character recognition (MICR) is another medium for reading characters by computer. Here the characters are printed on paper in magnetized ink. An MICR reader can examine the shape of the magnetic-ink characters and convert

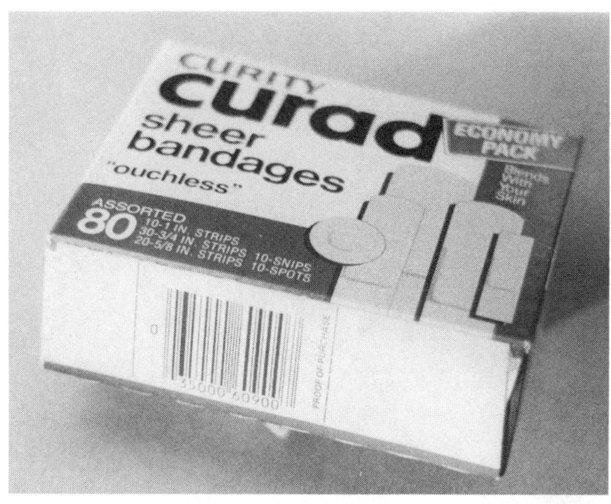

FIG. 3-10. Bar codes on medical supplies.

them into binary code for computer input. The most common example of an MICR is the magnetized characters imprinted on bank checks. Most banks use the MICR method (Fig. 3-12).

Magnetic Media

The various types of magnetic media used primarily for auxiliary memory storage are also used as input. They include magnetic tape, cassette tape, magnetic disk, floppy disk, and hard disk. (See the discussion on auxiliary memory storage for descriptions.) When used as input, these media use a tape or disk drive to read and input data into computer memory.

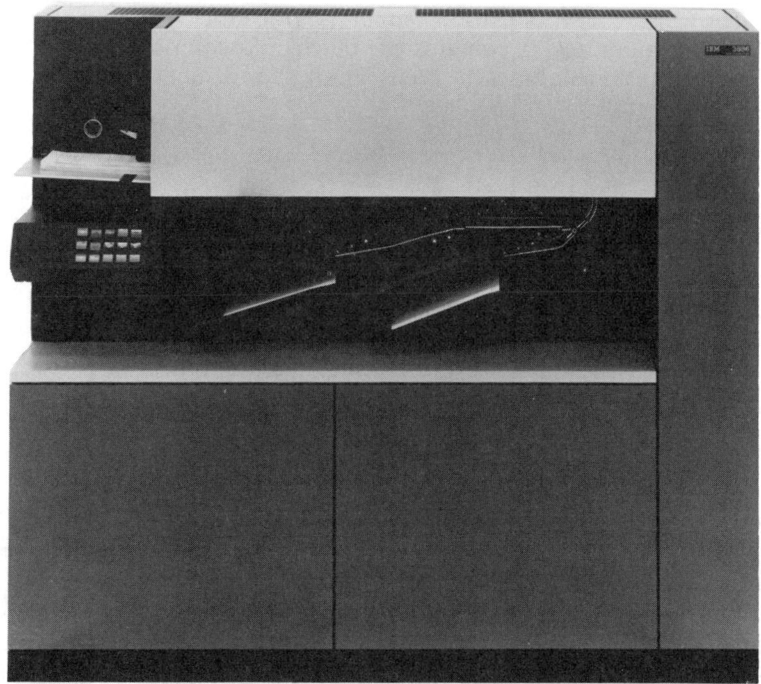

FIG. 3-11. Optical character reader. (Courtesy IBM)

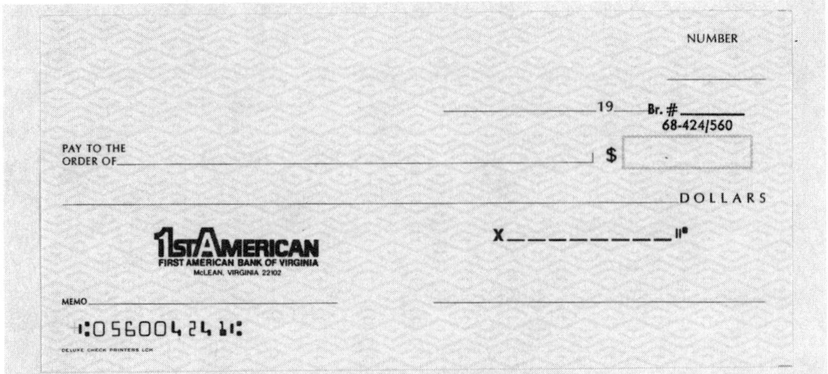
NUMBER
19 Br. #
68-424/560
PAY TO THE
ORDER OF
$
DOLLARS
1ST AMERICAN
FIRST AMERICAN BANK OF VIRGINIA
McLEAN, VIRGINIA 22102
X
MEMO
⑆056004246⑆

FIG. 3-12. An example of magnetic-ink recognition medium.

Voice/Image

Other input devices include those for voice and image input. Voice input requires a special audio input device. Although automatic recognition of the human voice is not yet perfected, voice input is used in situations requiring only a few spoken words. It may eventually become a common medium for all computer systems.

Several different types of image input devices are available, which primarily transform images from various types of graphics into a form that the computer can process. Many graphic images on paper or microfilm can thus become computer input (Necas, 1983).

Central Processing Unit

The CPU, which controls and supervises the entire computer system, is the "brain" of the computer. It contains the electronic components essential for computer operation and includes the control unit, the arithmetic and logic unit, and the main memory unit.

Control Unit

The control unit supervises and monitors all computer system activities. Controlling and coordinating the machine's devices and data required to perform and process a computer program, it also selects the input/output devices needed to process data, controls the movement of data to and from memory, and performs the instructions of a computer program. Further, it oversees and schedules data processing operations. It is analogous to a telephone exchange, in which controlling instruments ring phones and connect and disconnect circuits.

Arithmetic/Logic Unit

The arithmetic/logic unit, the "workhorse" of the computer, is the simplest component to understand. It performs all operations as directed by the control unit. This unit contains the electronic circuitry essential for performing arithmetic calculations and logical operations and comparisons; the arithmetic calculations include addition, subtraction, multiplication, and division. Calculating the inpatient census of a hospital, for instance, would require that admissions be added and discharges subtracted from the previous day's census.

The logical operations can be reduced to three basic comparisons—equal to, less than, and greater than—in which the arithmetic/logic unit compares the values of data being processed. These logical operations are based on the true–false propositions set forth by George Boole, the founder of boolean algebra. In 1854 he developed his sets of algebralike rules or truth tables to facilitate describing logical functions. Boole's rules for manipulating the true–false propositions rely on the logical connectives *and, or*, and *not* (Korfhage, 1983) (Fig. 3-13).

The computer performs these three basic comparisons, or their combinations, to process data. For example, the question whether a patient's temperature is within normal range requires several comparisons:

1. Equal to (=): Comparison in which one data element is equal to another data element. (The patient's temperature is normal at 98.6°F or equal to 98.6°F)
2. Less than (<): Comparison in which one data element is less than another data element. (The patient's temperature is subnormal at 95.2°F or less than 98.6°F).
3. Greater than (>): Comparison in which one data element is greater than another data element. (The patient's temperature is elevated at 101.8°F or greater than 98.6°F).

Main Memory Unit

The main memory unit, also called primary storage, stores computer software, including the data and instructions that the computer will process. Memory, logically organized and arranged so that stored data are located and accessed easily, uses specific addresses, similar to a post office, to store and locate data. Every coded character being stored has its own address (mailbox). The addresses do not move but data can be moved from address to address.

Memory Media. In most computers, memory consists of electronic components, thousands of microminiaturized circuits etched on tiny silicon chips that are only several square millimeters in size. The chip, which has revolutionized the computer industry, is compact, extremely reliable, and longlasting, and it uses little electricity and is relatively inexpensive to produce. The number of circuits etched on a chip continues to increase, which in turn decreases computer size and increases computer power.

The "And" Function

True (1) and True (1) = True (1)
True (1) and False (0) = False (0)
False (0) and True (1) = False (0)
False (0) and False (0) = False (0)

The "Or" Function

True (1) or True (1) = True (1)
True (1) or False (0) = True (1)
False (0) or True (1) = True (1)
False (0) or False (0) = False (0)

The "Not" Function

True (1) not False (0) = True (1)
False (0) not True (1) = False (0)

FIG. 3-13. Boolean true–false propositions.

The electronic circuits or "logic gates" can sense the absence or presence of electronic impulses, which represent data stored in memory. Absence (off) is represented by the binary digit 0, and presence (on) by the binary digit 1. The 0 or 1 is called a *bit,* which is the accepted abbreviation for *bi*nary digi*t*. (The binary numbering system uses a base of two, unlike the decimal numbering system, which uses a base of ten.)

Storage Types. Memory has two types of storage:

- Read only memory (ROM)
- Random access memory (RAM)

Read Only Memory. Read only memory (ROM) refers to the permanent storage of data, meaning that data may be read but not written on or altered. ROM generally contains the programs, called firmware, used by the control unit of the CPU to oversee computer functions. In microcomputers, this may also include the software programs used to translate the computer's high-level programming languages into machine language (binary code) (see Chap. 4). Further, it contains other software programs essential for computer function, such as the operating system. ROM storage is not erased when the computer is turned off. ROM is generally developed by computer manufacturers.

Random Access Memory. Random access memory (RAM) refers to memory used for primary storage. It is volatile and used as temporary storage. RAM can be accessed, used, changed, and written on repeatedly. It contains data and instructions that are stored and processed by computer programs called applications programs. The computer programs, which are not permanent, are read from or written by a user and may be altered. RAM is lost if the power is turned off in a microcomputer, unlike ROM.

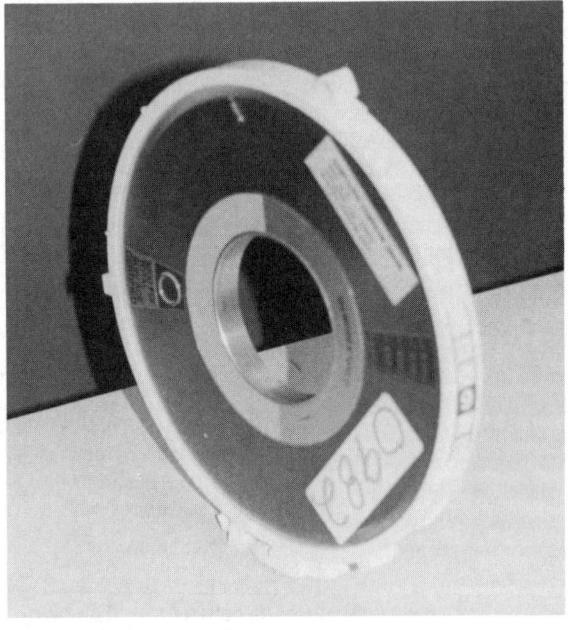

FIG. 3-14. Magnetic tape.

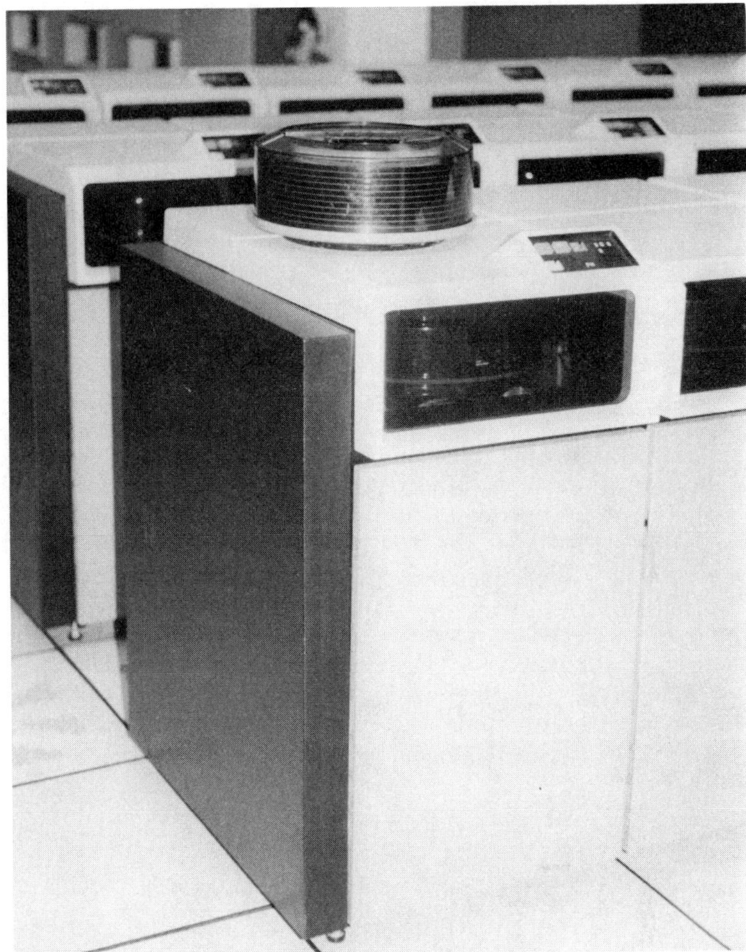

FIG. 3-15. Magnetic disk pack and disk drives.

Auxiliary Memory Unit. Auxiliary memory is used to expand the memory capacity of a computer system, since main memory has limited storage space. Auxiliary memory can be on line or off line. If on line, then the computer has immediate access; that is, it can read and retrieve data that are generally stored on magnetic disks. However, if the storage is off line, the computer must wait until a computer operator loads a magnetic tape containing the data needed for processing onto the computer.

Several more common types of auxiliary memory, called secondary storage, include the following:

- Magnetic disk/magnetic tape
- Floppy disk/diskette
- Hard disk

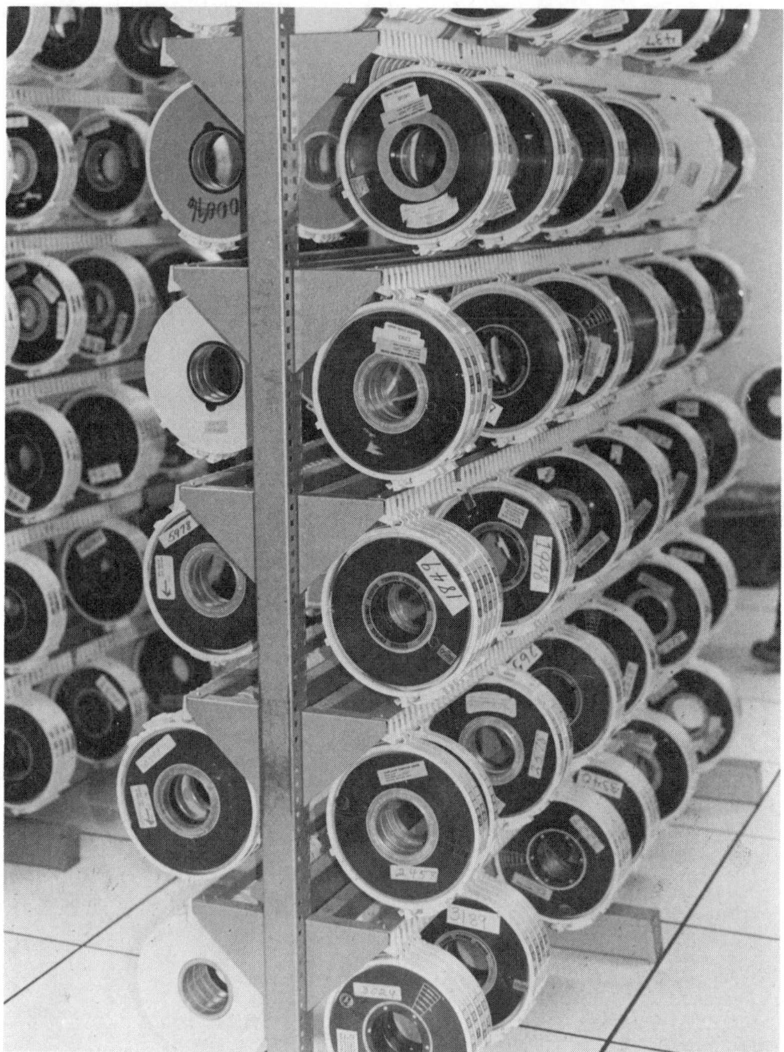

FIG. 3-16. Magnetic tapes off line.

Magnetic Disk and Magnetic Tape. Magnetic disk and magnetic tape are both used as auxiliary memory and as input/output media for mainframes and minicomputers. Magnetic disks, which are replacing magnetic tape, make it possible for computer systems to store large volumes of data at a relatively low cost.

Data are recorded onto magnetic disks and magnetic tapes from a keyboard, or a CRT/VDT, punched card, or as output from a computer system and converted into magnetized spots representing machine-readable binary code. They are read or written on through special input devices called magnetic disk or tape drives. Both these devices contain a read/write head that can sense, interpret, and convert the magnetized spots into electronic impulses the computer can understand.

The magnetic tape resembles a ½-inch reel of film strip (Fig. 3-14). The mag-

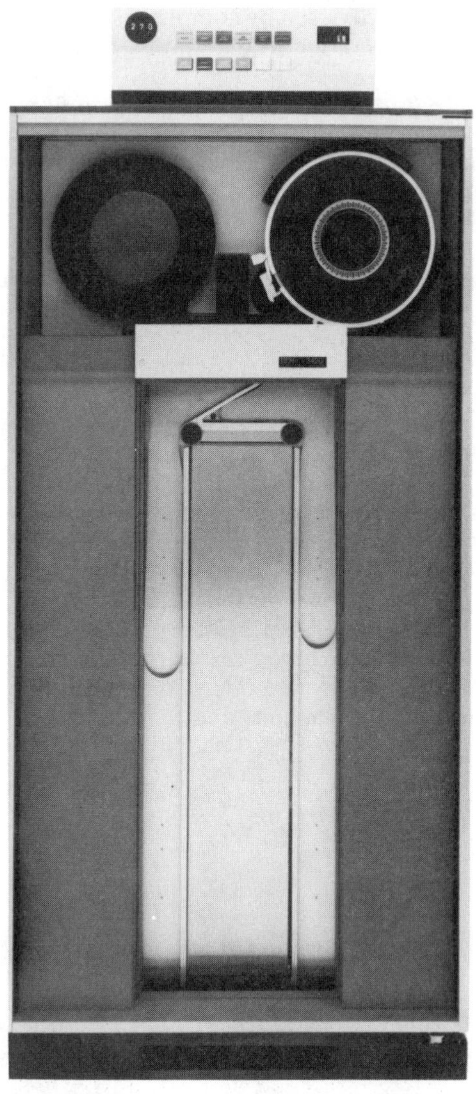

FIG. 3-17. Magnetic tape drive. (Courtesy IBM)

netic disk, a metal platter usually 14 inches in diameter, is generally found in a disk pack that contains a stack of eight or ten 12-inch high-fidelity records, all connected and enclosed in what resembles a large cake dish (Fig. 3-15). The magnetic tapes are stored on shelves and mounted onto devices called magnetic tape drives when needed as computer input (Figs. 3-16 and 3-17). Magnetic disks are either permanently installed or mounted onto magnetic disk drives. They are connected together and to the computer to provide on-line input and can be added as needed to allow for expanded data storage.

Magnetic disks make it possible for on-line interactive information systems in large health care facilities to store and process large volumes of data. Such systems permit many users direct access to the database. Magnetic tapes, on the other hand, are primarily used by computer systems to store data that are not essential for daily system operation. For example, records of discharged patients can be stored in an off-line mode.

Floppy Disk (Diskette). The floppy disk, commonly called a diskette, is another form of auxiliary memory. It is also used as input/output medium. The floppy disk is largely used by microcomputers and minicomputers. Data are read and written on, with disk drives, in the same manner as with magnetic tapes and magnetic disks (Fig. 3-18).

A diskette, which resembles a 45-rpm stereo record, is a flexible Mylar plastic-coated disk thinly covered with magnetic material. It is available in 8-, $5\frac{1}{4}$-, $3\frac{1}{4}$-, and 3-inch squares, as well as several other less common sizes, to accommodate various computer models. All disks are jacketed in a protective paper envelope. Each is sectioned into concentric rings or tracks and each track into sectors. Each floppy disk can store thousands of usable characters (bytes). Diskettes are available in various formats — single or double sided and single or double density. Such variations determine the number of characters the disk can store.

Hard Disk. The hard disk, commonly referred to as a "Winchester," is another form of auxiliary memory. It too is used as an input/output medium. A hard, metal, recordlike platter produced for use in some minicomputers and microcomputers, it was introduced by IBM in 1973 (Capron and Williams, 1984). Unlike the floppy disk, it is rigid and generally encased in a nonremovable sealed container. Its storage capacity is at least ten times that of the floppy disk. The Winchester, much faster to access than the floppy disk, is the most reliable mass storage for some minicomputers and microcomputers. It comes in various sizes depending on desired storage capacity and requirements.

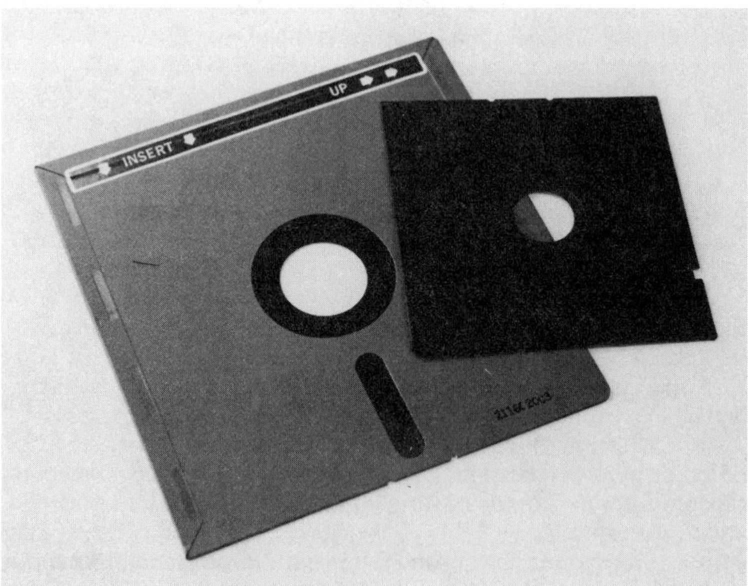

FIG. 3-18. Floppy disk/diskette.

Output Unit

The fifth functional component of a computer system, the output unit, functions in reverse of the input unit. It provides the information generated by the computer system, generally transmitting the processed information to users in an English-like form. The output unit can also transmit data to auxiliary memory as well as to other computer systems.

Output Devices/Media

In any computer system, the output is the final product of the data processing functions; several different output devices and media can be present, but most of the input and auxiliary memory devices are also used as output. The most common input device used for output is the CRT terminal; however, other types of terminals are also used as output devices, as are magnetic disks, magnetic tapes, floppy disks, and hard disks. Output devices consist of the following:

- CRT terminal
- Other terminals
- Magnetic media
- Printer
- Microfilm/microfiche
- Graphic display/copy
- Voice output
- Photographic material

Cathode Ray Tube Terminal

A CRT terminal, also called a VDT or monitor, can be used as output. This type of terminal displays the data processing actions without requiring a printer.

A CRT terminal has many uses as output. For example, it can display text being prepared when a word processing software package is used, allowing the user to view, create, and correct the text easily. It also allows a user to accent words by darkening or underlining them and to perform other options for printing hard copy. It can be used to scroll text or data around the screen and to display whole screens or pages of data at one time. The CRT terminal can also be used to prepare "windows," which are display screens divided into sections like window panes. This option allows data from different parts of the file to be viewed at one time.

Other Terminals

Other terminals used to communicate with the computer can also be considered output devices. They include the hard copy/teletypewriter and portable and hand-held terminals. They can produce output that is displayed on the terminal video screen or printed on paper. (See discussion on terminals.)

Magnetic Media

All magnetic media used for auxiliary memory (magnetic tape, cassette tape, magnetic disk, floppy disk, and hard disk) also act as output. These media, like input, use tape or disk drives to write and produce computer data. (See the discussion on auxiliary memory for a complete description.)

Printer

The printer, the most important output device, converts information generated by the computer system into printed form, rendering data in the binary code into readable English. The major types of printed output include printed hard copy (paper), microfilm (microfiche), photographs, and graphic copy (Necas, 1983; Capron and Williams, 1984).

Printed paper copy, known as ***hard copy,*** is output produced on paper, in contrast to ***soft copy,*** which refers to video displays. Paper is printed either by impact or nonimpact. The former uses a device similar to a typewriter to strike the paper; the latter uses heat, laser, ink jet, or photography to print. Nonimpact printers can print at very high speed and produce graphic displays.

The impact printer, either line printers or character printers, are the most common. A line printer, as its name indicates, prints an entire line of characters at one time; its speed is generally measured by the number of lines it can print per minute. It is essentially an output device for mainframes and minicomputers that generate large volumes of hard copy (paper) output (Fig. 3-19).

The character printer, which resembles a typewriter, prints one character at a time. Its speed is measured by the number of characters it prints per second. This type of printer is generally slower and costs less than the line printer; it is essentially an output device for some minicomputers and nearly all microcomputers.

Several types of character printers are currently available. One uses a "typewriter ball" similar to the one on the IBM Selectric Typewriter. Another employs the "daisy wheel," which produces letter-quality printing and is used for word processing and correspondence. A third type relies on a "dot matrix," which consists of small wires for producing characters composed from a series of dots.

Microfilm/Microfiche

Microfilm and Microfiche are two other output media. The computer output on microfilm (COM) is output that has been photographed from a special high-resolution display, producing a microfilm that contains miniaturized photographs on a film strip (Fig. 3-20). The COM can also be produced as small photographs on a 5- by 7-inch film sheet known as a ***microfiche.*** A microfiche saves space, since one sheet can store from 100 to 200 pages of filmed output (Fig. 3-21).

Graphic Display/Copy

The most common graphic displays are those produced from a graphic software package on a CRT terminal designed to display graphic as well as alphanumeric data. They generally include a line, bar, or pie chart graph. These graphs can be printed as hard copy using a dot matrix printer with graphic capability (Figs. 3-22 to 3-24). In addition, special graphic display terminals can display colored maps and charts, and ink-jet printers can produce graphic images in many colors. Finally, plotters can produce hard copy maps and charts.

Voice Output

Voice output devices, sometimes called voice synthesizers, are now available to vocalize data stored in main memory. It is currently easier for a computer system to produce voice output than to accept voice input. Voice output is generally used for short responses by telephone companies, automobile manufacturers, and several manufacturers of toys in promoting their products.

(Text continues on p. 70)

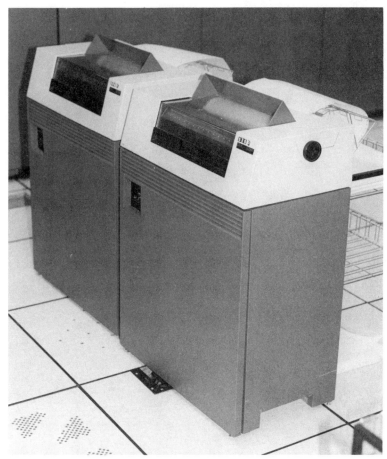

FIG. 3-19. Line printer.

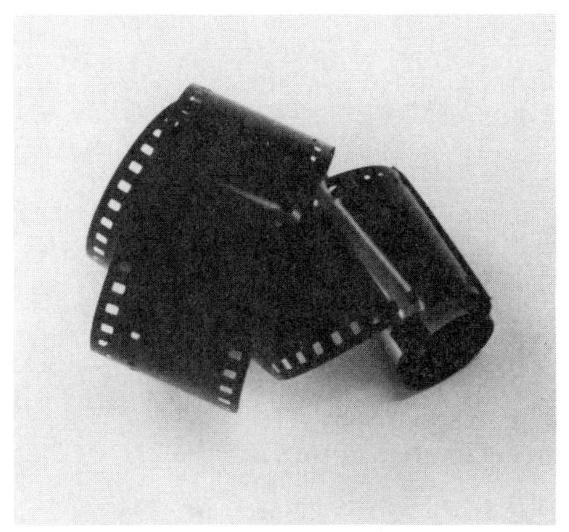

FIG. 3-20. Microfilm.

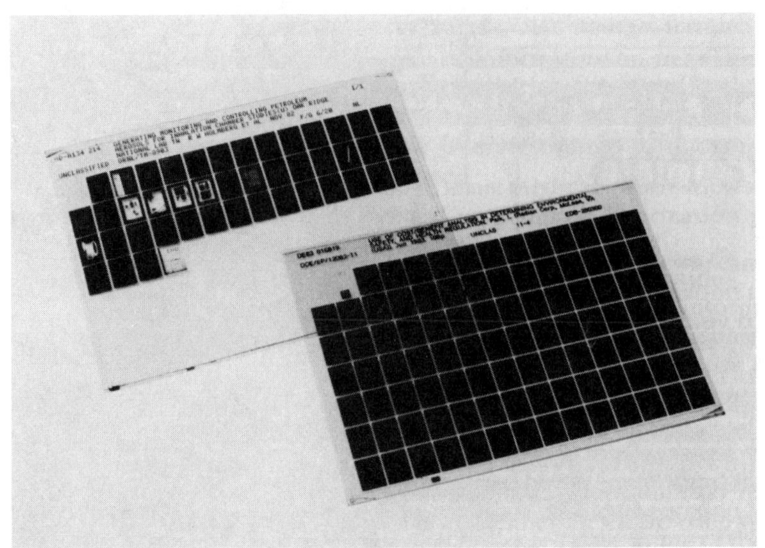

FIG. 3-21. Microfiche.

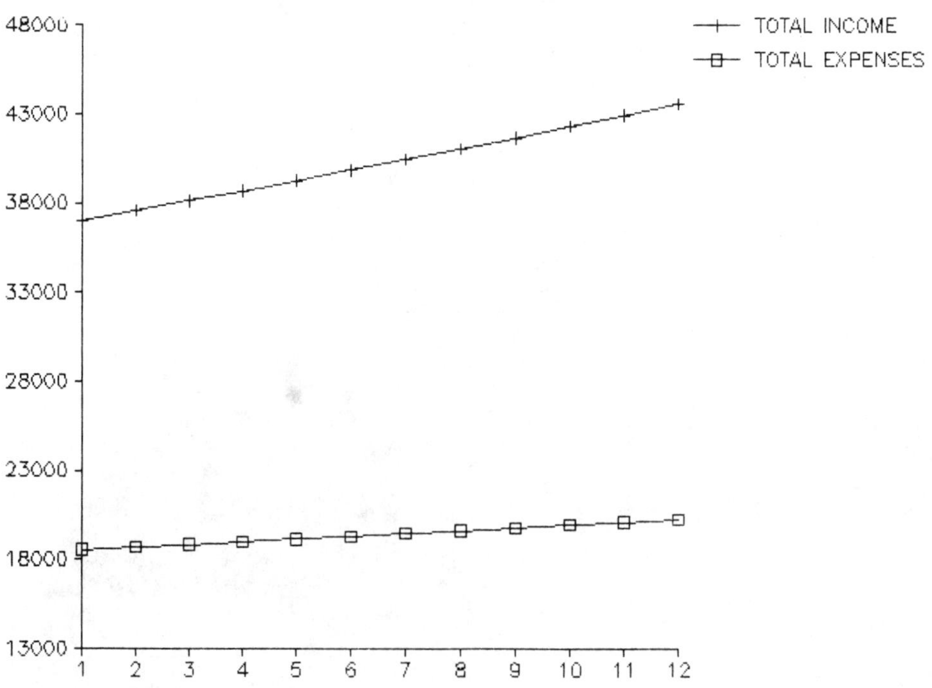

FIG. 3-22. Graphic line chart.

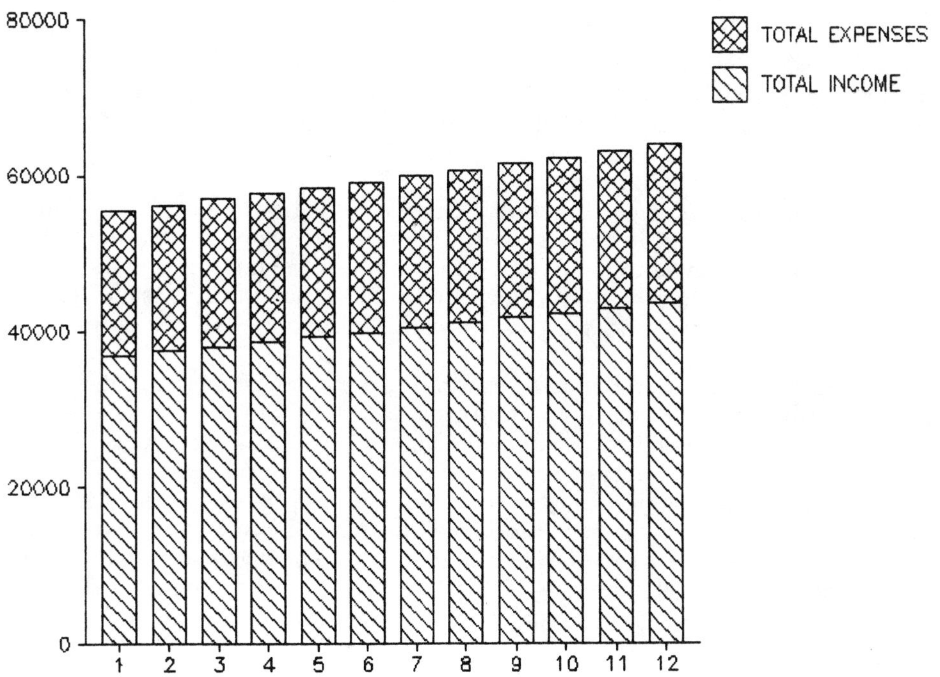

FIG. 3-23. Graphic bar chart.

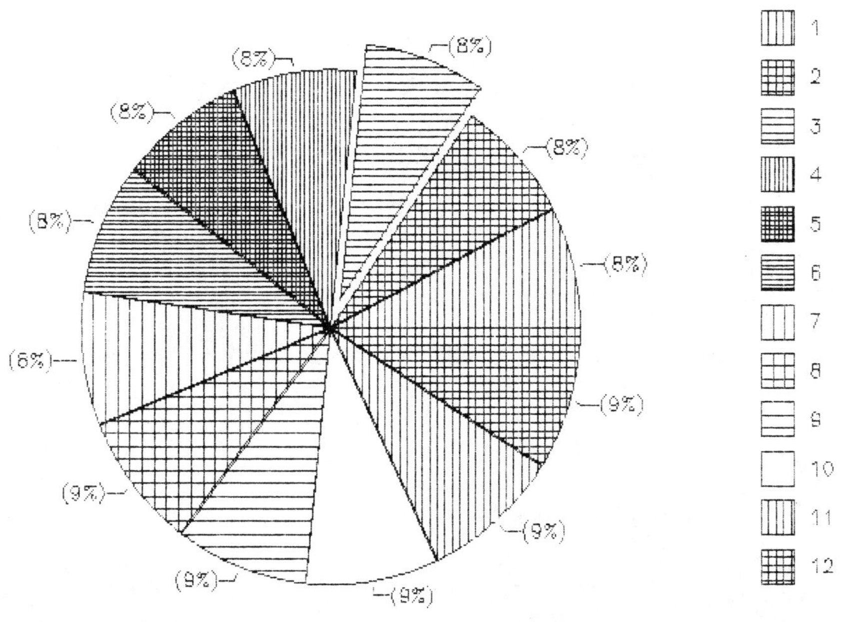

FIG. 3-24. Graphic pie chart.

SUMMARY

This chapter has described computer hardware, which consists of all tangible parts. It also describes computer classes, characteristics, and types. The computer classes are analog, digital, and hybrid. The computer characteristics are defined as automatic, electronic, general purpose, and digital. Computer types include the mainframe, minicomputer, and microcomputer.

It outlines the five major functional components of a computer—the input unit, the central processing unit (consisting of the control unit, the arithmetic and logic unit, and the main memory unit), the auxiliary memory unit, which is an extension of main memory, and the output unit. The input unit acts as the "reception desk," the central processing unit runs the computer, and the output unit produces information.

The different devices and media these units use are described in detail, and the most common input devices—the keyboard and the CRT/VDT terminals—are reviewed. The two different types of main memory, ROM (read only memory) and RAM (random access memory), are discussed; the former is for permanent storage and the latter for temporary storage. The major auxiliary memory storage devices are highlighted, including magnetic tapes, magnetic disks, floppy disks (diskettes), and hard disks. Finally, output unit devices and media are reviewed. These include not only the CRT and magnetic media, but the various types of printers, microfilm, microfiche, graphic displays and copy, and voice output.

STUDY QUESTIONS

1. What are the three broad classes of computers?
2. Name four major characteristics of a computer.
3. Name the three types of computers.
4. Name the five functional components of a computer.
5. Name the most common input device.
6. Name the two types of terminals.
7. Name the input media for the early computers.
8. Name the three units in the CPU.
9. What are the two operations that the arithmetic and logic unit performs?
10. What are the three basic comparisons the arithmetic logic unit performs?
11. Name the two types of memory units.
12. Name the two types of memory storage.
13. Name the four types of auxiliary memory (secondary storage) media.
14. Name two auxiliary storage media used by the microcomputer.
15. Name six major output devices.

REFERENCES

Capron HL, Williams BK: Computer and Data Processing, 2nd ed. Menlo Park, CA, Benjamin/Cummings, 1984

Finkelstein CB: IBM Card. In Ralston A, Reilly ED Jr (eds): Encyclopedia of Computer Science and Engineering, 2nd ed, pp 706–709. New York, Van Nostrand Reinhold, 1983

Garfield J: Buying your first modem. inCider, pp 58–60, August 1984

Hopper GM, Mandell SL: Understanding Computers. New York, West Publishing, 1984

Korfhage RR: Boolean algebra. In Ralston A, Reilly ED Jr (eds): Encyclopedia of Computer Science and Engineering, 2nd ed, pp 179–184. New York, Van Nostrand Reinhold, 1983

Libes S: Editor's page. Microsystems 4(5):8–9, 1983

Morris GJ: Digital computers: General principles. In Ralston A, Reilly ED Jr (eds): Encyclopedia of Computer Science and Engineering, 2nd ed, pp 524–533. New York, Van Nostrand Reinhold, 1983

Necas J: Input-output devices. In Ralston A, Reilly ED Jr (eds): Encyclopedia of Computer Science and Engineering, 2nd ed, pp 735–766. New York, Van Nostrand Reinhold, 1983

Rosen S: Digital computers: History: Contemporary and future. In Ralston A, Reilly ED Jr (eds): Encyclopedia of Computer Science and Engineering, 2nd ed, pp 540–554. New York, Van Nostrand Reinhold, 1983

BIBLIOGRAPHY

Bernstein J: When the computer procreates. The New York Times Magazine, pp 34–38, February 15, 1976

Boraiko AA: The chip: Electronic minimarvel that is changing your life. National Geographic 162(4):421–458, 1982

Bonner P: Hard disks made easy. Personal Comput, pp 66–73, November 1983

Bronzino JD: Computer Applications for Patient Care. Reading, MA, Addison-Wesley, 1982

Covvey HD, McAlister NH: Computers in the Practice of Medicine, vol I, Introduction to Computing Concepts. Reading, MA, Addison-Wesley, 1980

Davis RM: Evolution of computers and computing. Science 195(4283):1096–1102, 1977

Doletta TA: Terminals. In Ralston A, Reilly ED Jr (eds): Encyclopedia of Computer Science and Engineering, 2nd ed, pp 1489–1495. New York, Van Nostrand Reinhold, 1983

Encyclopedia Britannica Educational Corp: Understanding Computers. Skokie, IL, Encyclopedia Britannica Educational Corp, 1982

Enlander D: Computers in Medicine: An Introduction. St Louis, CV Mosby, 1980

Frankenhuis JP: How to get a good mini. Harvard Business Review, pp 139–149, May–June 1982

Freeman DN: Memory: Auxiliary. In Ralston A, Reilly ED Jr (eds): Encyclopedia of Computer Science and Engineering, 2nd ed, pp 955–956. New York, Van Nostrand Reinhold, 1983

Grobe SJ: Computer Primer and Resource Guide for Nurses. Philadelphia, JB Lippincott, 1984

Hedberg A: Choosing the best computer for now. Money, pp 68–117, November 1982

Heller RS, Martin DC: Bits'n Bytes About Computing: A Computer Literacy Primer. Rockville, MD, Computer Science Press, 1982

IBM Corp: Introduction to IBM Data Processing Systems. Poughkeepsie, NY, IBM Corp, 1981

IBM Corp: More About Computers. Armonk, NY, IBM Corp, 1974

McGlynn DR: Personal Computing: Home, Professional and Small Business Applications, 2nd ed. New York, John Wiley & Sons, 1982

McLeod R Jr, Forkner I: Computerized Business Information Systems: An Introduction to Data Processing. New York, John Wiley & Sons, 1982

Prichard K: Computers. I. An introduction. Nurs Times 78(5):355–357, 1982

Ralston A, Reilly ED Jr (eds): Encyclopedia of Computer Science and Engineering, 2nd ed. New York, Van Nostrand Reinhold, 1983

Rinder RM: A Practical Guide to Small Computers for Business and Professional Use. New York, Monarch Press, 1981

Sanders DH: Computers in Business: An Introduction, 4th ed. New York, McGraw-Hill, 1968

Shea T: Personal computer graphics: Pushing technology to the limit. InfoWorld 5(51):34–36, 1983

Shelly GB, Cashman TJ: Introduction to Computers and Data Processing. Brea, CA, Anaheim Publishing, 1980

Stern RA, Stern N: An Introduction to Computers and Information Processing. New York, John Wiley & Sons, 1982

Vacroux AG: Microcomputers. Sci Amer 232(5):32–40, 1975

Walsh ME: Understanding Computers: What Managers and Users Need to Know. New York, John Wiley & Sons, 1982

Zak R: Your First Computer: A Guide to Business and Personal Computing. Berkeley, CA, SYBEX, 1980

4 Computer Software

Objectives

- Define and describe computer software.
- Describe the difference between system programs and application programs.
- List the three levels of programming languages.
- List the common high-level programming languages.
- Describe the different steps in programming.

Computer software makes the computer run and controls computer hardware. In a sense, computer software comprises all the computer components that are not considered hardware and are not visible, although it primarily refers to the various types of computer programs and their programming languages.

Computer programs consist of sets of instructions organized in sequence and stored in the computer memory. The computer follows these step-by-step instructions to perform the functions required to make it run. The term *software* includes not only computer programs written by computer programmers but already prepared ones called *software packages.*

Software packages, which are designed to carry out a specific application or solve a specific problem, are usually structured to make computer programs easier to use and adapt.

Programming languages, the specially designed languages used to communicate with the computer, consist of a set of symbols and rules, allowing the user to interface with the computer.

This chapter describes several significant aspects of computer software. First, it discusses the different uses and types of computer programs, including software packages. It then describes programming languages, highlighting several of the common ones. Finally, it describes programming, the writing of a program. The three major areas of software include the following:

- Computer programs
- Programming languages
- Programming

COMPUTER PROGRAMS

The idea of the stored computer program was first considered by Charles Babbage for his analytical engine in the 1880s. His friend Ada, Countess of Lovelace and Lord Byron's daughter, described the use of repetitious arithmetic operations—the *loop* concept. She advocated that this loop would be performed by the analytical engine. Ada is considered the first programmer in computer history (Wilkes, 1983; Hopper and Mandell, 1984). However, it was not until 1946 that Von Newmann proposed that both data and instructions be stored in the computer and that instructions be automatically carried out. This concept was subsequently implemented as a major feature of the computer.

Definition

A computer program is a set of stored instructions enabling the computer to perform a function or procedure or to solve a problem. It can be further described as a series of instructions written in proper sequence that adhere to the rules of a programming language.

Generally, computer programs are described according to how they function; two major categories exist:

- Systems programs
- Application programs

System Programs

System programs refer to any program that runs the computer system. These stored programs, which carry out, maintain, supervise, and control all automatic functions of a computer system, are generally not visible or accessible to users. They generally are written by manufacturers and come with the computer hardware. Developed to ensure the smooth functioning of the computer system, they include the programs stored in read only memory (ROM).

All computer systems have system programs. The mainframes and minicomputers require more system programs to carry out their many functions than the microcomputers because they are larger and more complex. In these machines, system programs must supervise and schedule the concurrent processing of many programs for many users. Microcomputers, need fewer such programs, since they generally process one program at a time.

System programs can be further described by the different functions they perform:

- Operating systems
- Translation programs
- Utility programs

Operating Systems

Operating systems are sets of programs that act as "traffic cops" by supervising and controlling computer resources, managing data, and performing computer programs. They schedule and control all input and output devices and functions, manage data flow in and out of memory, and assign data to storage locations. They also control computer programs that run concurrently. The operating systems thus control multiprogramming, timesharing, and other special automatic features found in large computer systems without computer users being involved.

Most operating systems come with computers and were developed either by special vendors or by manufacturers. They are specifically tailored to fit a certain type of computer hardware and ensure its efficient operation. All computers, regardless of type or size, require an operating system.

Translation Programs

The major function of translation programs is to translate programming language into machine language. Translation programs, called compilers, interpreters, or assemblers, are machine dependent, which means that a computer must have a specific compiler, interpreter, or assembler to translate the general programming language of the computer program into the language specific for the machine. For example, if a program is written in the language FORTRAN, the computer must have a compiler to translate FORTRAN into machine language.

Utility Programs

The utility programs are primarily designed to handle the computer's housekeeping procedures. They take care of repetitive tasks and are used to streamline computer operations. For example, they can update files or convert the use of one type of input/output medium to another (*e.g.,* paper copy to microfilm).

Application Programs

Application programs process data. Unlike system programs, they are written by or for system users. Generally written by computer programmers in a programming language to solve a problem, perform a task, or produce some type of result, they can be used in several different computer models. However, any computer used must have a translation program to translate the programming language into machine language. Such programs are stored in random access memory (RAM).

Software Packages

Application programs are also written as software packages, which are already prepared sets of computer programs developed for a specific function for many computer users. Generally written in an English-like computer language, they require little or no programming knowledge and are ready to use.

Software packages, available for all sizes of computers, are being developed and marketed by an increasing number of software vendors. Vendors generally retain ownership rights, thus limiting the making of copies for resale. Some of these software packages are also referred to as systems.

Some of the more popular software packages include database management systems developed to manage and monitor the data in databases. Authoring systems allow authors to use the computer to develop computer-assisted lessons and computer-based instructional materials. Statistical packages are designed to perform various mathematical calculations. Software packages found in hospital nursing departments are used to process patient classification in order to determine nurse staffing and scheduling. Other software packages do word processing, spelling verification, editing, and electronic spreadsheets.

Many software packages are written with a convenient high-level programming language, allowing users to interact with the computer with what is called a *query language.* A query language consists of English-like words and sometimes is refered to as *user friendly.* This means that users, authors, and other nonprogrammers can follow and run the programs with little or no programming knowledge. Most software packages have their own query language.

Generally, these software packages are designed so that different types of displays are visible on a cathode ray tube (CRT)/video display terminal (VDT) screen. The two most common variations are as follows:

- Menu
- Template

Menu

The menu, a list of choices, leads the user through a sequence of steps. It does not change until an option is selected or carried out. Depending on the selection, other menus may automatically be displayed. This process continues until the computer program is completed. The menu for a word processing software package might include the options *type, print, get, save, remove,* and *exit.*

Template

The template, a display used to enter data into the computer, can be a list of questions requiring an answer or merely headings or terms needing completion. For example, a template for a new admission into a hospital information system (HIS) might display a list of demographic headings and terms requiring completion, such as name, address, sex, race, religion, physician's name, and insurance company. Opposite each heading is a space for information; once keyed in, data are entered into the system.

PROGRAMMING LANGUAGES

A programming language, a language used to communicate with the computer, is defined by the American National Standards Institue (ANSI) as "a language used to prepare computer programs" (Sammet, 1969). It contains a defined set of characters (symbols) and rules (semantics); the rules clearly define how to use the symbols.

Computer programming languages have a history of their own. With the invention of the computer in 1946, machine languages emerged, followed by assembly languages. High-level programming languages followed in the 1950s as the computer industry advanced. Instrumental in this development was Commodore Grace Hopper, USN, who with associates developed one of the first automatic coding system or high-level languages—COBOL (*CO*mmon *B*usiness *O*riented *L*anguage). COBOL is used primarily for business applications (Johnson, 1982; Rosen, 1983).

The three levels of computer programming languages are as follows:

- Machine language
- Assembly language
- High-level languages

Machine Language

The machine language, a low-level language, is the true language of the computer. Any program must be translated into machine language before the computer can execute it (Fig. 4-1). The machine language consists only of the binary numbers 0 and 1, representing the *on* and *off* electronic impulses. All data—numbers, letters, and symbols—are represented by combinations of binary digits. For example, the number 3 is represented by eight binary numbers (0000 0011), and 6 is represented by 0000 0110. Machine languages are machine dependent and thus dissimilar. Thus, each machine has its own unique machine language.

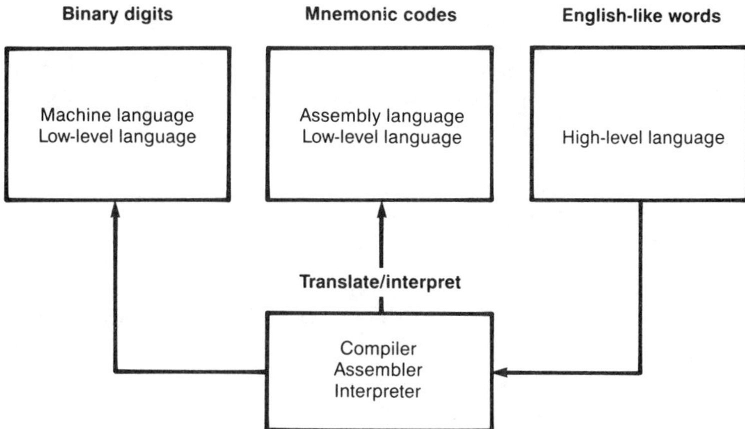

FIG. 4-1. The three levels of computer programming languages.

Assembly Language

The assembly language, another low-level language, was developed to make writing computer programs less burdensome. Assembly languages use abbreviations or mnemonic codes for computer programs instead of binary codes; symbols are used for programming instructions. For example, A or AD might be used for add, and S might be used for subtract.

Assembly language is written on a one-to-one basis, as is machine language. For each line of assembly language code an equivalent line of machine language code exists. To code the instruction "ADD 6 and 3," the assembly language might read "AD 6, 3." One line of code is used for the instruction.

An assembler program translates assembly language into machine language. Like machine language, assembly language is machine dependent.

High-Level Languages

Like assembly language, high-level languages were developed to make writing programs easier. Approximating language used to state or solve a problem, high-level languages resemble English and use English-like words to code programs. Scientific problems are therefore more readily understood, since mathematical formulas can be expressed clearly in the coding; by the same token, business terms are more readily understood, since their common terms are used for naming variables. Over 200 programming languages are considered to be high-level languages.

High-level languages have many advantages over low-level machine and assembly languages. They are not written for a specific machine but for programmers, thus requiring little or no knowledge of a specific computer; however, they do require learning the rules of the language. A programmer can write a program with little or no knowledge about the specific computer the program will be "run" on. Generally, program instructions are relatively easy to write, since they are written in terms similar to those used for solving the problem. Each instruction is translated into several lines of machine language code. For example, the instruction to read two variables, "READ A, B," will be translated into several separate instructions of machine language code.

All high-level languages are machine independent. The instructions cannot be executed unless the computer translates them into machine language; all high-level languages thus require the use of a compiler program or interpreter program.

High-Level Language Selection

Selecting a high-level language is based on several factors. First, the language must be able to resolve the problem, be easy to use, and be easily transportable to other machines. Next, a compiler or interpreter for the specific computer must be available. Also, the language should have potential for other applications. Described below, in aphabetical order, are several major high-level programming languages in current use (Shelly and Cashman, 1980; Capron and Williams, 1984; IBM, 1981).

ADA

Named for Ada, Countess of Lovelace, ADA was developed for the Department of Defense. Completed in 1984, it is designed to meet the department's high technical, management, and cost criteria requirements. Designed to provide greater reliability and efficient maintenance of computer programs, ADA is structured to be used for scientific, business, and command and control applications.

ALGOL

ALGOL (the *ALGO*rithmic *L*anguage) is an international algebraic language. Introduced in 1960 by European and American scientists, it was developed primarily for scientific applications and is thus similar to FORTRAN (see below).

BASIC

BASIC (*B*eginners *A*ll-purpose *S*ymbolic *I*nstruction *C*ode), introduced in 1965 at Dartmouth College under the direction of Professor John Kemeny, is an interactive English-like language that is easy to learn and use. Developed for use on a timesharing system by students, it is mathematical but also allows for freeform text. It has become one of the major languages used for the microcomputer.

COBOL

COBOL (*CO*mmon *B*usiness *O*riented *L*anguage), the most widely used programming language for business applications, was developed in 1959 by the "Mother of COBOL," Commodore Grace Hopper, USN, along with associates, and is one of the earliest high-level languages. COBOL is officially sanctioned as the federal language for all business applications. Machine independent, it is translated and used by many different types of computer systems (Johnson, 1982; ICP, 1980; Washington Post Parade Magazine, 1982).

FORTRAN

FORTRAN (*FOR*mula *TRAN*slator), a programming language used primarily for scientific and mathematical applications, was introduced by IBM in 1954 and is the oldest of the high-level languages. Originally developed for scientists, engineers, and business statisticians, it has proved to be an excellent language for all scientific fields. A major advantage of FORTRAN is its applications for complex mathematical calculations and problems.

MUMPS

MUMPS (*M*assachusetts General Hospital *U*tility *M*ulti *P*rogramming *S*ystem), in use since 1965, was developed for clinical health care applications. Its hierarchical structure permits large volumes of data to be handled easily. MUMPS is primarily available on minicomputers. Because many computers did not have compilers or interpreters that could translate the language, it had limited use.

PASCAL

Named after Blaise Pascal, PASCAL, introduced in 1972, was developed by the Swiss professor Nicklaus Wirth for all types of applications and for applying structured programming. PASCAL is noted for its efficiency, portability, and all-around usability. A popular language for teaching, it is widely used on many microcomputers.

PLI

PLI (*P*rogramming *L*anguage *I*) is a symbolic general-purpose language developed by IBM in 1964 for a variety of business, engineering, and scientific applications. A powerful and flexible language, it incorporates the major advantages of both COBOL and FORTRAN.

RPG

RPG (*R*eport *P*rogram *G*enerator) appeared in 1964. Developed for use on IBM computers and relatively easy to use, it was designed to allow for rapid generation of business reports.

PROGRAMMING

Programming refers to the process of writing a computer program, which is a series of instructions written in proper sequence to solve a specific problem. A program primarily encompasses the program instructions and is generally written by a computer programmer.

The five major steps in writing any computer program are as follows:

- Problem definition
- Program design
- Program preparation
- Program testing
- Program implementation/documentation

Problem Definition

Problem definition is the most critical step in programming, since it requires a thorough understanding of the problem at hand. The definition must state what problem requires a solution, including relevant data and where to find them.

In essence, the problem definition must analyze and outline in detail the scope of the problem and all the elements needed to solve it. For example, a very simple problem definition for the cost of a nursing visit might read as follows: "Calculate the cost of nursing visit C by totaling cost of nurse A and cost of supplies B."

Program Design

The Program design is the plan designed to solve the problem, preliminary to actual preparation and coding. The plan must be detailed enough to outline how to produce the desired output. The problem must be analyzed and broken down into a

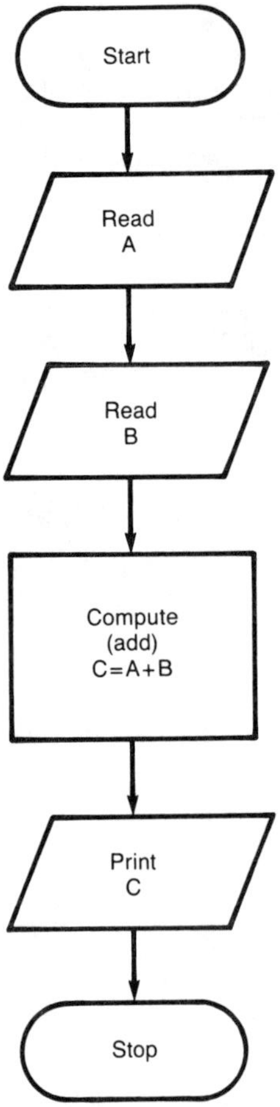

Start

Read
A

Read
B

Compute
(add)
C=A+B

Print
C

Stop

FIG. 4-2. Example of a flowchart. Problem: To read values A and B to find their sum, C.

set of logical sequential steps called an algorithm. An algorithm is actually the procedure or "recipe" that solves the problem. The steps of the algorithm are generally listed and illustrated with a flowchart (Fig. 4-2).

Flowchart

A flowchart employs a series of symbols to illustrate graphically the logical solution to a problem. It specifies the sequence of instructions or groups of instructions in a computer program. Such an illustration clarifies essential details and their relationships in the computer program. Various operations, data, tasks, and the flow process are presented graphically.

Flowcharts are characterized by sequence, symbols, and loops. The sequence of the program instructions is indicated by a line between symbols that depicts the direction of the flow process, which is one way and cannot backtrack.

Symbols or boxes used are those established by ANSI to represent the various computer operations. One symbol may signify the start and end of a program or the input/output operations. The more common symbols are illustrated in Figure 4-3. The symbols are available as templates or rulers, as illustrated in Figure 4-4.

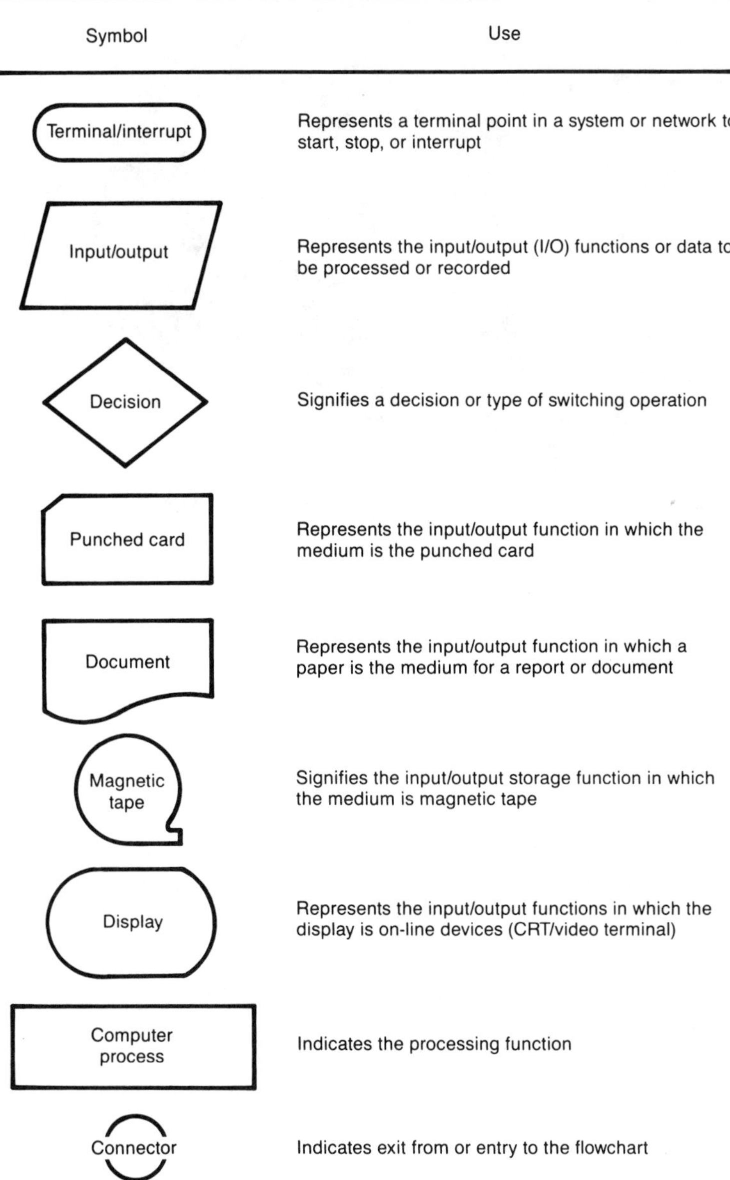

Symbol	Use
Terminal/interrupt	Represents a terminal point in a system or network to start, stop, or interrupt
Input/output	Represents the input/output (I/O) functions or data to be processed or recorded
Decision	Signifies a decision or type of switching operation
Punched card	Represents the input/output function in which the medium is the punched card
Document	Represents the input/output function in which a paper is the medium for a report or document
Magnetic tape	Signifies the input/output storage function in which the medium is magnetic tape
Display	Represents the input/output functions in which the display is on-line devices (CRT/video terminal)
Computer process	Indicates the processing function
Connector	Indicates exit from or entry to the flowchart

FIG. 4-3. Selected flowchart symbols. See Appendix for complete listing of flowchart symbols. American National Standards Institute (ANSI) system flowchart symbols are shown in the first column.

Loops represent graphically the repetitive operations or instructions in a computer program. A unique feature of programming and a major characteristic of a computer program, loops require both lines and symbols. Figure 4-5 illustrates a flowchart with a loop.

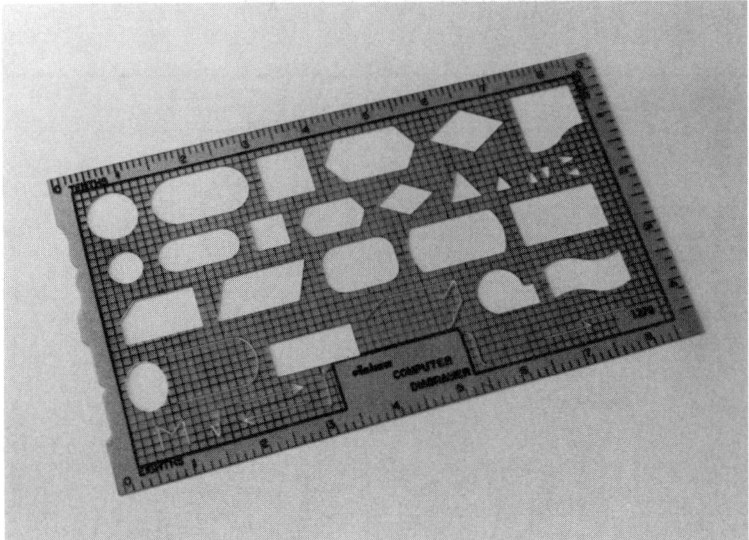

FIG. 4-4. Flowchart template.

Program Preparation

Program preparation, the actual writing of the program, entails coding the program with a programming language. The program instructions (algorithms) must be coded in detail and in logical sequence so that the program can be processed correctly. The programming language selected must not only be appropriate for processing the problem but must be translatable by the computer for which it is written. The language rules must be followed precisely, since a single coding error can stop the program from running or cause program malfunction.

A mathematical problem might be coded with a high-level language as follows:

```
START

READ A

READ B

COMPUTE C = A + B

PRINT C
```

Program Testing

Program testing occurs after coding. Actual data should be used to test the program to ensure correct output and program writing and coding. The program is also tested to determine if the programming language is correct, if the processing logic

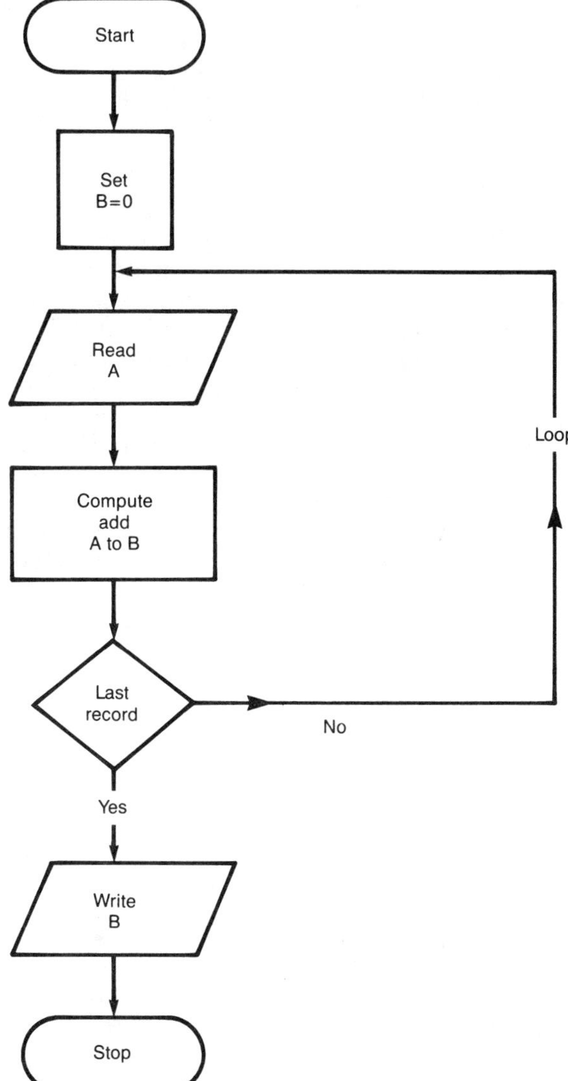

FIG. 4-5. Example of flowchart with loop. Problem: To read many values of A together and find their sum.

is sound, and if the program runs correctly. The program can be implemented after it has been judged correct.

A major activity in testing is debugging, which means checking the program to ensure that it is free of error. The term *debugging* was coined by Commodore Grace Hopper. In 1945, when working at Harvard on the MARK II, she removed a moth from the computer that had caused it to stop. As a result, the term was used to refer to any correction of a computer problem (Mace, 1983).

Program Implementation/Documentation

Program implementation/documentation is the final step in programming. Once the program has been tested and debugged, it is ready to produce the defined output; however, it requires detailed documentation (according to accepted standards) of each programming step. Documentation generally should be prepared to aid program users and programmers who will perform program maintainence (changes, revisions, updates). The program must be documented sufficiently to satisfy the reference needs of both groups.

SUMMARY

This chapter highlights computer software, which includes the various computer programs and their programming languages that run the computer.

Computer programs are sets of instructions stored in computer memory; sets of computer programs designed for many users and different computers are called software packages. They are frequently written in a query language using English-like words. Software packages generally require little or no programming expertise.

Programming languages, needed to communicate with the computer are reviewed, and the three levels of programming languages—machine, assembly, and high level—are presented. Several programming languages are highlighted.

Finally, the five major programming steps—problem definition, program design, program preparation, program testing, and program implementation/documentation—are described. This also includes a description of a flowchart.

STUDY QUESTIONS

1. What does computer software do?
2. A computer program is a set of organized instructions written in sequence and stored in computer memory. True or false?
3. Who first described the stored computer program?
4. Who proposed the stored program concept for the modern computer?
5. Name the two major categories of programs.
6. Name two functions performed by system programs.
7. Name the three translation programs.
8. Application programs are stored in what type of memory?
9. Name three types of software packages.
10. Name the two types of displays on a CRT screen.
11. Name the three levels of computer programming languages.
12. Which language consists of the binary digits 0 and 1?
13. What language requires an assembler?
14. Which language uses English-like words?
15. Name the most common business high-level language.
16. Name the language used primarily for scientific and mathematical applications.
17. Name the language developed for clinical health care applications.
18. Name the five steps in preparing a computer program (programming).
19. What is used to illustrate graphically the logical solution to a program?
20. What is used to represent graphically the repetitive operation in a computer program?

REFERENCES

Capron HL, William BK: Computers and Data Processing. Menlo Park, CA, Benjamin/Cummings, 1984

Hopper GM, Mandell SL: Understanding Computers. New York, West Publishing, 1984
IBM Corp: Introduction to IBM Data Processing Systems, 5th ed. White Plains, NY, IBM Corp, 1981
ICP Interview With Grace M. Hopper. ICP INTERFACE Administrative and Accounting, pp 18–23, Spring 1980
Johnson S: Grace Hopper—a living legend. All Hands, pp 3–6, September 1982
Mace S: Mother of COBOL—still thinkin', still workin'. InfoWorld 5(18):29–31, 1982
Rosen S: Software. In Ralston A, Reilly ED Jr (eds): Encyclopedia of Computer Science and Engineering, 2nd ed, pp 1346–1348. New York, Van Nostrand Reinhold, 1983
Sammet JE: Programming Languages: History and Fundamentals. Englewood Cliffs, NJ, Prentice-Hall, 1969
Shelly GB, Cashman TJ: Introduction to Computers and Data Processing. Brea, CA, Anaheim Publishing, 1980
Washington Post Parade Magazine: The first lady of computers, pp 21, November 14, 1982
Wilkes MV: Charles Babbage. In Ralston A, Reilly ED Jr (eds): Encyclopedia of Computer Science and Engineering, 2nd ed, pp 157–158. New York, Van Nostrand Reinhold, 1983

BIBLIOGRAPHY

Davis RM: Evolution of computers and computing. Science 195(4283):1096–1102, 1977
Denning PJ: Third generation computer systems. Comput Surv 3(4):175–213, 1971
Denning PJ: Operating systems. In Ralston A, Reilly ED Jr (eds): Encyclopedia of Computer Science and Engineering, 2nd ed, pp 1053–1075. New York, Van Nostrand Reinhold, 1983
Encyclopedia Britannica Educational Corp: Understanding Computers. Skokie, IL, Encyclopedia Britannica Educational Corp, 1982
Enlander D: Computers in medicine: An Introduction. St Louis, CV Mosby, 1980
DATAPRO Research Corp: An Evaluation of the MUMPS Language. Delron, NJ, DATAPRO Research Corp, 1981
Frenzel LE: Understanding personal computer software. onComputing, pp 17–25, 77–99, Winter 1979
Harm LW: Software packages. In Ralston A, Reilly ED Jr (eds): Encyclopedia of Computer Science and Engineering, 2nd ed, pp 1364–1370. New York, Van Nostrand Reinhold, 1983
Heller RS, Martin DC: Bits 'n Bytes about Computing: A Computer Literacy Primary. Rockville, MD, Computer Science Press, 1982
Kemeny JG: Man and the Computer. New York, Charles Scribner, 1972
Morris RA: Comparison of some high-level languages. BYTE 5(2):128–139, 1980
Pogue RE: The authoring system: Interface between author and computer. J Res Devel Educ 14(1):57–68, 1980
Price D: Questions and answers on programming languages. Microcomputing, pp 82–85, June 1980
Pritchard K: Computers. I. An introduction. Nurs Times 78(5):355–357, 1982
Ralston A, Reilly ED Jr (eds): Encyclopedia of Computer Science and Engineering, 2nd ed. New York, Van Nostrand Reinhold, 1983
Sammet JE: Programming languages. In Ralston A, Reilly ED Jr (eds). Encyclopedia of Computer Science and Engineering, 2nd ed, pp 1228–1232. New York, Van Nostrand Reinhold, 1983
Stern RA, Stern N: An Introduction to Computers and Information Processing, 2nd ed. New York, John Wiley & Sons, 1982
Tropp HS: Hopper, Grace Murray. In Ralston A, Reilly ED Jr (eds): Encyclopedia of Computer Science and Engineering, 2nd ed, pp 685–686. New York, Van Nostrand Reinhold, 1983
The Washington Post Magazine: Grace M. Hopper: Programmer's programmer, pp 113–114, November 28, 1982

Zaks R: Your First Computer: A Guide to Business and Personal Computers. Berkeley, CA, SYBEX, 1980

Zin KL: Authoring languages and systems. In Ralston A, Reilly ED Jr (eds): Encyclopedia of Computer Science and Engineering, 2nd ed, pp 144–146. New York, Van Nostrand Reinhold, 1983

5 Data Processing

Objectives

- Describe the data processing cycle of input, process, and output.
- List the different common operations performed by the computer.
- Describe the organization and structure of data storage.
- Describe the various data processing methods and types.
- Discuss data security and privacy.

Computers essentially process data — raw material such as facts, figures, addresses, and temperatures. Once processed, data become the information that solves a specific problem. Computer hardware, the machine, processes data as instructed by computer software, making data processing the interaction between hardware and software that transfers data into information.

Chapters 3 and 4 have described computer hardware and software. This chapter discusses how the computer transforms data into information. It will describe several aspects of data processing, including the following:

- Data processing
- Data processing operations
- Data storage organization and structure
- Data processing methods
- Data processing types
- Data security
- Privacy

DATA PROCESSING

Data processing is the changing of raw data into information as instructed by computer programs.

Raw facts are data that must be analyzed. Examples include the height, weight, temperature, and blood pressure measurements of a given patient. Such data can be analyzed to determine if the patient has normal vital signs. Instructions are the sequence of steps that the computer performs to analyze (process) the raw data. The computer would analyze and compare the above patients' vital signs with normal measurements to determine if they are within acceptable ranges.

Data are always processed in the same manner, as directed by the control unit. First, the raw data and the computer program that will process them are entered, as input, into computer memory, where they remain until processing begins. When ordered, the program instructions and data are transmitted on a "data bus" (lines that send and receive data) to the arithmetic and logic unit for processing. Only in that unit are instructions carried out and data processed. Once completed, the processed data are sent back by "data bus" into memory. The processed data, now information, remain stored until instructed to be produced as output.

DATA PROCESSING OPERATIONS

A computer performs two types of data processing operations. First are the operations performed before and after data are actually processed. They include the following:

- Input
- Store
- Update
- Retrieve
- Output

Second are the operations that actually process the data. Some of the most common ones are as follows:

- Sort
- Classify
- Compare
- Compute
- Summarize

Those operations performed before data are processed deal with raw facts that are input, stored, and, if necessary, updated in computer memory. Once processed, data can be retrieved and produced as output. However, the actual data processing is based on the computer program. Data can be sorted in a particular sequence (*e.g.*, alphabetically or diagnostically); data can be classified according to a particular characteristic (*e.g.*, sex, age, or ethnic origin). Data can be compared to normal values, and data can be computed when calculations, such as doses of drugs, are needed. Finally, data can be summarized, as in the census report done at the end of each nursing shift (Capron and Williams, 1984).

DATA STORAGE ORGANIZATION AND STRUCTURE

Data in computer storage are organized into logical entities such as identification, data, medical data, billing data, and so on. Generally, all data are organized in a hierarchy so that they can be easily located. This hierarchy consists of the following:

- Bit
- Character/byte
- Field
- Record
- File
- Database

Bit

A bit (*BI*nary digi*T*) is the smallest unit of information used to code all stored data. Since it is too small to represent a letter or a number, combinations of bits are used to code characters (bytes).

Character (Byte)

A character, also called a byte, is the smallest logical entity stored in the computer. It is any number, letter, or symbol used to enter data into the computer. A character or byte is coded by combinations of seven or eight bits (see above). For example, the numeral 1 is represented by the eight bits 1111 0001, and the letter A is represented by the eight bits 1100 0001 in the EBCDIC binary coding scheme (see below).

Two standards are used to code characters in the computer industry.

- EBCDIC
- ASCII

The eight-digit or bit coding scheme called EBCDIC (*E*xtended *B*inary *C*oded *D*ecimal *I*nterchange *C*ode) was developed by IBM primarily to represent the letters of the alphabet. Eight bits represent a character or byte. The EBCDIC standard is used widely by the computer industry (Fig. 5-1).

The second coding scheme, ASCII (*A*merican *S*tandard *C*ode for *I*nformation *I*nterchange), was also developed to be the standard code for the computer industry. It uses either seven or eight bits to form a character.

Computer memory is characterized by its capacity and is described by the thousands of bytes it can store. This capacity is described by the letter K, which represents 1024 bytes and signifies 2^{10}. The 1024 bytes are generally rounded off to 1000 bytes and are described as 1000 bytes of data. A computer with a storage capacity of 128 K actually stores more than 128,000 characters of data. If storage capacity goes beyond 1000 K, megabytes are used to describe the millions of bytes of data the computer can store.

Decimal Number	Code	Symbol	Code
1	1111 0001	$	0101 1011
2	1111 0010	*	0101 1100
3	1111 0011	?	0101 1111
4	1111 0100	:	0111 1010
5	1111 0101	=	0111 1011
6	1111 0110	@	0111 1100
7	1111 0111	'	0111 1100
8	1111 1000	Blank	0100 0000
9	1111 1001		

Letter	Code	Letter	Code
A	1100 0001	N	1101 0101
B	1100 0010	O	1101 0110
C	1100 0011	P	1101 0111
D	1100 0100	Q	1101 1000
E	1100 0101	R	1101 1001
F	1100 0110	S	1110 0010
G	1100 0111	T	1110 0011
H	1100 1000	U	1110 0100
I	1100 1001	V	1110 0101
J	1101 0001	W	1110 0110
K	1101 0010	X	1110 0111
L	1101 0011	Y	1110 1000
M	1101 0100	Z	1110 1001

FIG. 5-1. Binary numbering system using extended binary coded decimal interchange code (EBCDIC).

Field

A field generally represents a single piece of information, such as a patient's identification number:

Identification number—03363
Name—John Smith
Street address—120 N. Wayne St.
City—Arlington
State—MA
Zip code—01220

Identification number, name, street address, city, state, and zip code are each a separate piece of information. In this example, the patient's identification information is composed of six different fields (Fig. 5-2).

Record

A record, which is composed of several related data elements or fields, is a unit of information that contains several separate pieces. For example, the identification information for John Smith is a record, since it is composed of six fields that form one unit (record) (see Fig. 5-2).

A record may be fixed length or variable length depending on the computer and the method and type of storage media. The fixed length record allows a fixed number of spaces for a field or data element; the variable length record takes only the spaces it actually needs. For example, John Smith's name, identification number, and address require 43 spaces. If his record were stored as a fixed length record, 60 spaces might be set aside to accommodate different records, leaving 17 spaces empty in this instance. However, as a variable length record, it would use only 43 spaces.

These two different record structures affect computer processing capability, since fixed length records are not very flexible, even though programs written to process them are easier to write. It is easier to process variable length records but

Category	Data		
Field	Patient ID Number	—0 3 6 6 3*	Record (Name and Address of One Patient)
Field	Patient Name	—John Smith*	
Field	Patient Address Street	—120 N. Wayne St.*	
Field	City	—Arlington*	
Field	State	—MA*	
Field	Zip code	—10638*	
Record	Name and Address of John Smith		File (Names and Addresses of All Patients)
Record	Name and Address of Nancy Doe		
Record	Name and Address of Virginia Green		
Record	Name and Address of Dick Jones		
File	Names and Addresses of Patients		Database (Patients' Accounts)
File	Patients' Accounts		
File	Patient Drug Accounts		
File	Other Accounts		

* Each number, letter, or symbol is a character (byte).

FIG. 5-2. Illustration of data organization by category.

more difficult to write computer programs for them. Also, variable length records store data more efficiently but cost more to process.

File

A file, the next level of data storage, generally contains all related records. For example, the patient identification file would contain John Smith's record and those of numerous other patients (see Fig. 5-2).

A computer file is the key to efficient data processing; it resembles office files organized in file cabinets. Different file types, storage sizes, and processing methods are available, but organization is the crucial element in efficient data processing.

File Types

The many different types of files for various aspects of data processing include the following:

- Master files
- Transaction/update files
- Report/sort files

Master File. A master file contains all the permanent raw data for a specific application, such as the identification information records of all patients.

Transaction/Update File. A transaction/update file contains all the corrections and additions needed to update the master file, such as corrections on patient information and new admissions.

Report/Sort File. The report/sort file contains records needed for processing special data, such as the records of all patients with a particular diagnosis.

File Structure

Files are primarily organized as sequential, direct/random, or indexed files.

Sequential File. The sequential file, the simplest method of structuring files, organizes records sequentially; they may be arranged alphabetically or serially or by some type of special arrangement (*e.g.*, name or diagnosis).

Direct/Random File. The direct/random file allows files to be arranged randomly. They are identified with a label, called a key, allowing for direct retrieval.

Indexed File. The indexed file, also called the indexed sequential file, combines features of the sequential and the direct/random files. Generally, records are arranged sequentially but are also indexed so that they can be found either sequentially or directly. The index, which resembles a directory, contains a key to each record stored in the file (London, 1973; Capron and Williams, 1984).

Database

A database, the highest level of data storage, organizes and stores all related data. It generally refers to all data stored in the files and records that can be processed for more than one application. Such data are generally shared and, in theory, connected to each other, even though they are stored in several different files. A database usually requires directly accessible storage. For example, John Smith's data is in the patient identification file and in several other files stored in the patient accounts database as well (see Fig. 5-2).

Building a database is as critical for accessing data as is organizing files and records. Several different database structures are used, including the hierarchical, network, and relational databases. Data stored in databases are generally managed by a software package called the database management system (DBMS).

Hierarchical Structure

The hierarchical structure, also called the tree structure, arranges data in order of rank, with all elements connected to the same base. Beginning at the base, a record points to successive layers of branches (see below). Although in this structure all records are based on one particular "root," levels do occasionally exist. In the patients' accounts database, for example, John Smith's name or identification number could be the root for his identification information records in other accounting files. His nursing diagnosis, on the other hand, might be the root for a database containing nursing information.

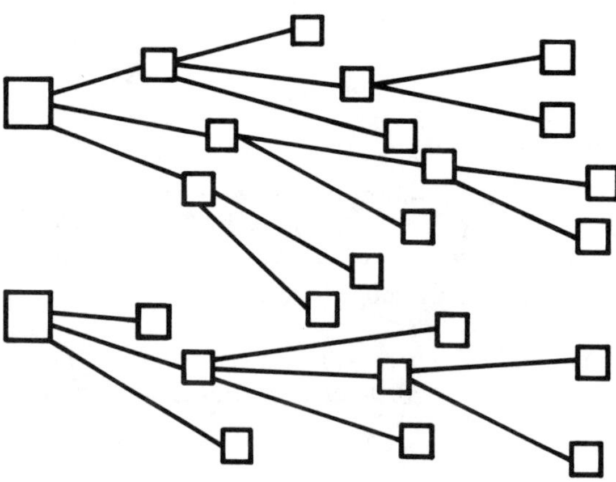

Network Structure

In the network structure records are linked together by "pointers" using some type of relationship (key), such as patient name, physician name, or diagnosis. Thus, John Smith's records in the different files can be linked on the basis of his diagnosis, his name, his physician's name, or any other variable.

Relational Structure

In the relational structure two or more records are interrelated by attributes that connect the records. This type of structure allows for easy access and manipulation of records.

Database Management Systems

A DBMS is a special software package containing a set of computer programs and a unique query (high-level programming) language. The programs are designed to create, access, manage, and monitor a database; the query language allows users to communicate easily with the database without having extensive programming skills. Most DBMSs have their own query language (Olle, 1983; Chorafas, 1983; Blasgen, 1982).

A DBMS is actually considered a tool used to manipulate a large database, since it allows a computer user to work with the database without having to write a program. Sometimes it can help a user design an efficient database more quickly and easily; it can also edit data being entered into the computer and provide computer security by controlling access to data. A DBMS is the key to an integrated computer system.

Usually developed by computer manufacturers and software vendors, DBMSs are available for all sizes of computers. Many of the large computerized information systems that contain patient data and that generate patient care reports use a DBMS. They are used in microcomputer systems to manage one specific database, such as personnel, patient classification, or nurse staffing and scheduling.

DATA PROCESSING METHODS

The methods by which data are accessed and processed depend primarily on how records, files, and databases are organized and designed as well as on whether data are stored on line or off line (Shelly and Cashman, 1980). The two major methods used to access data in memory for processing are as follows:

- Sequential access
- Random access

Sequential Access

In the sequential access method, data are organized sequentially (*e.g.*, alphabetically or serially). Sequential organization of files was the earliest and most common type of file organization, since magnetic tape could only store files sequentially. In this method, records are accessed one after the other, which means that access is slow and accessibility of data limited. For example, if John Smith's record were in alphabetical order, all records from A to S would have to be read before his record could be accessed.

Random Access

Random access, sometimes called direct access, allows data to be processed directly from the stored files in memory and to be retrieved at random without searching or reading the files. Such records are arranged and stored in any order and identified with labels or keys for easy direct access.

The random access method makes it possible to access data quickly. For example, John Smith's record, if organized randomly, could be instantly accessed with one key. This method is generally used to process data stored on a magnetic disk, which is the most common on-line storage device used today. With this type of storage, data are accessed on line and processed instantly. Such instant processing is sometimes called *real time* (Capron and Williams, 1984).

DATA PROCESSING TYPES

Data processing types, the different ways of processing data, include the following:

- On-line processing
- Interactive/real-time processing
- Batch processing

On-Line Processing

On-line processing directly connects a computer terminal to a computer. In such systems data are entered from a VDT or CRT terminal or other data input terminal. The data are transmitted directly to the computer and stored, to remain until needed. In this method, the terminal is used to transmit or receive data (Freeman, 1983; IBM, 1981).

An example of an on-line computer system may be found in patient care units where an on-line CRT terminal is used to process patients' bills. Patient care services are recorded by a clerk on a CRT terminal and data are transmitted directly to the accounting office. Similarly, in some public health and community health agencies, data on patient care services are transmitted on-line to an offsite service bureau computer for processing.

Interactive/Real-Time Processing

Interactive/real-time processing, the most common type of processing used for random access, generally refers to mainframes and minicomputers that process data immediately upon instruction. Data are entered through on-line CRT terminals directly connected to the computer's database. The data are processed and results are transmitted directly back to system users. Such computer systems allow the user at the CRT terminal to interact with the computer database (Shelly and Cashman, 1980).

This type of processing has many advantages. Using the CRT terminal, a user can prepare, edit, and correct data as they are entered into the terminal. This interactive processing can be used to update files, revise computer programs, and design outputs.

Different levels of interactive/real-time processing are available. They include the processing of a transaction, processing of a problem, or continuous processing. In the first instance, each transaction is completed before another one is initiated. In the second instance, the problem is formulated and executed and the results are retrieved on line. In continuous processing, computer applications are ongoing, such as those found in the processing of a space program flight (Capron and Williams, 1984; Head, 1983).

Interactive/real-time processing has been made possible by magnetic disk storage. This processing technique has expanded computer storage to an almost unlimited extent and is generally found in the newer hospital information systems (HISs) that use mainframes or large minicomputers. In such systems, nursing personnel may enter current information on any patient through the one or more on-line CRT terminals located in different hospital units. Simultaneously, the user interacts directly with the computer to maintain complete, up-to-date medical records.

Batch Processing

In batch processing data are assembled and processed at once or at specially designated times. Data are never processed as they enter the computer but are stored for processing later. Batch processing is used in any system where data are processed at fixed intervals, such as for a hospital payroll. The computer program and data to be processed are generally stored off line on magnetic tapes or magnetic disks and mounted onto the computer when the computer programs are run.

DATA SECURITY

A major consideration for any computer system is data security, which involves protecting data against deliberate destruction, accidental access, or loss by unauthorized persons. Data security involves protecting the hardware and software as well, including the physical security of the computer system equipment (input/

output devices, storage units, and central processing unit) and protecting the data itself (Brewer, 1983; IBM, 1981).

Physical Security

A computer system requires protection from natural disasters such as fire and floods and from deliberate destructive acts. Physical security can be maintained by limiting access only to authorized personnel and by installing door locks, card-key systems, and closed-circuit television. A duplicate computer system installed in a second location can provide a backup for any loss of physical equipment.

Data security also refers to the secure use of the computer system. CRT terminals can be secured by limiting their access through the use of passwords or security codes. Database design can limit access to specific users by giving different groups of hospital personnel different security codes. For instance, the nurse's aide's security code might allow access to certain items in the database such as vital signs but deny access to other information, such as medication orders or laboratory results.

Data Protection

Protection of data during transmission to and from the computer system is also part of data security. Wiretapping and eavesdropping are security threats that computer users can take measures to prevent. Data being transmitted over telecommunication lines can be protected by scrambling; that is, the data are encoded by the sender, sent, and decoded by the authorized receiver.

Data security involves methods to ensure that all data input, processing, and output are accurate. Assorted checks and audits enable users to ensure that data are not lost, altered, or used incorrectly. One type of check is the automatic recording of all uses and transactions performed by the computer system; such a method can detect any unlawful user or unauthorized transaction. Another is the use of audit trails to ensure that computer programs process data correctly and that they have not been tampered with.

Data security can be costly, but every computer system requires some level of security.

PRIVACY

Privacy of a computer system ensures people that personal data is protected against improper access. Such protection is critical to the integrity of any computer system. As computer systems multiply in number and increase in size and scope, data on individuals is also increasingly available.

Several legislative acts have been passed in an effort to protect people's privacy. The Fair Credit Act of 1970 gives people access to their credit records, and the Freedom of Information Act of 1970 gives them access to data collected by federal agencies.

The Privacy Act of 1974 (PL 93-579), one of the most significant acts, established safeguards for protecting records the government collects and keeps on citizens. It stipulates that federal agencies cannot maintain any secret files on citizens and that citizens have the right to know what government files say about them. A Privacy Commission set up as a result of this act formulated and published a basic document on protecting the privacy of citizens that recommended six basic principles for the private sector: "(1) all personal records should be made public;

(2) individuals must be allowed to find out when information is stored about them and how it is used; (3) personal information should be used only for its intended purpose; (4) individuals must be able to amend records about themselves; (5) personal information must be obtained in such a way so as to ensure that it is complete, accurate, relevant, timely, and secure; and (6) all uses of personal information should be accounted for by a responsible manager" (Capron and Williams, 1984). It also recommended that Social Security numbers be used only in connection with official government business and that any new private sector computer systems not use them for identification purposes.

As a result of this commission, several states and local governments passed similar legislation protecting the privacy of data on their residents. These laws affect what data on individuals can be stored in computer systems.

SUMMARY

This chapter describes data processing, which is essentially what computers do. It highlights the various operations possible with data processing and describes the organization and structure of data, including the logical entities organized in a hierarchy—bit, character, field, record, file, and database.

Data structure and organization and how data are accessed and processed are described. The differences between on-line, interactive/real-time, and batch processing are reviewed. Finally, the various types of data security methods are outlined. The differences between physical security of the system and the security of the data are stressed, and how data on individuals are protected is discussed.

STUDY QUESTIONS

1. What does data processed by the computer produce?
2. Name five common operations the computer performs.
3. Name the six logical entities in which data are organized and stored in the computer.
4. How many numbers are used in the binary numbering system?
5. A bit can have what two values?
6. What is another name for a character?
7. Code the number 2 using the binary numbering system with eight bits.
8. What are the two standards the computer uses to code bytes?
9. How many bytes are described by the letter K (kilobyte)?
10. Name the two types of record lengths.
11. A field represents a single piece of information. True or false?
12. Name three types of files.
13. Name three different file structures.
14. Name the three different database structures.
15. Name two major characteristics of a DBMS.
16. What are the two methods of data processing?
17. Name three types of data processing.
18. How are data entered into the computer in interactive/real-time processing?
19. Card-key methods to access the computer are installed for what purpose?
20. Can the Social Security number of citizens be used in any nongovernment computer system?

REFERENCES

Blasgen MW: Database systems. Science 215(4534):869–872, 1982
Brewer SC: Data security. In Ralston A, Reilly ED Jr (eds): Encyclopedia of Computer Science and Engineering, 2nd ed, pp 493–497. New York, Van Nostrand Reinhold, 1983
Capron HL, Williams BK: Computer and Data Processing, p 387. Menlo Park, CA, Benjamin/Cummings, 1984
Chorafas DN: DBMS for Distributed Computers and Networks. New York, Petrocelli Books, 1983
Freeman DN: Processing modes. In Ralston A, Reilly ED Jr (eds): Encyclopedia of Computer Science and Engineering, 2nd ed, pp 1217–1218. New York, Van Nostrand Reinhold, 1983
Head RV: Real-time applications. In Ralston A, Reilly ED Jr (eds): Encyclopedia of Computer Science and Engineering, 2nd ed, pp 1265–1272. New York, Van Nostrand Reinhold, 1983
IBM Corp: Introduction to IBM Data Processing Systems. Poughkeepsie, NY, IBM Corp, 1981
London KR: Techniques for Direct Access. Philadelphia, Auerbach Publishing, 1973
Olle TW: Database management. In Ralston A, Reilly ED Jr (eds): Encyclopedia of Computer Science and Engineering, 2nd ed, pp 441–447. New York, Van Nostrand Reinhold, 1983
Shelly GB, Cashman TJ: Introduction to Computers and Data Processing. Brea, CA, Anaheim Publishing, 1980

BIBLIOGRAPHY

Boraiko AA: The chip: Electronic minimarvel that is changing your life. National Geographic 162(4):421–458, 1982
Bronzino JD: Computer Applications for Patient Care. Reading, MA, Addison-Wesley, 1982
Brown WF, Jacobsen RV: Security of computer installations, physical. In Ralston A, Reilly ED Jr (eds): Encyclopedia of Computer Science and Engineering, 2nd ed, pp 1308–1310. New York, Van Nostrand Reinhold, 1983
Carroll JM: Computer Security. Boston, MA, Butterworth Publishing, 1977
Covvey HD, McAlister NH: Computers in the Practice of Medicine, vol I, Introduction to Computing Concepts. Reading, MA, Addison-Wesley, 1980
Encyclopedia Britannica Educational Corp: Understanding Computers. Skokie, IL, Encyclopedia Britannica Educational Corp, 1982
Enlander D: Computers in Medicine: An Introduction. St Louis, CV Mosby, 1980
Frankenhais JP: How to get a good mini. Harv Bus Rev pp 139–149, May–June 1982
Fry JP, Sibley EH: Evolution of data-base management systems. Comp Surv 8(1):7–42, 1976
Heller RS, Martin DC: Bits 'n Bytes About Computing: A Computer Literacy Primer. Rockville, MD, Computer Science Press, 1982
Hopper GM, Mandell SL: Understanding Computers. New York, West Publishing, 1984
Hume JNP: Data security. In Ralston A, Reilly ED Jr (eds): Encyclopedia of Computer Science and Engineering, 2nd ed, pp 493–497. New York, Van Nostrand Reinhold, 1983
MacLeod RJ, Forkner I: Computerized Business Information Systems: An Introduction to Data Processing. New York, John Wiley, 1982
Martin J: Introduction to Teleprocessing. Englewood Cliffs, NJ, Prentice-Hall, 1982
National Bureau of Standards: Guidelines for Security of Computer Applications (Fips pub. no. 73). Washington, DC, National Bureau of Standards, 1980
Report of the Secretary's Advisory Committee on Automated Personal Data Systems: Records Computers and the Rights of Citizens (DHEW pub. no. OS 73-94). Washington, DC, U.S. Government Printing Office, 1973
Sanders DH: Computers in Business: An Introduction. New York, McGraw-Hill, 1979
Sibley EH: The development of data-base technology. Comp Surv 8(1):1–5, 1976

Stern RA, Stern N: An Introduction to Computers and Information Processing. New York, John Wiley & Sons, 1982

Yovits MC: Information and data. In Ralston A, Reilly ED Jr (eds): Encyclopedia of Computer Science and Engineering, 2nd ed, pp 714–717. New York, Van Nostrand Reinhold, 1983

Walsh ME: Understanding Computers: What Managers and Users Need to Know. New York, John Wiley & Sons, 1982

PART C

Computer Systems

6 Systems Theory and Systems

Objectives

- Explain systems theory and systems.
- Describe the configuration of a computer system.
- List the different types of information systems.
- Discuss the focus and purpose of a management information system.
- Provide an overview of a hospital information system.

Chapter 3 described hardware, Chapter 4 software, and Chapter 5 data processing. Added together, these components make a system. The use of systems in computer technology is based on systems theory; both are essential for an understanding of the computer. Systems theory provides the basis for viewing a computer system, and the concept of systems provides a framework for understanding the relationships of all parts of the computer system. Together, these two concepts explain computer technology.

This chapter discusses systems theory and systems. It gives an overview of systems, including various types, elements, and characteristics, and focuses on computer systems, information systems, management information systems (MISs), and hospital information systems (HISs).

Specifically, this chapter describes the following:

- Systems theory
- Systems
- Computer systems
- Information systems
- MISs
- HISs

SYSTEMS THEORY

Systems theory is the conceptual basis for any system, especially a computer system. When applied to describe the computer, with all its interrelated parts, it explains how many parts can achieve a desired result when put together. The interaction of the parts is essential in making the computer run; without it, the sophisticated hardware of the computer is useless (Optner, 1975).

General systems theory was introduced in the 1930s and developed in 1950 by the biologist Ludwig von Bertalanffy (1968), who formulated it as a framework for integrating and interpreting scientific knowledge. Stating that to understand all living organisms it is necessary to view them as parts of a whole, he advocated that his theory be used to view the empirical world as one whole made up of varying interrelated parts. He argued that all living organisms interact with their environment and, as such, are open systems (Shoderbek and colleagues, 1980).

In the 1950s, Kenneth Boulding, also a biologist, produced his classification of general systems theory, which provided a framework of nine levels in a complex progressive hierarchy (Boulding, 1956). The levels ranged from a static closed one used to classify the lowest structure of elements to the most complex transcendental level for describing changing structures and relationships among elements. This classification was proposed as a means of bridging the gap between theoretical models and empirical knowledge.

During World War II, systems theory, then called systems analysis, emerged as a holistic approach for solving problems. It was first applied by British scientists in the area of radar technology. They pioneered in combining the skills of many experts to deal with unresolved mathematical problems. They also used this technique by integrating different classes of people and pooling all types of resources to resolve the problem of saving their cities.

In the United States, systems theory was also first applied during World War II. Here again, the military used it to facilitate the development of improved weapons. Systems theory was also used to research the development of other military projects, such as the supersonic bomber (Optner, 1975).

After World War II, the systems theory concept was used to develop computer hardware and software. Systems theory influenced computer design, enabling computers to solve specific problems.

During this time, systems theory applications also expanded into other areas of computer science and into social sciences, medicine, and nursing. Systems theory influenced the development of nursing theory, which first evolved during the 1960s (Newman, 1972; Donnelly and colleagues, 1980). At that time, nurse theorists began to view nursing practice as unique and to separate it from the traditional medical model. Nurses began to use systems theory concepts found in other disciplines to analyze nursing practice in terms of a holistic approach and created several conceptual systems of nursing theory.

SYSTEMS

A system is a concept describing a unit composed of interrelated subunits or parts. Each part works independently but is essential to the whole system. The unit is greater than any of its parts, but if any one part changes, all other parts are affected. In short, a system describes sets of interrelated elements (Ackoff, 1971; Optner, 1968; Kaufman, 1972).

A description of systems includes the following:

- System types
- System elements
- System characteristics

Types

Because the term *systems* is used to describe many concepts, many types have developed, including mechanical, organizational, or human structure or combination of structures. For example, a computer, a hospital, and the nursing profession are all systems.

To illustrate, consider the mechanical structure of an automobile. Its parts work together to make it move; the automobile is thus a mechanical system. Then consider the organizational structure of a community health care delivery system. The health care facilities (parts) work together to produce health care services in a community. These parts may include a hospital, a nursing home, a public health agency, and a health maintenance organization (Fig. 6-1). Each facility has its own goals and is a system, yet each facility is also part of a larger system.

Next, examine the human structure of the nursing department in a large health care facility. The department is composed of nursing personnel in different nursing units (parts)—several patient care units, a research unit, and an education unit (Fig. 6-2). All the nurses work together to achieve the overall goal of the health care facility, yet the nurses in each unit must also achieve the goal of their respective unit. The nursing department is thus a system consisting of various subsystems that are themselves systems.

Elements

A system is generally described by the following five major elements (Optner, 1975):

- Input
- Process
- Output
- Feedback
- Control

Input

Input, the start-up force that puts a system into operation, consists of the raw facts and other requirements the system needs to operate.

Process

Process, the activity that transforms input into output, is the mode of operation. It can be modified in response to feedback and control.

Output

Output, the result of process, is the final product of the operation.

Feedback and Control

Feedback and control are two interrelated elements that control the system. Feedback, which allows adjustments to be made to control the system, is also used to monitor, evaluate, and direct the system. Control regulates the functions of input, process, and output and provides the rules and procedures for their operations. Control over input checks, validates, and verifies data. Control over process se-

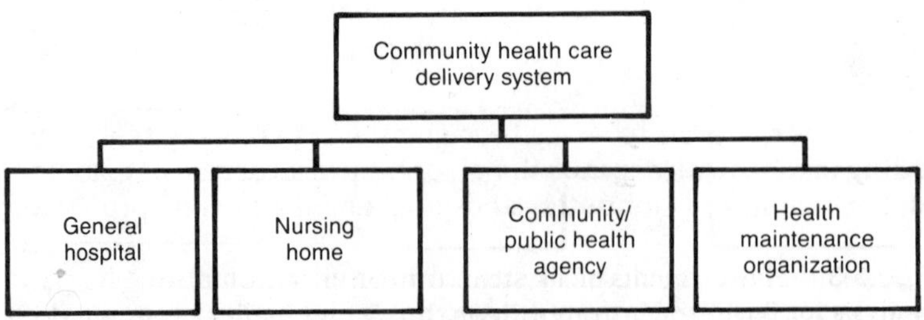

FIG. 6-1. An example of an organizational system.

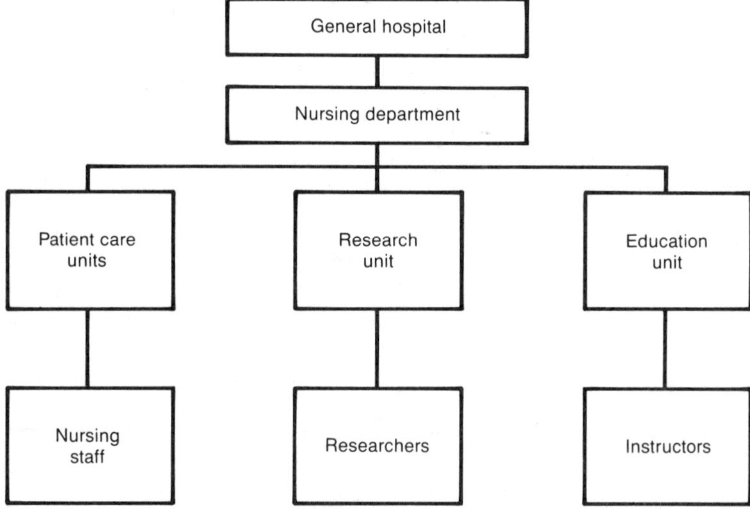

FIG. 6-2. An example of a human system.

quences and completes the operations and detects errors, and control over output ensures conformity, checks validity of content, and corrects errors. Certain restrictions may impose boundaries on a specific problem and, as such, operate as an additional control.

• • •

These elements make up the framework of a computer system, which is essentially an open system that allows for all types of adjustments based on feedback and control (Fig. 6-3).

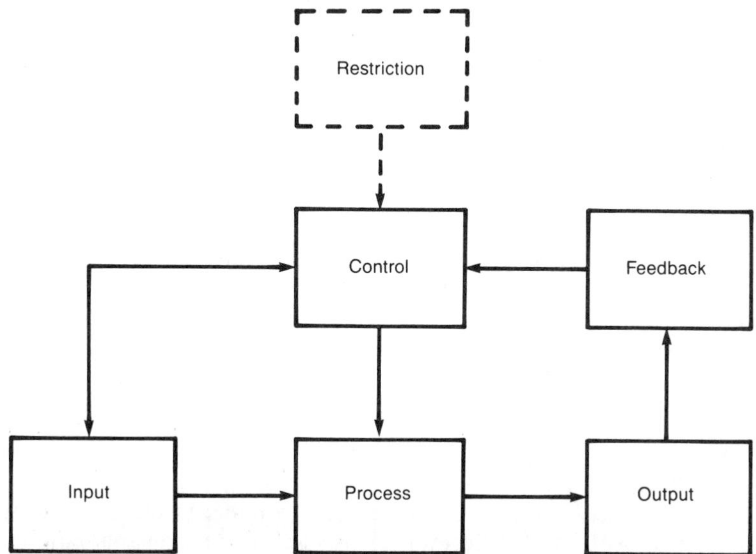

FIG. 6-3. Five elements of a system. (After Optner SL: Systems Analysis for Business Management, 3rd ed. Englewood Cliffs, NJ, Prentice-Hall, 1975)

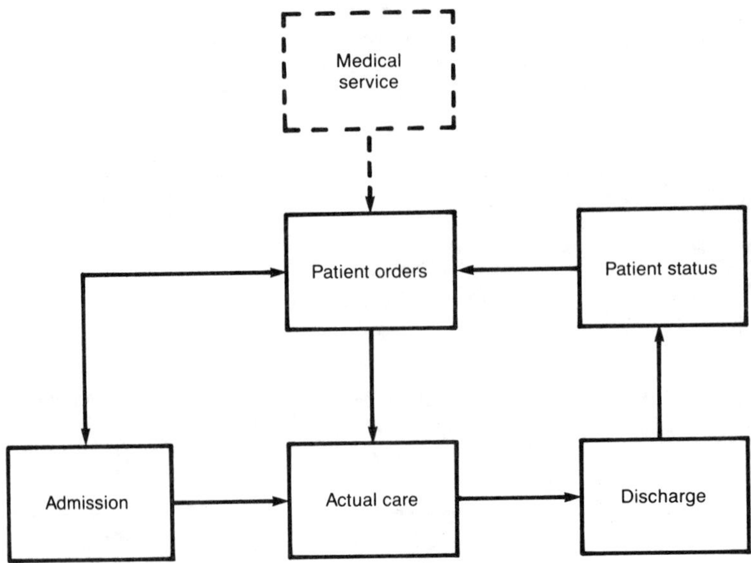

FIG. 6-4. An example of the five elements of a system.

A general hospital system can illustrate these various elements (Fig. 6-4). The admission of a burn patient is the input into a general hospital. The actual medical and nursing care are the process. Once care is completed, the patient is discharged, which is the output. The feedback is information on the patient's progress, and control refers to orders and actions taken based on information and feedback. Feedback and control thus affect the care process. The restriction for the patient might be the medical service responsible for the care. The protocols used affect how the patient is treated.

Characteristics

Systems are characterized in many ways, the most common being as follows:

- Closed system
- Open system

Closed System

A closed system is generally one with complete, fixed, unchanging elements (Optner, 1975; Shoderbek and colleagues, 1980). It does not interact with its environment; it therefore does not change. It is self-contained and automatically controls its own operation. An example of a closed system is a physiological monitoring unit, which contains an alarm that is set off automatically when a patient's heart rate deviates from normal.

Open System

An open system is dynamic. Because its elements are affected by and respond to external forces, and it therefore allows for change and adaptation. An example of an open system is a hospital census system; the number of discharges influences the number of admissions.

COMPUTER SYSTEMS

A computer system is simply the application of systems theory to the computer. It refers to the hardware and software that interact to process data into meaningful information. This interaction is essential to make the computer function, since without it sophisticated computer hardware is useless.

A computer system consists of a complex configuration of components. The hardware includes the main computer and all the peripheral equipment—terminals, storage devices, communication devices—and refers to any size of computer—mainframe, minicomputer, microcomputer—and any type of computer—analog, digital, hybrid. The software refers to all necessary computer programs that are needed to make the computer run.

A computer system is characterized by its high speed and reliability in processing data for many applications. It is capable of storing large volumes of data that are readily accessible for processing (Hellerman and Smith, 1983). Thus, a computer system is composed of equipment (hardware) and programs (software) that together process data into information.

INFORMATION SYSTEMS

A modern information system is also the application of systems theory to the computer. Sometimes called an information processing system or a data processing system, it uses computer hardware and software to process data into information required to solve a problem (Teichroew, 1983). Designed for human-machine interaction, an information system consists of computer programs written for a specific purpose and a database containing raw facts.

The computer solves a problem by accepting data into a database, processing the data according to a specific program, and generating the results as output. An information system thus refers to the processing of data into information.

Data Versus Information

In an information system, data are distinguished from information, the end product (Schoderbek and colleagues, 1980). *Data* is derived from the Latin verb *do, dare,* meaning "to give," and refers to unstructured raw facts. These facts, even though they lack structure, are accepted by the computer as input in preparation for processing.

The term *information* is derived from the Latin verb *informo, informare,* meaning "to give form to." Information is data that have been given form or structure and are organized. Thus, unstructured data (facts) are processed to produce a structured form (information) as the result of processing (Yovits, 1983).

Information System Types

The information systems found in health care delivery systems vary widely depending on how they are described. Some systems are described by purpose or focus of application; others are described by the type of use or service they provide. Some are described as tools for developing information systems; still others are combinations of various types. Information systems are also described by how they process information—on-line, interactive/real-time, and batch processing (see Chap. 5).

These various types of information systems are found in hospitals, community health agencies, research facilities, and educational institutions. The most common systems, listed below, encompass many nursing applications, components, and functions:

- Dedicated systems
- Transaction systems
- Retrieval systems
- Monitoring systems
- Word processing systems

Dedicated Systems

A dedicated system, sometimes called a special purpose system, is one dedicated to a single application or function (Yourdin, 1972; Teichroew, 1983). Most dedicated systems are described by their purpose. For example, airline reservation, banking, or hospital information systems have an evident purpose. Special purpose systems are also found in such hospital specialty departments as pharmacy, laboratory, and radiology. The patient classification and nurse staffing/scheduling systems, for example, are special purpose, or dedicated, systems in the nursing department.

Another type of dedicated system processes a single application, such as a survey or a one-time problem. In this type of system, computer programs are written to process survey data that have been input and stored in a database. Once the survey results are processed and reports generated as output, the system has fulfilled its purpose and the programs and data are no longer necessary.

Transaction Systems

A transaction system, sometimes called a reporting system, is used to process predefined transactions and produce predefined reports. It is thus designed for repeated applications using a fixed list. From this list, displayed on a CRT terminal, a user selects the names of transactions to be processed. The computer programs are written so they can be used repeatedly to process the same type of transactions and generate the same type of reports or products. The computer programs and the list of transactions are retained in storage and are available as needed.

A nursing department payroll system falls into this category, since paychecks are repeatedly processed in the same manner (the same computer programs are used) at regular intervals for all hospital employees. The same list of items used to order and reorder supplies is another example of a transaction system. Reporting systems in community health agencies designed to produce monthly patient services bills or annual statistical reports are also transaction systems. In these systems the computer programs do not change and are stored in the computer. The only change is the raw data.

Retrieval Systems

A retrieval system, sometimes called an information and storage system or a document retrieval system, is used to store and retrieve information. The narrative input stored is available for retrieval in the same format. Many retrieval systems are applications used to research the literature; they are designed to provide bibliographic data on journal articles, books, and narrative reports. Such systems may contain not only citations to documents but keywords, abstracts, and other descriptive facts in their databases (Teichroew, 1983; Salton, 1983).

Monitoring Systems

A monitoring system, sometimes called a control system, is often used to assist in the nursing care of patients by monitoring specific situations and providing alarm signals from sensors for predefined emergency conditions. Monitoring systems in hospitals are found primarily in intensive care units, critical care units, and emergency rooms.

Physiological monitoring systems are being used more frequently to measure and monitor continuous automatic physiological findings such as heart rate, blood pressure, and other vital signs. This monitoring provides an alarm to detect significant abnormal findings when personnel are needed to provide patient care and save lives. (Several applications are presented in Part D.)

Word Processing Systems

A word processing system consists of a software package or set of programs designed to process words in text. The term *word processing* was coined by IBM in 1964 to mean an electronic way of creating, editing, storing, and printing text (Wohl, 1983; Capron and Williams, 1984). Originally, word processing systems were computer systems dedicated to a single purpose, but they are now available as software packages for all sizes of computer systems. They are primarily found in office systems that require the creation of narrative text.

Word processing systems are generally written with a query language using English-like words requiring minimal or no programming knowledge. They use "menus" to display the various options or "templates" to enter data (see Chap. 3). Word processing systems make it possible to create, revise, and rearrange text with minimal keying. They can add, delete, and transfer text words. Many word processing systems offer options such as text editing to manipulate text, spelling verification, and dictionaries.

An example of a menu from a word processing system might look like the display screen below. The options lead the user through the computer program. Each option has a number that, when keyed/typed, initiates the action or activates other displays. This process continues until the instructions are completed.

```
1.   TYPE     4.   SAVE

2.   PRINT    5.   DELETE

3.   GET      6.   EXIT
```

An example of a template from a word processing system might look like the display on page 108. The template terms actually determine the way data are entered into the computer system, since data are keyed/typed in next to the term. Once the terms on the template are completed, other displays appear. The process continues until the instructions are completed.

Menus and templates, found in many of the on-line interactive information systems, simplify the use of computer systems.

MANAGEMENT INFORMATION SYSTEMS

A management information system (MIS) processes information to support management activities and functions. It can affect the nursing department in any health care facility; in fact, it can be designed as a special system for the nursing department in a hospital, community health agency, educational institution, or research facility.

NAME	....	SEX	....
ID NUMBER	....	RACE	....
ADDRESS	....	MD NAME	....
	....	INSURANCE CO.	....
	....	NUMBER	....

A MIS is defined as an organized standardized system for managing the flow of information in an organization in a timely manner; it therefore assists in the decision-making process. When properly designed and implemented, it helps an organization analyze and manage its information logically (Kennevan, 1970; Saba, 1974). It can effectively meet organizational objectives, be responsive to decision-making functions, and provide relevant feedback for short- and long-range planning.

A MIS is based on the structure and functions of any organization and provides the information needed to satisfy these components. The structure of an agency refers to the three levels of management—top, middle, and lower—and to their three functional areas of control—strategic planning, management control, and operational control (Anthony, 1965) (Fig. 6-5).

Strategic planning in a nursing department generally refers to the policy decisions made by the top-level nursing administrator. The administrator requires sum-

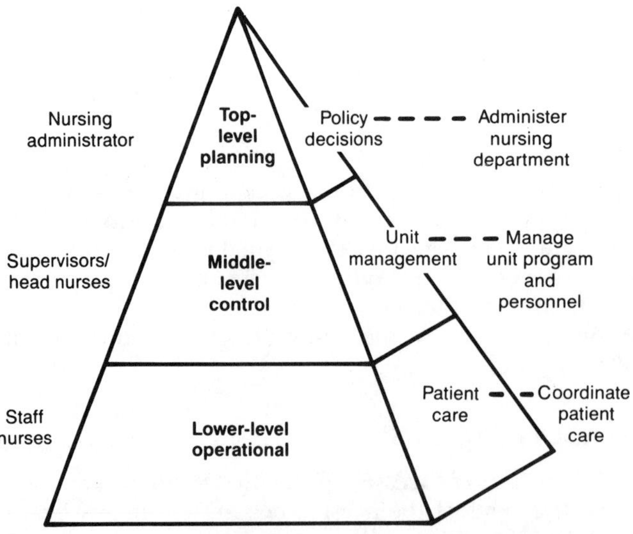

FIG. 6-5. Functional levels of a management information system in a nursing department of a health care agency.

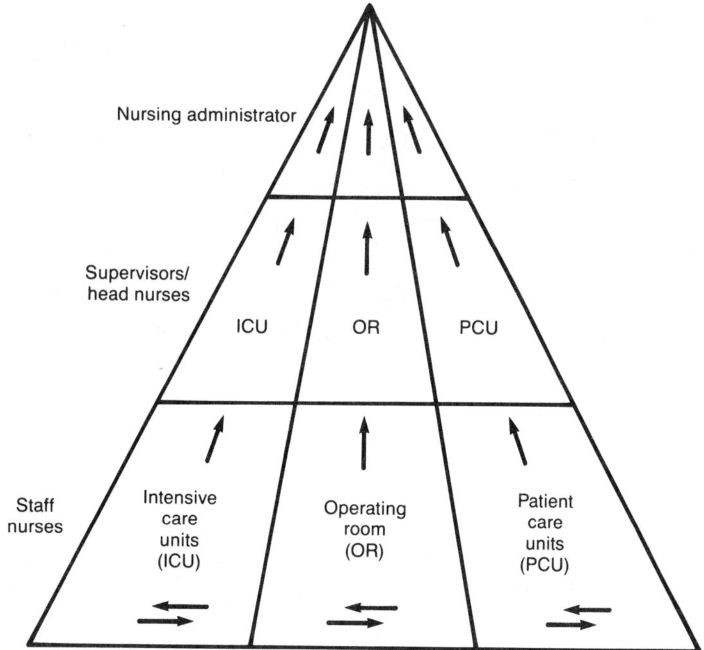

FIG. 6-6. Vertical and horizontal flow of information for a management information system in a nursing department of a health care facility.

mary information to administer the department, plan the agency program, and forecast future needs that meet agency goals. The management control function refers to the program and personnel decisions made by middle-level managers, supervisors, and head nurses. They need information to measure performance standards and to control, plan, and allocate resources. The operational functions are made by the lower-level nursing staff to manage, coordinate, and provide patient care. They need information so that they can effectively and efficiently carry out patient care (Hopper and Mandell, 1984).

A MIS therefore gives personnel at the three functional levels the necessary information for them to perform activities and make decisions. A carefully structured MIS also provides the essential management information so that it flows vertically and horizontally. In a MIS, information flows upward. Data collected at the operating level are processed by the MIS; the information produced is used by the nursing staff to coordinate patient care. Then the MIS generally provides selected information for the supervisors and head nurses to manage their units, and finally it provides summary information for the nursing administrator. Information also flows across departmental units—patient care units to intensive care units to operating rooms. Such information is shared so that units function consistently (Fig. 6-6).

Most MISs in health care agencies are separate from the hospital information systems (HISs) or other systems in the agency. Dr. Morris Collen, an authority on HISs, advocated that the subsystems in an integrated hospital information system be used to support management (Collen, 1983a). He indicated that from a HIS, a user could get information on patient registration and tracking, quality assurance, utilization review, education, and research. In other words, a great deal of information can be shared between the HIS's extensive database and the MIS.

HOSPITAL INFORMATION SYSTEMS

A HIS, sometimes called a medical information system, focuses on hospital functions, including the documentation required for patient care services; it should facilitate daily hospital operations (Veazie and Dankmyer, 1977, 1980). It generally refers to the large integrated information systems used in the delivery of patient care services. Hospitals may also have other separate information systems for special purposes, such as processing medical records or carrying on research studies.

A discussion of HISs includes a review of the following:

- Definitions
- Types
- Configurations

Definitions

According to Collen, a HIS is "the dedicated use of a computer with associated hardware, software and terminals to collect, store, process, retrieve and communicate relevant patient care and administrative information to support primarily the professional specialty group providing direct patient care within a hospital and its associated clinical departmental subsystems, and its outpatient services" (Collen, 1983b, p 61). He also stated that the major functions of a HIS are to communicate and integrate the subsystems or components as well as to provide management support.

Austin, another authority on HISs, restates Collen's points and stresses the need for data files in the system to be integrated (Austin, 1983). Both authors concur that the major purpose of any HIS is to facilitate the communication and integration of data necessary to deliver patient care and associated services.

Types

HISs vary widely, but most consist of various applications centering around services, including nursing, provided to and received by patients (Collen, 1983a). They are designed to incorporate administrative and clinical applications and special applications to satisfy medical, nursing, and other departments' requirements. (Several HISs are described in Part D.)

Administrative and Clinical Applications

Administrative applications include budgeting and payroll, cost accounting, patient billing, inventory control, bed census, and medical records. Clinical applications may include order entry and order transmission, vital signs, shift report, nursing care plans, nurses' notes, and other areas pertinent to patient care.

Special Applications

Special applications refer to the services other than medical and nursing that a patient receives (*e.g.*, laboratory tests, medications, and x-ray studies).

Configurations

HISs can use several different computer system configurations, the most common ones being the stand-alone systems, the large on-line interactive systems, and the network systems. Also emerging are systems that combine the various computer types.

Stand-Alone Systems

The stand-alone systems are the special-purpose systems generally found in different hospital departments. Generally small, these systems are designed to meet specific requirements of a single department (*e.g.*, laboratory, pharmacy, nursing, or dietary). A stand-alone system in a nursing department might be used only for nurse staffing and scheduling.

On-Line Interactive Systems

The large on-line interactive systems are designed to communicate patient information throughout the hospital. Generally consisting of on-line CRTs located in various departments, all of which are connected to a main computer, these HISs have two different levels (Ball and Hannah, 1984).

Level 1 merely transmits and communicates patient care services data (orders) to the accounting, pharmacy, and pathology departments, among others. This type of HIS acts as a messenger service.

Level 2 is used not only to communicate but also to interact with the main computer. This type of system includes various degrees of documentation of patient records and can integrate data in a real-time mode. As well as communicating and transmitting orders, the system can process and generate information needed to provide care and document the care process. It allows for both real-time and batch processing and generally has a large secondary storage (Fig. 6-7).

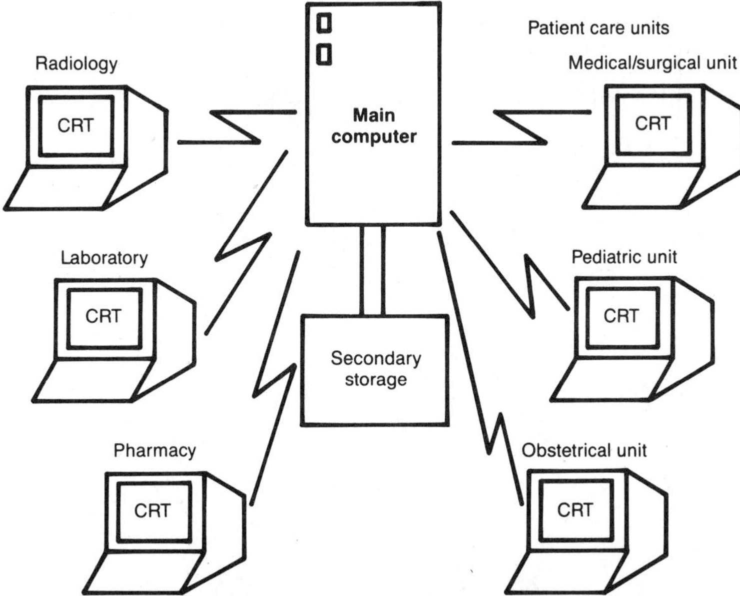

FIG. 6-7. An integrated/real-time hospital information system using a mainframe and minicomputer with CRT terminals.

Network Systems

In network systems several computers support a main computer, as when several departmental minicomputers are connected to a main computer to form a special network. In this arrangement, each minicomputer shares a common integrated database maintained by the main computer and yet has its own departmental database. This type of configuration allows the HISs to remain small and relatively inexpensive and yet to perform functions similar to those of a large integrated system (Fig. 6-8).

Combination Systems

The newest configurations of HISs combine two different types of computers. In one such combination, microcomputers support a main computer, allowing data processing at different levels and for different purposes. This combination allows each department to carry out a variety of computer applications.

In these systems microcomputers replace CRTs for two reasons. Like CRTs, they are connected on line with the main computer, but as terminals, they can communicate and interact in a real-time mode with the computer's database. In addition, they are used as stand-alone microcomputers; as such, they too can store and process data and generate information. Such information may not require processing by the main computer and may not be an integral part of the HIS. The processed information, however, may become input to the main computer system.

For example, a microcomputer application that is not an integral part of a HIS can be a separate computer-assisted instruction (CAI) software package for patient education. Another can be a word processing software package for carrying out secretarial requirements. Still another can be a patient classification system to determine staffing requirements; once determined, this information is communicated to the main computer to generate nursing schedules.

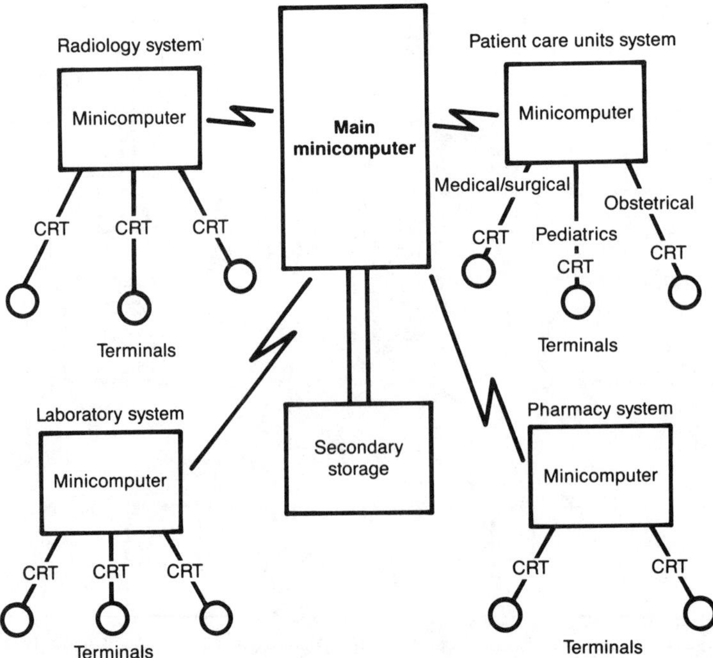

FIG. 6-8. An integrated/real-time hospital information system using a network of minicomputers.

SUMMARY

This chapter discusses when and how general systems theory was introduced. It describes the concept of systems, including types, elements, and major characteristics. A computer system is then defined, followed by a discussion of major types of information systems—namely, dedicated, transaction, retrieval, monitoring, and word processing.

The review of MISs highlights how the three levels of management in any organization can benefit from these systems. Finally, HISs are defined and various types discussed. The basic configurations of several HISs are presented.

STUDY QUESTIONS

1. Who first introduced general systems theory?
2. What event caused systems theory to emerge?
3. What is a system?
4. Name four types of systems.
5. What are the five major elements of a system?
6. Name two characteristics of systems.
7. Define a computer system.
8. Name the five common types of information systems.
9. What is the purpose of a menu in a word processing system?
10. What is the purpose of a template in a word processing system?
11. What are the three functional levels addressed in a MIS?
12. Name the three personnel levels in an organization.
13. What is the purpose of a HIS?
14. Name the three types of HIS applications.
15. Several minicomputers connected together form what system configuration?

REFERENCES

Ackoff RL: Toward a system of systems concepts. Manage Sci 17(11):661–671, 1971

Anthony RN: Planning and Control Systems: A Framework for Analysis. Cambridge, MA, Harvard University Press, 1965

Austin CJ: Information Systems for Hospital Administration, 2nd ed. Ann Arbor, MI, Health Administration Press, 1983

Bertalanffy L von: General Systems Theory. New York, George Braziller, 1968

Ball MJ, Hannah KJ: Using Computers in Nursing. Reston, VA, Reston Publishing, 1984

Boulding KE: General systems theory—the skeleton of science. Manage Sci 2:197–208, 1956

Capron HL, Williams BK: Computers and Data Processing. Menlo Park, CA, Benjamin/Cummings, 1982

Collen MF: The Function of a HIS: An Overview. In Fokkens O, et al (eds): MEDINFO 83 Seminars, pp 61–64. Amsterdam, North-Holland, 1983a

Collen MF: General requirements for clinical departmental systems. In Van Bemmel JH, Ball MJ, Wigertz O (eds): MEDINFO 83, pp 61–64. Amsterdam, North-Holland, 1983b

Donnelly GF: Mengel A, Sutterley DC: The Nursing System: Issues, Ethics and Politics. New York, John Wiley & Sons, 1980

Hellerman H, Smith IA: Computer systems. In Ralston A, Reilly ED Jr (eds): Encyclopedia of Computer Science and Engineering, 2nd ed, pp 370–375. New York, Van Nostrand Reinhold, 1983

Hopper GM, Mandell SL: Understanding Computers. New York, West Publishing, 1984

Kaufman RA: Educational System Planning. Englewood Cliffs, NJ, Prentice-Hall, 1972

Kennevan WJ: Management information systems—MIS universe. Data Manage, September 1970

Newman MA: Nursing's theoretical evolutions. Nurs Outlook 20(7):449–453, 1972
Optner SL: Systems Analysis for Business Management, 2nd ed. Englewood Cliffs, NJ, Prentice-Hall, 1968
Optner SL: Systems Analysis for Business Management, 3rd ed. Englewood Cliffs, NJ, Prentice-Hall, 1975
Saba VK: Basic consideration in management information systems for public health/community health agencies. In National League for Nursing (ed): Management Information for Public Health/Community Health Agencies: Report of the Conference, pp 3–13. New York, National League for Nursing, 1974
Salton G: Information retrieval. In Ralston A, Reilly ED Jr (eds): Encyclopedia of Computer Science and Engineering, 2nd ed, pp 719–725. New York, Van Nostrand Reinhold, 1983
Shoderbek CG, Shoderbek PP, Lefales AG: Management Systems: Conceptual Considerations. Dallas, Business Publishers, 1980
Teichroew D: Information systems. In Ralston A, Reilly ED Jr (eds): Encyclopedia of Computer Science and Engineering, 2nd ed, pp 726–729. New York, Van Nostrand Reinhold, 1983
Veazie S, Dankmyer T: HISs, MISs, and DBMSs: Sorting out the letters. Hospitals 51(20):80–84, 1977
Wohl AD: Word processing. In Ralston A, Reilly ED Jr (eds): Encyclopedia of Computer Science and Engineering, 2nd ed, pp 1573–1574. New York, Van Nostrand Reinhold, 1983
Yourdin E: Design of On-Line Computer Systems. Englewood Cliffs, NJ, Prentice-Hall, 1972
Yovits MC: Information and data. In Ralston A, Reilly ED Jr (eds): Encyclopedia of Computer Science and Engineering, 2nd ed, pp 714–717. New York, Van Nostrand Reinhold, 1983

BIBLIOGRAPHY

Ball MJ: Medical data processing in the United States. Hosp Finan Manage 28(1):10–30, 1974
Blum BI (ed): Information Systems for Patient Care. New York, Springer-Verlag, 1984
Bocchino WA: Management Information Systems: Tools and Techniques. Englewood Cliffs, NJ, Prentice-Hall, 1972
Bronzino JD: Computer Applications for Patient Care. Reading, MA, Addison-Wesley, 1982
Collen MF: Hospital Computer Systems. New York, John Wiley & Sons, 1974
Covvey HD, McAlister NH: Computers in the Practice of Medicine, vol II, Issues in Medical Computing. Reading, MA, Addison-Wesley, 1980
Davis GA: Management information systems. In Ralston A, Reilly ED Jr (eds): Encyclopedia of Computer Science and Engineering, 2nd ed, pp 910–915. New York, Van Nostrand Reinhold, 1983
Dayhoff RE (ed): Proceedings: The Seventh Annual Symposium on Computer Applications in Medical Care. New York, IEEE Computer Society Press, 1983
Fitzgerald J, Fitzgerald AF, Stalling WD Jr: Fundamentals of Systems Analysis, 2nd ed. New York, John Wiley & Sons, 1981
Fokkens O, et al (eds): MEDINFO 83 Seminars. Amsterdam, North-Holland, 1983
Giebink GA, Hurst LL: Computer Projects in Health Care. Ann Arbor, MI, Health Administration Press, 1975
Gillies DA: Nursing Management: A Systems Approach. Philadelphia, WB Saunders, 1982
Hannah KJ: The computer and nursing practice. Nurs Outlook 24(9):555–558, 1976
Hazzard ME: An overview of systems theory. Nurs Clin North Am 6:385, 1971
Kiley M, Holleran EJ, Weston JL, et al: Computerized nursing information systems (NIS). Nurs Manage 14(7):26–29, 1983
Lindberg D: The Growth of Medical Information Systems in the United States. Lexington, MA, Lexington Books, 1977

MacEachern MT: Hospital Organization and Management. Chicago, Physicians' Record, 1946

McWilliams PA: The Word Processing Book. Los Angeles, Prelude Press, 1982

Mintzberg H: The Structuring of Organizations. Englewood Cliffs, NJ, Prentice-Hall, 1979

Murdick RG, Ross JE: Information Systems for Modern Management. Englewood Cliffs, NJ, Prentice-Hall, 1971

National League for Nursing: Management Information System for Public Health/Community Health Agencies: Report of the Conference. New York, National League for Nursing, 1974

Ralston A, Reilly ED Jr (eds): Encyclopedia of Computer Science and Engineering, 2nd ed. New York, Van Nostrand Reinhold, 1983

Van Bemmel J, Ball MS, Wigertz O (eds): MEDINFO 83, vols I and II. Amsterdam, North-Holland, 1983

Walsh ME: Understanding Computers: What Managers and Users Need to Know. New York, John Wiley & Sons, 1982

Wiederhold G: Hospital information systems. In Ralston A, Reilly ED Jr (eds): Encyclopedia of Computer Science and Engineering, 2nd ed, pp 686–688. New York, Van Nostrand Reinhold, 1983

Young EM (ed): Automated Hospital Information Systems Workbook, vol II, Guide to AHIS Suppliers. Los Angeles, Center Publications, 1980

Wilson IG, Wilson ME: Information, Computers, and System Design. New York, John Wiley & Sons, 1965

Yura H, Walsh MB: The Nursing Process: Assessing, Planning, Implementing, Evaluating, 2nd ed. New York, Appleton-Century-Crofts, 1973

Zielstorff R (ed): Computers in Nursing. Wakefield, MA, Nursing Resources, 1980

7 Nursing Information Systems

Objectives

- Describe and define a nursing information system specific for the nursing profession.
- Discuss how different nurse theorists describe patient care, which in turn affects the nursing information system.
- List the various organizational structures where nursing information systems exist.
- Describe the four major areas where nursing information systems are found—namely, nursing administration, practice, research, and education.

Nursing information systems (NISs) are systems that use computers to process nursing data. They appeared on the horizon over a decade ago and are becoming part of everyday life for an increasing number of nurses. Most of the existing NISs are computerized versions of paper-based systems, long used in hospitals, community health agencies, research facilities, and educational institutions. To understand NISs therefore requires knowledge of computers, systems theory, other systems specific to nursing, and nursing and nursing systems.

Basically, a NIS uses a computer to process data into information to support all types of nursing activities or functions. It is an invaluable aid for administering hospital and community health agencies, assisting nursing practice, retrieving information for research, and educating students. As stated in Chapter 6, information systems are described according to their purpose, focus, use, service, and so on and thus encompass many nursing applications, components, and functions. Some of their uses in nursing departments have been cited in previous chapters.

This chapter will concentrate on NISs specific to the nursing profession. It will discuss the factors that have influenced their development and provide an overview of their applications. (See Part D for an in-depth description.) Specifically, this chapter includes the following:

- Background
- Overview of applications

BACKGROUND

One must understand the background of the factors that influence NISs in order to understand the systems. Many NISs are used in conjunction with larger systems that may be based on a particular definition or theory of nursing, on the organizational unit affected, or on the specific focus of the system. This section thus includes the following:

- Nursing definitions
- Nursing system theories
- Organizations where NISs exist
- NIS definitions

Nursing Definitions

Certain definitions of nursing expand the scope of a NIS. Nursing is a profession responsive to the changing needs of society, patient care, and the nursing profession itself. Definitions of nursing vary depending on the focus of nursing practice. Most nursing departments uphold the hospital definition of nursing, a definition that generally affects the focus of a NIS for nursing practice.

The American Nurses' Association (ANA), in its social policy statement, says: "Nursing is the diagnosis and treatment of human responses to actual or potential health problems" (ANA, 1980). Another definition of nursing comes from Henderson, who states that nursing "assist[s] the individual, sick or well, in the performance of those activities contributing to health or its recovery (or to peaceful death) that he would perform unaided if he had the strength, will, or knowledge, and to do this in such a way to help him gain independence as rapidly as possible" (Henderson, 1964, pp 63–68; Flynn and colleagues, 1984).

A NIS developed from the ANA definition would differ from one developed from Henderson's definition. The nursing diagnosis would be a part of the nursing database in the ANA system but not in Henderson's system. Each of the two definitions, however, describes nursing practice. Note that these definitions do not encompass the nursing activities and functions of administrators, educators, and researchers in the practice of nursing, which must be recognized before a NIS is described.

Nursing Systems Theories

Primarily used to describe nursing by the different ways patient care is provided, nursing systems theories also describe the organizational structure in which nurses function. These theories dictate the focus of and provide the framework for NISs.

Many nursing theorists, leaders, and authors have described nursing systems. For example, Rogers, a nurse theorist, identified "four building blocks" as the key elements for the conceptual framework of a nursing system (Rogers, 1970; Fordyce 1984, p 248). Orem, another theorist, described three nursing systems by the level and degree of patient involvement (Orem, 1971; Fordyce, 1984). Yura and Walsh (1973) affirmed that the nursing process illustrates the nursing system. The nursing process is composed of the assessment, planning, intervention, and evaluation components involved in patient care. However, Goodwin and Edwards (1975) illustrated that the nursing process was a systems model that could be computerized; Ozbolt revised this model in 1983 (Fig. 7-1).

In 1978 Putt wrote on how systems theory can be used to design and describe nursing care plans. Viewing nursing systems in terms of patients' physiological care needs, she provided a guideline for recording patient care, which has been used as a tool in nursing audits (Putt, 1978). Donnelly and colleagues (1980) outlined the issues, ethics, and politics of the professional nursing system. Gillies (1982) described the nurse manager as one working among a variety of systems in an organiza-

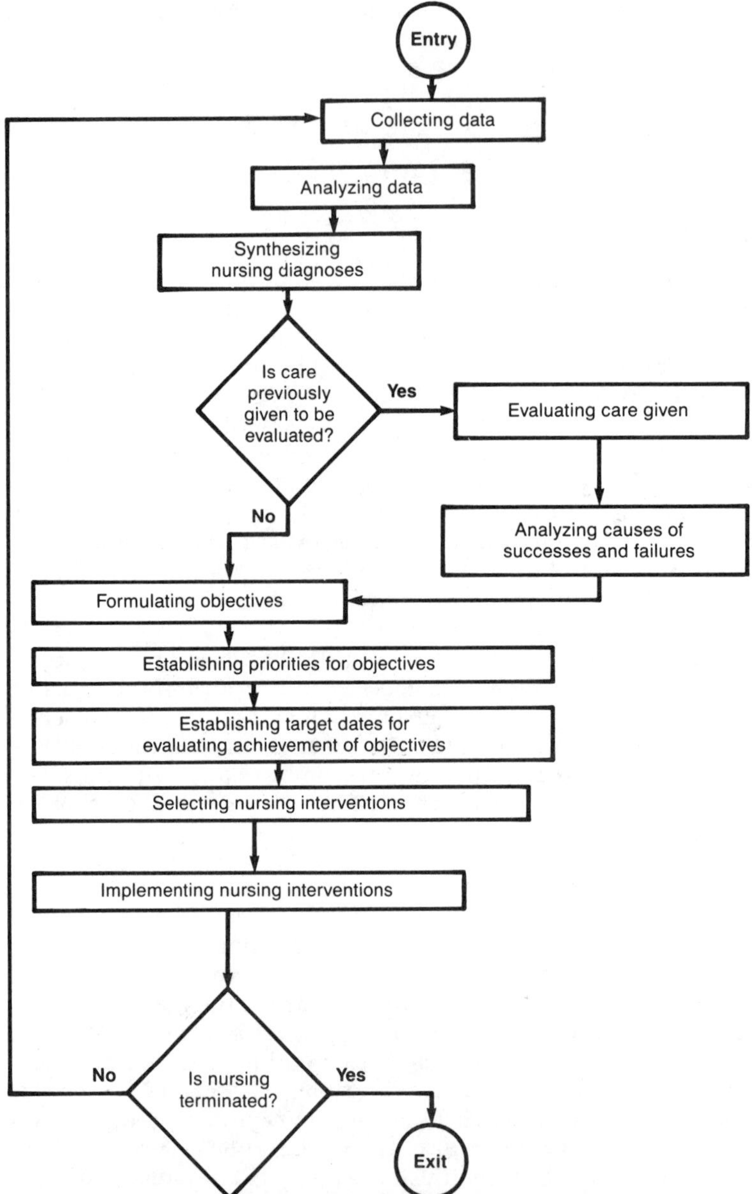

FIG. 7-1. General model of the nursing process. (Ozbolt J: A prototype information system to aid nursing decision. In Blum B (ed): Proceedings of the Sixth Annual Symposium on Computer Applications in Medical Care, pp 653–657. New York, IEEE Computer Society Press, 1983)

tion. McFarland and colleagues (1984) related systems to strategies for nursing leadership and management.

Each of these nursing theories or systems can act as the focus or purpose of a NIS. For example, a NIS based on Rogers's theory of four building blocks would require data elements relevant to that framework. Data elements for the nursing process outlined by Yura and Walsh would depict assessment, planning, intervention, and evaluation components.

Organizations Where Nursing Information Systems Exist

Describing the organizations where NISs exist is relatively easy, since they are primarily found in facilities where nurses are employed. Hospitals, community health agencies, and educational institutions employ the greatest number of nurses.

Generally, most hospitals have or are implementing some type of hospital information system (HIS) or medical information system (MIS), sometimes called a patient care system (PCS). Such systems generally are implemented with subsystems or components specifically for nursing; hence these subsystems are called NISs. Such NISs are generally implemented and expanded to assist nurses in documenting and processing data needed for patient care. NISs may also be found in hospitals as stand-alone systems specifically designed for the nursing department; these are generally implemented to process special nursing applications.

Hospitals may have many information systems, including NISs, all dedicated to specific applications. Hospitals are beginning to share and establish a communication network with other hospitals for certain applications. The emerging NIS stand-alone systems, which use minicomputers or microcomputers for specific nursing applications, are designed to generate timely statistics for managing and allocating nursing personnel and resources.

NISs are also found in community and public health programs, where they are used to assist nurses in managing and delivering patient care. These NISs generally are components of information systems restricted within the agency, city, county, or state. Some of these systems have developed communication networks within their organizational structure, that is, linkages between units throughout the agency, city, or state.

NISs also exist in educational institutions, where they are usually restricted to nursing departments. Generally, most large educational institutions have a central computer system that supports student and faculty management, teaching, and research. It usually consists of a large mainframe computer with cathode ray tube (CRT) terminals that link the different academic departments and offices within the university to the computer center. Generally, such a system is not linked to any outside institution. Used by management to process the institutions' business applications, such a system is used by students and faculty to study computer technology, to carry out coursework, and to conduct research.

Emerging in large educational institutions are computer learning resources centers, which departments such as nursing install or share with other departments. These centers contain several CRTs or microcomputers. The CRTs are connected to the institution's mainframe and used for applications that cannot be run on the microcomputer.

Both mainframe and microcomputer systems are used for many NIS applications. Mainframes, used to store large nursing databases, can also run statistical software packages where research study data must be analyzed. Microcomputers are primarily used as stand-alone systems; students run computer-assisted instruction (CAI) software packages, develop nursing care protocols, or develop and test nursing research theories on them. They are also used by faculty members to run computer-managed instruction (CMI), software packages to manage student programs, and by the dean to run specific managerial applications or administer the requirements of the office.

NIS Definitions

Definitions of NISs vary depending on whether a system is interpreted according to purpose or by what it encompasses. The Study Group on Nursing Information Systems (1983, p 101) described a NIS as a system that "applies to the automated processing of the data needed to plan, give, evaluate, and document patient care, as well as to collect the data necessary to support the delivery of nursing care, such as staffing and cost."

Collen (1983, p 736), on the other hand, in describing clinical departmental systems (CDS) for hospitals, implies but does not specify that nursing can be considered a CDS. He describes a CDS as a system that "is a direct patient care subsystem within a hospital or medical information system, but it may be a separate stand-alone system serving one professional specialty for the care of inpatients and/or outpatients."

Flynn and colleagues (1984, p 32) describe NISs as "a collection of computerized programs that contain nursing and selected patient and medical data. The system may or may not be a part of a larger medical information system used to record, review, monitor, and analyze these data."

However, in this book a NIS is defined as *a computer system that collects, stores, processes, retrieves, displays, and communicates timely information needed to do the following* (Fig. 7-2):

Administer the nursing services and resources in a health care facility
Manage standardized patient care information for the delivery of nursing care
Link the research resources and the educational applications to nursing practice

OVERVIEW OF APPLICATIONS

NISs are found in many situations and encompass various nursing activities. They can be stand-alone systems, subsystems, or system components. Generally, as components of a larger information system, they are found in a large hospital or community health agency information system. They can also be part of a medical information system, patient care system, or management information system. As stand-alone systems, sometimes called freestanding systems, they are designed for a specific purpose. For example, a patient classification, nurse staffing, and scheduling system may be an integral part of a hospital information system or may be a stand-alone dedicated system that runs on its own minicomputer or microcomputer.

Most NISs are found in four major nursing areas in which other computer systems are also used to help nurses administer nursing departments, provide patient care, and link research and education to patient care. This section provides an overview of these nursing areas:

- Nursing administration
- Nursing practice
- Nursing research
- Nursing education

Figure 7-2 presents a model of the state of the art of NISs and other related applications that will be described in Part D.

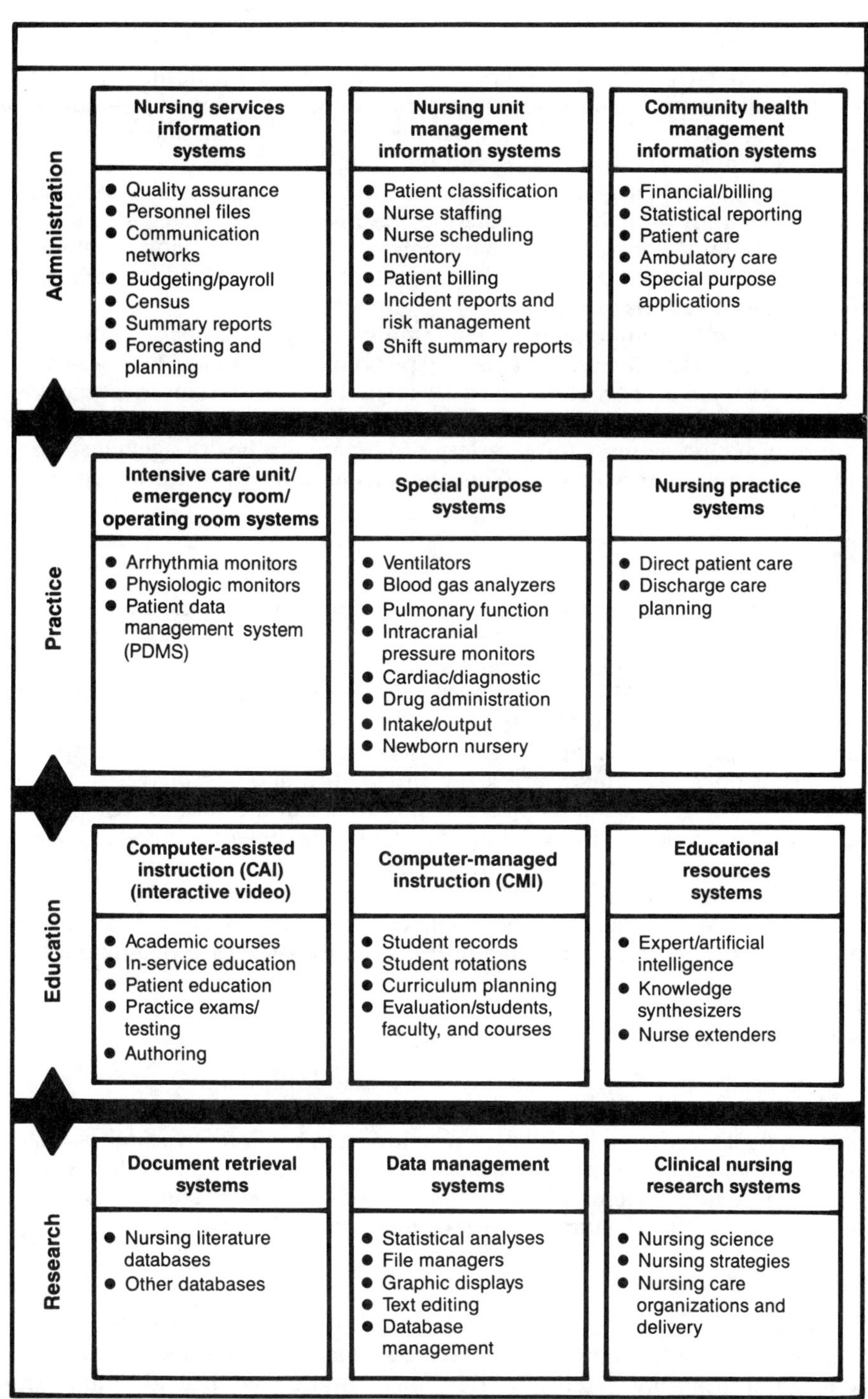

Administration
Nursing services information systems
• Quality assurance
• Personnel files
• Communication networks
• Budgeting/payroll
• Census
• Summary reports
• Forecasting and planning
Nursing unit management information systems
• Patient classification
• Nurse staffing
• Nurse scheduling
• Inventory
• Patient billing
• Incident reports and risk management
• Shift summary reports
Community health management information systems
• Financial/billing
• Statistical reporting
• Patient care
• Ambulatory care
• Special purpose applications
Practice
Intensive care unit/ emergency room/ operating room systems
• Arrhythmia monitors
• Physiologic monitors
• Patient data management system (PDMS)
Special purpose systems
• Ventilators
• Blood gas analyzers
• Pulmonary function
• Intracranial pressure monitors
• Cardiac/diagnostic
• Drug administration
• Intake/output
• Newborn nursery
Nursing practice systems
• Direct patient care
• Discharge care planning
Education
Computer-assisted instruction (CAI) (interactive video)
• Academic courses
• In-service education
• Patient education
• Practice exams/ testing
• Authoring
Computer-managed instruction (CMI)
• Student records
• Student rotations
• Curriculum planning
• Evaluation/students, faculty, and courses
Educational resources systems
• Expert/artificial intelligence
• Knowledge synthesizers
• Nurse extenders
Research
Document retrieval systems
• Nursing literature databases
• Other databases
Data management systems
• Statistical analyses
• File managers
• Graphic displays
• Text editing
• Database management
Clinical nursing research systems
• Nursing science
• Nursing strategies
• Nursing care organizations and delivery

FIG. 7-2. Model of nursing information systems and other related applications.

Nursing Administration

NISs are generally found as subsystems in nursing administration, dedicated primarily to administering nursing services. Such subsystems encompass quality assurance, personnel files, communication network, budgeting and payroll, census, summary reports, and forecasting and planning.

Nursing unit management information systems are also considered to be NISs and are generally available as special-purpose systems, subsystems, or stand-alone systems. They deal particularly with patient classification, nurse staffing, nurse scheduling, inventory, patient billing, incident reports and risk management, and shift summary reports.

NISs exist as components of community and public health MISs, generally addressing the administration of nursing personnel and nursing care services. They too may be stand-alone systems in small agencies or subsystems in larger agencies. They primarily encompass finances and billing, statistical reporting, and patient care information systems for a variety of community health agencies. They also encompass ambulatory care systems and special purpose studies, programs, and project applications.

Nursing Practice

In the area of nursing practice, NISs focus on the intensive care unit, emergency room, and operating room systems. Computerized physiological monitoring systems assist nurses in observing patients' vital signs. Such systems may stand alone or be connected to a NIS that integrates the information from the monitors into patient data management systems (PDMS). Special-purpose systems, also found in the area on nursing practice, are generally stand-alone systems for specific applications. The major ones that nurses use are ventilators, blood gas analyzers, pulmonary function systems, intracranial pressure monitors, cardiac/diagnostic systems, drug administration systems, intake/output systems, and newborn nursery systems.

NISs are also subsystems in large on-line, integrated/real-time HISs and, in some cases, stand-alone systems. Such systems collect, store, process, display, retrieve, and communicate direct patient care information. Order entry, charting of vital signs, care planning, nursing notes, and discharge care planning all may be incorporated specifically for nursing documentation.

Nursing Research

Systems used in nursing research vary. They include the document retrieval systems and other databases that allow for searching the nursing literature. Data management systems also may be used to provide such tools for research as statistical analysis software packages, file managers, graphic displays, text editors, and database management systems. Finally, research NISs are used to study nursing science, nursing strategies, and nursing care organization and delivery.

Nursing Education

In the area of nursing education, CAI is being used to teach students and for in-service and patient education. NISs are also used for practice examinations and testing and authoring systems. In addition, computerized-management instruction (CMI) is used for student records and student rotations. CAI is also used to plan curricula and evaluate students, faculty, and courses. Both comprise computer-based education. Educational resources include expert systems that are a form of artificial intelligence, knowledge synthesizers, and nurse extenders.

• • •

In part D the various applications of NISs are described in detail.

SUMMARY

This chapter provides an overview of NISs. It presents several definitions of a NIS and lists factors that influenced the development of NISs, including nursing definitions and nursing systems theories. Places where NISs exist, that is, health care facilities where nurses are employed, are noted. Finally, the various NISs found in nursing are presented. The four areas where NISs are found—namely, nursing administration, practice, research, and education—are described. Included are other information systems that nurses use in providing patient care and carrying out nursing activities.

STUDY QUESTIONS

1. Define an NIS.
2. What organization defined nursing in its social policy statement?
3. Name three nurse theorists or authors who have described different ways patient care is provided.
4. In what organizational structures does nursing information exist?
5. List three major types of facilities where NISs exist.
6. Name the various groups that have defined a NIS.
7. Name the four major nursing areas where NISs are found.
8. In which two major in-hospital nursing areas are NISs generally found?
9. Name a system specific for nursing practice.
10. Name two areas in research where computers are used.
11. What is included in computer-based education?
12. An expert system is a form of artificial intelligence. True or false?

REFERENCES

American Nurses' Association: Nursing: A Social Policy Statement. Kansas City, MO, American Nurses' Association, 1980

Collen MF: General requirements for clinical departmental systems. In Van Bemmel JH, Ball MJ, Wigertz O (eds): MEDINFO 83, pp 736–739. Amsterdam, North-Holland, 1983

Donnelly GF, Mangel A, Sutterley DC: The Nursing System: Issues, Ethics, and Politics. New York, John Wiley & Sons, 1980

Flynn JB, Foerst H, Heffron PB: Nursing: Past and present. In McCann/Flynn JB, Heffron PB (eds): Nursing: From Concept to Practice, pp 31–88. Bowie, MD, Robert J. Brady, 1984

Fordyce EM: Theorists in nursing. In McCann/Flynn JB, Heffron PB (eds): Nursing: From Concept to Practice, pp 237–258. Bowie, MD, Robert J. Brady, 1984

Gillies DA: Nursing Management: A Systems Approach. Philadelphia, WB Saunders, 1982

Goodwin JO, Edwards BS: Developing a computer program to assist the nursing process. Nurs Res 24(4):299–305, 1975

Henderson V: The nature of nursing. Am J Nursing 64(8):62–68, 1964

McFarland GK, Leonard HS, Morris MM: Nursing Leadership and Management: Contemporary Strategies. New York, John Wiley & Sons, 1984

Orem DE: Nursing: Concepts of Practice. New York, McGraw-Hill, 1971

Ozbolt J: A prototype information system to aid nursing decision. In Blum B (ed): Proceedings: The Sixth Annual Symposium on Computer Applications in Medical Care, pp 653—657. New York, IEEE Computer Society Press, 1983
Putt AM: General systems theory: A guide for nursing. In Putt AM (ed): General Systems Theory Applied to Nursing, pp 25–29. Boston, Little, Brown & Co, 1978
Rogers ME: An Introduction to the Theoretical Basis of Nursing. Philadelphia, FA Davis, 1970
Study Group on Nursing Information Systems: Special report: Computerized nursing information systems: An urgent need. Res Nurs Health 6(3):101–105, 1983
Yura H, Walsh MB: The Nursing Process: Assessing, Planning, Implementing, Evaluating, 2nd ed. New York, Appleton-Century-Crofts, 1973

BIBLIOGRAPHY

Abbey JC: A general systems approach to nursing. In Putt AM (ed): General Systems Theory Applied to Nursing, pp 19–25. Boston, Little, Brown & Co, 1978
Ball MJ, Hannah KJ: Using Computers in Nursing. Reston, VA, Reston Publishing, 1984
Bronzino JD: Computer Applications for Patient Care. Reading, MA, Addison-Wesley, 1982
Edmunds L: Making the most of a message function for nursing services. In Dayhoff R (ed): Proceedings: The Seventh Annual Symposium on Computer Applications in Medical Care, pp 511–513. New York, IEEE Computer Society Press, 1983
McCann/Flynn JB, Heffron PB: Nursing: From Concept to Practice. Bowie, MD, Rober J. Brady, 1984
Grobe SJ: Computer Primer and Resource Guide for Nurses. Philadelphia, JB Lippincott, 1984
Henderson V: The Nature of Nursing. New York, Macmillan, 1966
Henderson V, Nite G: Principles and Practice of Nursing, 6th ed. New York, Macmillan, 1978
Kiley M, Halloran EJ, Weston JL, et al: Computerized nursing information systems (NIS). Nurs Manage 14(7):26–29, 1983
Pocklington DB, Guttman L: Nursing Reference for Computer Literature. Philadelphia, JB Lippincott, 1984
Pritchard K: Computers 3: Possible applications in nursing. Nurs Times 78(7):465–466, 1982
Pritchard K: Computers 4: Implication of computerization. Nurs Times 78(8):491–492, 1982
Putt AM (ed): General Systems Theory Applied to Nursing. Boston, Little, Brown & Co, 1978
Romano C, McCormick K, McNeely L: Nursing documentation: A model for a computerized data base. Adv Nurs Sci 4:43–56, 1982
Scholes M, Bryant Y, Barber B (eds): The Impact of Computers on Nursing: An International Review. Amsterdam, North-Holland, 1983
Sweeney MA, Olivieri P: An Introduction to Nursing Research. Philadelphia, JB Lippincott, 1981
Werley H, Grier M (eds): Nursing Information Systems. New York, Springer, 1981
Young EM (ed): Automated Hospital Information Systems Workbook, vol II, Guide to AHIS Suppliers. Los Angeles, Center Publications, 1980
Zielstorff RD (ed): Computers in Nursing. Wakefield, MA, Nursing Resources, 1980

8 Developing a Nursing Information System

Objectives

- Describe the five phases in developing a nursing information system (NIS).
- Describe the personnel responsible for developing a NIS.
- Identify the various tools of the trade used in developing a NIS.
- Describe the methods of evaluating a NIS.

A computerized nursing information system (NIS), which assists nurses with decision making and problem solving, may be designed for different purposes: to administer a nursing department, assist nursing practice, retrieve information for research, or assist in teaching. However, the NIS described in this chapter is designed primarily for a nursing department of a health care facility that provides patient care.

A NIS can be designed as a stand-alone system, a subsystem of a larger system, or a component of another system. It can be programmed for processing by a mainframe, minicomputer, or microcomputer, and it may share the same equipment that other systems in the facility use.

Regardless of what type of system is designed or what size computer it runs on, any NIS for a health care facility generally follows the five phases of development listed below and adheres to the problem-solving approach or the scientific method (Capron and Williams, 1982; Shelly and Cashman, 1980) (Fig. 8-1).

- Planning phase
- Analysis phase
- Design phase
- Development phase
- Implementation and Evaluation phase

COMMITTEE AND PROJECT STAFF

Before a NIS can be developed, administrators must appoint a NIS Committee and a project staff (Fig. 8-2). The NIS committee generally includes the following:

A representative from the facility's nursing administration to uphold the nursing department's commitments
A nursing representative from each of the major health care departments, programs, or units
A systems nurse
A computer consultant or systems analyst
Other appointed members

All must understand the nursing problem to be studied.

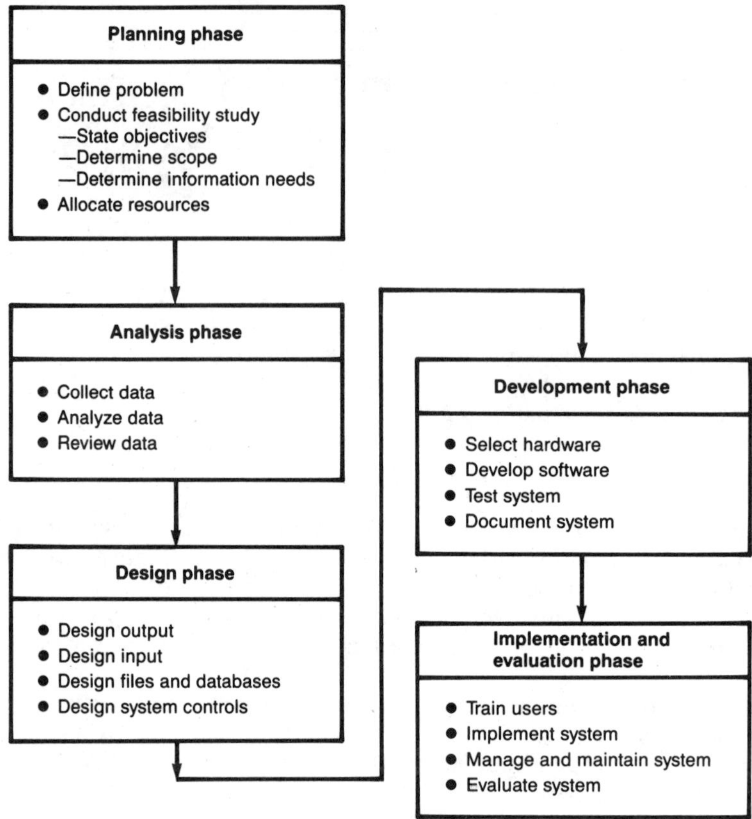

FIG. 8-1. Developing a nursing information system model.

The systems nurse must have had academic as well as practical training in computer technology; that is, the nurse must be computer literate. He or she must also thoroughly understand the facility's nursing department and be authorized to act on its behalf. The computer consultant or systems analyst should have experience in developing information systems for the particular type of problem or particular type of health care facility in question. The person may be a staff member or may be contracted from outside.

The NIS committee is responsible for coordinating the entire project. Committee members must see that all activities are performed; they are responsible for obtaining needed resources. They must look after the nursing department's interests and those of the system's potential users. The committee also must collaborate with any other information system committees in the facility. The committee, once established, initiates the system phases.

The project staff includes at least the key members of the committee—the systems nurse and the consultant or a systems analyst. They are responsible to the NIS committee but report to the management information systems department, if one exists. The project staff is responsible for carrying out the planning phase and determining how the system is proceeding. Project staff size will vary depending on the size and scope of the system being developed. Staff must coordinate their activities with any other information system committee in the facility.

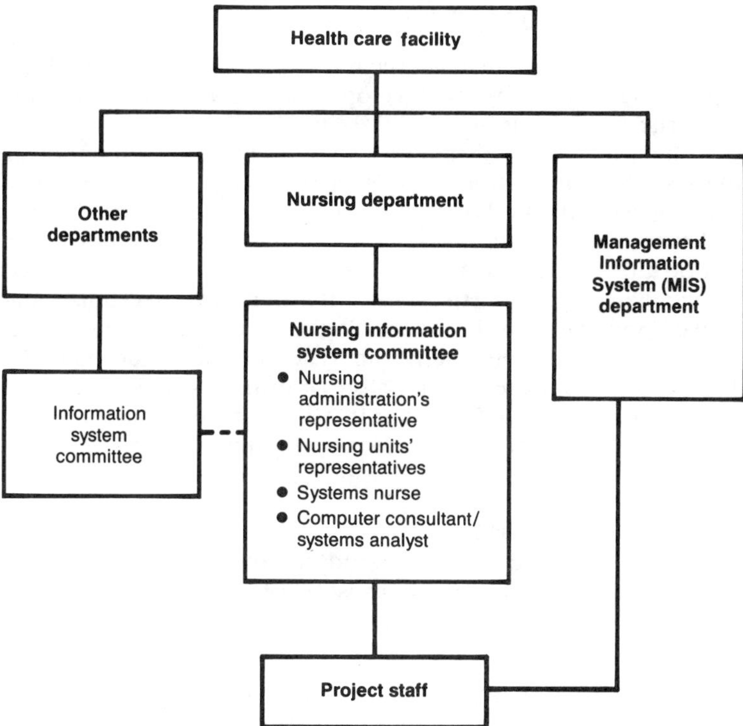

FIG. 8-2. An example of an organizational chart depicting a nursing information system committee.

PLANNING PHASE

Planning the system is critical, since during this initial phase the entire nursing problem is assessed. The planning phase involves the following steps.

- Define problem
- Conduct feasibility study
  - State objectives
  - Determine scope
  - Determine information needs
- Allocate resources

Define Problem

The first step in Planning, to define the problem precisely, is critical. It may not be easy, however, because the stated problem and the "real" problem may differ. Not until a problem is analyzed are its real characteristics revealed (Fitzgerald and colleagues, 1981).

For example:

1. The problem of unfair nurse staff assignments may relate to invalid patient classifications (inaccurate grouping of patients) rather than to workload measurements.
2. Unnecessary health department reports may result from inappropriate statistics instead of unreasonable reporting requirements.

Conduct Feasibility Study

The feasibility study analyzes the nursing problem to determine if the stated problem can be resolved by the development of a NIS. The study asks if the system will solve the problem or improve the situation.

The feasibility study not only clarifies the problem but determines the objectives, scope, informational needs (requirements), and functional requirements of the proposed NIS. In short, it highlights what the proposed system will encompass and provides the framework for its operation. This study identifies the types of information relevant to solving the problem and the types of computer resources essential for developing the system. It provides a cost estimate and presents ways to manage and maintain the system; it also gives a time frame for completion.

The feasibility study helps the NIS committee understand the real problem by analyzing it and presenting possible solutions. It highlights whether the system is worth what it costs and whether it will produce usable products. Thus, the study addresses the critical elements for developing a system and is, in a sense, a model of a "minisystem."

State Objectives

The first step in the feasibility study is to state the objectives for the proposed system, which constitute the purpose(s) of the system. All objectives must be stated in terms appropriate for computer processing.

For example:

1. An objective relating to nurse assignments might be stated as follows: "Develop a nurse staffing and scheduling NIS that uses valid and reliable patient classifications."
2. An objective relating to statistical reporting in a community health agency might be stated as follows: "Develop a system for reporting statistical information as required by local, state, and federal authorities."

Determine Scope

The scope of the proposed system establishes system constraints, including its controls and parameters, and outlining what the proposed system will and will not produce.

For example:

1. The scope relating to nurse staffing and scheduling might be stated as follows: "The system would only provide nurse staffing and scheduling requirements for general, not specialty, units."
2. The scope relating to community health statistical reporting might be stated as follows: "The system would collect only data needed for routine, and not one-time reports, that is, statistical reports required by local, state, and federal authorities."

Determine Information Needs

In this step, sometimes called a needs assessment, the information needs (requirements) system users will require are outlined. Identifying information needed helps clarify what users will expect from the system. Such knowledge is essential in designing system output, input, and processing needs.

For example:

1. The nurse staffing and scheduling system based on patient classification would need the following information:

- A valid patient classification for determing staffing requirements
- Number of nursing personnel required to staff each patient care unit
- Types of nursing personnel required to staff each patient care unit
- Method of scheduling nursing personnel

2. A statistical reporting system designed to meet local, state, and federal reporting would require the following information:
   - Time personnel spend making visits
   - Cost of visits by type of provider
   - Number of clients per program
   - Characteristics of active clients
   - Number of services provided to clients by nurses
   - Type of sites where services are provided

Allocate Resources

The last step in the planning phase is determining what is needed to make the NIS work. Generally, the functional requirements have been defined in the feasibility study, but a firm commitment of resources for development of the entire NIS is needed before the system can fulfill its stated objectives.

The following functional requirements must be considered:

- Personnel
- Time frame
- Cost/budget
- Facilities and equipment

Personnel

The additional staff needed to develop the system may be drawn from several sources, including the nursing department, an existing management information system unit, or a consultant firm or computer vendor.

The project staff appointed at the beginning of the investigation should, if possible, be retained for project duration. These persons, especially the systems nurse and the computer consultant or systems analyst, have worked closely with NIS committee members through the planning phase and the decision to proceed.

In all nursing matters related to developing a NIS, the systems nurse assumes leadership. He or she is directly responsible to the nursing department administrator and the nursing committee. The "key person" who understands the functions of the nursing department, the system nurse has the clinical expertise to implement the nursing requirements of the NIS and the ability to implement the training programs to educate nursing personnel about the system.

A successful NIS requires a capable systems analyst, one who has been vital in developing the information system for nurses. He or she must be able to design, develop, and implement an information system.

The systems manager may be selected from any of the above sources but must be a capable administrator. Such a person not only supervises developing the system but administers project staff personnel, time, budget control, and cost activities. This person is responsible to the NIS committee.

Time Frame

A time frame is needed to outline and synchronize all the steps in developing the NIS. A milestone chart or a Gantt chart can be useful for plotting, in sequence, the major tasks and accomplishments required in developing the NIS. The milestone chart consists of lines; the Gantt chart uses bar graphs to highlight activities and time of their completion (Fig. 8-3).

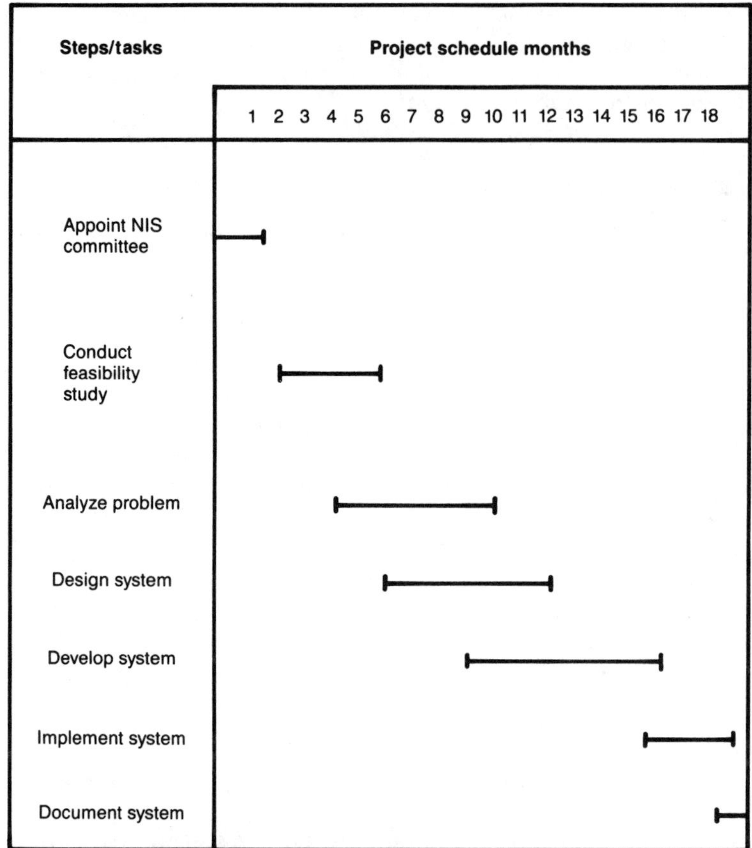

FIG. 8-3. An example of a milestone chart outlining selected steps in developing a nursing information system.

Cost/Budget

The cost/budget for developing a NIS must be established and approved "up front," since without it the system cannot be completed in a timely, cost-effective manner.

Funds are critical and must be set aside for developing, managing, maintaining, and evaluating the system. Funds are also needed for ongoing staff training. The budget for the system must be approved by the NIS committee, but continued budget control and auditing are the project manager's responsibility.

Facilities and Equipment

All computerized systems require facilities and equipment, that is, hardware, software, and peripheral equipment. A computer–information system unit may be needed to house the basic hardware and its components, especially if a mainframe or large minicomputer system is considered. Such a unit must be large enough to store all relevant working materials and equipment. The computer unit staff must also be organized with lines of authority and established formal communication channels.

Summary Report

The results of the planning phase are generally summarized in a report for review by the NIS committee. The report should contain the planning phase findings as outlined in this section and should make recommendations on whether the existing information system should be upgraded, a new system instituted, or the proposed system incorporated into an existing larger system. It recommends the kind of system, subsystem, or components appropriate for solving the problem and whether the system should be developed in-house or through contract services (see the discussion on the development phase). Finally, it estimates both cost and benefits. This report must be approved by the NIS committee before the project staff can develop the NIS.

ANALYSIS PHASE

The analysis phase, the second phase of developing a NIS, is the fact-finding phase. All data related to the problem are collected and analyzed in order to understand what exists and what is needed. This analysis is essential to the actual system design. Also examined are the objectives and scope as written in the feasibility study, the informational and functional requirements, the dataflow procedures, and the scope (boundaries, interfaces, and decision points). Current costs and resources required for processing the data are compared with estimates for a new system (Capron and Williams, 1984; Hopper and Mandell, 1984; Shelly and Cashman, 1980).

The analysis phase consists of the following three steps:

- Collect data
- Analyze data
- Review data

Collect Data

Collecting data is a fact-finding activity. Assisting in the analysis of the existing nursing problem, data collection reveals the full scope of the problem at hand. The major sources of data essential for this activity are as follows:

- Written documents
- Questionnaires
- Interviews
- Observations

Written Documents

Written documents, collected to ascertain different aspects of the nursing problem, must be carefully reviewed. They include standards, orders, procedures, operating manuals, routine reports, and forms used to collect data. Further, the raw facts (data elements) themselves must be analyzed, including their processing, a flowchart of the process, and the resultant reports.

Questionnaires

Questionnaires, another source of information, provide useful information without being too time-consuming. They can ascertain the needs of the system users.

Interviews

Interviews are one of the best sources of information on an existing nursing problem. Interviews with selected personnel at all organizational levels can elicit very specific information on how, when, where, and in what kinds of situations data are processed. Moreover, standard form interviews help to document, in a logical sequence, the kinds of information used.

Observations

Observations, another excellent way to understand staff views, can reveal how staff members relate to each other, how they manage the information they handle, and how they use that information. This may include a time study to determine, for example, the time spent on various nursing activities.

Analyze Data

To analyze data is to correlate all collected data. This process provides a complete overview of the nursing problem in order to better understand its scope.

Several tools of the trade, that is, methods of documentation, are necessary to help review and gain perspective on all collected data. Some of the more common tools are as follows:

- Data flowchart
- Grid chart
- Decision table
- Organizational chart
- Model

Data Flowchart

A data flowchart, one of the most important tools in data analysis, graphically illustrates the sequential steps found in processing the nursing problem. In a sense it provides a "road map" of the flow of information. A data flowchart is an excellent tool for tracing where and when the flow of information begins and where it goes (Fig. 8-4).

Grid Chart

A grid chart, also called a data analysis chart, analyzes the interrelationships of the data used to process the nursing problem. It generally includes a listing of all the data elements collected as input that are processed and generated as output. A grid chart can also be used to list the kinds of information generated as output, including purpose and recipient (Fig. 8-5).

Decision Table

A decision table, sometimes called a decision–logic table, illustrates the logical decisions and possible alternatives for solving the nursing problem. It provides a tabular display of all relevant data, lists all possible choices, and highlights the logical rules used for processing the data (Fig. 8-6).

Organizational Chart

An organizational chart depicts the levels of authority and the formal lines of interorganizational communication. Helping to distinguish line personnel from staff personnel, the chart also depicts the reporting relationships among various positions and shows various jobs. It helps clarify who is responsible for what and how current data are processed (Fig. 8-7).

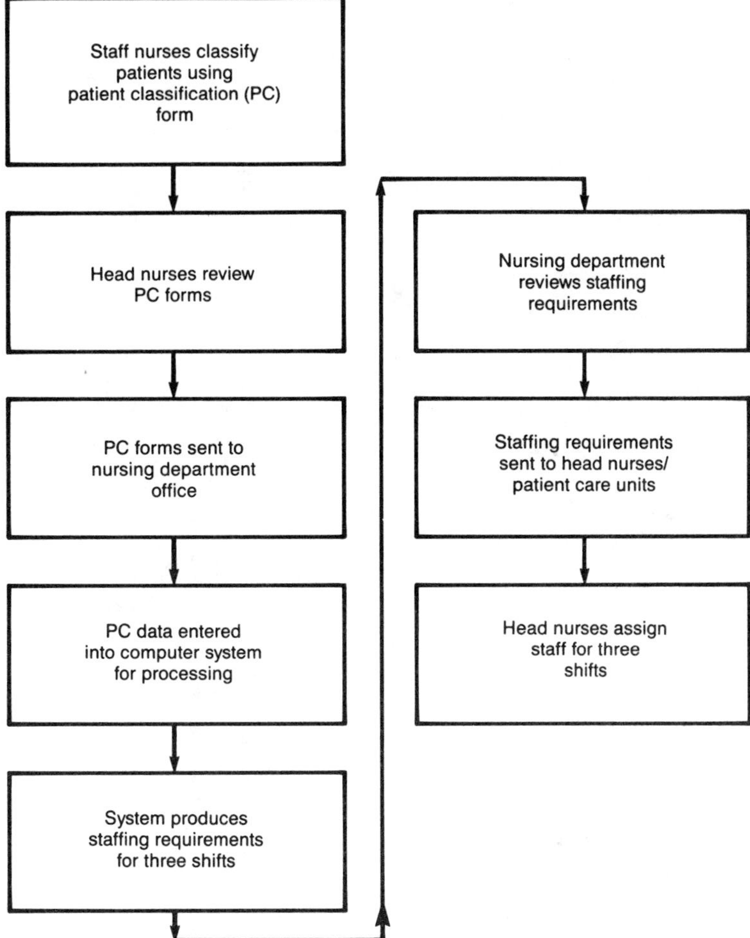

FIG. 8-4. An example of a data flowchart outlining the flow process of a patient classification nurse staffing system.

Model

A model provides an abstraction of a real situation, thus helping to analyze circumstances too complex for actual presentation. Moreover, it is far more economical to develop a model that graphically displays the proposed system than to present the real-life situation (Fig. 8-8).

For example:

1. It can outline the various nurse staffing patterns for the different care units.
2. It can display the flow process of statistical data from origin to termination.

The two major types of models relevant to data analysis are forecasting and simulation. Forecasting helps with decision making. For example, it may be used to predict future staffing needs based on certain assumptions. Simulation, on the other hand, presents an abstraction of reality. Simulations can be used to present how different staffing needs will vary based on different ground rules. Both models can be used to determine the best method of predicting staffing.

Data elements	Reporting requirements					
	Third party payer	**Federal government**	**State government**	**Agency director**	**Agency supervisor**	**Agency staff**
Patients served (demographic/biographic data)	Determine eligibility requirements	Determine federal funds	Determine state funds required	Determine resource requirements	Determine workload; supervise staff	Assess patients
Type of services	Arrange certification eligibility payment		Obtain state approval	Supply guidelines; establish billing rates	Determine patients' quality of care/acuity levels	Plan and perform patient care
Reason for services	Determine reason for service	Appraise cost of care	Determine need for new sites	Establish new sites	Determine if patients' needs are being met	Evaluate quality of care
Costs of services	Determine payment sources	Plan health care costs	Plan state allocation	Determine budget/billing rates	Plan services based on cost	Determine costs of care

FIG. 8-5. Example of a data analysis/grid chart outlining the statistical reporting requirements for a community health nursing agency.

Activity type	Patient activity (Yes or no)							
Bath—assist Position—assist Observe—every 1 to 2 hours	No No No	Yes No No	No Yes No	No No Yes	Yes Yes No	No Yes Yes	Yes No Yes	Yes Yes Yes
Patient classification level*	I	II	II	II	III	III	III	IV

* Patient classification is determined by the number of patient activities requiring nursing assistance ("yes") plus one.

FIG. 8-6. An example of a decision table outlining patient classification levels for three patient activities.

Other types of models are available. Network planning models can highlight resources, time, materials, and major activities relevant to a given process. Both the program evaluation review technique (PERT) and the critical path method (CPM) are network models for planning, scheduling, and controlling a system's activities. The latter generally highlights a time frame and sometimes cost for completing

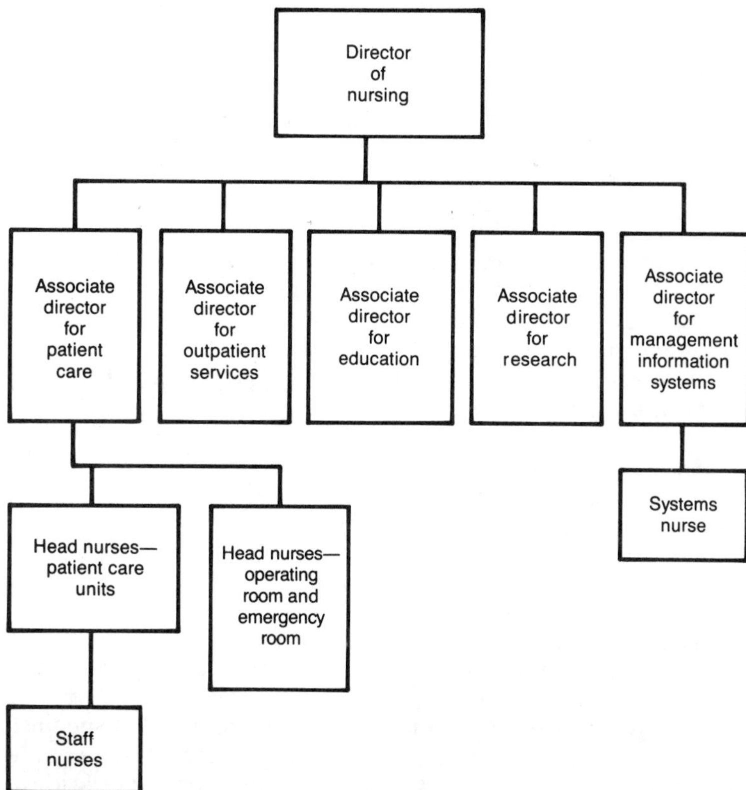

FIG. 8-7. An example of an organizational chart outlining a hospital nursing department.

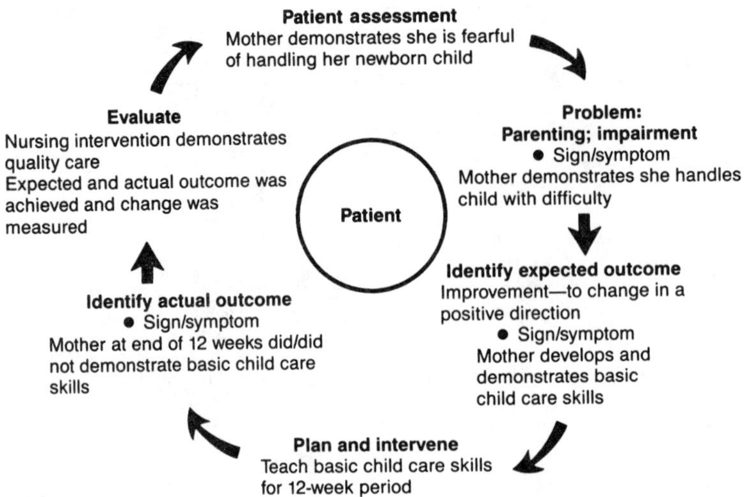
Patient assessment
Mother demonstrates she is fearful of handling her newborn child
Problem:
Parenting; impairment
• Sign/symptom
Mother demonstrates she handles child with difficulty
Identify expected outcome
Improvement—to change in a positive direction
• Sign/symptom
Mother develops and demonstrates basic child care skills
Plan and intervene
Teach basic child care skills for 12-week period
Identify actual outcome
• Sign/symptom
Mother at end of 12 weeks did/did not demonstrate basic child care skills
Evaluate
Nursing intervention demonstrates quality care
Expected and actual outcome was achieved and change was measured
Patient

FIG. 8-8. An example of a community health nursing care process model.

certain critical project activities; PERT predicts the probable time requirements for completing certain critical activities (Fig. 8-9).

Review Data

The final step in the analysis phase is reviewing the data. All pertinent information on the nursing problem is summarized in a report that is sent to the NIS committee. This final review furnishes the basis for recommendations concerning the proposed NIS and raises the question: "How well will the proposed NIS correct or eliminate the existing nursing problem?"

Carefully managed, data review can be beneficial. In a sense, it clarifies what *can* be done and what *should* be done. It can help develop better standards, documentation, and procedures for better management control, and it sets forth the requirements for the new system design.

As a result of this review, a model that graphically displays the major components of the proposed system is produced. In addition to displaying the major components, the model outlines what information is required and what resources (functional requirements) are needed to carry out the stated objectives. In addition, the model shows system controls. Finally, the model presents the actual time and costs needed to make the system work.

DESIGN PHASE

In the design phase the existing nursing problem is solved with a better system. It is possible to design a new system because the nursing problem has been defined, analyzed, and reviewed.

The system design produces the complete detailed specifications of the proposed system. The outline indicates how the system functions and explains how it will look and what it will offer its users. The major steps leading to such a design include the following:

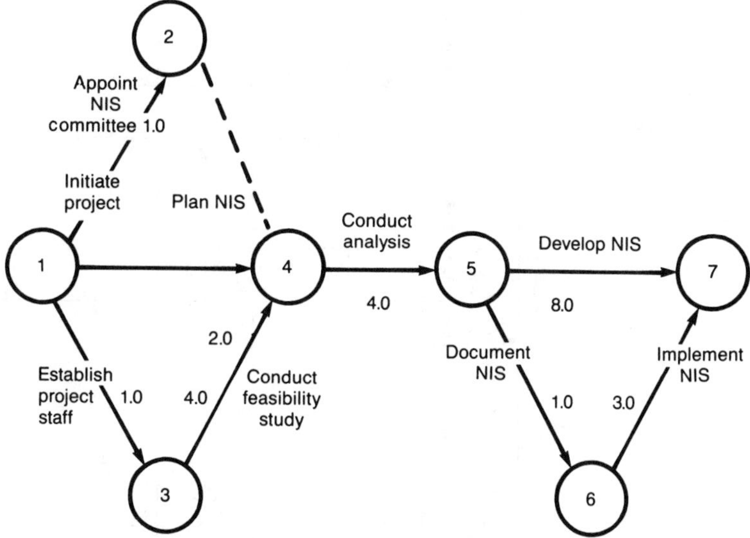

Solid arrow represents an activity that uses a resource. Broken arrow represents an activity that requires no resources. Circles represent events in the sequence from completion of one activity to start of the next. Each activity generally includes a time factor that estimates the time (in weeks) required to complete it. CPM (critical path method) indicates the longest path (time) the project will take from beginning to end.

FIG. 8-9. An example of a PERT chart.

- Design outputs
- Design inputs
- Design files and databases
- Design system controls

Design Outputs

Designing the NIS outputs is the first step in the design phase. They must be completed before or when the inputs are designed because they identify the data required as input. The outputs provide the information the users need and basically justify the system (Austin, 1983).

The design of the outputs is critical to the success of the NIS. Good output design requires an understanding of users' (*i.e.,* nurses') needs. The following factors must be considered:

Content
Format
Medium
Estimated volume
Frequency
Distribution

The content and purpose of each output must be specified in detail, and each

(Text continues on p. 140.)

(138)

Hospital: **Unit:**
Shift: **Type of unit:** **Date of Study:**

Area of activity	Head nurse		RN		LPN		Aide		Student		WC		Total	
	Minutes	%	Minutes	%	Minutes	%	Minutes	%	Minutes	%	Minutes	%	Minutes	%
1. Communication with patient and/or family														
2. Medication, IV (administering)														
3. Nutrition and elimination														
4. Patient hygiene														
5. Patient movement														
6. Positioning, exercising														
7. Rounds: assist M.D. or other with patient														
8. Nursing rounds, checks, symptom observation														
9. Specimen gathering and testing														
10. Treatment and procedures														
11. Vital signs														

11A. Total direct care														
21. Charting														
22. Communication about patient														
23. Preparing medication														
24. Transcribing orders														
24A. Total indirect care														
31. Housekeeping														
32. Clerical														
33. Communication with others														
34. Errands														
35. Meetings														
36. Supplies														
36A. Total unit-related														
40. Total personnel														
Total all activities														

FIG. 8-10. An example of an output form. The table presents average number of minutes and percent distribution of time by unit, level of personnel, and activity for all study days from the work sampling form. (Methods for Studying Nurse Staffing in a Patient Unit. PHS contract no. 1-NU-340481. Washington, DC, U.S. Department of Health, Education and Welfare, 1978)

output should be in a meaningful and easy-to-understand format. For example, the format of a report may increase its effectiveness if numbers appear with clarifiers such as percentages.

Next to be considered is what type of medium will best present the output. An output can be a report produced on paper, microfilm, or microfiche, a display on a cathode ray tube (CRT) terminal, or as a graphic representation from a graphic output device. Sometimes output may be a product from any of the other computer output media (Figs. 8-10 to 8-12).

The estimated volume, frequency, and distribution of the outputs should be based on potential users' expected needs. Who the users are, what outputs they require, and at what time must be spelled out in detail.

Design Inputs

Designing the inputs is another major step in system design. Inputs (data) make up the computer files and databases. What type of inputs to design depends largely on how data will be processed (*e.g.,* on-line, real-time/interactive, or batch processing) and on the required outputs (Figs. 8-13 to 8-15).

Like output design, input design requires the following factors:

Content
Data source
Scope
Format
Medium
Coding scheme
Editing rules
Testing
Estimates of volume
Frequency

(Text continues on p. 144.)

Adams Medical Care Unit							
Patient classification levels	**No. of patients census**	**Registered nurse hours**			**Aide hours**		
		Days	**Evening**	**Nights**	**Days**	**Evening**	**Nights**
I	4	2.4	2.0	1.8	0.4	0.4	0.3
II	5	6.3	2.0	4.3	1.1	0.9	0.6
III	3	6.2	5.2	4.2	1.4	1.4	0.7
IV	4	7.0	6.1	5.1	1.4	1.4	0.9
Total	16	21.9	15.3	15.4	4.3	4.1	2.5
Total staff per 8-hour shift		2.7	1.9	1.9	0.5	0.5	0.3
Staff required		3	2	2	1	1	0

FIG. 8-11. An example of an output report that recommends staff for a hospital medical patient care unit based on a patient classification scheme.

Date prepared 03/08/84
Municipality total

Public Health Nursing Service
Patient visits by program by location
for period 01/01/84 – 01/31/84

Management report
no. HHA-05
Page no. 0034

	Location							
Program	Home	Office	Clinic	Hospital	Nursing home	Other	Not stated	Total
Ante partm	4							4
Post partm	18							18
Premature	3		1					4
Newborn-28	6		1					7
Newbn-1yr	38		13					51
WC 1-4yrs	51	1	32					84
WC 5-1yrs	12							12
OT cld hth	14							14
Adult hth	40		39					79
TB detect	22	9			1	1		33
TB active	10							10
TB inact	17	4			8			29
TB contact	37	3				12		52
Arthritis	83							83
Cancer	215							215
Chest/resp	29	1						30
CVD	532					1	1	534
CVA	600		11				2	613
Cere palsy			8					8
Diab/metab	66							66
Vision	5		5					10
Injury/acc	253							253
Mental ill	26					4		30
Mental ret	2	9						11
Mult scler	106							106
Orthopedic	158	2	45				1	206
OT non-cum	4							4
OT chronic	762	12				7	1	782
Alcoholism	2							2
Total	3115	41	155		9	25	5	3350

FIG. 8-12. An example of an output report produced from a community health information system. (Courtesy New Jersey State Department of Health)

(142)

Hospital: ______________________ Day of study: ______________ Observer: ______________
Type of unit: ______________________ Shift: D E N Date: ___/___/___
Unit: ______________________ Hour: ______________

	Area of activity	1. Head/ charge nurse					2. RN					3. LPN					4. NA/ orderly					5. Student					6. Ward clerk					
		Q1	Q2	Q3	Q4	T	Q1	Q2	Q3	Q4	T	Q1	Q2	Q3	Q4	T	Q1	Q2	Q3	Q4	T	Q1	Q2	Q3	Q4	T	Q1	Q2	Q3	Q4	T	
1	Communication with patient and/or family																															1
2	Medications, IV (administering)																															2
3	Nutrition and elimination																															3
4	Patient hygiene																															4
5	Patient movement																															5
6	Positioning, exercising																															6
7	Rounds or assist M.D. or other with patient																															7
8	Routine checks, patient rounds, symptom observations—nursing personnel only																															8
9	Specimen gathering and testing																															9
10	Treatments and procedures—nursing only																															10
11	Vital signs																															11

21	Charting, checking, chart, or Kardex																															21
22	Communications about specific patient with others																															22
23	Medications, IV—preparing																															23
24	Transcribe orders, charge slips																															24
31	Cleaning—housekeeping tasks																															31
32	Clerical																															32
33	Communication with others—unit related																															33
34	Errands off unit																															34
35	Meetings, inservice, unit reports																															35
36	Supplies, check restock																															36
40	Personnel																															40
	Other																															

FIG. 8-13. An example of an input form (work sampling data collection form). (Methods for Studying Nurse Staffing in a Patient Unit. PHS contract no. 1-NU-340481. Washington, DC, U.S. Department of Health, Education and Welfare, 1978)

Patient classification form

Hospital: __________ Date: __/__/__

Type of unit: __________ Bed no.: __________

Unit: __________

Day of study: __________ Patient ID:

Shift: D E N __________

Patient Classification	I	II	III	IV
Activity, independent	( )			
Bath, partial assist		( )	( )	
Position, partial assist		( )	( )	
Position, complete assist			( )	( )
Diet, partial assist		( )	( )	
Diet, feed			( )	( )
IV added q 6 h or more or TKO		( )	( )	( )
Observe q 1–2 h			( )	( )
Observe, almost constantly				( )
	(✓)	(✓)		
Total			0.5	

Comments:

FIG. 8-14. An example of an input form (patient classification form).

The content of each input (data element) must be specified in detail to meet output requirements. Each data element that is an input should be processed for an output. The source, definitions, rules, and codes of the data elements, must be fully spelled out. Data collected repeatedly, such as patient identification information, should only be collected and entered once.

The scope of the data inputs should always be the smallest definible data elements. For example, the birthdate and not the age of a patient should be entered as an input. Each input must also be in a format that users will readily understand. For example, temperature, pulse, and respirations, when collected, should be entered in that order.

The medium for entering data also requires consideration. Data can be entered directly, using a CRT keyboard at the source, as they occur, or inputs may be selected from CRT video displays. However, data can also be collected on a precoded form and keyed into a CRT at any time. How data are entered is related to hardware and software selection and determines input design and affects output.

If precoded forms are used to collect data for input, then their design must be considered and a simple, easy-to-complete form must be devised. It should have a specific coding scheme and editing rules and checks so that errors may be easily identified.

Finally, all types of input must be tested to ensure that essential data elements needed for outputs are logical and have been collected. They should be revised and

DEPARTMENT OF HEALTH

PATIENT ADMISSION, RE-ADMISSION, SERVICE AND DISCHARGE RECORD

ACTION AND IDENTIFICATION (Always complete this section)

Agency Code: 0 1 3

Patient Identification Number: Ø Ø

Date of Birth: MO · DAY · YR

Date of Action (today's date): MO · DAY · YR

Record Number: 050005

Check type of Record(s)
1 ☐ Admission
2 ☐ Re-admission
3 ☐ Service
4 ☐ Discharge

Name ______
Address ______

County | Municipality | Center/District

Employee Code | Employee Name ______

ADMISSION OR RE-ADMISSION (Complete only to admit or re-admit)

Patient Last Name | First Name | Initial

SEX: 1 ☐ Male 2 ☐ Female RACE: 1 ☐ White 2 ☐ Black 3 ☐ P.R. 4 ☐ Other REFERRAL CODE

SERVICE (Complete only to record visit data)

DIAGNOSIS/PROBLEM (Check one only)		SERVICES PROVIDED (Check one only)	PAYMENT PLANS (Check maximum of three)
01 ☐ Family Planning	25 ☐ Arthritis	01 ☐ Physical Care	01 ☐ Medicare "A"
02 ☐ Ante Partum	26 ☐ Cancer	02 ☐ Health Ed. & Guide.	02 ☐ Medicare "B"
03 ☐ Post Partum	27 ☐ Chest/Respiratory	03 ☐ Supervision of Aide	03 ☐ Med. "B" Outpatient
04 ☐ Well Child Premature	28 ☐ CVD	04 ☐ Detection & Screening	04 ☐ Medicaid
05 ☐ W.C. Newborn to 28 days	29 ☐ CVA	05 ☐ Detec. & Screen Follow-up	05 ☐ Blue Cross
06 ☐ W.C. 28 days to 1 year	30 ☐ Cerebral Palsy	06 ☐ Epidem. Investigation	06 ☐ Am. Cancer Society
07 ☐ W.C. 1 year thru 4	31 ☐ Diabetes/Metab.	07 ☐ Evaluation	07 ☐ Crippled Child. Program
08 ☐ W.C. 5 years thru 19	32 ☐ Drug Abuse	08 ☐ Consultation	08 ☐ Veteran's Admin.
09 ☐ Other Child Health	33 ☐ Dental	09 ☐ Immunization	09 ☐ Multiple Sclerosis
10 ☐ Adult Health Promot.	34 ☐ Hearing	10 ☐ Not Home/Not Found	10 ☐ Migrant Program
11 ☐ ______	35 ☐ Vision	11 ☐ Other	11 ☐ Patient Full Fee
12 ☐ ______	36 ☐ Injury/Accident	12 ☐ ______	12 ☐ Patient Part Fee
13 ☐ ______	37 ☐ Lead Poisoning	13 ☐ ______	13 ☐ Certified Hlth. Serv.
14 ☐ T.B. Detection	38 ☐ Mental Illness	14 ☐ ______	14 ☐ Family Planning
15 ☐ T.B. Case	39 ☐ Mental Retardation	15 ☐ ______	15 ☐ Private Ins. Cos.
16 ☐ T.B. Reactor	40 ☐ Multiple Sclerosis	LOCATION OF SERVICE	16 ☐ Schools
17 ☐ T.B. Suspect	41 ☐ Orthopedic	01 ☐ Home	17 ☐ United Fund
18 ☐ T.B. Contact	42 ☐ Other Non-Commun.	02 ☐ Office	18 ☐ Other Contract/Agree.
19 ☐ Venereal Disease	43 ☐ Other Chronic	03 ☐ Clinic	19 ☐ No Charge Visit
20 ☐ Hepatitis	44 ☐ ______	04 ☐ Hospital	20 ☐ ______
21 ☐ Other Communicable	45 ☐ ______	05 ☐ Nursing Home	21 ☐ ______
22 ☐ ______	46 ☐ ______	06 ☐ Other	22 ☐ ______
23 ☐ ______	47 ☐ ______	ACTIVITY TIME	23 ☐ ______
24 ☐ ______	48 ☐ ______	Service Hrs. / Service Min. / Travel Hrs. / Travel Min.	24 ☐ ______

DISCHARGE (Complete only to discharge)

RELATED DATE of Admission or Re-Admission: Mo · Day · Yr

Method of Discharge	Reason/Condition of Discharge			
01 ☐ With Visit	01 ☐ Expired	02 ☐ Service Not Required	03 ☐ Referral Other Agency	04 ☐ Self Sufficient
02 ☐ Without Visit	05 ☐ Enter Institution	06 ☐ Moved/Can't Locate	07 ☐ ______	08 ☐ ______

H1922

FIG. 8-15. An example of an input form that collects data for a community health information system. (Courtesy New Jersey State Department of Health)

retested, if necessary, to guarantee that they are correct. Also, both estimated volume and frequency must be addressed. The number of input forms that will be completed establishes certain input requirements. Likewise, how often nurses use a CRT determines how many terminals the system will require.

Design Files and Databases

Good file and database design ensure efficient data processing and help ensure prompt responses to users' informational needs.

Several areas of concern must be explored:

Content
Record format
File organization
File access
Storage requirements

The size of each file and database, including content and format of records, must be specified in detail. Both are essential to avoid redundancy in filed data. Also, the data elements themselves must be organized in the records, files, and databases to enhance processing.

File organization is also important, since it determines if files and databases will be developed according to the "top down" or "bottom up" approach. The "top down" approach starts with the end product and proceeds to analyze its data elements. The "bottom up" approach starts with the data elements and builds them up for processing into the end product. For example, a patient classified by one number (level) reflects the "top down" approach. However, a patient classified by combining activities reflects the "bottom up" approach.

Finally, storage requirements are affected by users' needs. Files that must be accessed by on-line or real-time/interactive processing will require random access storage devices. However, files accessed off line for batch processing, for example, can use off-line storage devices. Storage is also affected by file size and volume of and frequency of use.

Another aspect of file storage is their updating and purging. This activity requires special rules for retaining and destroying data. What data and how long they are stored are questions that must be resolved. Data used for analysis such as audit, quality assurance, and research will also affect storage requirements.

Design Controls

Design controls ensure that input data are duly processed, that output information is complete and accurate, and that no data have been lost or stolen. In other words, system controls help minimize and eliminate system errors.

Adequate controls can be established with several different methods. It is possible, for example, to determine the accuracy of the source documents being input by balancing the input totals against the output totals. Controls of data input may be achieved through automatic checking of data limits to ascertain that they are within normal ranges. Audit trails can also check and trace transactions from input to output. The matching of computer-processed outputs with manually processed ones can help ascertain that data are being processed correctly.

Still another type of system control calls for backup files. They allow the NIS to remain intact even if its current data files are damaged or destroyed.

System controls also imply that the files are secure and protected (see Chap. 4). The security of the files must be maintained; every effort must be made to protect the privacy of patients' files. Procedures must be followed to ensure system integrity and security.

DEVELOPMENT PHASE

In system development, the design is completed and the system is ready for preparation. Generally, a system is developed in-house, as described later in this chapter, or through a contract with a computer vendor or system supplier.

Selecting contract services is time-consuming. It requires the following activities:

Request for proposal
Evaluate responses
Negotiate contract

Initially, a request for proposal (RFP), sometimes called a solicitation bid, is circulated among the prospective bidders. A formal statement of the specifications of the system, it outlines the design requirements for the system. The prospective bidders generally respond with a response called a request for contract (RFC) (Young, 1981).

Next, the bidders' RFCs are evaluated by the NIS committee and the financial or contract officers of the agency. An evaluation form is used to score the vendors' capabilities for fulfilling the system requirements (Figs. 8-16 and 8-17). The evaluation scores help to identify the eligible system suppliers. Once a bidder's proposal is selected, the NIS committee should make site visits to view the proposed system in operation and check out other facilities that use the suppliers' systems. Such visits allow the committee members not only to see the system but also to question nurses using the system.

The final step in this process is to select the supplier and negotiate a contract. The successful bidder is contracted to develop a system, provide an already developed system, or adapt another facility's system to meet the NIS committee's specifications. Whichever system is chosen for purchase must be described in the negotiated contract between the supplier and the buyer.

On the other hand, if the NIS committee decides to develop its own system, the project staff must proceed with the development phase of the system, which includes the following:

- Select hardware
- Develop software
- Test system
- Document system

Select Hardware

Selecting the correct hardware for the system depends on its design, application, and software requirements. These conditions dictate whether to select a mainframe, a minicomputer, a microcomputer, or a combination.

Computer hardware is obtained in several different ways. Mainframes and minicomputers may be purchased or leased from a vendor for in-house use. However, if cost is a factor, then timesharing with other facilities should be considered. Since microcomputers are small, they may be the most economical for some applications. Input, output, and processing media, including secondary storage, must also be selected, and all hardware must be installed and able to test the computer programs at the appropriate time.

Information system application	Vendor/supplier costs					
	A	B	C	D	E	F
Admission/patient registration	$	$	$	$	$	$
Master patient census	$	$	$	$	$	$
Order-entry network	$	$	$	$	$	$
Patient care plans/protocols	$	$	$	$	$	$
Patient accounts	$	$	$	$	$	$
Patient classification	$	$	$	$	$	$
Nurse staffing	$	$	$	$	$	$
Nurse scheduling	$	$	$	$	$	$
Nurse personnel payroll	$	$	$	$	$	$
Total	$	$	$	$	$	$

FIG. 8-16. An example of an evaluation worksheet comparing the cost of vendor/supplier information system applications.

Develop Software

Developing software requires careful consideration of the system design. Software must suit the hardware and the specific application, making it necessary to choose the correct programming language and write the computer programs.

System vendor/ supplier name	Vendor/supplier functional requirements	
	Total points (100 maximum)	Rank
A	72	5
B	65	6
C	80	2
D	85	1
E	77	3
F	75	4

FIG. 8-17. An example of an evaluation worksheet listing the rankings of vendor/supplier system functional requirements.

The composition of the computer hardware and the programming needs of the NIS must be examined before an appropriate programming language can be selected. For example, COBOL is used for business applications, FORTRAN for scientific applications, MUMPS for medical applications, and BASIC for various microcomputer applications.

A programmer must write the computer program, which generally follows a logical sequence. First, a narrative description of the system is prepared. Second, flowcharts showing program codes are developed. The actual programs are then written, including the programs needed to process all inputs, design the files and databases, and generate all outputs. The computer programs are then tested and debugged until considered free of errors.

Test System

The system must be tested to ensure that all data are processed correctly and generate the desired outputs. Testing helps verify that the computer programs are written correctly and ensures that, when implemented, the system will run as planned.

The computer programs are tested first to determine if the programming language is used correctly. Each computer program is then tested to determine if it is correct. Next, live data (real facts) are used to test the overall computer programs. After the tests are completed, the programs are debugged or revised and retested until proved reliable and valid. Such a process provides a review of all test inputs, test files, and test outputs to ensure that all data are entered, stored, and processed correctly.

The procedures needed to implement the system are also tested, including all procedures that users will follow to "run" the system.

Document System

Documentation, the preparation of documents to describe the system for all users, must be an ongoing activity that is written as the various system phases and steps are developed. It must give detailed specifications on what information the system requires and what makes the system function, and it must include detailed information on the design and coding structure of inputs, outputs, and flowcharts and file layouts (Fitzgerald and colleagues, 1981).

Several manuals are usually prepared, the major ones being a user's manual, an operator's manual, and a maintenance manual. These manuals provide guides to the system components and outline how the entire system has been "put together."

User's Manual

The user's manual highlights the features of the system and describes what outputs the system can produce.

Operator's Manual

The operator's manual instructs operators on how to run the system. It describes what data are input, how they are processed, and the way in which particular outputs are generated.

Maintenance Manual

The maintenance manual enables programmers to keep the system "alive" by providing the specifications needed to upgrade, revise, and correct the system.

• • •

Proper documentation is directed to system users, operators, and programmers who will maintain it. Manuals must be written in sufficient detail to help all of these people understand how the system was developed, how it operates, and how it can be maintained, updated, and repaired.

IMPLEMENTATION AND EVALUATION PHASE

The final phase of developing a computerized NIS, the implementation and evaluation phase, ensures that once the system is installed it will run smoothly. During this phase the system is evaluated to determine whether it has accomplished the stated objectives.

To implement the system, the project staff and NIS committee must coordinate their efforts and conduct the following steps:

- Train users
- Implement system
- Manage and maintain system
- Evaluate system

Train Users

It is essential to train nurses how to use the system properly. Usually the systems nurse does this training. A NIS will function only as well as its users understand its operation. Nurses must understand the capabilities of the system; training should take place before, during, and, as needed, after system implementation.

Training generally consists of lectures on system use. Training guides or manuals explain the system. Computer-assisted instruction (CAI) in a special training room can be used, and CRTs can provide hands-on experience.

Training should be offered at two levels: one to provide a general overview of the system and one to explain the system in detail. The first presentation is aimed at NIS committee members or others needing an introduction to system objectives and capabilities. The second presentation, directed at nursing personnel using the system, must explain the system in detail and provide in-depth information on how to use it. These users will also require "on-the-job" assistance. The user's manual, described above, should be retained for all users.

Implement System

Implementation means installing the system and then getting it to operate correctly after the computer programs have been tested, debugged, revised, and retested, users trained, procedures established, and the total system rechecked.

The conversion from old method to new depends on available personnel and equipment, system complexity and size, and users' needs. Four approaches are possible:

Parallel
Pilot
Phased
Crash

In the parallel approach, the new system runs parallel with the existing method until users can adjust. In the pilot approach a few users try out the new system to see how it works and help others to use it. In the phased-in approach the system is implemented one unit at a time. In the crash approach the old system is stopped abruptly and the new one is installed (Hopper and Mandell, 1984).

System implementation includes procedures that must be established to operate the system, including time frames and deadlines for receiving and entering data and generating outputs and reports. Accepted procedures for correcting errors and checking data also are important. Decisions on how long data files will be stored and when they will be purged or destroyed must be resolved. In short, all procedural activities must be put in final form.

Manage and Maintain System

System success depends on management and maintenance. Management of a NIS is a continuous process; a separate unit in the agency may be needed to administer the system. Such a unit requires not only a clear line of authority but adequate staffing, an office, and a budget. Special procedures and operating policies must be established to guide the unit. The unit staff, generally consisting of the project staff, oversees the management of the system and ensures that the operating procedures are followed. They must be able to respond properly and assist system users.

The system also needs continuous maintenance and monitoring by the unit staff. Maintenance activities include keeping the hardware in working order, monitoring system security, updating and revising computer programs as needed, and instituting cost-saving measures.

Evaluate System

Evaluating the system is the final step in implementation and evaluation. The system must be assessed to determine whether it meets the stated objectives satisfactorily.

Evaluation generally takes place not less than 6 months and preferably 1 to 2 years after the system has been implemented. The evaluation should be conducted by an outside evaluation team so that it will be objective.

The evaluation process involves a review of the entire system—hardware, software, and actual applications. The entire computer operation, including users, procedures, quality of equipment, and the scope and validity of databases, are examined. Functional performance and technical performance are evaluated thoroughly, and system costs and benefits are assessed (Anser, 1982; McCormick, 1983).

Evaluation of the functional performance of the system requires methods and tools that compare operations before and after system implementation. Such tools should be designed to identify what effects the NIS has on the nursing components of patient care.

For example:

1. Did nurses improve their documentation of patient care by system use?
2. Did their documentation take less time than previously and thus leave more time for providing patient care?
3. Did system use increase their awareness of patients' problems?

If so, the system may be considered an aid to improve the quality of patient care (Kelly and Hanchett, 1977).

Hospital ID# ____________

Codes	Item
☐☐☐	Patient: study no.
☐☐	Age
☐	Sex
☐☐☐	Study day admitted
☐☐☐	Study day discharged
☐	Record reviewed by ____________ 1. Doris Adamson 4. Mary Thom 7. Diane Elson 2. Rosemary Vale 5. Suki Subin 3. Effie Han 6. Sandy Palm
☐	Time to complete ____________ 1. 0–30 minutes 4. 121–240 minutes 2. 31–60 minutes 5. >241 minutes 3. 61–120 minutes
☐☐	No. of active problems on permanent problem list
☐☐	No. of temporary problems on temporary problem list
☐	Nursing database by ____________ 1. Clinical specialist 2. RN 3. LPN 4. NA

Date ____________

FIG. 8-18. An example of a record review form for collecting identifying information. (Courtesy Medical Center Hospital of Vermont)

Various methods and tools can evaluate a system's functional performance:

- Record review
- Time study
- User satisfaction

Record Review

A record review assesses how comprehensive is documentation of nursing care activities. The manual record can be compared with the output of the computerized system to determine if there is a difference. Other variables, such as the completeness of the database, as measured by the nursing audit, progress notes, statement of types of patient problems, nursing orders, listed interventions, interdisciplinary communications, and teaching plans, can be evaluated (Figs. 8-18 and 8-19).

Time Study

A time study can be conducted both before and after system implementation to compare the time staff take to provide specific patient care activities under the old and new systems. Such a study can also include the time nursing staff spend in other activities required in the old versus the new system (Figs. 8-20 and 8-21).

Time studies can also be conducted, once the computer system is in place, to determine system use by nursing staff. For example, a time study can show how often nursing personnel use the CRT (*i.e.,* document patient care). It can highlight whether the system increased or decreased the time spent in providing patient care. Time studies can also help estimate the cost of resources as well as other factors needed to run the system.

User Satisfaction

A questionnaire or a checklist can assess users' reactions and perceptions of the system. A questionnaire can assess the degree to which a user is satisfied with overall system performance; a checklist can identify system strengths and weaknesses. It can measure whether the system improves the nurses' understanding of patient problems and thus affects patient care, and it can assess the usefulness and contributions of the system. Some specific questions to assist in this evaluation and criteria for appraising the system's technical performance are listed below (Figs. 8-22 and 8-23).

Other approaches to evaluating the functional performance of a system exist. Investigating such functions as administrative control, medical/nursing orders, charting and documentation, and retrieval and management reports can assess system benefits. Each of these areas can be appraised through time observations, work sampling, operational audits, and surveys.

Finally, system functional performance can be assessed by examining patient care, nurses' morale, and nursing department operations (Anser, 1982; McCormick, 1983).

Documentation of care must be assessed if patient care benefits are to be evaluated. The following questions must be answered:

- Does the system assist in improving the documentation of patient care?
- Does the system reduce patient care costs?
- Does the system save lives?

To evaluate nurses' morale requires appraising nurses' satisfaction with the system. The following questions must be answered:

(Text continues on p. 157.)

Study ______

Instructions: Circle all of the codes that apply and write in record information where indicated.

Item	Code	Content
		Area no. ______
24	☐	Problem(s) listed: (0 = no, 1 = yes) # 24–26
	☐	Listed: permanent problems list
25	☐	Listed: temporary problems list
26		Listed: nursing assessment/plan
27	☐	Initial goals—if present, please write in 0. None, absent 1. Present (write in) ______ 5. Initial plans for nursing care by M.D. only—skip to # 32
28	☐	Initial plans: 0. None—go to 32 1. Present—if present, complete # 29–31 5. M.D.—nursing
29	☐	Initial plans: A 0. None listed below 1. Complete database, gather further information 2. Monitor, observe for, check (VS, S&A, I&O) 4. Give medications, treatments as ordered

Item	Code	Content
34	☐	Plan for this area included in discharge note/plan
35	☐	Referral to visiting nurse or home health agency 0. None 1. Referral made, information about this area included

B. Written interdisciplinary communication

Item	Code	Content
36	☐	0. None present regarding this area 1. Present—if present, complete III, C as indicated

C. Status of patient problem

Item	Code	Admission severity	Type
73–74	☐☐	0. None or NA	0. None or NA
		1. Mild	1. Threat to life
		2. Moderate	2. Threat to limitation of function
		3. Severe	4. Discomfort, pain
		9. ND	9. Other ______

Item	Code	Content
75	☐	Source of information 1. M.D. 2. RN, LPN 4. Other

30 ☐ Initial plans: B
0. None listed below
1. Encourage or discourage activity and/or rest
2. Emotional support and/or intervention
4. Patient education

31 ☐ Initial plans: C
0. None listed below
1. Specific to unique patient-preference/experience
2. Refer
4. Other (write in) ______

32 ☐ Progress notes, this area
0. Absent
1. Present—if present, complete III, B

33 ☐ Flowsheet parameters recorded (circle any or all)
0. None
1. Patient condition (*i.e.*, VS, S&A, I&O)
2. Medications given
4. Treatment given

76–77 ☐☐

Discharge severity	Type
0. None or NA	0. None or NA
1. Mild	1. Threat to life
2. Moderate	2. Threat to limitation of function
3. Severe	4. Discomfort, pain
	9. Other ______

78 ☐ Source of Information
1. M.D.
2. RN
4. Other

Comments ______

Form #889-004 (2/77)

FIG. 8-19. An example of a record review form for collecting problem identification and follow up. (Courtesy Medical Center Hospital of Vermont)

Time ________________

Starting point (check one)

1. ________ Solarium
2. ________ Nurses' station
3. ________ Office

Name of observer ______________________________

Time: 7 AM–11 AM ________ 3 PM– 7 PM ________
11 AM– 3 PM ________ 7 PM–11 PM ________

Date ______________________________

I	HN, RN, LPN				VI
	II	III	IV	V	
		Activity			Description:
Time	Person observed	Content	Skill	Location	What is being done

FIG. 8-20. An example of a time study form (nursing activity study observer's record). (Courtesy Medical Center Hospital of Vermont)

Unit: Name of Observer: M. Jones Date:
Shift: Morning X Afternoon ______ Night ______ Page of pages

I	II	III	IV	V
Time	Person observed	Area	Level*	Activity Description: What was being done
8:00	HN		A	Assessing patient before assigning staff
	RN_1		N	Preparing of preoperative medications
	RN_2		N	Assisting physician with a spinal tap
	PN_1		N	Giving a cleansing enema
	PN_2		N	Charting nursing notes on new admission
	NA_1		D	Distributing breakfast trays
	NA_2		D	Distributing breakfast trays
	CI		C	Phoning x-ray to inform them of patient's transfer to another unit

* A, administration; n, nursing activity; c, clerical; d, dietary; h, housekeeping; m, messenger; u, unclassified.

FIG. 8-21. An example of a time study form (nursing activity study observer's record data). (Courtesy Medical Center Hospital of Vermont)

- Does the system facilitate nurses' documentation of patient care?
- Does it reduce the time spent in such documentation?
- Is it easy to use?
- Is it readily accessible?
- Are the video display "screens" easy to use?
- Do the video displays capture patient care?
- Does the system enhance the work situation and contribute to work satisfaction?

To evaluate the nursing department's benefits requires determining if the NIS helps improve administrative activities. The following questions must be answered:

- Does the new system enhance the goals of the nursing department?
- Does it improve department efficiency?

I. Biographical data

Nurse's name ______________________

Level of nursing: Personnel (check one)
{ } Head nurse
{ } Staff nurse
{ } LPN
{ } Aide

ID number ______________________

Number of years { } { }

Birthdate { } { } { } { } { } { }
Day Mo Yr

Experience with computer { } no { } yes

Hours of formal instruction on system { } { }

II. Questions

1. Has your amount of work { } increased { } stayed the same { } decreased?
2. Has your amount of time with patients { } increased { } stayed the same { } decreased?
3. Has your understanding of the patient as a person { } become better { } stayed the same { } become worse?
4. Has your care { } become more effective { } stayed the same { } become less effective?
5. Has your understanding of patient care { } become better { } stayed the same { } become worse?
6. Is entering patient data { } easy { } confusing { } hard?
7. Does the system help you document patient care? { } helps { } hinders { } makes no difference
8. Do you get help if you have a problem using the system? { } yes { } no { } sometimes
9. Do you rely on a CRT terminal or Kardex? { } CRT { } Kardex
10. Will you miss the system if it is removed? { } yes { } no { } makes no difference

FIG. 8-22. An example of a user satisfaction questionnaire that evaluates the nurse's satisfaction with a computerized information system.

- Does it help reduce the range of administrative activities?
- Does it reduce clerical work?

Other criteria are necessary to evaluate technical performance, including reliability, maintainability, use, responsiveness, accessibility, availability, and ability to meet changing needs. These areas must be examined from several different points; the technical performance of the software as well as the hardware must be appraised. The following questions must be answered:

- Is the system accurate and reliable?
- Is it easy to maintain at a reasonable cost?
- Is it flexible?
- Is the information consistent?
- Is the information timely?
- Is it responsive to users' needs?
- Do users find its inputs and outputs satisfactory?
- Are input devices accessible and generally available to users?

Finally, a cost-benefit analysis is necessary to determine if the system is "worth" its price. The cost-benefit analysis relates system cost and benefits to system design, level of use, timeframe, and equipment costs. Each of these costs must be assessed in relation to benefits derived. Such an evaluation can help determine the future of the system.

• • •

An evaluation study attempts to describe and assess, in detail, system perform-

Nurse's name ______________________ Patient care unit ______________________
ID number ______________________

Performance area	Satisfaction level				
	Very satisfied	Satisfied	Neutral	Dissatisfied	Very dissatisfied
1. Accuracy	1	2	3	4	5
2. Timeliness	1	2	3	4	5
3. Reliability	1	2	3	4	5
4. Training	1	2	3	4	5
(a) Routine task	1	2	3	4	5
(b) Full system potential	1	2	3	4	5
5. Manuals	1	2	3	4	5
6. Ease of use	1	2	3	4	5
(a) Data entry	1	2	3	4	5
(b) Information retrieval	1	2	3	4	5
7. Legibility	1	2	3	4	5
8. Completeness	1	2	3	4	5
(a) Data entry	1	2	3	4	5
(b) Information retrieval	1	2	3	4	5
9. Flexibility	1	2	3	4	5
(a) Data entry	1	2	3	4	5
(b) Information retrieval	1	2	3	4	5
10. Conciseness	1	2	3	4	5
(a) Data entry	1	2	3	4	5
(b) Information retrieval	1	2	3	4	5
11. Overall performance	1	2	3	4	5

FIG. 8-23. Example of a user satisfaction checklist that evaluates nurses' satisfaction with information system performance.

ance. It summarizes the system, thus identifying any weaknesses. A sound evaluation study can sometimes lead to a revised, and better, system.

SUMMARY

This chapter describes the process of developing a NIS for nursing departments in health care facilities. It outlines and describes the five phases of the process—planning, analysis, design, development, and implementation and evaluation.

The planning phase determines the problem scope and outlines the entire project to show if the system is feasible and worth developing for the allocated resources. The analysis phase assesses the problem being studied. The design phase produces detailed specifications of the proposed system. Development involves the actual preparation of the system. Implementation and evaluation involve system installation and assessment, including training users and managing, maintaining, and evaluating the system.

STUDY QUESTIONS

1. Name the three ways a NIS is designed.
2. Name the five phases in developing a NIS.
3. Name the two groups of people needed to begin developing a NIS.
4. What is another name for the planning phase?
5. List one critical step in the planning phase.

6. What factors are considered in allocating resources?
7. Name the three major steps in the system analysis phase.
8. What are the four major sources of data for the fact-finding activity?
9. What five tools of the trade are used to analyze data?
10. What four major steps are carried out in the design phase?
11. Name three factors that must be considered in designing outputs.
12. Name the scope of data inputs.
13. What two approaches are used in developing data files?
14. What are the three major steps in selecting a system contract service?
15. Name the four steps in the system development phase.
16. What dictates the type of hardware selected?
17. Who writes the computer software programs?
18. What type of data are used to test the system?
19. Name the three manuals that should be prepared to document the system.
20. Name the four steps in the implementation and evaluation phase.
21. What are the four possible approaches to implement the system?
22. Name two levels of training.
23. Who manages and maintains the system?
24. Name three tools that can be used to evaluate a system.
25. Name four approaches that can be used to evaluate a system.

REFERENCES

Anser Analytic Services: Evaluation of the Medical Information System at the NIH Clinical Center, vol 1, Summary of the Findings and Recommendations (contract no. NO1-CL-0-2117). Arlington, VA, Anser Analytic Services, 1982

Austin CJ: Information systems for hospital administration, 2nd ed. Ann Arbor, MI, Health Administration Press, 1983

Capron HL, Williams BK: Computers and Data Processing, 2nd ed. Menlo Park, CA, Benjamin/Cummings, 1984

Fitzgerald J, Fitzgerald AF, Stallings WD: Fundamentals of Systems Analysis, 2nd ed. New York, John Wiley & Sons, 1981

Hopper GM, Mandell SL: Understanding Computers. New York, West Publishing, 1984

Kelly PA, Hanchett ES: The impact of the computerized problem-oriented record on the nursing components of patient care (contract no. No1-NU-44126). Hyattsville, MD, Division of Nursing, Department of Health and Human Services, 1977

McCormick KA: Monitoring and evaluating implemented HIS. In Dayhoff RE (ed): Proceedings: The Seventh Annual Symposium on Computer Applications in Medical Care, pp 507–510. New York, IEEE Computer Society Press, 1983

Shelly GB, Cashman TJ: Introduction to Computers and Data Processing. Brea, CA, Anaheim Publishing, 1980

Young EM (ed): Automated Hospital Information, vol 1, Guide to Planning, Selecting, Acquiring. Implementing and Managing an AHIS. Los Angeles, Center Publications, 1981

BIBLIOGRAPHY

Ball MJ: Fifteen hospital information systems available. In Ball M (ed): How to Select a Computerized Hospital Information System, pp 10–27. Basel, Switzerland, S. Karger, 1973

Ball MJ, Hannah KJ: Using Computers in Nursing. Reston, VA, Reston Publishing, 1984

Battele Columbus Laboratories: Evaluation of a Medical Information System in a Community Hospital (NCHSR Research Digest Series) (DHEW pub. no. (HRA) 76-3144). Rockville, MD, National Center for Health Services Research, 1976

Birks EG: Requirements analysis and specification. In Cotterman WW, Couger JD, Enger NL, Harold F (eds): Statistical Analysis and Design: A Foundation for the 1980's, pp 58–74. Amsterdam, North-Holland, 1982

Blum BI (ed): Information Systems for Patient Care. New York, Springer-Verlag, 1984

Bocchino WA: Management Information System Tools and Techniques. Englewood Cliffs, NJ, Prentice-Hall, 1972

Bronzino JD: Computer Applications in Medical Care. Reading, MA, Addison-Wesley, 1982

Carlsen RD, Lewis JA: The Systems Analysis Workbook, 2nd ed. Englewood Cliffs, NJ, Prentice-Hall, 1979

Coffey RM: How a Medical Information System Affects Hospital Costs: The El Camino Experience (NCHSR Research Summary Series) (DHEW pub. no. 80-3265). Hyattsville, MD, National Center for Health Services Research, 1980

Cotterman WW, Couger JD, Enger NL, Harold F (eds): Systems Analysis and Design: A Foundation for the 1980's. Amsterdam, North-Holland, 1982

Covvey HD, McAlister NH: Computers in the Practice of Medicine, volume II, Issues in Medical Computing. Reading, MA, Addison-Wesley, 1980

Drazen E, Metzger J: Method for Evaluating Costs of Automated Hospital Information Systems. (NCHSR Research Summary Series) (PHS pub. no. 81-3283). Hyattsville, MD, National Center for Health Services Research, 1981

Drazen EL: Planning for purchase and implementation of an automated hospital information system: A nursing perspective. J Nurs Admin 8(9):9–12, 1983

Enger NL: Classical and structured systems life cycle phases and documentation. In Cotterman WW, Couger JD, Enger NL, Harold F (eds): Statistical Analysis and Design: A Foundation for the 1980's. Amsterdam, North-Holland, 1982

Farlee C: System evaluation: Problems and challenges. In National Institutes of Health: Computer Technology and Nursing: First National Conference (NIH Pub. No. 83-2142), pp 34–41. Bethesda MD, National Institutes of Health, 1983

Farlee C, Goldstein B: A role for nurses in implementing computerized hospital information systems. Nurs Forum 10(4):339–357, 1971

Fokkens O, et al (eds): Medinfo 83 Seminars. Amsterdam, North-Holland, 1983

Giovannetti P, Thiessen M: Patient Classification for Nurse Staffing: Criteria for Selection and Implementation. Edmonton, Alberta, Canada, Association of Registered Nurses, 1983

Hartman W, Matthes H, Proeme A: Management Information Systems Handbook. New York, McGraw-Hill, 1968

Houser ML, Rieder KA, Barlow J, Tedeschi R: How to prepare for your hospital information system. Computers in Health Care, pp 24–39, August 1984

Houser ML, Rieder KA, Barlow J, Tedeschi R: How to prepare for your hospital information system. Part II. Computers in Health Care, pp 42–50, September 1984

Landers TJ, Myers JG: Essentials of School Management. New York, McGraw-Hill, 1977

Lucas HC: The Analysis, Design and Implementation of Information Systems, 2nd ed. New York, McGraw-Hill, 1981

McLeod R, Forkner I: Computerized Business Information Systems: An Introduction to Data Processing. New York, John Wiley, 1982

Methods for Studying Nurse Staffing in a Patient Unit. PHS contract no. 1-NU-340481. Washington, DC, U.S. Department of Health, Education and Welfare, 1978

Murdick RG, Ross JE: Information Systems for Management. Englewood Cliffs, NJ, Prentice-Hall, 1971

National Center for Health Services Research: Demonstration and Evaluation of a Total Hospital Information System (NCHSR Research Summary Series) HRA pub. no. 77-3188). Rockville, MD, National Center for Health Services Research, 1977

National Institutes of Health: Computer Technology and Nursing: First National Conference. (NIH pub. no. 83-2142). Bethesda, MD, National Institutes of Health, 1983

National League for Nursing: Selected Management Information Systems for Public Health/Community Health Agencies. New York, National League for Nursing, 1978

National League for Nursing: State of the Art in Management Information Systems for Public Health/Community Health Agencies: Report of the Conference. New York, National League for Nursing, 1976

National League for Nursing: Management Information Systems for Public Health/Community Health Agencies: Report of the Conference. New York, National League for Nursing, 1974

National League for Nursing: Management Information Systems for Public Health/Community Health Agencies: Workshop papers. New York, National League for Nursing, 1975

Optner SL: Systems Analysis for Business Management, 3rd ed. Englewood Cliffs, NJ, Prentice-Hall, 1975

Pocklington DB, Guttman L: Nursing Reference for Computer Literature. Philadelphia, JB Lippincott, 1984

Pritchard K: Computers. II. Systems analysis. Nurs Times 78(6):414–415, 1982

Saba VK: Basic considerations in management information systems for public health/community health agencies. In National League for Nursing: Management Information Systems for Public Health/Community Health Agencies: Report of the Conference, pp 3–13. New York, National League for Nursing, 1974

Saba VK: A guide to understanding management information systems. In National League for Nursing: State of the Art in Management Information Systems for Public Health/Community Health Agencies: Report of the Conference, pp 93–105. New York, National League for Nursing, 1976

Sanders DH: Computers and Management. New York, McGraw-Hill, 1970

Sanders DH: Computers in Business: An Introduction, 4th ed. New York, McGraw-Hill, 1979

Scholes M, Bryant Y, Barber B (eds): The Impact of Computers on Nursing. Amsterdam, North-Holland, 1983

Somers JB: Information systems — the process of development. J Nurs Admin 9(1):53–59, 1979

Stern RA, Stern N: An Introduction to Computers and Information Processing. New York, John Wiley & Sons, 1982

Tomaski EA, Lazarus H: People-oriented Computer Systems: The Computer in Crisis. New York, Van Nostrand Reinhold, 1975

Van Bemmel JH, Ball MJ, Wigertz O (eds): Medinfo 83 (2 vols). Amsterdam, North-Holland, 1983

Viers VM: Introducing nurses to computer world. Nurs Manage 14(7):24–25, 1983

Werley HH, Grier MR (eds): Nursing Information Systems. New York, Springer, 1981

Zielstorff RD (ed): Computers in Nursing. Wakefield, MA, Nursing Resources, 1980

Zielstorff RD: The planning and evaluation of automated systems: A nurse's point of view. J Nurs Admin 5(6):14–16, 1976

PART D

Nursing Applications

9 Administrative Applications

Objectives

- Describe the basic categories of administrative applications.
- Describe the essential components of nursing services information.
- Describe the essential components of nursing unit management information.
- Understand how nurse administrators and unit managers use computers.
- Understand the administrative applications available on mainframes, minicomputers, and microcomputers.
- Identify the issues confronting administrative applications.

In order to determine the available administrative computer applications, nurses can read at least a 10-year history of computer use in nursing and hospital administration journals. Today's nurse can also visit the exhibits at any major nursing or computer conference worldwide or check his or her financial or personnel file.

This chapter presents an overview of administrative applications on mainframes, minicomputers, and microcomputers. (Integrated systems for prospective payment mechanisms are discussed in Chap. 10.)

Specifically, this chapter will discuss the use of computerized information for the following:

- Nursing services
- Nursing unit management

In this chapter the director of a nursing service is considered an administrator who requires nursing services information to run a nursing service. A head nurse or supervisor of several nursing units or stations is considered a manager who requires nursing unit management information. Classification schemes described in other textbooks do not apply to computer applications for nursing. The tools that administrators in community health and educational settings use are described in other chapters.

The purpose of both systems is to help nurse administrators and unit managers maximize their effectiveness with timely and appropriate information. Whether administrators use mainframes, minicomputers, microcomputers, or a combination of computer resources, the key to successful administrative applications is the management and analysis of volumes of information to maintain quality control and cost control (O'Connor, 1983). The key to successful nursing unit management is the management of efficient records and operations.

NURSING ADMINISTRATIVE INFORMATION: AN OVERVIEW

Approximately 150 functions for administrative information are available on a mainframe hospital information system (HIS) (Table 9-1). Technical applications for processing data and special-purpose functions for housekeeping services, safety and environmental records, medical records, and other departments are available. This information is presented first so that nurses can appreciate the communication networks available through the HIS as well as the variety of applications within HIS capabilities. Some of the applications can also be special-purpose ones available on a minicomputer or microcomputer (Young and colleagues, 1981).

ESSENTIAL COMPONENTS OF NURSING SERVICES INFORMATION

Table 9-2 lists the essential components of a nursing services administration information system. In this chapter, nursing services administration information will be explained as it concerns the following:

- Quality assurance
- Personnel files
- Communication networks within the nursing department
- Budgeting and payrolls
- Census
- Summary reports
- Forecasting and planning

Quality Assurance

The nursing profession evaluates the impact of the health care it delivers to the consumer. Since health care encompasses many variables, some assessment method for evaluating structure, actions, outcomes, process, and competency levels of the nurse provider and patient consumer is considered a monitor of quality assurance. Nursing has dedicated over a decade to the issue of quality assurance; many frameworks and methods have been described. Some, especially the Medicus Systems Corporation and Rush-Presbyterian – St. Luke's joint project, focus on the computer for compilation and scoring of worksheets. Potentially all quality assurance worksheet forms can be set up to be computerized.

In 1979 the American Nurses' Association (ANA) sponsored an invitational conference to identify what was needed to assess quality of nursing care. Participants agreed that establishing nursing information systems (NISs) would facilitate a quality assurance system and that establishing a taxonomy or classification nomenclature system such as nursing diagnosis would facilitate the standardized database for nursing. Continued studies on the impact of nursing on patient outcome as well as the structural variables affecting the nursing process and outcomes of nursing care were also deemed necessary.

Figure 9-1 shows a computer system model for processing all information related to quality control in an institution, an application that is practical. However, computer systems have not solved the issue of identifying valid and reliable criteria on which to input information. These systems have the potential for producing the same information and problems existing in the manual mechanism of monitoring quality assurance.

Even the Joint Commission on Accreditation of Hospitals (JCAH) uses computers to monitor adherence to its quality assurance standards. The only difference is that the Commission uses computers to analyze the volumes of data that standard compliance reviews accumulate annually. The JCAH designed a system to summarize the findings on each of 1156 hospitals surveyed in 1982 in an automated data file. Preliminary data revealed that most hospitals comply with most of the stan-

TABLE 9-1 *Major Functions of a HIS*

1. Budget preparation
2. Equipment inventory
3. Hospital manuals and procedures
4. Laundry management
5. Message exchange
6. Salary budget control
7. Salary budget preparation
8. Space use planning and control
9. Supplies budget preparation
10. System security and access control
11. Telephone lists for patients/religion classification
12. Word processing
13. Forecasting
14. Policies manual preparation
15. Admission/discharge/transfer notifications
16. Addressograph plate generation
17. Bed assignment and status
18. Label generation
19. Newborn registration with mother's data
20. Patient database
21. Patient identification number assignment
22. Patient name retrieval
23. Patient number retrieval
24. Registration reports and form printing
25. Transfer status to other facilities
26. Death certificates
27. CCU arrhythmia monitoring
28. ECG historical base line on patients
29. ECG interpretation
30. Echocardiography
31. Impedance cardiography
32. Dietary master list
33. Menu forecasting
34. Patient menus
35. Special diet list
36. Emergency registration/database linkage
37. Emergency room statistics
38. Emergency service roster
39. Patient allergy/drug incompatibility
40. Risk patient tracking
41. Trauma registry
42. Organ bank registry
43. Antibiotic use reporting
44. Detection of bacterial infection
45. Infection notices
46. Laboratory culture screening
47. Communication routing
48. Retrieve/update housekeeping bed record
49. Room assignments for housekeeping
50. Intensive care patient monitoring
51. Diagnostic equipment monitoring
52. Patient medication profile retrieve/update
53. Patient plan of care/length of stay
54. Update problem/diagnosis for patient
55. Analog signal acquisition
56. Blood bank management
57. Blood donor file management
58. Clinical laboratory result quality control
59. Clinical laboratory specimen control
60. Results reporting
61. Laboratory historical report by patients
62. Laboratory current cumulative report by patients
63. Pathology/cytology comparative result file retrieval
64. Pathology/cytology reporting
65. Schedule clinical laboratory tests
66. Specimen pickup schedule
67. Worksheets
68. Drug distribution monitoring
69. Nonsterile supplies inventory
70. Office supplies inventory
71. Pharmacy central inventory
72. Purchasing storeroom inventory
73. Sterile supplies inventory/expiration dates/renewal
74. Narcotic distribution monitoring
75. Equipment maintenance schedules
76. Discharge summary information
77. Medical record number assignment
78. Literature searches
79. Patient diagnosis
80. Nurse index
81. Nursing meeting schedules
82. Telephone lists for nurses
83. Assign/update nursing care plans
84. Charge compilation
85. Inpatient census/reports
86. Nurses' notes
87. Vital sign update chart
88. Nursing staffing management
89. Nursing scheduling automatic reminders
90. Nursing staff rosters
91. Order format tailoring
92. Order transmission
93. Pharmacy floor stock inventory
94. Medication administration charts
95. Transfer notes
96. Discharge care plan
97. Summary reports

TABLE 9-1 *(Continued)*

98. Special procedures
99. Patient classification
100. Quality assurance worksheets
101. Personnel profiles
102. Training and education reports
103. Incident reports
104. Workload management
105. Message exchange
106. Medication instructions
107. Education resources
108. Specimen collection
109. Perinatal risk assessment
110. Radiation therapy management
111. Tumor registry
112. Ambulatory therapy scheduling
113. Outpatient assignment and status
114. Outpatient scheduling
115. Outpatient visit recording
116. Hours and wage reports
117. Personnel history
118. Personnel surveys
119. Wage and salary studies
120. Cumulative inpatient drug profile
121. Drug/drug incompatibility
122. Drug/laboratory incompatibility
123. Formulary (pharmacy)
124. Generic name cross-reference (pharmacy)
125. Narcotic use
126. Patient medication profile
127. Pharmacy manufacturing reports
128. Prescription issues/labels
129. Solutions
130. Computerized poison identification
131. Poison control and antidotes
132. Automated MMPI interpretation
133. X-ray jacket control
134. Pulmonary function studies
135. Discharge care plan communicated to community
136. Anesthesiology monitoring
137. Operating room/recovery room log
138. Operating room/recovery room management
139. Surgery scheduling
140. Utilization review
141. Volunteer services
142. Labor cost distribution
143. Labor time collection
144. Accounts payable
145. Budget/actual expense reports
146. Capital equipment accounting
147. Capital equipment depreciation
148. Cost allocation by cost centers
149. Coordination of insurance benefits
150. Medicare billing

(After Young E, Brian E, Hardy D: Automated Hospital Information Systems Workbook, vol 1, Guide to Planning, Selecting, Acquiring, Implementing and Managing an AHIS. Los Angeles, Center Publications, 1981)

dards; however, the computer system could identify those standards that were not in compliance with JCAH standards. From the first review of 1982 surveys, it appears that half the hospitals received some type of contingency accreditation. Further, 61.6% of all contingencies attached to accreditation awards were the result of quality assurance deficiencies. Nursing services received only 7% of the total contingencies. Further examination of the quality assurance standards suggest that ten areas of these standards had a disproportionate number of contingency

TABLE 9-2 *Essential Components of a Nursing Services Administration Information System*

Quality assurance
Personnel files
Communications networks within the nursing department
Budgeting and payroll
Census
Summary reports
Forecasting from unit management and planning the use of services

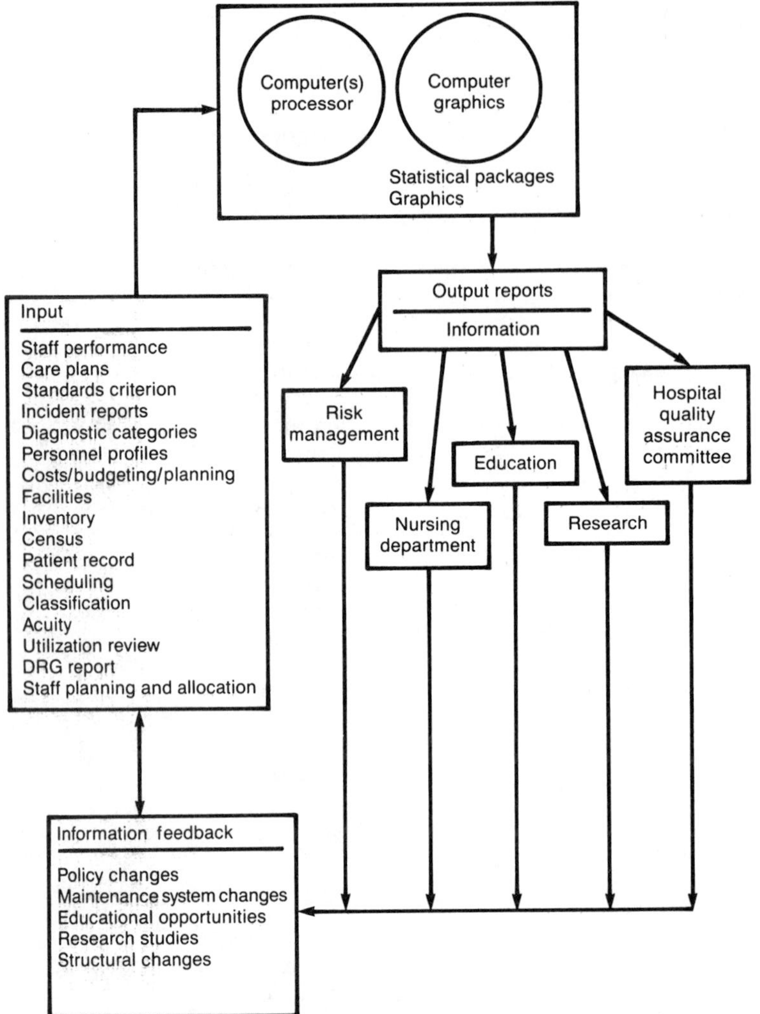

FIG. 9-1. Model for computerization of quality assurance.

recommendations (Table 9-3). Many of these deficiencies could most likely be corrected if updated summaries and reviews through computerized documentation and quality assurance programs were provided (Downey and colleagues, 1983).

Personnel Files

Because computers can help organize information, they are being used to assist administrators in personnel planning and productivity analysis. Such systems maintain and update employees' permanent files, provide ready access to personnel profiles, and allow for employee quality control. These systems generate reminders for various personnel actions, such as license renewal or position change, and they produce reports on labor costs, employee analysis, and forecast requirements (Austin, 1979).

TABLE 9-3 *JCAH Quality Assurance Deficiencies that Computerization Could Correct: Contingency Findings by Quality Assurance Standard*

STANDARDS	NO. OF CONTINGENCIES	QA CONTINGENCIES (%) (N = 7511)
Review and document antibiotic use	781	10.4
Review/evaluate/document rehabilitation services	466	6.2
Surgical case review and follow-up action	386	5.1
Document care and treatment	286	3.8
Review drug utilization and effectiveness	237	3.2
Review/evaluate/document special care	240	3.2
Review/evaluate/document anesthesia care	213	2.8
Review/evaluate/document emergency care	192	2.6
Review/evaluate/document respiratory care	187	2.5
Delineate clinical privileges	180	2.4
Total	3,168	42.2

(After Downey J, Walczak R, Hohri W: Evaluating hospital compliance with JCAH quality assurance standards. In Dayhoff R [ed]: Proceedings of the Seventh Annual Symposium on Computer Applications in Medical Care, pp 94–97. Silver Spring, MD, IEEE Computer Society Press, 1983)

An example of the data that can be collected to provide regular reports on nursing personnel is given in Table 9-4. A personnel file of this type can be used to do the following:

- Generate mailing lists
- Plan educational programs
- Determine promotion eligibility, census of personnel, personnel budget expenditures, locations of personnel with particular preparation, validation of license, and certification updates in order to prepare for hospital standard reviews
- Prepare profile analysis of nursing personnel

Communication Networks

Computer systems that facilitate communication are designed to transmit information from point to point in a computer terminal network. In these systems, messages are not usually processed but are transmitted from one terminal (entry) to another (receiver).

The computer is a communication integrator, which is also an integral part of any HIS or management information system (MIS). The computerized communication system affects work patterns, thus reducing nurses' clerical functions. These systems also enhance interhospital communication networks. (Schmitz and colleagues, 1976).

Communication systems have many functions. Figure 9-2 is a common communication network that has the following features (Filosa, 1978):

- Send notices of patient appointments, admissions notification, discharges, and hospital census
- Provide summary information on laboratory tests, medications, and other orders
- Locate patients

TABLE 9-4 *Personnel File Information Elements Available on Computers*

Name				
Social security number				
Sex				
Marital status				
Identification number				
Date of birth				
Number of children				
Date entered on duty				
Status of employment (full or part time)				
Telephone number				
Mailing address				
Person to contact in case of emergency				
RN/LN license number			State	Expiration date
Educational preparation			Degrees	
Current enrollment				
Practice experience			Certifications	
Professional membership				
Vacation credits				
Sick leave				
Awards				
Assignment	Location			
	Status			
	Salary code			
Publications				
Consultations				
Languages spoken				
Specific specialty preference			Shift preferences	
Unique skills				
Last performance evaluation (date)			Completed by	
			Rating	
Continuing education update		Courses attended	Date	No. of continuing education credits
Cardiopulmonary resuscitation certification		Date		
Safety certification		Date		
Benefits received				

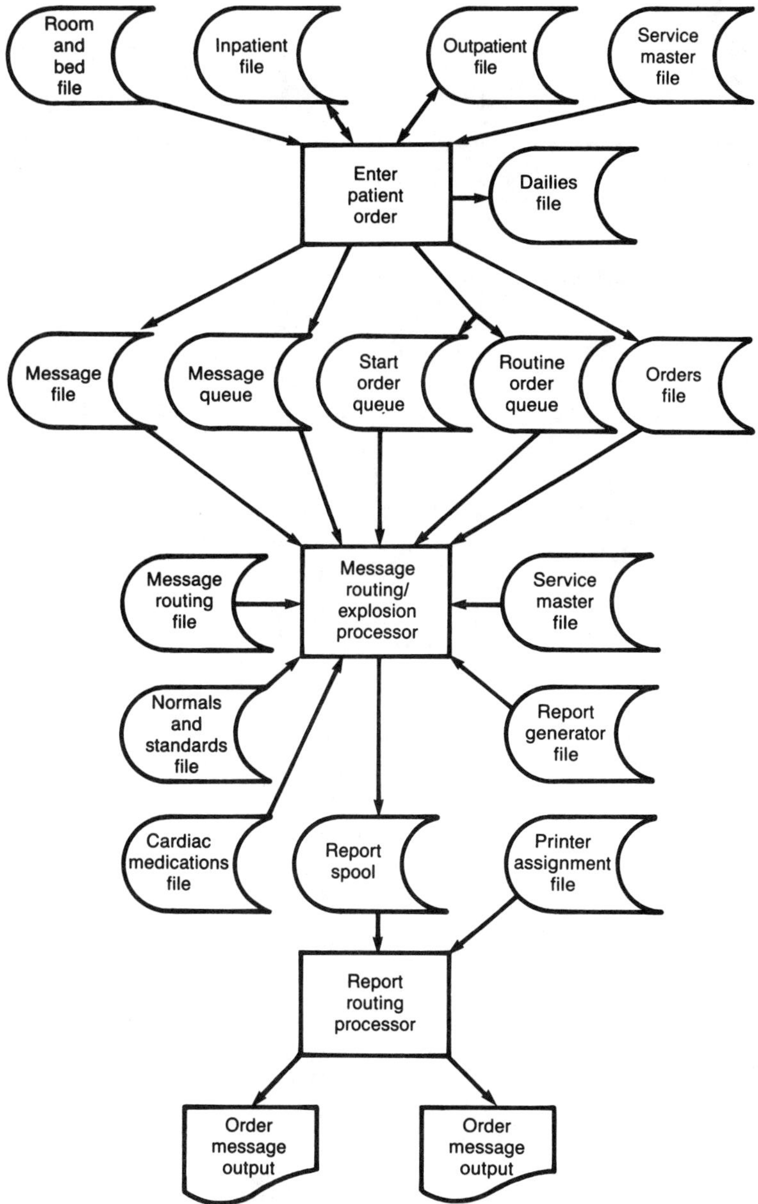

FIG. 9-2. Communication network—NCR/MEDNET.

- Identify current charges and patient needs
- Provide accurate billing

Computer communication systems eliminate searches through procedure manuals and expedite delivery of requisitions for services and procedures, thus reducing clerical tasks. Such systems reduce the need for couriers to hand carry reports and forms from the nursing department to the nursing unit, thus serving as efficient message centers.

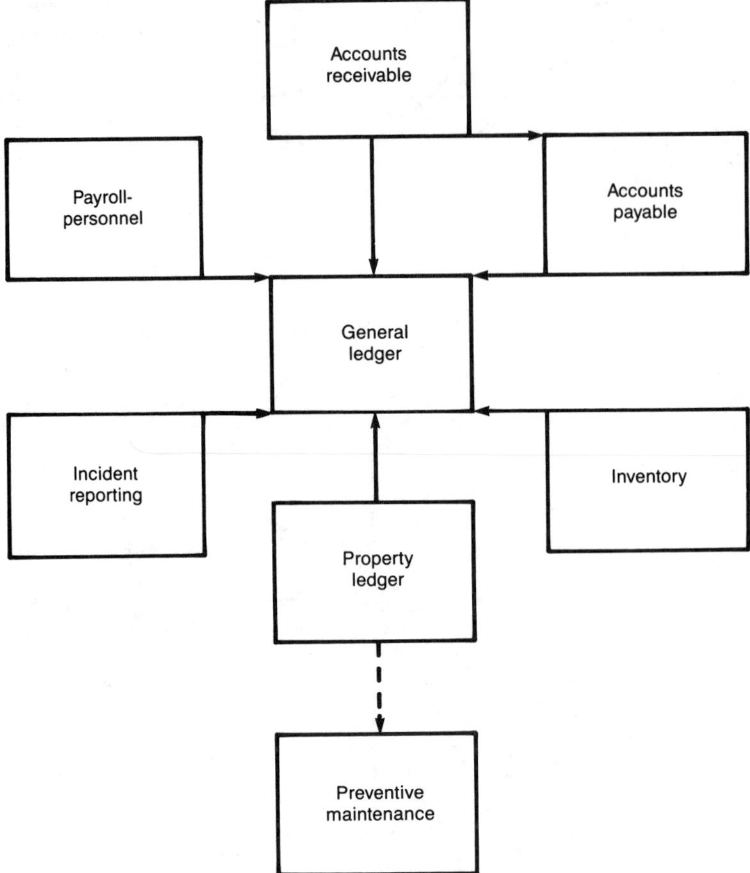

FIG. 9-3. Financial system used by Hospital Data Center of Virginia.

Budgeting and Payrolls

One of the greatest advantages of computers for nursing administrators is in budgeting, a complex process that includes many layers of cost analysis. Figure 9-3 summarizes financial systems and their relationships. Included below is a list of financial functions with which computer systems provide administrators:

- Accounts receivable
- Patient accounts
- Accounts payable
- General ledger
- Property ledger accounting
- Debts
- Collections
- Preventive maintenance costs
- Medicare/Medicaid patient profiles
- Cost allocation
- Cash control

Intimately related to the central budget are the information reports that come from payroll systems, inventory records, incident reports, length of stay reports, the nursing record, and quality care information.

Because nursing is a central activity in the delivery of health care, the ability to assess the adequacy of care and determine the cost of care is vital. Criteria frequently used in evaluating nursing productivity include nursing hours per patient day, staff : patient ratios, and cost per patient day. Formulas for analyzing the cost of nursing care have also been developed. Since these reports require information, computers have been used to process summary reports. An example of a computer-generated budget report is shown in Figure 9-4.

Census

Census systems provide users with the capability of entering information on patient admission, discharge, birth, death, or transfers. A master file of available beds and bassinets is maintained with the appropriate legal information on occupancy.

A census is a registration of inpatients and the beds they occupy. Many hospitals may do the census on a microcomputer. The census application is also the heart of most HISs; newer HISs usually allow on-line control of the census function. The census report is needed at all times in order to account for patients in the hospital, emergency room, or outpatient clinics. All hospital areas must have continuous access to the computer system in order to determine a patient's status related to preadmission, admission, transfer, discharge, or death. The census systems usually provide immediate information on bed availability. Standard reports, usually a part of a census system, can provide statistical analysis and forecasting information, such as which units have reduced census between April and July or September and December. Figure 9-5 shows a computer-generated census report.

Summary Reports

Several types of summary reports might facilitate JCAH accreditation standards. If a hospital has a HIS or a microcomputer, some summary reports might include the following:

- Incident reports
- Poison control
- Allergy and drug reactions
- Error reports
- Infection control reports
- Unit reports including census, patient status, activities, procedures, and patients at risk
- Utilization review information

Most of these reports originate on the nursing unit and are filled out by staff nurses, head nurses, unit managers, or supervisors. (These reports are described in detail later in the chapter.) If a nursing service administrator neglects to include the summary reports into nursing service information, however, this important information may not receive adequate attention.

Forecasting and Planning

Systems have been designed to predict staff needs, determine trends in patients' nursing care needs, and forecast departmental budgetary compliance. They can

DRG	Description	Number of cases	Hospital rank	State rank	Average length of stay	Total nursing cost (all patients)	Average nursing cost per case	Percent nursing cost of DRG	Nursing rank all DRGs
039	Lens OR, procedure	310	6	9	3.34H 3.25S	37,897.H 34,747.S	122.25H 112.09S	24.69	15
243	Back disorder, medical	208	21	21	8.50H 8.75S	76,641.H 65,099.S	368.47H 312.98S	49.09	1
122	Circulatory disorder with AMI, D/C alive s̄ cardiovascular complications, medical	144	10	14	13.13H 14.67S	199,943.H 208,224.S	1,388.00H 1,446.00S	78.63	2
441	Hand procedure for injury	6	252	219	1.50H 2.20S	729.H 966.S	122.00H 161.00S	33.47	253
177	Ulcer s̄ complications, age 70+, medical	14	157	145	9.43H 8.85S	10,640.H 7,686.S	760.00H 549.00S	64.80	104
202	Cirrhosis and/or alcoholic hepatitis	23	97	114	12.13H 11.00S	20,360.H 16,652.S	885.00H 605.00S	63.98	50

FIG. 9-4. An example of a budget report. (Toth RM: DRGs: Imperative strategies for nursing service administration. Nurs Health Care 4:197–203, 1984)

BED CONTROL

DOCTOR#: 1
DOCTOR-NAME: ANDERSON, ROBERT T

PAGE 1 16:57 1/01/90
DOCTOR CENSUS FOR ANDERSON, ROBERT T

ROOM-BED NUMBER	PATIENT NUMBER	PATIENT NAME	NRS STA	DAYS IN HOSP	SERV	AGE	SEX/ MAR	
3100-02	00000310	JONES, MARY	3CEN	1	SUR	37	F-S	ADMITTING
3101-02	00000311	ALLEN, SAMUAL B.	3CEN	1	MED	67	M-M	ADMITTING
3102-02	00000312	SMITH, JOHN	3CEN	1	MED	55	M-M	ADMITTING
3103-02	00000313	LOWER, JAMES T	3CEN	1	MED	55	M-M	ADMITTING
3104-02	00000314	MARKUS, GEORGE	3CEN	1	MED	33	M-M	ADMITTING
3027-02	00000303	MCFARLAN, JOHN S.	3SWG	4	SUR	49	M-M	ADMITTING
3002-02	00000306	SIMMS, JIMMY	3WST	5	MED	30	M-M	ATTENDING
2143-02	00000210	HICKS, FRED W	ICU	1	MED	44	M-W	ADMITTING
2149-02	00000212	PLOTZ, LENARD C	ICU	4	MED	56	M-D	ADMITTING

FIG. 9-5. An example of a census report (NCR/MEDNET).

also make predictions for effective management of float personnel and interunit exchange of personnel. Nurse administrators can use computers to define monitoring tasks and to establish what variables nurses must monitor in patients requiring different care patterns.

Many types of systems are available for planning schedules, hospital expansions, financial planning, and preventive maintenance planning. A patient scheduling system can provide the accuracy, flexibility, and timeliness of on-line outpatient and inpatient scheduling. Visit codes can be described, and length of visits and number of assigned professional staff can be controlled. Summary reports can facilitate planning for clinic and inpatient staffing.

Hospital expansion can be facilitated with data from other systems, including census, staffing, scheduling, and financial information. Similarly, hospital programs that need to be eliminated can be identified.

Financial planning can be done with many available systems. To date, planning has come from retrospective information; the need for prospective financial information is becoming greater (see Chap. 10).

Preventive maintenance planning includes systems that aid in organizing and scheduling maintenance. This type of planning system provides for more reliable equipment and reduces equipment failure. Even the computer needs a maintenance planning system to determine "downtime" as well as scheduled maintenance.

Planning systems can be used to determine what information is needed for what services. When special services are audited periodically, particular services may prove to be unnecessary or may need to be used by different groups of patients. For example, an audit of the use of lodgings for parents of pediatric patients with terminal cancer may show that the services are underused. However, spouses and relatives of geriatric patients need such a facility. Computerized planning systems can provide the information to accommodate these decisions.

Systems can help administrators determine where space is available both within the hospital and on hospital grounds. These advantageous systems can also categorize space by type, location, amount, and other criteria.

ESSENTIAL COMPONENTS OF NURSING UNIT MANAGEMENT INFORMATION

Several computers facilitate nursing unit management. The essential components of a nursing unit management systems, listed in Table 9-5, include the following:

- Patient classification
- Staffing based on patient acuity and nurses' experience and level of competence
- Staff schedules and rosters
- Inventories
- Patient billing
- Incident and other reports
- Shift summary reports

A staff nurse can generate the above reports when computerized management applications are available. Summary sheets may be used by the head nurse or unit supervisors. Many of these reports are sent to the nurse administrator for nursing service administration applications, but it is usually the staff nurse who interacts with these systems.

Patient Classification Systems

An approach to management efficiency is the patient classification system—a scheme by which patients' needs for nursing services can be assessed (Jelinek and colleagues, 1974, 1973). Such systems are ultimately used to plan nurse staffing assignments.

A stated aim of patient classification and its methodology is to match staffing to patient requirements, resulting in the following:

TABLE 9-5 *Essential Components of a Nursing Unit Management System*

1. Data entry for patient classification
2. Nursing staff assignment based on acuity, nursing experience, and level of competency
3. Staff schedules and rosters
4. Inventory lists
5. Patient bills for supplies used
6. Incident reports, risk management, infection control reports, error reports, and other reports
7. Shift reports of patients' conditions and census, new admissions, transfers, and deaths

Optimum use of personnel
Improved quality of care
Savings from prevention of overstaffing

Further, the patient classifications systems represent a methodological approach unique to the nursing profession. By devising a method to assess patients' needs for nursing care and thus the hours of care required during each 24-hour period and the category of personnel needed, a quantitative statement of patients' requirements for nursing care can be established.

In 1978, the government published reports on methods for studying nurse staffing in a patient unit. The project recommended that staffing needs be established by comparing the service level with care estimates based on patient classification and the head nurse's perception of adequate care. The model also provides a conceptual framework for evaluating personnel skills or different staffing patterns (Department of Health and Human Services, 1978).

Many issues exist in choosing a patient classification system, including whether a staffing formula based on patient classification is reliable and which method of patient classification is best for a particular institution. Major classification schemes have been computerized and are described below.

Staffing Based on Acuity Systems

Acuity values reflect the relative proportion of nursing time required for each classified patient type. Classification translated into workload equals acuity. Staffing is based on patient types.

Software programs, interchangeable with programmable calculators, can compute staffing needs, allocate staff, and construct management reports. In addition, they provide a unit profile that adjusts for illness/and absences, overtime, and other factors.

Staffing and Scheduling Systems

Computer applications for staffing and scheduling have existed for over 10 years; an early description of computer applications in nursing staffing rosters was written in 1970. Computers were used to allow objective and consistent staffing assignments (Dominick, 1970).

Staff rosters and scheduling systems are available on mainframes, minicomputers, and microcomputers. A staff roster can operate on the hospital's patient acuity system or census. Daily staffing worksheets, productivity sheets, and assignments based on qualifications, unit preference, and skills are available through these systems. These systems boast of saving 90% time in staffing and scheduling and six full-time equivalents (FTEs) or more in improved staff control. The scheduler systems create customized schedules and automatically incorporate workload, work preferences, special requisitions, and assignments to continuing education programs.

Inventory

An inventory is a record of pharmacy items and other supplies that have been received and disbursed; it shows what is in stock on nursing units. These applications provide necessary information for auditing and analyzing use of unit stock and maintenance files on unit stock activity. Nursing unit managers are often accountable for records related to storeroom and sterile supplies. Computerized supply inventories provide them with the capability to account for stock items, track expired lots, and bill patients for supplies used.

A special type of inventory is the narcotic usage inventory, which produces special records that describe the receipt, disbursement, and amount of narcotic drugs on a nursing unit. These systems can produce summary reports acceptable for legal documentation of narcotic usage.

Patient Billing

Computers allow nurse managers to enter charges for services rendered or supplies used. More important, computers can record charges and transmit them to patient files to be compiled and entered into the patient's overall bill. Two stages of compilers are common:

Recording the charges for compilation and changing incorrect charges to correct ones

Transmitting unit charges to a central automated record that is compiled with the patient's total hospital bill

Incident and Other Reports

Many nursing unit management reports can be recorded and transmitted to the appropriate hospital department. Such reports cover the following:

- Incident reports
- Poison control
- Allergy and drug reactions
- Error reports
- Infection control reports
- Unit reports, including census, patient status, activities, procedures, and identification of patients at risk
- Utilization review

Incident Reports

Incident reports identify patient, visitor, or personnel accidents. A documented record of incidents can be summarized regularly, and corrective policies, education, or research programs can be initiated. When incident reports are printed in the risk management office as they occur, corrective actions may be taken. For example, if a nurse receives a needle puncture, the nurse administrator might inform that nurse to seek corrective treatment immediately, assign a float nurse to cover, and inform the head nurse of an emergency sick leave request.

When incident report summaries indicate statistically significant occurrences of particular problems (*e.g.*, patient falls and medication errors), the incidents may precipitate policy changes, new documentation requirements, or in-service education programs. If patients fall frequently on geriatric services, nurse administrators may want to determine if the nursing assessment for documentation on the computer includes a category for "mobility" or "potential for trauma." If nursing personnel are not using that category either before or after an incident, in-service education, policy changes, and documentation requirements might be considered.

Poison Control

Poison control systems have also been described. Capable of maintaining files that report accidental poisoning, these systems also include information on the most common toxic substances and appropriate antidotes or therapy.

Allergy and Drug Reactions

Allergy and drug reaction lists include not only patients with particular allergies but those patients receiving medications known to have incompatibilities. These lists can be produced regularly, and logs can be compiled indicating the number of patients who have come in contact with drugs they are allergic to or medications that are incompatible with other drugs.

Error Reports

Error reports can be summarized and transmitted to a nurse administrator for review on a regular basis. They may include medication or documentation errors. Some error systems track errors on line, alerting nurse administrators to take quick corrective action.

Infection Control

Infection control reports recognize patterns of bacterial or viral spread throughout a hospital or nursing unit. These systems integrate infection reports, incident reports, and laboratory culture screening reports over time to describe patterns of probable infection in the hospital. Often the area of contamination can be recognized from these reports. Computerized monitoring provides summary information.

Unit Reports

Unit reports, including census, patient status, and activities and procedures have been computerized in several hospitals nationwide. They provide timely information that the unit nurse can enter into the terminal and send to the nursing administrator's office. In some hospitals, these shift reports are no longer collected, photocopied, and distributed by the evening and night supervisors; these supervisory personnel have been relieved of this secretarial function. Since the secretarial function is no longer required, many hospitals have eliminated this level of supervision.

Patients at risk can be automatically and rapidly identified through computer systems. In addition, when special procedures or medications are ordered for patients at risk, alert notices are printed at the nursing station. If emergencies occur, emergency procedures can be printed on the unit.

Utilization Review

A utilization review summary report includes information on the concurrent review of all patients. Information is available to certify each patient for admission and length of stay. Patient demographic information is combined with the diagnosis and operative information to determine length of stay data. Daily summary reports may then be produced for the utilization review. The summary report lists all patients who must be reviewed for admission certification and extension of length of stay.

Shift Summary Reports

Computers allow a summary of patient classifications, acuity/staffing information, and nursing personnel information to be produced. These cumulative shift reports integrate the information of other nursing unit reports and are then transmitted to the nursing administrator to integrate with nursing service information. These records are also integrated with the hospital or nursing department budgeting system.

SELECTED ADMINISTRATIVE APPLICATIONS

Table 9-6 lists suppliers and administrative applications; it was produced from suppliers' descriptions of their systems. Many systems have multiple applications. The applications included below are available on both mainframes and minicomputers:

- Technicon Medical Information System
- IBM Patient Care System
- Medicus Nursing Productivity and Quality System
- Hospital Data Center of Virginia
- National Cash Register
- Shared Medical Systems
- GRASP (Grace Reynolds Applications and Study of PETO)
- Systems Architecture
- HELP (Health Evaluation Through Logical Processing)
- Medical Information Technology

Mainframes and Minicomputers

Technicon

Computerized quality assurance programs in hospitals can be done from standard nursing care plans on a MATRIX MIS from Technicon (Mayers, 1974).

An instrument for measuring care given to patients in an extended care facility that relied on the ANA standards was developed and used in conjunction with the

TABLE 9-6 *Mainframe and Minicomputer Administrative Applications*

SUPPLIER	NURSING SERVICES INFORMATION							NURSING UNIT MANAGEMENT INFORMATION						
	QUALITY ASSURANCE	PERSONNEL FILES	COMMUNICATION NETWORKS	BUDGETING AND PAYROLLS	CENSUS	SUMMARY REPORTS	FORECASTING AND PLANNING	CLASSIFICATIONS	STAFFING/ACUITY	SCHEDULES	INVENTORY LISTS	PATIENT BILLINGS	INCIDENT AND OTHER REPORTS	SHIFT SUMMARY REPORTS
Technicon	X		X		X					X		X		
IBM	X		X		X			X	X	X	X	X		
HELP				X			X				X	X		
Systems Architecture					X				X	X	X	X		
NCR					X				X	X	X	X		
Shared Medical Systems	X	X	X	X	X				X		X		X	
Medical Information Technology	X			X	X			X	X			X		
Medicus	X	X	X	X	X	X	X	X	X	X		X		
HDCV	X	X	X	X	X	X	X				X	X	X	
GRASP	X			X		X		X	X					

Technicon MIS. Through the computerized framework, categories, problems, and desired outcomes were identified (Table 9-7). This design integrated nursing documentation of patient care with a quality assurance audit framework so that the nursing actions most often leading to desired patient outcomes could be identified. A separate section allowed nursing actions related to physicians' orders to be separated from nursing actions related to patient outcomes (Howe, 1980).

IBM

The IBM HIS, known as the Patient Care System (PCS), allows quality assurance data to be managed as it is at Duke University Hospital (Peter, 1977). A computer-assisted quality assurance model was developed and implemented manually for this system. A five-tier framework of patient conditions evaluates quality by means of the nursing record, observations, interviews, and physical assessment. The modular design incorporates patient care standards, structure, process, outcome criteria, and interrelated standard criteria coding (Edmunds, 1983).

At the Brigham and Women's Hospital in Boston, where an IBM PCS is used for nursing care plans and laboratory orders and results, the system was expanded to include patient classification, staffing, and patient acuity levels. The nurse could select indicators for patients in the following categories:

1. Admission, transfer, discharge
2. Physical activity—partial or complete
3. Elimination needs—partial or complete
4. Nutritional needs (level 1 or 2)
5. Fluid and electrolytes (level 1, 2, or 3)
6. Special medications
7. Learning needs (level 1 or 2)
8. Emotional needs—complex or crisis
9. Respiratory needs (level 1 or 2)
10. Dressings—simple or complex
11. Isolation—simple or complex
12. Special integumentary needs
13. Assessment and observation (level 1 or 2)

These selected categories were weighted, resulting in a staffing sample based on patient acuity (Fig. 9-6) (Gebhardt, 1982).

Medicus

Medicus offers a manageable computerized system based on validity and reliability studies for monitoring quality assurance. Its nursing productivity and quality system (NPAQ) is automated on a microcomputer or minicomputer or can be added to a mainframe.

NPAQ automates eight components of nursing services and nursing unit management applications (Medicus Systems, 1983):

Patient classification
Staff planning and allocation
Quality monitoring
Personnel data management
Scheduling

TABLE 9-7 *A Framework for Integrating Patient Care Documentation With Quality Assurance*

CATEGORIES	PROBLEMS	GOALS
A. Ingestion of food, fluid, and nutrients	Feeding self (The ability to manage utensils, containers, and get food to mouth without spilling. The ability to ingest fluids and solids to a prescribed volume)	Feeds self independently Understands and follows prescribed diet Adequate fluid intake Adequate nutrition
	Swallowing (Ability to chew, clear mouth, propel food and fluids into esophagus without choking or drooling)	Swallows without choking
	Task performance (Ability to perform specified tasks safely, consistently, and within prescribed regime) Preparing meals Gastrostomy care Tube feedings	Performs specified tasks safely
B. Elimination of body waste	Urination (Ability to void sufficient volume of urine in appropriate container)	Continent of urine Adequate urinary output
	Defecation (Ability to eliminate stool in sufficient volume and desired consistency in appropriate container)	Continent of stool Establishes regular elimination pattern
	Task performance Colostomy care Ileostomy care Ileoloop care Nephrostomy care Catheter irrigation Self-catheterization	Performs specified tasks safely
C. Relating with environment	Skin integrity (Ability to maintain skin as flexible, soft, and intact with ordinary care)	Maintains skin integrity
	Vision (Ability to see and identify objects and people within the immediate environment)	Maintains safe environment
	Orientation (Ability to know where you are, who you are, in what time reference, and for what reasons)	Promotes orientation
	Perception of sensation (Ability to recognize and distinguish variations in temperature and feelings of pressure)	Maintains safe environment Promotes comfort Maintains correct position
	Sleeping (Ability to naturally suspend consciousness for 7 to 10 uninterrupted hours)	Promotes sleep
	Task performance Hygiene Grooming Dressing Skin care Wound care Smoking on own Wearing eyeglasses Denture care	Performs specified tasks safely

TABLE 9-7 *(Continued)*

D. Purposeful movement and exercise	Ambulation (Ability to walk on level surfaces, curbs, and stairs)	Walks independently
	Position (Ability to turn over, stand, and sit)	Maintains correct position
	Transfers (Ability to move from one surface to another)	Transfers independently
	Task performance Using assistive devices Using total hip precautions	Performs specified task safely
E. Relating with others	Communication (Ability to send and receive verbal, graphic, nonverbal messages)	Communicates needs and wants Understands directions and explanations
	Hearing (Ability to hear conversation, speak at normal volume)	Maintains safe environment Promotes orientation Understands directions and explanations
	Task performance Caring for own hearing aid Using communication device	Performs specified task safely
F. Relating with self	Self-image (Ability to describe and use body and/or affected body parts realistically)	Promotes realistic self-image
	Self-concept (Ability to describe assets and limitations realistically and to participate in prescribed regime)	Promotes self-concept

DRG reporting
Budget planning
Executive reporting

An integrated system based on a patient classification instrument and a quality monitoring methodology, NPAQ is automated on a powerful microcomputer. Quality is intertwined with nurse productivity and workload distribution, patient classification, and acuity levels. The tool uses critical indicators of patient care needs to define patient types and to yield valid measures of nursing workload.

The tool is a preprinted "mark sense" form collected manually and transmitted to a "mark sense reader" to be classified and scored (Fig. 9-7). The results are two indexes (Fishman, 1983):

Workload based on a weighted census generated by multiplying the number of patients in a category by weighting factor; for example, a type II patient would be classified as requiring 3 to 5 nursing hours.

Average acuity, which is a value representing the overall mix of patients on a unit. It is determined by dividing the workload index by the census for a given unit.

The Medicus tool evaluates quality of care issues; it was developed by Medicus

```
07/16/81                                                                14.09.30
                         **NURSING STATION MASTER**
                     NURSING STATION:  14A                 STATUS: A
                         DESCRIPTION:  FLOOR 14 POD A
                                UNIT:  1 LOCATION: P
                          FIRST ROOM:  14AV01 AUTHORISED BEDS: 018
                     FTE STAFF REQUIRED PER CASE LEVEL
        CARE LEVEL: 1    STAFF REQUIRED/SHIFT — 1: 00.200   2: 00.090   3: 00.080
        CARE LEVEL: 2    STAFF REQUIRED/SHIFT — 1: 00.300   2: 00.250   3: 00.160
        CARE LEVEL: 3    STAFF REQUIRED/SHIFT — 1: 00.450   2: 00.400   3: 00.325
        CARE LEVEL: 4    STAFF REQUIRED/SHIFT — 1: 00.750   2: 00.750   3: 00.650
        CARE LEVEL: 5    STAFF REQUIRED/SHIFT — 1: 01.000   2: 01.000   3: 01.000

PFK = 1 UPDATE     2-ADD     3-NEXT     4-PREVIOUS     9-DELETE     LAST-UPD =
```

FIG. 9-6. An example of staffing/acuity on an IBM computer. (Gebhardt A: Computers and staff allocation made easy. Nurs Times 78:1471–1474, 1982)

and several client hospitals under government funding. It is based on 367 criteria within a framework of 6 major objectives and 32 subobjectives. The major objectives measure the following components:

Nursing process, including care planning, physical care delivery, nonphysical care delivery, and nursing care evaluation
Management
Support services.

Subobjectives serve as monitors of performance (Fishman, 1983).

The tool can be used on medical, surgical, obstetric, pediatric, labor and delivery, psychiatric, nursery, emergency room, and recovery units. The quality score is achieved when approximately 10% of monthly admissions on any unit are monitored. Observations are made by trained nurses, who must achieve an 85% interrater reliability (*i.e.,* two persons making observations have the same results 85% of the time). Output is quality index scores for each objective and subobjective analyzed (Fishman, 1983).

Data on quality monitoring are intertwined with patient classification/and acuity and staffing component data. Staffing levels are calculated based on the workload index and the average acuity. Three parameters facilitate staffing projections:

1. A productivity target, that is, hours per unit of workload, provides a common comparative basis for all nursing units, since workload index is weighted census.
2. The skill mix parameter weights patient care needs with the level of personnel (a philosophical weight that can vary with each hospital).
3. The shift mix parameter summarizes the amount of care delivered on each shift for each patient category.

Staffing parameters are correlated with quality monitoring to determine if staffing is appropriate. Output is a daily report comparing recommended, scheduled, and actual staffing by unit, service, shift, and skill level. The advantages of a three-tiered system such as this are listed in Table 9-8 (Fishman, 1983).

PAGE ____ OF ____ UNIT ____________

SIGNATURE ____________

MONTH	JAN FEB MAR APR MAY JUN JUL AUG SEP OCT NOV DEC
DAY	0 1 2 3
	0 1 2 3 4 5 6 7 8 9
UNIT CODE	0 1 2 3 4 5 6 7 8 9
	0 1 2 3 4 5 6 7 8 9

PATIENT CLASSIFICATION

* FOR ITEMS BRACKETED ONLY ONE MAY BE MARKED *

Item	No.	Marks	No.
{ Admission or Transfer In	1	1 2 3 4 5 6 7 8 9 10 11 12	1
{ Discharge or Transfer Out	2	1 2 3 4 5 6 7 8 9 10 11 12	2
{ Less Than 2 Years	3	1 2 3 4 5 6 7 8 9 10 11 12	3
{ Age 2 - 6 Years	4	1 2 3 4 5 6 7 8 9 10 11 12	4
{ Unconscious	5	1 2 3 4 5 6 7 8 9 10 11 12	5
{ Confused/Disoriented	6	1 2 3 4 5 6 7 8 9 10 11 12	6
Sensory Deficits	7	1 2 3 4 5 6 7 8 9 10 11 12	7
{ Partial Immobility	8	1 2 3 4 5 6 7 8 9 10 11 12	8
{ Complete Immobility	9	1 2 3 4 5 6 7 8 9 10 11 12	9
{ UP AD LIB	10	1 2 3 4 5 6 7 8 9 10 11 12	10
{ Up with Assistance	11	1 2 3 4 5 6 7 8 9 10 11 12	11
{ Bed Rest	12	1 2 3 4 5 6 7 8 9 10 11 12	12
{ Bath with Assistance	13	1 2 3 4 5 6 7 8 9 10 11 12	13
{ Bath Total	14	1 2 3 4 5 6 7 8 9 10 11 12	14
{ Assistance c̄ Oral/Tube Feed	15	1 2 3 4 5 6 7 8 9 10 11 12	15
{ Total Oral/Tube Feed	16	1 2 3 4 5 6 7 8 9 10 11 12	16
{ I & O Simple	17	1 2 3 4 5 6 7 8 9 10 11 12	17
{ I & O Complex	18	1 2 3 4 5 6 7 8 9 10 11 12	18
IV's & Site Care	19	1 2 3 4 5 6 7 8 9 10 11 12	19
{ Specimen Collection — Simple	20	1 2 3 4 5 6 7 8 9 10 11 12	20
{ Specimen Collection — Complex	21	1 2 3 4 5 6 7 8 9 10 11 12	21
Isolation	22	1 2 3 4 5 6 7 8 9 10 11 12	22
Incontinent/Diaphoretic	23	1 2 3 4 5 6 7 8 9 10 11 12	23
{ Simple Wound and/or Skin Care	24	1 2 3 4 5 6 7 8 9 10 11 12	24
{ Extensive Wound and/or Skin Care	25	1 2 3 4 5 6 7 8 9 10 11 12	25
Tube Care	26	1 2 3 4 5 6 7 8 9 10 11 12	26
Oxygen Therapy	27	1 2 3 4 5 6 7 8 9 10 11 12	27
Respirator	28	1 2 3 4 5 6 7 8 9 10 11 12	28
Trach/ET Tube	29	1 2 3 4 5 6 7 8 9 10 11 12	29
{ Vital Signs, Q1½ - 2 Hr.	30	1 2 3 4 5 6 7 8 9 10 11 12	30
{ Vital Signs, Q1 Hr. or More Often	31	1 2 3 4 5 6 7 8 9 10 11 12	31
{ Monitoring — Non-Invasive	32	1 2 3 4 5 6 7 8 9 10 11 12	32
{ Invasive Monitoring	33	1 2 3 4 5 6 7 8 9 10 11 12	33
Prep. for Test/Procedure	34	1 2 3 4 5 6 7 8 9 10 11 12	34
Special Teaching Needs	35	1 2 3 4 5 6 7 8 9 10 11 12	35
Special Emotional Needs	36	1 2 3 4 5 6 7 8 9 10 11 12	36
Multi-System Instability	37	1 2 3 4 5 6 7 8 9 10 11 12	37
	38	1 2 3 4 5 6 7 8 9 10 11 12	38

BED NO.	PATIENT NAME	PATIENT I.D. NO.
1		
2		
3		
4		
5		
6		
7		
8		
9		
10		
11		
12		

SCHEDULED STAFF
DATE: ____/____

DAY	1	
	2	
	3	
	4	
	5	
EVE	1	
	2	
	3	
	4	
	5	
NITE	1	
	2	
	3	
	4	
	5	

ACTUAL STAFF
DATE: ____/____

DAY	1	
	2	
	3	
	4	
	5	
EVE	1	
	2	
	3	
	4	
	5	
NITE	1	
	2	
	3	
	4	
	5	

← FEED THIS DIRECTION →

SCAN-TRON® FORM NO. 2546-MMS

830520-999

FIG. 9-7. An example of a MEDICUS "mark sense tool." (Copyright ©, Medicus Systems Corporation, 1985)

The NPAQ has a patient classification module that enables administrators to define quantity, mix, and distribution of workload based on critical indicators of patient needs. This module has had extensive testing for validity over the past 10 years (Medicus Systems, 1983).

The Medicus model of nursing scheduling and the mathematical formulas governing it have also been described. The advantage of this system is that it balances staffing needs with schedule preferences. By 1975 this system had been evaluated in a 40-nursing-unit hospital with 900 nursing personnel (Miller and colleagues, 1975).

A centralized staffing system for nursing units has been described. Such a system can do the following (Ballantyne, 1979):

Facilitate precise staffing based on preceding staffing
Ensure adequate staff
Provide for employee satisfaction
Relieve professional nurses of staffing functions
Provide personnel efficiency and effectiveness
Provide reports for budgetary analysis

The system also offers a personnel scheduling component designed to save time in developing unit schedules and rosters. Based on the concept that each employee has particular work cycles, the system generates staffing schedules after taking needs, budget restraints, and employee preferences into account (Medicus Systems, 1983).

A personnel data management module that sorts information on all personnel is available on NPAQ. It provides nurse administrators with reports on licensure status, continuing education, skills, hire and termination history, and other data. It can supplement an already existing payroll personnel system (Medicus Systems, 1983).

TABLE 9-8 *Advantages of a Three-Tiered NPAQ System*

1. Allocates resources objectively, consistently, and efficiently
2. Reconciles quantity and quality of nursing care
3. Tracks performance against goals
4. Plans programs for enhancing quality of care
5. Understands and influences the cost of care on a per case basis
6. Bills for care on a patient-specific basis
7. Reduces the time and paperwork associated with staffing, scheduling, budgeting, and personnel management
8. Compares performance with other hospitals nationwide
9. Justifies staffing levels to reimbursement authorities
10. Meets JCAH requirements for patient classification and quality of care assessment

Hospital Data Center of Virginia

The census is the core component of the Hospital Data Center of Virginia (HDCV), with its patient data management systems (Fig. 9-8). The nursing station worksheet can easily be integrated with the census reporting system. HDCV also has an incident reporting application within its financial system to provide hospital reports of incidents involving patients, visitors, or employees. The reports are used in the risk management program to document trends in specific occurrences. The summary report includes the specific incident and the number of persons involved. Hospital areas can be designated as high or low incident–generating areas; for instance, mental health and retardation areas may be high-incident areas.

A HDCV HIS system also includes in its security subsystem the ability to track errors on line. If a medication error is entered on a nursing unit, the printer in the central nursing department may report it. A nurse administrator may interview the nurse who has made the error, and together they may consult with the pharmacy department to see what corrective actions are appropriate. This subsystem also provides cumulative error statistics so that hospital administrators may schedule in-service education or change policies to address error incidents. For example, if the number of errors in blood administration rose, hospital policies for administering blood may need to be analyzed. An in-service education program might be required, and communication with the blood bank administrator might be necessary.

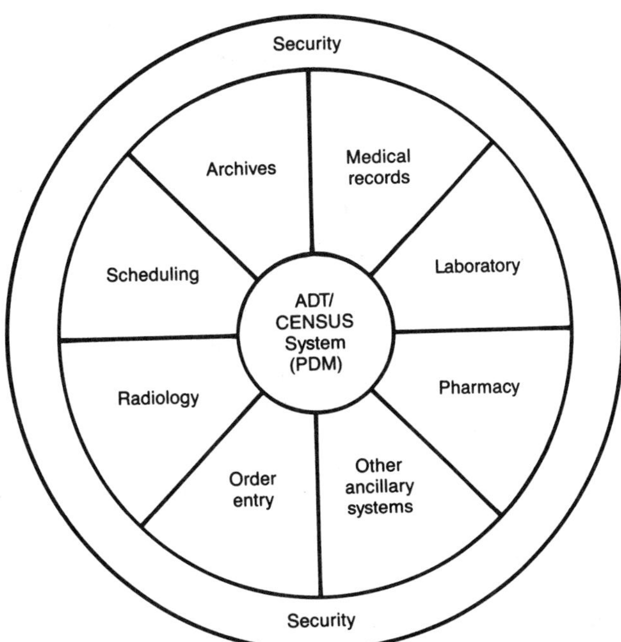

FIG. 9-8. Hospital Data Center of Virginia system components, of which census is the core. (Hospital Data Center of Virginia, Norfolk, VA, 1983)

National Cash Register

The National Cash Register (NCR) hospital information system, NCR/Mednet, is a mainframe system that can accomplish order entry, patient admission, transfer and discharge, census, bed allocation, and nursing care plans at bedside.

Shared Medical Systems

Another mainframe computer system, Shared Medical Systems (SMS), allows nurse administrators and managers to integrate patient care information from nurses' notes with the following (Shared Medical Systems, 1983):

- Automated acuity and staffing modules
- Communication through order entry formats
- Retrospective staffing analysis
- Quality assurance, problem-oriented identification
- Infection control
- Risk management, reporting
- Computer-assisted instruction
- Procedure manuals produced through a word processing module
- Personnel files
- Budget reports

Utilization Review. SMS has a HIS called COMMAND that includes a utilization review subsystem as a part of the PCS. Reports are available 5 days a week to identify patients who are near the end of their certified stay and who need continued stay review. The report includes up-to-date patient information, including diagnoses, procedures, previous certification detail, and reviewer comments. The utilization review is sequenced by the nursing station identified, hospital service and bed, or last review coordinator and bed review. Daily summaries are provided when needed, and current and future review loads are predicted. To indicate future staffing needs, the system provides summaries of future patient loads. Each month the summary reports review each patient's admitting diagnosis to provide information to establish cost rates for each diagnosis, to examine the effectiveness of the review mechanism, and to support more effective discharge scheduling. This subsystem can provide either diagnosis or procedure reviews.

Census. The census system is the cornerstone of COMMAND. It is one of seven subsystems available from the SMS financial management system. In addition, the COMMAND information system involves a five-component resource management subsystem, a 15-component patient care system, and two levels of communication subsystems. The census system provides monthly statistical analysis of patient admission by hospital service, sex, and age. The detailed census statistics include patient days for each sex and age category within hospital services and is used to analyze hospital services and to determine variations in time in patient mix for each hospital service.

Minicomputers

GRASP

The GRASP System is an acuity system based on nursing workload measurement. GRASP is an acronym for the *G*race *R*eynolds *A*pplication and *S*tudy of *P*ETO. Grace is the name of a hospital in North Carolina where the PETO system was tested and modified. The Kate B. Reynolds Health Care Trust provided initial funding.

The GRASP System is proprietary to MCS, Inc., Morganton, North Carolina, which developed and made the system available for use at other health care facilities. The measurement tool that must be customized for each health care facility and specialized nursing unit consists of the nursing actions that typically represent 85% of the physical care required by patients. Also included are teaching and emotional support needs of patient and family, indirect care, and nursing process activities. Table 9-9 shows these interventions in a sample tool and their corresponding time requirements expressed in tenths of an hour. The measurement document is called a PCH (Patient Care Hour) Chart. It is directly linked to the nursing process of assessment, planning, implementation, and evaluation. The GRASP Tool is also used for care planning and retrospective documentation for charting, quality assurance, and costing of nursing care.

The efficiency and popularity of the computerized versions of the GRASP System have been attributed to the fact that the system has been proven to work well manually. The minicomputer system is supplemental to a Hospital Information System (Zak, 1984; Meyer, 1978, 1981).

The computer scans the nursing documentation per day or per shift and produces the following reports:

- Number of patient care hours per location
- Number of patient care hours per patient
- Number of staff required
- Number of actual staff
- Lists of float personnel
- Variance
- Utilization percentages (from patient care and nursing care hours)
- Staff mix
- Total patient care days
- Total patient care hours
- Total patient care hours per patient day
- Number of required nurses per patient day
- Number of actual nurses per patient day

Several HIS vendors have introduced systems that fully integrate GRASP acuity assessment and reporting. Some also include automated care planning modules and DRG costing. Automated staffing, scheduling, and management reporting software, based on GRASP input data, is also available for microcomputers (Meyer, 1984). In microcomputer programs, PCH totals are input to produce the reports similar to those mentioned above, including nursing costs and budget variances each day.

Systems Architecture

The automated hospital integrated system from Systems Architecture has four major modules:

Patient care/patient accounting
General ledger/budgeting
Purchasing/accounts payable/inventory
Payroll/personnel management

TABLE 9-9 *The GRASP System*
24° Patient Care Hour Chart
M/S Nursing Record (© MCS/GRASP 1985. Reproduced with permission)

DATE: ________ DIET: ________

RESTRICTIONS: ________

ADDRESSOGRAPH

"COLUMN A"		E	N	D
Assessment				
• Initial	5	___	___	___
• Update/revise assessment	1	___	___	___
Planning				
• Initial care plan development	2	___	___	___
• Update/revise care plan (daily)	1	___	___	___
Implementation				
Teaching/Support				
• Daily planned education/support	2	___	___	___
• Planned teaching	4	___	___	___
• Additional emotional support	1	___	___	___
Nutritional Needs				
NPO/ice only	1	___	___	___
Self feed	1	___	___	___
Family feed	1	___	___	___
Assist feed/super. feed	7	___	___	___
• Total feed	13	___	___	___
• Intermittent tube feed	10	___	___	___
• Continuous tube feed ql° check	10	___	___	___
Supplemental feedings/HS snack		___	___	___
• Teaching feed		___	___	___
Elimination Needs				
Bathroom privileges I & O	1	___	___	___
BRP with assistance	7	___	___	___

"COLUMN B"		E	N	D
Mobility Needs				
• Walk with assistance QD	2	___	___	___
• Walk with assistance bid/tid	5	___	___	___
• Bedrest turn every 2° w/skin care	9	___	___	___
• Teaching mobility		___	___	___
Suctioning/Resp. Aids				
• Tracheal suction every 4° (trach care)	10	___	___	___
• Tracheal suction every 2° (trach care)	15	___	___	___
• Cough deep breath/leg exer/spiro care	4	___	___	___
Other Direct Nursing Care				
Diagnostic enemas	13	___	___	___
Isolation technique (strict)	3	___	___	___
• Specimen collection	1	___	___	___
• Ventilator care	16	___	___	___
• Peritoneal dialysis	40	___	___	___
Oral Care		___	___	___
Indirect Care	10	___	___	___
Evaluation				
• Review/Evaluate/Document care given	1	___	___	___
Sub Total "Column B"	☐	___	___	___
"Column A & B" Total Patient Care Hours	☐	___	___	___

Item	Value	E	N	D
• Incontinent care	10	___	___	___
Voiding sufficient quantity		___	___	___
Bowel movement		___	___	___
Vital Signs and Measurements				
• Routine vital signs QD/BID	1	___	___	___
• Vital signs every tid/qid	2	___	___	___
• Vital signs every 4° (inc. post op)	5	___	___	___
• Neuro checks every 4°	3	___	___	___
• Neurovascular circulation checks 4°	3	___	___	___
• Post procedure vital signs	12	___	___	___
Hygiene/Skin Care Needs				
Bath without help/HS care	2	___	___	___
Partial bath or but/shower w/check	4	___	___	___
Complete bath	8	___	___	___
• Simple dressing either/or debcubitus care	3	___	___	___
• Complex dsgs. either/or decubitus/ostomy	13	___	___	___
• Restraint care	8	___	___	___
• Teaching hygiene/skin care		___	___	___
Med/Fluid Administration				
• Oral, gtts, suppos, oint (inc. prn) 1–6QD	2	___	___	___
• Oral, gtts, suppos, oint (inc. prn) 7–12+QD	4	___	___	___
• Injections (inc. prns) 1–6QD	2	___	___	___
• I.V. medications 1–4 × QD	4	___	___	___
• I.V. medications 5 or more QD	9	___	___	___
• I.V. continuous/hyperalimentation	11	___	___	___
• Transfusions—blood/blood products	10	___	___	___
• Hickman catheter care	4	___	___	___
• Teaching medications		___	___	___
Sub Total "Column A"	☐	___	___	___

• Requires Documentation on reverse side (narrative nursing notes) or elsewhere as designated.

Note: Time values have been increased to account for unlisted/unpredicted nursing care interventions.

IV Therapy		E	N	D
NO-New Order	B-Butterfly			
RES-Restart	C-Catheter			
INF-Infiltration	N-Needle			
OCC-Occlusion				
16G–18G–19G–20G–21G–22G–23G				
CVC-Central venous catheter				
HC-Hickman catheter				
Specify entry site				
TC-Tubing change				
DC-Dressing change				
F-Flush				
SC-Site check				
INITIALS		___	___	___

Treatments	E	N	D
______________________	___	___	___
______________________	___	___	___
______________________	___	___	___
______________________	___	___	___
______________________	___	___	___

Signatures

E	______________________	LPN/NT RN	Side Rail Bed
N	______________________	LPN/NT RN	Side Rail Bed
D	______________________	LPN/NT RN	Side Rail Bed

This system, which provides medical, financial, and management information, is a subsystem of a master system that structures the information for easy retrieval. Personnel files, budgeting, forecasting, and planning modules are available. Its potential for nursing is great.

HELP

An innovative patient acuity system has been generated with the alert components of the HELP (*H*ealth *E*valuation Through *L*ogical *P*rocessing) system's nursing documentation component. It is used at the Latter Day Saints Hospital, Salt Lake City, Utah, in the critical care, medical-surgical, maternity, newborn, and other specialties units. This system quantitates the time spent on specific nursing activities, including the following:

Admission, transfer, discharge
Vital signs
Fluid intake/and diet
Drainage tubes
Daily hygiene
Respiratory care/aids
Medications
Turning or assisted activity
Laboratory work
Miscellaneous

When a nurse enters a routine care activity into the computer, it is assigned a time factor through an acuity program. At the end of a shift, the computer provides the acuity measurement, which correlates directly with what is documented. When a test or procedure has been ordered but a nurse has not documented it and the acuity score is low, the computer informs the nurse to document care given. Items on the care plan that have not been documented also receive an alert printout. Nurses can thus be assigned to the unit based on acuity outcomes (Killpack, 1984).

Microcomputers

Several other administrative applications are available on microcomputers (Table 9-10). Microcomputers are being used more frequently to include both nursing services information and nursing unit management information.

The following microcomputer applications are described:

- NURSystem
- Janna+
- Micro-budget systems
- Micro-planning systems
- Micro-personnel systems
- Automated nurse staffing office system (ANSOS)

NURSystem

A powerful microcomputer made by Digital Equipment Corporation (DEC) runs NURSystem, which accomplishes the following 15 administrative and management functions:

Tour of duty schedules
Ad hoc schedules
Daily staffing adjustments
Daily activity reports
Daily staffing reports
Daily adjustment summary (overtime)
Nursing hours/patient day comparisons
Statistical summaries of staffing for 2 weeks including job titles
Spending rate analysis for previous pay periods
Labor turnover summary
Position control that lists vacancies
Attendance report including vacations, sick leave, holidays
Shift staffing report to plan upcoming shift coverage
Annual holiday report
Personnel profiles

The following reports are generated from this system:

Patient classification
Nursing hours per patient day
Advance duty schedule
Position control
Employee attendance
Monthly spending rate analysis
Employee profile
Labor turnover statistics

TABLE 9-10 *Microcomputer Administrative Applications*

SUPPLIER	NURSING SERVICES INFORMATION							NURSING UNIT MANAGEMENT INFORMATION						
	QUALITY ASSURANCE	*PERSONNEL FILES*	*COMMUNICATION NETWORKS*	*BUDGETING AND PAYROLLS*	*CENSUS*	*SUMMARY REPORTS*	*FORECASTING AND PLANNING*	*CLASSIFICATIONS*	*STAFFING BASED ACUITY*	*SCHEDULES*	*INVENTORY LISTS*	*PATIENT BILLINGS*	*INCIDENT AND OTHER REPORTS*	*SHIFT SUMMARY REPORTS*
NURsystem		X		X			X		X	X		X		X
Janna+	X	X		X	X		X	X	X	X		X		
ANSOS		X		X	X	X	X		X	X		X		
Personnel systems		X												
Micro-planning							X							
Micro-budget				X			X							

Janna+

Janna+ offers two patient classification options:

Patient care plan
Patient acuity classification

The patient care plan option allows a patient's nursing orders to be evaluated objectively. The matrix of nursing care tasks is used to create a plan that is translated into numbers or units of care required. A daily care plan is a secondary gain from this classification scheme. Patient acuity classification allows a patient's condition to be characterized. The degree of illness (acuity) is determined according to the number and type of characteristics recorded on an evaluation form. These data are translated into numbers to establish an acuity classification (Janna Medical Systems, 1983).

Janna+ also has a staffing component based on acuity. Number and professional level of staff are calculated for each unit and each shift from information obtained in the patients' needs assessment modules. Staff levels are then optimized by comparing the results to the available staff and making adjustments to create an adequate balance of care required with available staff and budget. The computer displays costs of proposed staffing configurations so that alternatives within the nursing department's operating budget can be chosen if needed (Janna Medical Systems, 1983).

Janna+ has a scheduling component that prints out all schedules available. This module compiles information from staffing patterns, personnel changes, staff

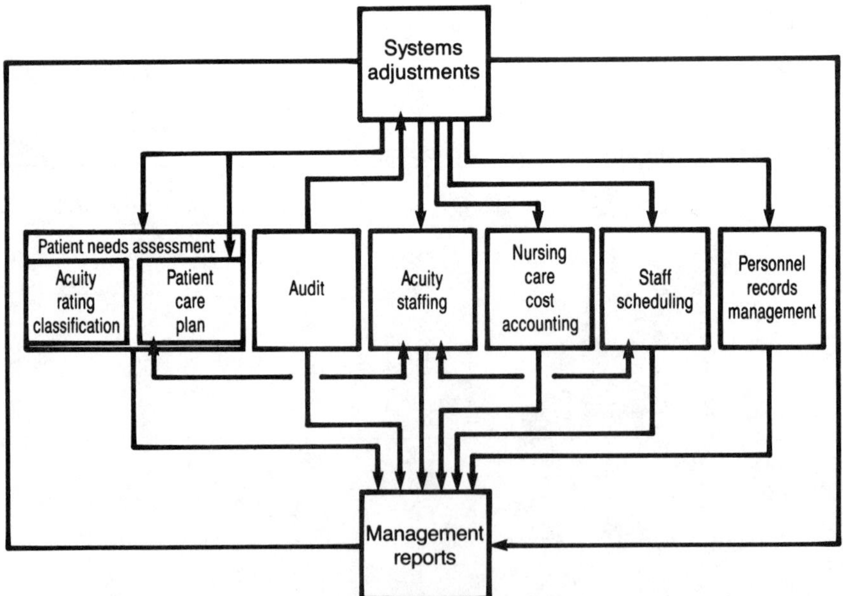

FIG. 9-9. Seven program components of JANNA+. (Janna Medical Systems, Inc., Nursing Division: JANNA+. St. Louis, MO, Janna Medical Systems, 1983)

scheduling requests, and census and acuity projections with budget adjustments. The computer system report facilitates forecasting (Janna Medical Systems, 1983).

Finally, Janna+ is an integrated system consisting of seven program components (Fig. 9-9):

Patient needs assessment (patient care plan and patient acuity classification)
Acuity-based staffing
Nursing care hours cost accounting
Staff scheduling
Personnel records management
Internal nursing audit
Management reporting and system adjustment

Janna+ offers a microbased computer system installed in the nursing department that can be transposed to any computer system.

In addition to the components described above, this model allows for internal nursing audit to validate acuity data and patient needs assessment options, nursing care hours delivered, and charges billed. Data regularly collected from audits are entered into the computer to produce comprehensive reports on operational variances. These reports are used to improve and refine the four areas validated. This component is used to promote nursing accountability and peer review information, detect documentation problems, and identify trends in patient care. The management reporting component consists of printed reports (figures, graphs, and schedules) for each of the preceding components. The system adjustment component allows flexible changes to be made in the programs without additional programming needs (Janna Medical Systems, 1983).

Micro-Budget

A microcomputer has also been used to process data in a nursing department to project anticipated salary expenditures of nursing personnel based on nursing care hour standards, patient days or visits, and the ratio of staff by title. The program calculates required direct and indirect patient care and also analyzes available staff compared to calculated requirements. The variance is designated as the funding requirements for new personnel or the justification for supplemental staffing. Monthly reports help administrators determine if decreased or increased spending was based on changes in patient days, salaries, or hours of care per patient (O'Donohue and Ramshorn, 1983).

Micro-Planning

Planning can also be facilitated by a software package called sys/PLANR that runs on a microcomputer. It can do the following:

Automate the ranking of potential projects using consistent, objective criteria
Specify interproject scheduling and constraints
Estimate personnel and hardware use for a potential project
Estimate the type and magnitude of a project's benefits
Simulate the scheduling of a project based on priorities and estimate availability of personnel integrated with information about projects in process

Forecast aggregate future personnel needs, disk storage, terminal, and hardware requirements
Generate equipment and personnel acquisition forms and budgets
Forecast the impact of the new system on future cash flow
Compute the return on investments for a new project or group of projects

This planning system is designed to assist medical information systems management by doing the consulting needed in planning information system changes (Systems Research Services, 1983).

Micro Personnel

An IBM personal computer has been used to describe nursing personnel files. Up to 33 items of information have been entered, including demographic, education, and employment data. Standard output reports include summaries of personnel by division and title, name lists by cost centers, salary expenditures by title, validation of license expirations, continuing education, cardiopulmonary resuscitation updates needed, and annual evaluations. Personnel files have been used to compare the profiles of long-term employees with those who resign shortly after starting. Some administrators find personnel files more helpful in making information available for decision making than for saving time (O'Donohue and Ramshorn, 1983).

ADMINISTAR is one software package available for various microcomputers to store information on nursing department personnel. The system allows storage and retrieval in up to 10 categories with up to 12 variables in each category (Mosbystar, 1983):

Staff records
Categorized filing system
Automatic pagination
Mailing list
Comprehensive data reports
Easy editing
Past permanent records
Multiple data entry
Interactive reporting
Automatic sorting
Easy-to-read reports
Automatic data file creation

ANSOS

ANSOS (*A*utomated *N*urse *S*taffing *O*ffice *S*ystem) integrates staffing, scheduling, and personnel productivity. The software package, used with an IBM personal computer in a nursing office, provides 4-week schedules based on staff nurse preference, automates the daily staffing allocation and reporting functions, and generates management reports such as productivity, sick leave, license renewal, and turnover. It can operate from the hospital's acuity system, census, or staffing components. It prints daily staffing worksheets and allows staffing assignments based on qualifications, preference, and skills. It also provides information on productivity, comparing target to actual hours worked by staff nurses on units,

ATWORK MEMORIAL HOSPITAL

TURNOVER ANALYSIS

PERIOD 2 08-01-82 TO 08-28-82

	TOTAL		RATE		SERVICE		REASON1		REASON2		REASON3		REASON4		REASON5		REASON6		REASON7	
	PER	YTD	PER	YTD	PER	YTD	PER	YTD	PER	YTD	PER	YTD	PER	YTD	PER	YTD	PER	YTD	PER	YTD
6-W	3	4	100	80	9	11	2	3	0	0	1	1	0	0	0	0	0	0	0	0
6-E	0	1	0	18	0	22	0	0	0	1	0	0	0	0	0	0	0	0	0	0
7-W	1	1	32	16	17	17	0	0	1	1	0	0	0	0	0	0	0	0	0	0
7-E	2	2	62	31	11	11	0	0	0	0	2	2	0	0	0	0	0	0	0	0
FLT	0	1	0	22	0	23	0	0	0	1	0	0	0	0	0	0	0	0	0	0
TOT	6	9	48	36	11	14	2	3	1	3	3	3	0	0	0	0	0	0	0	0

REASON 1, PROMOTION; REASON 2, FAMILY RELOCATION; REASON 3, TO ANOTHER HOSPITAL; REASON 4, OTHER VOLUNTARY; REASON 5, INACTIVE; REASON 6, TERMINATED; REASON 7, OTHER

FIG. 9-10. Turnover analysis report from ANSOS. (ATWORK Corporation: An untitled marketing handout. Santa Clara, CA, Atwork Corp, 1983)

tracks sick leave days taken, continuing education units taken, or special staff nurses requests, and license renewal, turnover analysis, anniversary, position control, and other reports. Figure 9-10 shows an example of an ANSOS report (Atwork, 1983).

SUMMARY

Many nurse administrators and managers now have computer systems for administrative activities. This chapter has described these systems, which serve as tools to monitor the administrative activities of quality assurance, payrolls, communications, budgeting, census, summary report, forecasting and planning. Patient classification, nurse staffing systems, schedules, inventories, patient bills, incident and other reports, and shift summary reports also served to help nursing managers use their personnel according to standardized workload requirements. Examples of computer applications are included.

Although many hospitals have developed their own methods of patient classification, the conversion of patient classification data for predicting nurse staffing by computer processing is relatively new (Giovannetti, 1981). The wave of the future in administrative computer applications is the integrated system. Although the hospital administrative and unit management functions were separated in this chapter for purposes of discussion, single-function systems will not provide sufficient information for tomorrow's administrator.

ISSUES

- Nursing must know what items are put into budget analysis. If inventories, drugs, and sterile supplies are added to nursing budgets, they may inappropriately count as nursing costs.

- No single system can include all the information an administrator or unit manager needs. Similarly, no adequate studies on the efficacy of mainframe or microcomputer systems alone or in sequence to collect and integrate this vast amount of information exist.
- If nursing unit management reports and hospital administrative reports were consolidated in a central nursing office, the hierarchical structure of nursing might be flattened. A nursing department could potentially become managed by a single person.
- The computerization of administrative applications provides more timely information for nurse administrators and managers.
- Computerized administrative applications allow nurses to spend more time in direct patient care and less time in administrative and management duties.
- Computers help nurse administrators with administrative applications more than they help staff nurses with direct patient care applications.
- Evaluative studies comparing the use of unit managers who are not nurses to those who are nurses in generating the computerized reports to nursing administrators are necessary.
- Potential administrative applications are almost limitless.
- The acquisition of commercially prepared software will allow nurse administrators to make comparisons and monitor nursing trends.
- As more staff nurses are informed about management reports, and more administrators are informed about hospital administrative reports, more nurses will request sophisticated additions to hospital mainframes, minicomputers, and microcomputers.
- Nurse administrators can access most HIS or develop their own computer resources through microcomputers.
- Enthusiasm for using administrative applications should not preclude a thorough evaluation of any system considered.
- Could the data generated from administrative applications be put to better use in hospitals?
- National planning could ensure the compatibility of databases nationwide.

SUGGESTIONS FOR HANDS-ON EXPERIENCES

1. Most of the administrative applications are available in hospitals, in the nursing service administrator's office, or on the nursing unit. Therefore, one hands-on experience can be a visit to a hospital, the nursing service administrator's office, or the nursing unit to examine input and output forms generated.
2. Visit a hospital computer department and evaluate the type of communication networks or systems that exist to support nursing administration.
3. Visit another hospital and compare the systems described to support administrative applications.
4. Visit the exhibit area of any major nursing convention or convention or symposium on computer applications and ask the sales representative for a hands-on experience, a copy of input and output reports, and evaluate literature about the system being described to support nursing administrative applications.
5. Invite a sales representative or educational representative from any of the companies described to visit a class and provide a hands-on experience.

6. Determine from the computer department what hardware is available to run a temporary software package during a specified time.
7. Invite a company to send a software package under a temporary license agreement for education and evaluation.
8. Invite a company to send a complementary demo disk to use on a microcomputer.

STUDY QUESTIONS

1. What are the two main categories of administrative applications?
2. What are the essential components of a nursing services administration information system?
3. What are the essential components of nursing unit management systems?
4. Describe a quality assurance system in which the computer is the central processor.
5. List important information that can be provided on payroll systems.
6. Define a patient classification system.
7. How is patient classification converted by computers to workload measures?
8. List the components of a budget system.
9. What types of unit reports can be generated with computers?
10. How many mainframe and minicomputer systems have all the administrative and management applications?
11. How many microcomputer systems have all the administrative and unit management applications?
12. Discuss one issue confronting the administrative applications of computers.

REFERENCES

Atwork Corporation: An untitled marketing handout. Santa Clara, CA, Atwork Corp, 1983

Austin C: Information Systems for Hospital Administration. Ann Arbor, MI, Health Administration Press, 1979

Ballantyne D: A computerized scheduling system with centralized staffing. J Nurs Admin 9:38–45, 1979

Department of Health and Human Services, Division of Nursing: Methods for Studying Nurse Staffing in a Patient Unit: A Manual to Aid Hospitals in Making Use of Personnel. (DHHS pub. no. 78-3). Washington, DC, U.S. Government Printing Office, 1978

Dominick V: Automation of nursing staff allocation. Superv Nurse, 43:20, 1970

Downey J, Walczak R, Hohri W: Evaluating hospital compliance with JCAH quality assurance standards. In Dayhoff R (ed): Proceedings of the Seventh Annual Symposium on Computer Applications in Medical Care, pp 94–97. Silver Spring, MD, IEEE Computer Society Press, 1983

Edmunds L: A computer assisted quality assurance model. J Nurs Admin 13:36–43, 1983

Filosa L: Automated communication saves time, money. Hosp Prog 49:115–118, 1978

Fishman R: Computers in nursing administration and practice: An information system for managing nursing productivity and quality patient care: NPAQ. Computers in Nursing 1(5):1–3, 1983

Gebhardt A: Computers and staff allocation made easy. Nurs Times 78:1471–1474, 1982
Giovannetti P: The distributed processing approach to providing a combined staffing and word processing system for nursing service. In Heffernan H (ed): Proceedings of the Fifth Annual Symposium on Computer Applications in Medical Care, pp 783–787. Silver Spring, MD, IEEE Computer Society Press, 1981
Howe M: Developing instruments for measurement of criteria: A clinical nursing practice perspective. Nurs Res 29(2):100–103, 1980
Janna Medical Systems, Inc., Nursing Division: Janna+. St. Louis, MO, Janna Medical Systems, 1983
Jelinek R, Zinn T, Brya J: Tell the computer how sick the patients are and it well tell how many nurses they need. Mod Hosp 121:81–85, 1973
Jelinek R, Haussman D, Hegyvary S, Newman J: A Methodology for Monitoring Quality of Nursing Care. (DHEW pub. no. HRA 74-25). Washington, DC, U.S. Government Printing Office, 1974
Killpack A, Budd M, Chapman R, et al: Automating patient acuity from nursing documentation. In Cohen G (ed): Proceedings of the Eighth Annual Symposium on Computer Applications in Medical Care, pp 709–711. Silver Spring, MD, IEEE Computer Society Press, 1984
Mayers M: Standard Nursing Care Plans. Palo Alto, CA, K. P. Co Medical Systems, 1974
Medicus Systems: NPAQ. Evanston, IL, Medicus Systems, 1983
Meyer D: GRASP: A Patient Information and Workload Management System. Morganton, NC, 1978
Meyer D: GRASP TOO: Applications and Adaptations of the GRASP Nursing Workload Management System. Morganton, NC, 1981
Miller H, Pierce F, Pierskalla W: Implementation of Nurse Scheduling Using Mathematical Programming. (NTIS Pub. No. HRP-0010314). Washington, DC, U.S. Government Printing Office, 1975
Mosbystar: ADMINISTAR. St. Louis, MO, CV Mosby, 1983
O'Connor, F: Nurse management systems and budget control. In Fokkens O, Haro A, Vanderwerff A et al (eds): MEDINFO 83 Seminars. Amsterdam, North-Holland, 1983
O'Donohue N, Ramshorn M: The microcomputer as a management tool for nurse executives. In Dayhoff R (ed): Proceedings of the Seventh Annual Symposium on Computer Applications in Medical Care p 506. Silver Spring, MD, IEEE Computer Society Press, 1983
Peter M: Duke Hospital's quality assurance program in nursing—background, organization and evolvement. Nurs Admin Q 1:9–25, 1977
Schmitz H, Ellerbrake R, Williams T: Study evaluates effects of new communication system. Hospitals 50:129, 1976
Shared Medical Systems: An untitled marketing handout. King of Prussia, PA, Shared Medical Systems, 1983
Systems Research Services: Sys/PLANR. McLean, VA, Systems Research Services, 1983
Young E, Brian E, Hardy D: Automated Hospital Information Systems Workbook, vol I, Guide to Planning, Selecting, Acquiring, Implementing and Managing an AHIS. Los Angeles, Center Publications, 1981
Zak E, Chastain C: Computerization of the GRASP system to determine patient care requirements. Comp Healthcare 34:3, 1984

BIBLIOGRAPHY

Ball M, Hannah K: Using Computers in Nursing. Reston, VA, Reston Publishing, 1984
Carpenter C: Computer use in nursing management. J Nurs Admin 13:17–21, 1983
Cook M, McDowell W: Changing to an automated information system. Am J Nursing, 75(1):46–51, 1977
Edmunds L: Computer-assisted nursing care. Am J Nursing 82:1076–1079, 1982
Finlayson H: Numbers approach to nursing management. Dimensions Health Serv 53:39–44, 1976

Freund L, Mauksch I: Optimal Nursing Assignments Based on Difficulty: Final Project Report. (NTIS pub. no. HRP-0011346), June 1975
Froment A, Michaud P, Milon H, et al: Computer-assisted patient care management. Med Info 4:119–125, 1979
Gabbert C, Kuydendall L, Swanke F, Simpkins D: Nursing Utilization Management Information System. Ann Arbor, MI, CSF, 1975
Giebink G, Hurst L: Computer Projects in Health Care. Ann Arbor, MI, Health Administration Press, 1975
Giovannetti P: Patient Classification Systems in Nursing: A Description and Analysis (DHEW pub. no. HRA 78-22). Washington, DC, U.S. Government Printing Office, 1978
Grobe S: Computer Primer Resource Guide for Nurses. Philadelphia, JB Lippincott, 1984
Halloran E: Analysis of variation in nursing workload by patient medical and nursing conditions. Diss Abstr Intl 41:3385B, 1981 (University Microfilms no. 8106567)
Hannah K: The computer and nursing practice. Nurs Outlook 24:555–563, 1976
Haussman R, Hegyvary S, Newman J: Monitoring Quality of Nursing Care. II. Assessment and Study of Correlates (DHEW pub. no. HRA 76-7). Washington, DC, U.S. Government Printing Office, 1976
Haussman R, Hegyvary S: Monitoring Quality of Nursing Care. III. Professional Review for Nursing: An Empirical Investigation. (DHEW pub. no. HRA 77-70). Washington, DC, U.S. Government Printing Office, 1977
Holbrook F: Computerization aids utilization review. Hospitals 49:53–55, 1975
Hospital Data Center of Virginia: An untitled marketing handout. Norfolk, VA, Hospital Data Center of Virginia, 1983
Howland D: Approach to nurse-monitor research. Am J Nursing 77:556–558, 1966
Keliher P: Standardized form. Superv Nurse 6:40, 1975
Lee A: What computers can do for you . . . and what they're already doing for the lucky few. RN 45:43–44, 121–127, 1982
Lehman M, Friesen Q: Centralized control system cuts costs, boosts morale. Hospitals 51:75, 1977
Martin K: A client classification system adaptable for computerization. Nurs Outlook 30:515–517, 1982
Medical Systems Research: An untitled marketing handout. Gainesville, FL, Medical Systems Research, 1983
Minnetti R, Hutchinson J: Systems achieves optimal staffing. Hospitals 49:1–62, 1975
Murray D: Computer makes the schedules for nurses. Mod Hosp 117:104–105, 1971
NCR Corporation: An untitled marketing handout. Dayton, OH, NCR Corp, 1983
Nordy R, Freund L: Model for nurse staffing and organizational analysis. Nurs Admin Q 1:1–13, 1977
NURSystem: An untitled marketing handout. Totowa, NJ, NURSystem, 1983
Pocklington C, Guttman L: Computer Technology in Nursing: A Comprehensive Bibliography—Nurse Planning Information Series #16 (DHHS pub. no. HRA 80-65). Hyattsville, MD, Department of Health and Human Services Division of Nursing, 1980
Reeves D, Underly N: Computerization of nursing. Nurs Manage 13:50–53, 1982
Roehrl P, Nickel L, Lake W: Nurse staffing through patient classification. In Blum B (ed): Proceedings of the Sixth Annual Symposium on Computer Applications in Medical Care, pp 551–556. Silver Spring, MD, IEEE Computer Society Press, 1982
Scholes M, Bryant Y, Barber B: The Impact of Computers on Nursing: An International Review. Amsterdam, North-Holland, 1983
Smith D, Wiggins A: Computer-based nurse scheduling system. Comp Oper Rev 4:195–212, 1977
Sylvester D, Shipley S, Long R: Tapping computer resources for quality assurance: Research and program development. In Heffernan H (ed): Proceedings of the Fifth Annual Symposium on Computer Applications in Medical Care, pp 730–733. Silver Spring, MD, IEEE Computer Society Press, 1981
SysteMetrics, Inc: Data Resources Workstation. Santa Barbara, CA, 1983

Systems Architecture: An untitled marketing handout. Boca Raton, FL, 1983

Toth RM: DRG's: Imperative strategies for nursing service administration. Nurs Health Care 4:197–203, April 1984

Werley H, Grier M (eds): Nursing Information Systems. New York, Springer, 1981

Zielstorff R: Computers in nursing administration. In Heffernan H (ed): Proceedings of the Fifth Annual Symposium on Computer Applications in Medical Care, pp 717–721. Silver Spring, MD, IEEE Computer Society Press, 1981

10 Prospective Payment Applications*

Objectives

- Describe prospective payment and diagnosis related groups as used by the largest payer of health care services.
- Identify uses for integrated computer systems in managing nursing resources.
- Describe several computerized applications.
- Understand the impact of prospective payment and computerization on nursing staff and management.
- Identify issues related to incentive payment systems.

Prospective payment applications can be effective because information provided through automated systems is timely. This chapter describes how computers help influence data needed for prospective payment systems, contain costs, and provide timely information while maintaining quality control.

Although most technologies were deemed the cause of high health care costs in the 1960s and 1970s, computers may be seen as the most useful technology to contain costs in the 1980s, according to preliminary data evaluating the impact of the diagnosis related groups (DRGs) in New Jersey. Preliminary reports on DRGs did not mention computers *per se*, but 96% of New Jersey hospitals have invested in new or improved information systems since the prospective payment system was introduced (Wasserman, 1982).

PROSPECTIVE PAYMENT: AN OVERVIEW

Cost containment efforts in health care, especially prospective payment, are major forces influencing the increased demand for and potential use of computerized information systems, but they are not new. Research and demonstrations, experiments with mandatory and voluntary controls, and public and political debates on this subject have existed for over a dozen years. The major event, however, was the enactment of the 1983 Social Security Amendments (PL 98-21), placing Medicare Part A, which covers hospital services for 30 million beneficiaries, on a prospective payment system.

This law was enacted unusually quickly; rising federal deficits and the impending insolvency of the Medicare trust fund worked to consolidate opinion and push Congress and federal officials into action. Although the 1983 amendments apply only to Medicare beneficiaries receiving inpatient hospital services, Medicare pur-

* This chapter was co-written by Maureen Rothermich Miller, M.P.H., R.N., Special Assistant to the Administrator, Health Care Financing Administration, Washington, DC. This chapter was written by Ms. Miller in her private capacity. No official support or endorsement by the Health Care Financing Administration is intended or should be inferred.

chases more health care, including more hospital services, than any other payer. As a result, the actions of Medicare are important for the whole health industry (Shaffer, 1984). Further, the Health Care Financing Administration (HCFA), which administers the Medicare and Medicaid programs, is planning prospective payment systems for other services, including skilled nursing care (in nursing homes) and home health care.

Retrospective Versus Prospective Systems

The retrospective or cost-based reimbursement system that Medicare used previously had several disadvantages (Schweiker, 1982):

1. The system paid hospitals whatever they spent, giving them no incentive to operate efficiently. This inflated costs in the hospital sector and compromised the federal government's ability to fund other health programs.
2. Different payments could be made for the same hospital service (*e.g.*, cataract removal could be billed at $450 in one area and $2800 in another).
3. The system was burdensome and intrusive because of the many regulations, forms, and reports required.

A prospective payment, simply stated, establishes a rate of payment for a service or product that is set in advance. Prospective payment systems may take various forms. To establish a system, the unit of payment and the method or mechanism for price setting must be decided. The unit for paying providers may be made as follows:

- Per diem
- Per service
- Per capita
- Per discharge
- Per case (type of discharge)

Prices may be set in advance through one of the following mechanisms:

- Cost finding, which requires detailed accounting of each hospital's budget
- Negotiated rates with each hospital
- Competitive bidding to select the most cost-effective providers
- A formula approach in which base year costs are established and future year amounts are set by proxy

After extensive deliberations, federal officials recommended that Medicare hospitals be placed on a prospective payment system that pays per case using a formula approach (Davis and Esposito, 1984).

Diagnosis Related Groups

Assisting policymakers with decisions was a classification system that placed patients in hospitals into clinically coherent groups called DRGs. This system was developed and refined at Yale University. In it, major diagnostic categories are subdivided into medically meaningful subgroups by principal diagnoses, secondary diagnoses, surgical procedures, age, sex, and discharge status; 468 DRGs represent not only clinically coherent groups but categories of patients with similar resource use. With like cases (or types of discharges) organized in this reasonable fashion, an index of weights was developed to reflect the relative resource consumption of each DRG. Stated another way, these weights reflect the relative cost of treating patients in each DRG in all hospitals (Federal Register, 1984). When specially adjusted and updated cost data are used with the DRG weights (the Medicare formula), a payment rate or price can be calculated.

DRGs are an advancement in knowledge and technology that allow the hospital's product or output to be determined (Shaffer, 1983). For the first time, prices can be set for like products with hospital payment reflecting the mix of cases in individual institutions. Because the weights and cost data are calculated and set in advance of the federal fiscal year, the pricing system is *prospective.*

The Medicare Prospective Payment System

Under Medicare's new payment system, the price set in advance is considered payment in full, thus altering the incentive under which inpatient care is provided. Hospitals able to provide care within or under their total annual DRG payments may keep the difference. Those hospitals that incur costs beyond their DRG payments are at risk for those costs. The incentive from this system is to provide only what is necessary to treat patients and manage hospital resources efficiently.

All hospitals participating in the Medicare program were placed on prospective payment during the federal fiscal 1983 year according to their individual cost reporting period. Certain specialty hospitals (*e.g.*, psychiatric, pediatric, long-term care, and rehabilitation) were excluded from the system and will continue to be paid based on the old cost-based system until DRGs or other forms of prospective payment are suitably developed for national implementation. Likewise, certain hospital units (*e.g.*, psychiatric and rehabilitation) can be excluded from the new payment system. Eventually, however, all hospitals and all special units will be part of the Medicare prospective payment system.

By law, provisions are made for hospitals with special circumstances that influence their ability to maximize resources. For example, isolated rural hospitals, regional referal centers, and hospitals primarily involved in cancer research and treatment may qualify for special payment provisions.

Implementation

Prospective payments for hospitals are being implemented over a 3-year period. During this time, Medicare payments will blend each hospital's own cost experience and DRG amounts. In each of the successive transition years, a larger portion of the hospital's payments will be based on the DRG amount; less will be based on the hospital-specific amount. Beginning with cost reporting periods on or after October 1, 1986, Medicare will pay hospitals by national DRG rates. The only difference taken into account will be whether hospitals are urban or rural.

The statute and regulations also recognize that atypical cases may require long hospital stays or unusually high costs. Cases that reach "outlier" criteria will have a formula for additional payment applied to them. Long stays that occur because a nursing home bed is unavailable likewise will receive additional payment. Provisions are also made for transfer cases; transfering hospitals may receive up to the full DRG payment, and receiving hospitals are paid a full DRG amount. Quality of care will be monitored through peer review organizations and computerized programs. The system will periodically be reviewed and evaluated, and the program will be modified to incorporate new knowledge and technology.

Trends

A DRG type of payment system may soon be adopted by other large payers. Several Blue Cross plans are now implementing DRG-based payment plans, and eventually all payers may use a DRG system for hospital payments (Coleman, 1983). However, as other providers join an incentive payment system, the "form" of the system may differ. For example, Medicare has a prospective payment system for the dialysis of end-stage renal disease patients. Rates are set in advance for dialysis treatment, and therefore the unit of payment is per service. Prospective payment systems for long-term care and home health care probably will not use DRGs. Whatever the payment mechanism or patient setting, however, incentives for efficiency and prudent use of health care resources will be common characteristics.

COMPUTER SYSTEMS: FACILITATING NURSING INFORMATION MANAGEMENT UNDER COST CONTAINMENT EFFORTS

Computer systems, when used in response to demands for cost containment and efficiency, can help nursing and hospital administrators by linking patient care, financial, and management information. When integrated systems are used to analyze nursing components of costs for each patient within a DRG, useful management information that a nurse administrator could obtain includes the following (Table 10-1):

1. Skill and patient mix by unit (patient classification and acuity)
2. Staffing patterns (workload)
3. Absenteeism
4. Patient occupancy patterns (census)
5. Nursing costs by unit
6. Costs of other services by unit
7. Quality assurance information (documentation against standards)
8. Discharge planning
9. Staff recruitment

TABLE 10-1 *Fifteen Useful Management Information Areas for Nurse Administrators*

1. Skill and patient mix by unit
2. Staffing patterns
3. Absenteeism
4. Patient occupancy patterns
5. Nursing costs by unit
6. Costs of other services by unit
7. Quality assurance information
8. Discharge planning
9. Staff recruitment
10. Performance and productivity evaluation
11. Risk management and incident reports
12. Payment mechanisms
13. Nursing orders
14. Transfer notes
15. Patients' DRG status

10. Performance and productivity evaluation
11. Risk management and incident reports
12. Payment mechanisms
13. Nursing orders
14. Transfer notes
15. Patients' DRG status

The major benefit of computers in this area is that they provide timely information so that the cost of each case can be monitored during the patient's stay, departmental costs and productivity can be reviewed, quality can be maintained, and information can justify an appeal for additional money when unique nursing care problems occur. Now more than ever the computerized information shared between professional, financial, and administrative personnel will force interdisciplinary planning and dismantle the boundaries between components in the provider setting. Each should be motivated to deliver ethical quality care in a cost-effective manner.

All hospital administrators may need to develop a cost-simulation computer software model in order to survive. It can be developed from currently existing data on a hospital information system (HIS), with integrated computers in different departments, or with a microcomputer. Some of the necessary software can be obtained by contacting a certified public accounting firm. Computer and financial savvy are quickly replacing the management savvy popular in the 1970s.

AVAILABLE COMPUTERIZED SYSTEMS

Software packages can do the following (Coleman, 1983):

Perform product-line costing
Develop case cost accounting and reporting systems
Profile physician admissions, costs, and resource consumption rates
Manage the total cost per case

Some systems and tools are described below. They are available for mainframes, microcomputers, or part of information systems for hospitals, hospice facilities, and ambulatory care settings.

Essential Computer System Components

Ideally, an integrated HIS might provide clinical, financial, and administrative reporting information for prospective payment. The essential components are listed in Table 10-2 and include the following:

- Planning
- Budgeting
- Medical and nursing performance evaluation
- Marketing
- Staff recruitment
- Quality assurance
- Utilization review
- Discharge planning
- Payment mechanism
- Other management reports (*e.g.*, risk management and incident reports)
- Census

TABLE 10-2 *Twenty Essential Components of an Integrated Computer System for Prospective Payment*

1. Planning
2. Budgeting
3. Medical and nursing performance evaluation
4. Marketing
5. Staff recruitment
6. Quality assurance
7. Utilization review
8. Discharge planning
9. Payment mechanism
10. Management reports
11. Census
12. Patient bills
13. Accounts receivable
14. Order entry
15. Case mix
16. Patients' conditions
17. DRG assignment
18. Communications
19. Results reporting
20. Litigations

- Patient bills
- Accounts receivable
- Order entry
- Case mix
- Patients' conditions
- DRG assignment
- Communications
- Results reporting
- Litigations (malpractice suits)

However, only the few systems described below are available.

Planning, Budgeting, and Clinical Management System

The Hospital Research and Educational Trust Planning, Budgeting, and Clinical Management system (PBCS) is a case-mix information system that integrates clinical and financial data, incorporates case-mix classification systems, and produces reports to assist hospitals for planning, budgeting, and clinical management activities.

The reports this system provides include the following (Hulm, 1983):

Historical information for trend analysis
Group comparison data to aid in setting internal standards
Educational materials explaining the system
A report mechanism
A methodology to enable forecasting

The PBCS provides information that allows administrators to make decisions on reimbursement, budgeting, performance assessment, marketing, planning, staff recruitment, quality assurance, and utilization review. The system separates operations data from management information. Reporting information includes case-mix data, clinical and financial performance indicators, patient origins and profiles, comparisons, and population (census) information through the following:

Group comparison data
Payer analysis reports by case-mix groups
Special reports on problem areas
Up to 6 years of historical information for trend analysis
A methodology enabling forecasting

This system makes use of information already available in hospitals' financial and information systems or run on microcomputer diskettes. By coordinating existing data and applying a carefully designed reporting system, this system provides the information that tomorrow's managers will need. Tested in six demonstration hospitals in the Carolinas and Michigan, the system has been implemented in 65- to 500-bed hospitals (The Hospital Research and Educational Trust, 1983).

The Hospital Patient Management System

Some New Jersey hospitals that have used computers for over 5 years have a database management system from Dynamic Control Corporation (DCC) that extends the capabilities of DCC's hospital patient management system (HPMS) so that clinical and financial information are integrated with information needed for DRGs. This occurred because the intricacies of the DRGs required complex, integrated, on-line, interactive, in-house administrative information systems that could continuously access a broad range of patient records throughout the hospital without redundancy. With this system, members of the administrative staff have been able to project case mix, determine payment amounts, charges, and costs, and, on demand, perform comparative analyses of different factors and conditions to manage patient care and financial affairs effectively. The essential components of the system are shown in Table 10-3 (McIlvane, 1983).

The HPMS covers the essential elements of a patient's hospitalization:

Admission
Discharge
Transfer
Census
Outpatient registration
Patient billing
Accounts receivable
Order communications
Results reporting

An essential feature of this system that facilitates DRG categorization is that on admission, data on a patient are entered into the database and assigned a DRG. This eliminates human coding errors, which can be as high as 30%. This information is readily available on line for the billing department to access. Within this system is a DRG grouper that increases the accuracy of determining a DRG assignment. Patients are categorized, and on-line service charges are captured to determine their status.

Another advantage is that the physician discharge diagnosis can be made more timely, allowing billing- and revenue-producing information to be supplied. The

TABLE 10-3 *Components of the Dynamic Control Corporation Hospital Patient Management System*

1. Admissions
2. Discharge
3. Transfer
4. Census
5. Outpatient registration
6. Patient billing
7. Accounts receivable
8. Order communications
9. Results reporting
10. DRG grouper
11. Medical records
12. Patient demographics
13. Reimbursement amounts

(McIlvane M: How a data base management system integrates patient care and financial data to manage diagnosis related groups. In Dayhoff R [ed]: Proceedings of the Seventh Annual Symposium on Computer Applications in Medical Care, pp 610–612. Silver Spring, MD, IEEE Computer Society Press, 1983)

most important advantage of this system is its ability to adjust to administrative changes easily. Since the DRG system may change annually over the next few years, a system must be flexible (McIlvane, 1983).

MediFlex

MediFlex includes a rate setting, financial modeling, budgeting, and DRG component. It can be used through timesharing or is available in-house to hospitals that have a mainframe. Some of its unique features also under development to run on a microcomputer are as follows:

Helps long-range planning with forecasting techniques
Quickly determines third-party settlements and precise contractual allowances
Generates approved formats for Medicare, Medicaid, or Blue Cross annual settlements
Integrates hospitals' internal and external reports
Helps management cost finding by analyzing fixed and variable hospital costs
Performs wage and salary projects in dollars or hours
Quickly evaluates union proposals
Prepares budgets and gives summary reports that are more flexible than general ledgers
Describes budget variance by department
Automatically pinpoints a budget exception

MediFlex has three basic modules:

Budgeting
Reimbursement
DRG case-mix analysis

They can be used separately or as an integrated system. The components of each module are listed in Table 10-4 (MediFlex Systems Corporation, 1983).

The Hospital Workstation

The Hospital Workstation from SysteMetrics Inc., is an integrated decision support system to merge financial, clinical, case-mix, and medical record information in a computerized form. It combines the power of large computers and on-line databases with local, user-friendly microcomputers. In addition, this system produces numbers, text, color graphics, and models that can be used in reporting information inside and outside of the hospital. It has four principal components:

A series of integrated databases
A standard set of hard copy reports
On-line versions of databases, with large computers
A microcomputer component

The first line of information for the system can come from the hospitals financial database or from external vendors. These databases generally include billing data, discharge abstract data, Medicare cost reports, and similar cost information. Once the data tapes are acquired by SysteMetrics, they are placed onto a large computer for editing, processing, and integration. The processing involves computing standard lengths of stay, assigning a DRG and stage of disease for each patient, calculat-

TABLE 10-4 *Three Basic Components of the MediFlex System*

BUDGETING MODULE	REIMBURSEMENT MODULE	DRG ANALYSIS MODULE
Custom tailored	Custom tailored	Tailored to reimbursement environment
Hospital chart of accounts	Cost-finding routines	Statistics used as cost-allocation basis
Hospital budgeting philosophy	Settlement Calculations	Demographic analyses of hospital cases
Flexible budgeting	100% accurate bottom line information	Patient origin
Fixed/variable	Complete audit trails	Payer mix
Unlimited department/Subaccounts	Sensitivity analysis through reimbursement	Age, sex, and discharge
History/Actual/Forecast	Income	Status analyses
Wage and salary projection	Expense	Income analyses
Unlimited statistics/Rates	Procedural sensitivity	By program
Standard inflation factor	Expense reclassification analysis	By DRG
Overrides	Medicare routine limit analysis	By physician
Statistical spreads	Reclassification analysis	By payer
Complete variance reporting	HCFA-approved Medicare reporting	By any combination of the above
Forecasting (15 methods)	Feasibility studies	
Tape input capabilities	Forecasting	
Data interface with MediFlex reimbursement	Variance reporting	
Total user control	Tape input capabilities	
	Data interface with MediFlex budgeting	
	Total user control	

(Courtesy MediFlex Systems Corporation, Shared Services Division, Atlanta, GA)

ing patient-specific costs using cost-to-charge allocations, and making other calculations for analytical use. Finally, complete reports are produced. The standard reports are as follows (SysteMetrics, 1983):

Service area and market reports
Utilization
Reimbursement/profitability
Case mix
Medical staff review

Nursing Productivity and Quality System

Nursing productivity and quality system (NPAQ), from Medicus Systems, now includes a DRG reporting component that enables nurse administrators to track acuity and nursing costs over the course of each patient's stay. Upon discharge this information is transmitted to medical records and patient accounting for their use in abstracting the acuity-based bill. A database can be retained for nursing to analyze nursing costs per DRG (Medicus Systems, 1983). Figures 10-1 to 10-3 show printouts from the NPAQ cost management module.

Janna+

Janna+ offers a nursing care hours cost accounting module within its microcomputer-driven system. This module produces documentation and exact amounts and costs of nursing care hours provided for patients on a daily basis and also provides 14-day reports. This cost information is useful for third party payer reports. In addition, the computer calculates skill mix activities and internal quality assurance controls and provides nurse administrators with the tools for precise budget planning with the DRG system. (Janna Medical Systems, 1983). Figures 10-4 and 10-5 show Janna+ nursing cost reports.

GRASP System

The GRASP System collects information on the patient's nursing care needed in the areas of mobility, diet, hygiene, elimination, frequency of medication, observations, treatments, and teaching and support. These needs are often related to staffing. The acuity, expressed in hours of nursing care required, is then used to calculate the charge for nursing care based on the cost of an hour of nursing. The patient's daily nursing charge directly reflects the hours of care that were required. Audits verify charges and are based on care given (Meyer, 1981). At one hospital, patients' needs are assessed using 50 specific nursing interventions related to the above-mentioned elements of nursing care. The actual nursing charges are computed from nursing care hours and correlated to four charge levels weighted by skill:staff ratio. This system, which has gained the approval of third-party payers, has been in effect since 1983. The system also lends itself to a DRG-based assignment of costs to nursing care by merging GRASP hours by patient with the other clinical and financial data in the hospital's cost accounting software programs (Meyer, 1983, 1984).

Relative Intensity Measures

Relative intensity measures (RIMS) have been proposed by the State of New Jersey to allocate nursing costs as a supplement to the current DRGs. Nine nursing clusters are important data elements in this system; included in these clusters, which vary

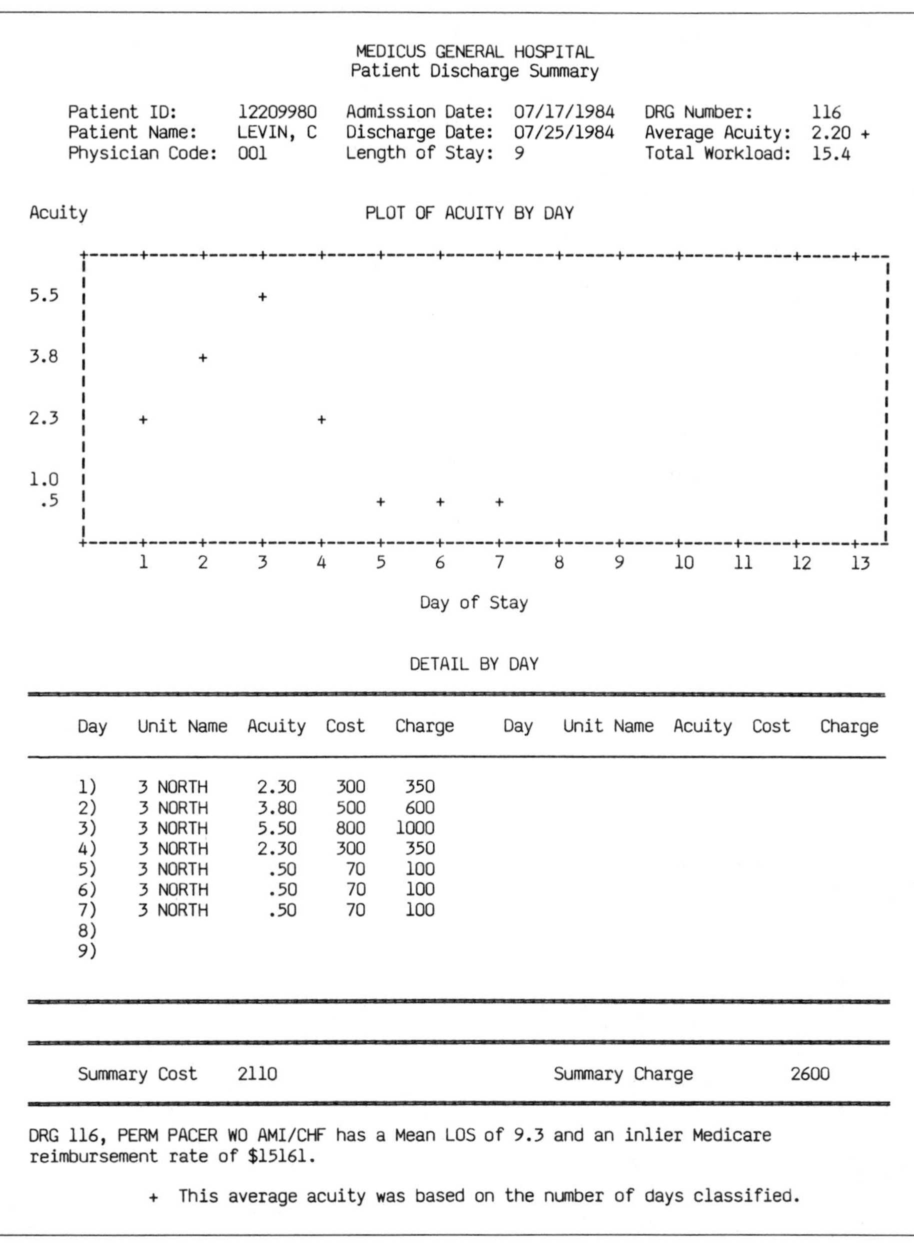

MEDICUS GENERAL HOSPITAL
Patient Discharge Summary

Patient ID:	12209980	Admission Date:	07/17/1984	DRG Number:	116
Patient Name:	LEVIN, C	Discharge Date:	07/25/1984	Average Acuity:	2.20 +
Physician Code:	001	Length of Stay:	9	Total Workload:	15.4

DETAIL BY DAY

Day	Unit Name	Acuity	Cost	Charge	Day	Unit Name	Acuity	Cost	Charge
1)	3 NORTH	2.30	300	350					
2)	3 NORTH	3.80	500	600					
3)	3 NORTH	5.50	800	1000					
4)	3 NORTH	2.30	300	350					
5)	3 NORTH	.50	70	100					
6)	3 NORTH	.50	70	100					
7)	3 NORTH	.50	70	100					
8)									
9)									

Summary Cost 2110 Summary Charge 2600

DRG 116, PERM PACER WO AMI/CHF has a Mean LOS of 9.3 and an inlier Medicare reimbursement rate of $15161.

+ This average acuity was based on the number of days classified.

FIG. 10-1. Patient Discharge Summary. (© Copyright, Medicus Systems Corporation, 1985. Reproduced by permission)

NURSING COSTS BY PATIENT

Medicus General Hospital
NURSING COSTS BY PATIENT

DRG 134
Average reimbursed cost: $2129.75

Accumulated from 7/01/83 to 12/31/83

Patient ID	Units	LOS	Avg Acuity	Cost Per Case Recomm	Cost Per Case Actual
104312	1, 2	8	1.40	561.79	564.00
188212	3	5	1.20	300.96	321.00
124431	3	7	1.10	386.23	392.10
143317	3	6	1.50	451.44	475.45
144482	1, 2, 3	16	2.40	1926.14	1850.20
147638	1, 6, 2	7	1.20	421.34	430.10
136201	1, 3, 6	4	1.40	280.89	210.15
042052	1, 3	6	1.38	415.32	610.10
Average		7.4	1.60	593.01	606.64

FIG. 10-2. An example of another Medicus NPAQ cost management module. (© Copyright, Medicus Systems Corporation, 1985. Reproduced by permission)

depending on the DRG, are information related to length of stay, surgical procedures, complications, comorbid conditions, and type of admission (Joel, 1983).

Nursing Diagnosis

Nursing diagnosis, now computerized and used in some hospitals to identify nursing problems, is being studied by the American Nurses' Association (ANA) with support from the HCFA. It remains to be determined whether nursing diagnosis schemes can effectively provide data on staffing, cost, and payment for nursing services. The North American Nursing Diagnosis Association lists at least 51 nursing diagnoses; the New Jersey RIMs study used 27 diagnoses.

Medical Diagnosis and Procedure-Based Systems

California relative value studies (CRVS), developed by the California Medical Association, and current procedural terminals (CPT-4), published by the American Medical Association, are two versions of a procedure-based system. CPT-4 is essentially a dictionary of terms for procedures. Staging and generalized patient management paths (GPMP) are two disease-based classification systems. The systems combine information on diagnosis and treatment. The earliest type of system to be computerized, the *International Classification of Diseases,* is in its ninth revision with clinical modification (ICD-9-CM). It lists over 1000 categories of diseases and 83 major diagnostic categories (MDCs) that generally correspond to the eighth revised ICD coding system. These latter coding schemas served as the basis for the original DRG categories (Plomann, 1983).

NURSING COSTS BY DRG

Medicus General Hospital
NURSING COSTS BY DRG

Accumulated from 7/01/83 to 12/31/83

DRG	Description	Cases	ALOS	Avg Acuity	Cost Per Case Recomm	Cost Per Case Actual	Avg Total Reimburs
1	Craniotomy Age >17, except trauma	128	21.0	2.31	2433.26	2250.77	10136.02
39	Lens Procedure	145	2.9	1.20	174.56	313.55	1513.69
42	Intraocular Procedure	316	3.4	1.64	279.69	300.67	1784.40
105	Cardiac Valve Procedure w/Pump	129	12.8	3.87	3160.33	2484.73	15801.66
107	Coronary Bypass w/o Cardiac Cath	950	13.0	3.55	2314.88	2604.24	12052.47
125	Circulatory Disorders except AMI w/Cardiac Cath	1104	4.8	4.10	980.12	1200.00	4971.63
133	Atherosclerosis Age <70 w/o Cardiac Cath	410	5.6	1.99	479.12	489.10	2598.06
134	Hypertension	8	8.2	1.38	567.04	652.00	2129.75
243	Medical Back Problem	110	7.5	1.26	474.00	480.00	4800.16
410	Chemotherapy	410	3.5	1.70	297.50	295.20	1065.63
462	Rehabilitation	22	18.0	1.40	1264.00	1232.43	5519.40

FIG. 10-3. An example of a Medicus NPAQ cost management module. (© Copyright, Medicus Systems Corporation, 1985. Reproduced by permission)

PAGE 4 OF 4 NURSE ASSIGNMENT/UTILIZATION REVIEW REPORT 05/04/85

05 MED/SURG

NAME	ROOM	ID	AGE	TOTAL	DAY	EVENING	NIGHT
ROSE, D	514B	325-22-4923 M	67	8.839	4.027	2.966	1.846
		RN		4.477	2.020	1.435	1.022
		LPN		2.678	1.200	0.892	0.586
		NA		1.234	0.577	0.419	0.238
		UC		0.450	0.230	0.220	0.000

FIG. 10-4. An example of a JANNA+ report. (© Copyright 1983, Janna Medical Systems, Inc.)

Patient Severity of Illness/Nursing Intensity Index

Another type of system includes a severity of illness index that measures stage of disease, responsiveness to therapy (rate and residual), complications, interactions, dependency, and procedures (Horn, 1983). These seven characteristics are then categorized into four levels of severity. This model has been proposed as a supplement to the DRG system and is currently being evaluated (Hartley and McKibbin, 1983).

In addition to the patient severity of illness index, a nursing intensity index has been developed to reliably indicate actual nursing care requirements of patients during their hospital stays. This index uses 11 functional health parameters to measure the degree, complexity, or magnitude of nursing input into patient care. These areas are as follows:

- Nutrition
- Elimination
- Sensory information
- Structural integrity

OPERATING SUMMARY

PAGE 2 OF 2 01/31/84

3 MED/SURG – JANNA GENERAL DEMO

ACTUAL HOURS VS. GOAL 01/30/84 CENSUS = 29

	HOURS	EQUIV. HOURS	EQUIV. GOAL	VARIANCE		COST OF VARIANCE
DAY	64.000	96.160	85.260	10.900	$	54.50
EVENING	56.000	84.960	74.530	10.430	$	52.15
NIGHT	40.000	61.440	53.360	8.080	$	40.40
TOTAL	160.000	242.560	213.150	29.410	$	147.05

ACTUAL HOURS VS. GOAL , 7 DAYS TO DATE TOTAL CENSUS = 203

	HOURS	EQUIV. HOURS	EQUIV. GOAL	VARIANCE		COST OF VARIANCE
DAY	456.000	690.880	596.820	94.060	$	470.30
EVENING	384.000	582.400	521.710	60.690	$	303.45
NIGHT	280.000	426.880	373.520	53.360	$	266.80
TOTAL	1120.000	1700.160	1492.050	208.110	$	1040.55

FIG. 10-5. An example of a JANNA+ nursing cost report. (Copyright © 1983 Janna Medical Systems, Inc.)

- Neurologic/cerebral function
- Circulatory function
- Respiratory function
- Emotional response
- Social system
- Cognitive response
- Health management pattern.

These health parameters are ranked with a four-point scale ranging from 1, which indicates a minor nursing resource consumption, to 4, indicating an extreme nursing resource consumption (Reitz, 1984).

IBM Microcomputer Version

An innovative review system that has been used by a private foundation runs with an IBM personal computer (PC) microcomputer. The system was developed to identify those areas of practice where most cost-effective measures could be introduced, particularly during hospitalization. Length of stay and level of ancillary service charges were analyzed and reported. An additional goal was to bring "peer pressure" on physicians to adopt cost-effective practices. A unique result of this system was that "peer pressure" was changed to "data pressure"; that is, a physician's patterns of practice were identified, and alterations in costly behaviors were mandated. The early result from 6 months of use was that 1386 fewer hospital days were used, resulting in annualized savings of more than $1.1 million dollars in hospital charges (Kincaid, 1983).

Hospice System Model

The DRG model as a case-mix management tool and the use of computer resources has been primarily described for hospitals. In the quest for a valid case-mix measure and the construction of an information system that would support case-mix investigations, a minicomputer was used to analyze the cost and effectiveness of DRGs in an inpatient hospice facility and in cancer patients' homes. The system not only provided an analysis of costs for different types of patients but provided the information that cancer patients who do not have surgery are less represented by current DRG groups and subdivisions (Johnson-Hurzeler and colleagues, 1983).

An Ambulatory Care System

Case-mix-based prospective payment methods are now applied to inpatient areas, but case-type classification methods are being developed for ambulatory care settings. Computer resources are especially important in ambulatory care for the following reasons:

The number of visits made per year to an active clinic can be in the millions.
Substantial costs are associated with ambulatory care visits.
An important structural and functional relationship exists between inpatient and outpatient care.

Providing ambulatory care with case-mix methods for classifying patients necessitates that large case-oriented databases that combine inpatient and outpatient methods into an integrated case-mix method of tracking resources be developed (Rogerson, 1983).

One approach to using a database to study case mix in ambulatory care was to categorize patients by primary diagnosis or primary diagnosis with secondary problems. This approach, however, requires that patients return to the *same* outpatient clinic or health maintenance organization (HMO) setting for treatment in a given year (Rogerson, 1983).

Another approach is the visit-oriented method, which characterizes ambulatory care in terms of given visits and associated primary diagnoses. The ambulatory care setting can be reimbursed for treatment, but acute conditions, stabilizing conditions, follow-up treatments, or monitoring deterioration of a patient's condition are not categorized (Fetter, 1980).

• • •

Although the content for an ambulatory care database is described above, the type of computer system that could implement these classification schemes is not described.

Alternate Payer Systems

Even Blue Cross is involved in computer applications for cost management through the development of patient classification systems to differentiate case mix among hospitals. This is another method to integrate case mix with quality assurance. A group of physicians prepared patient management categories and specified the components of care required for patients in each *ICD-9-CM* category. Two versions were computerized. The former included information describing the patient's chief problem necessitating hospitalization and elective surgery procedures. The other included routine information abstracted from a patient's medical record. This method provides a product diversity index that is valuable for payment as well as for effective facility planning and quality assurance (Schuchert, 1983).

Military System

Numerous quality assurance committees have begun to use the DRG groups to study the appropriateness of hospital use and length of stay patterns in the military. In fact, the 36 U.S. Navy hospitals have conducted utilization reviews using the DRGs. DRGs were found to be significantly more valid in grouping cases than previous methods (Kay, 1982).

International System

The DRG concept has also had an impact internationally. For over 3 years the Dutch have implemented it to integrate and manage financial and medical information. They have determined that the DRG indicators can be linked with costly diagnostic equipment and resource consumption produced within a hospital department. This cost-effectiveness data can be used to plan new facilities, new departments, and new staffing patterns.

Because of the benefits that nursing and medical personnel gain from the DRG information base, it has been recommended that nurses and physicians pay close attention to the computerized systems their hospitals are implementing. The Dutch feel that the DRG may be the panacea to integrate the information gap between patient records and financial management. The DRG also has been linked through the discharge care plan to the country system held in a national institute, the Foundation for Medical Registration (Hofdijk and DeJager, 1983).

IMPACT OF COMPUTERIZED PROSPECTIVE PAYMENT SYSTEMS ON NURSING ADMINISTRATORS

The implementation of prospective payment systems has already demanded innovative and comprehensive changes in health care information requirements. First, payment systems have shown that health care systems require more efficient, effective, valid information readily available at reasonable cost. To maintain financial survival, health care systems have had to comply with integrated information strategies to meet their information needs. Without accurate information at reasonable costs, health care institutions will have difficulty complying with the mandates of prospective payment mechanisms.

A predictable change as a result of computer use is that more managers will need new skills to exercise control. This will not necessarily lead to dehumanization, however. Daily computer-generated reports will allow managers to monitor their hospitals with thoroughness, which may be perceived as "iron-hand" monitoring. The vast access to knowledge that computerization bestows will enable fewer managers to exercise more control than is now feasible. It will be possible to see small hospitals manage as "one-man shows," with more precise staffing. More people are becoming familiar with computers, and the challenge will become less how to use the computer and more how to maximize its capabilities.

Tomorrow's managers may need new capabilities. New organizations may evolve because of the computer. Today's task forces, project teams, and ad hoc committees may be replaced by information. Power and authority will be redistributed; horizontal disbursement, with a shift of decisions sideways and downward, will occur. More emphasis will be placed on group competence. Complex problems will become nonroutine challenges, and new intraorganizational relationships will develop.

Now more than ever, nurses will be challenged as patient advocates using ethical judgment to balance efficiency. Collaboration and cooperation will do away with the need for autonomy in nursing as efficiency reports from all departments will be known to all department heads. Collaboration in designing creative ways to control costs efficiently will be necessary, and individual accomplishments will become less important than group accomplishments. Group success will help ensure the nursing department's success in the hospital. The ability to work with others will become more important than the ability to exercise authority over staff nursing personnel. Hierarchy will be diminished, since those who can recommend more productive and effective procedures will reach higher levels. The benefits of success will become more important to nursing personnel than the threats of failure. If the computer can be used to produce computer reports to help those who are managed to reach their goals, then the nurse administrator can be more assured of meeting administrative goals.

Even with the aid of computers, a nurse administrator must pay attention to four characteristics in order to achieve efficiency:

- How the nursing department's product is defined and measured
- The absence of information that relates services provided to costs or resources used
- The segregation of the nursing department's administrative and financial activities and decisions from its clinical activities and decisions
- The nursing department's relationship with the hospital's governing board and its focus on operational rather than strategic issues (The Hospital Research and Educational Trust, 1983)

In the long run, new computer capabilities will mandate that the nurse administrator will need sensitivity, ethical judgment, and encouragement. These qualities will be necessary so that staff do not feel dehumanized. Additionally, administrators must analyze situations using data, understand cost-benefit analysis and financial management, and be able to tackle problems and negotiate. Enthusiasm, warmth and caring—qualities that no computer can provide—will always be needed, however.

SUMMARY

This chapter began by describing the regulatory policies influencing prospective payments systems. It contrasted the old retrospective or cost-based reimbursement system with the prospective payments system. The classification system that was employed to place patients in hospitals into clinically coherent groups uses DRGs. In this system, major diagnostic categories are subdivided into 468 medically meaningful subgroups by principal diagnosis, discharge diagnosis, surgical procedures, age, sex, and discharge status. Medicare is now under a prospective payment system, and other large payers are considering using a similar system.

Fifteen ways that computers can facilitate nursing information management and contain costs were listed. Four basic types of software packages for these systems have been developed and were discussed. The 20 essential components an effective hospital system should include were described.

Applications included a description of a number of systems that have been described as facilitating administrators in the management of information related to prospective payments systems. Essentially these systems included PBCS, HPMS, MediFlex, The Hospital Workstation, NPAQ, Janna+, GRASP, Rims, Nursing Diagnosis, medical diagnosis and procedure systems, a microcomputer version, a hospice system, an ambulatory care system, another payer system, a military system, and an international system. Long term care facilities and nursing homes are only in the experimental stages and were excluded from the description of potential computer applications.

The most significant impact the computerized prospective payment systems will have on nursing administrators were inclusive of more timely, efficient, effective, and valid information. A predictable change is the need for nurse administrators to have new skills in financial systems and computer systems. New qualities will bring new challenges to administrators. Of the unique new qualities, the ability to balance efficiency with ethical judgment, will be of great importance. Even with the aid of computers a nurse administrator will be challenged to scrutinize (1) the way the nursing department's products are defined and measured, (2) the absence of information that relates services provided to costs or resource use, (3) the segregation of the nursing department's administrative and financial activities and decisions from its clinical activities and decisions, and (4) the nursing departments relationship with the hospital's governing board and its' focus on operations rather than strategic issues.

Finally, changes in the role of nurse administrators were discussed.

ISSUES

- To propose the use of computer-generated classification schemes is one thing; it is quite another to use these tools without testing their validity and reliability to generate cost data in a complex hospital environment.

- Will nursing personnel document using these computer systems if their salary depends on it?
- How will nurses respond if computers document a need for reduced nursing numbers because of more efficient management?
- How will society respond if computers document a need for more nurses to provide efficient, quality care?
- How will hospital nursing administrators respond if computers document that nurses with higher educational backgrounds can provide less costly care?
- If computers can provide a nurse administrator with all the information necessary to administrate a nursing service, could a one-administrator hospital be demonstrated with head nurse management? Could this result in the loss of intermediate supervisory personnel and flatten the administrative pyramid? Would this reduce or increase costs?
- What type of education will nursing administrators and managers need to respond to developing computer software that will integrate the cost and care components of nursing? Will this preparation be available through nursing schools at the graduate or undergraduate level?
- How can administrators acquire the skills necessary to evaluate available systems, determine hospital needs, and develop appropriate systems?
- As nursing's budget becomes known to nurse managers and administrators, hospital administrators, and physicians, will nursing have to change its attitudes on autonomy and collaborate and cooperate more with other departments?
- If computer documents demonstrate that nursing generates revenue, will nurses be able to command more authority on boards of directors or trustees?
- Can nursing justify through computers that costs of care previously defined in the nursing budget do not belong there (*e.g.*, laundry, housekeeping, unit building supplies)?
- Is prospective payment the panacea of health care payments?
- How have international health care providers from other countries defined their minimum data sets and integrated patient care with costs?

STUDY QUESTIONS

1. Which public law placed Medicare beneficiaries on a prospective payment system? In what year did this occur?
2. What unit of payment and method or mechanism for price setting was established by HCFA?
3. What advantages do computers have with nursing information under cost containment efforts?
4. Useful nursing management information can be obtained from what 15 areas?
5. What is the major benefit of computerized information for prospective payment?
6. How could existing software packages be classified?
7. Identify 20 essential components of an integrated hospital system for prospective payment.
8. Name a case-mix information system that integrates clinical and financial data, incorporates case-mix classification systems, and produces planning, budgeting, and clinical management reports.
9. What is the name of the Dynamic Control Corporation system?

10. Which system provides rate setting, financial modeling, budgeting, and DRG grouping?
11. Which system combines mainframes with microcomputer terminals?
12. Which system integrates nursing-based patient acuity ratings with costs?
13. Which system offers nursing care hours cost accounting within a microcomputer?
14. What, if any, system examines nursing procedures?
15. What New Jersey system supplements DRGs with nursing costs?
16. Has nursing diagnosis been computerized?
17. Name one medical diagnosis or procedure-based system.
18. Discuss one nursing management change that computerized prospective payment will have on future nurse administrators.

REFERENCES

Coleman J: Case-mix and DRG reporting. In Dayhoff R (ed): Proceedings of the Seventh Annual Symposium on Computer Applications in Medical Care, p 595. Silver Spring, MD, IEEE Computer Society Press, 1983

Davis CK, Esposito A: Research and Demonstrations in Prospective Payment Health Care: An International Perspective. Virgo JM (ed). Edwardsville, IL, International Health Economics Management Institutes, 1984

Federal Register, Part 4: Medicare programs; Prospective payments for medicare inpatient hospital services; Interim final rates. Washington, DC, U.S. Government Printing Office, 1984

Fetter R: Ambulatory Patient Related Groups. Institution for Social and Policy Studies, Yale University, New Haven, CT, 1980

Hartley S, McKibbin R: Hospital Payment Mechanisms, Patient Classification Systems, and Nursing: Relationships and Implications. Kansas City, MO, American Nurses' Association, 1983

Hofdijk W, DeJager K: Will the DRG system become a panacea for internal management? In Van Bemmel, Ball M, Wigertz O (eds): MEDINFO 83, pp 77–79. Amsterdam, North-Holland, 1983

Horn S, Sharkey PD, Bertram DA: Measuring severity of illness: Homogenous case mix groups. Med Care 21:14–31, 1983

The Hospital Research and Educational Trust: Planning, budgeting, and clinical management system (pamphlet). Chicago, Hospital Research and Educational Trust, 1983

Hulm C: Case mix information to assist the hospital management team. In Dayhoff R (ed): Proceedings of the Seventh Annual Symposium on Computer Applications in Medical Care, p 620. Silver Spring, MD, IEEE Computer Society Press, 1983

Janna Medical Systems, Inc., Nursing Division: Janna+. St. Louis, MO, Janna Medical Systems, 1983

Joel L: Case mix reimbursement; DRGs, RIMs. Mass Nurse 52:5–6, 1983

Johnson-Hurzeler R, Leary R, Hill C: Diagnosis related groups as a case mix/management tool of hospice patients. In Dayhoff R (ed): Proceedings of the Seventh Annual Symposium on Computer Applications in Medical Care, pp 595–598. Silver Spring, MD, IEEE Computer Society Press, 1983

Kay T: Using DRG's to conduct utilization review in Naval Hospitals. In Blum B (ed): Proceedings of the Sixth Annual Symposium on Computer Applications in Medical Care, pp 599–601. Silver Spring, MD, IEEE Computer Society Press, 1982

Kincaid W: Private review—running a medical care foundation with a microcomputer. In Dayhoff R (ed): Proceedings of the Seventh Annual Symposium on Computer Applications in Medical Care, pp 613–615. Silver Spring, MD, IEEE Computer Society Press, 1983

McIlvane M: How a data base management system integrates patient care and financial data to manage diagnosis related groups. In Dayhoff R (ed): Proceedings of the Seventh Annual Symposium on Computer Applications in Medical Care, pp 610–612. Silver Spring, MD, IEEE Computer Society Press, 1983

Medicus Systems: NPAQ. Evanston, IL, Medicus Systems, 1983

MediFlex Systems: MediFlex. Atlanta, GA, MediFlex Systems, 1983

Meyer D: Fourth and Fifth GRASP Users Conference Proceedings. Morganton, NC, MCS, 1983, 1984

Meyer D: GRASP—A Patient Information and Workload Management System. Morganton, NC, MCS, 1981

Plomann M: Nine Patient Classification Schemes: Development, Description, and Testing. Chicago, The Hospital Research and Educational Trust, 1983

Reitz J: Development and testing of a nursing intensity index, doctoral dissertation, The Johns Hopkins University School of Hygiene and Public Health, February 1984, pp 1–160

Rogerson C: Applying case-mix methods to ambulatory care. In Dayhoff R (ed): Proceedings of the Seventh Annual Symposium on Computer Applications in Medical Care, pp 606–608. Silver Spring, MD, IEEE Computer Society Press, 1983

Schuchert J: The computerization of patient management categories: Clinical basis for a case mix applications. In Dayhoff R (ed): Proceedings of the Seventh Annual Symposium on Computer Applications in Medical Care, pp 606–608. Silver Spring, MD, IEEE Computer Society Press, 1983

Schweiker RS: Report to Congress: Hospital Prospective Payment for Medicare. Department of Health and Human Services, 1982

Shaffer F: DRG's: Changes and challenges. New York, National League for Nursing, 1984

Shaffer F: DRG's: History and overview. Nurs Health Care 4:388–396, 1983

SysteMetrics, Inc, A Division of Data Resources, Inc: Workstation. Santa Barbara, CA, SysteMetrics, 1983

Wasserman J: DRG evaluation, vol I, Introduction and Overview. Princeton, Health Research and Education Trust of New Jersey, 1982

BIBLIOGRAPHY

Bickel R: The TRIMIS experience—an overview. In Blum B (ed): Proceedings of the Sixth Annual Symposium on Computer Applications in Medical Care, pp 209–211. Silver Spring, MD: IEEE Computer Society Press, 1982

Dowling W: Prospective rate setting: Concept and practice. Top Health Care Finan 3:7–37, 1976

Fetter R, Shin Y, Freeman J, et al: Case mix definition by diagnosis-related groups. Med Care 18:1–53, 1980

Grimaldi P, Micheletti J: Diagnosis Related Groups: A Practitioner's Guide. Trenton, New Jersey State Department of Health, 1983

Grimaldi P: DRG's & nursing administration. Nurs Manage 13:30–34, 1982

Simborg D: Rational staffing of hospital nursing service by functional activity budgeting. Pub Health Rep. 91:118–121, 1976

Simborg D: Technology in hospitals—the effects of prospective reimbursement. In Dayhoff R (ed): Proceedings of the Seventh Annual Symposium on Computer Applications in Medical Care, pp 19–22. Silver Spring, MD: IEEE Computer Society Press, 1983

Tri-Service Medical Information Systems: TRIMIS fact sheets. Bethesda, MD, Tri-Service Medical Information Systems, 1983

11 Community Health Applications

Objectives

- Describe computer systems available for community health and ambulatory care agencies.
- Describe the various types of computerized management information systems (MISs) found in community health nursing agencies.
- Describe the major ambulatory care systems.
- Describe the various types of special purpose computer applications used for community health studies, programs, and projects.

COMMUNITY HEALTH NURSING

Community health nursing focuses on care of all people in the community except those acutely ill persons who are hospitalized. Community health nursing practice, commonly known as public health nursing, combines nursing and public health practice to promote and preserve health. General and comprehensive, community health nursing is not limited to a particular age or diagnostic group and is continuing rather than episodic. Health promotion, health maintenance, health education, and coordinated continuity of care are used holistically with clients alone, families, and groups.

Today, national goals for health promotion and disease prevention deal with preventing major health problems at each principal stage of life: infancy, childhood, adolescence and young adulthood, adulthood, and older adulthood (U.S. Department of Health, Education and Welfare, 1979).

Nurses provide community health nursing services in homes, clinics, schools, and a variety of health care centers. Nurses are employed by state and local community health care agencies or official health departments, combination agencies, and nonofficial agencies such as visiting nurse associations. Also included in community health are home health agencies, which provide home care services, and health maintenance organizations (HMOs), which provide ambulatory care services.

The 1979 survey of community health agencies found approximately 5600 state and local community health agencies, excluding boards of education, employing some 63,000 nurses in the United States and its territories. Of this number, 54.9% were state and local official agencies, 22.9% were nonofficial agencies, including organized categorical programs, and 22.2% were organized home health agencies (U.S. Department of Health and Human Services, 1982). The number of agencies continues to grow, especially in the areas of home care and HMOs.

Background

Community health agencies have used computers for more than 20 years, primarily to process and generate statistics from patient to client visit data collected on punched cards. The Social Security Amendments of 1965 (PL 89-97), commonly referred to as Medicare and Medicaid, expanded the scope of community health care, including home health care services. Reimbursement for these services substantially increased, broadening the availability of community and home health services. In addition, the information required for reimbursement created a major demand for computerized information systems.

As a result of these amendments, the community and home health services available for homebound sick persons increased substantially, from 55.6% who used such services in 1963 to 91.8% in 1974 and 98.3% in 1979 (U.S. Department of Health and Human Services, 1982). Coverage increased as the number of community and home health agencies certified by the Social Security Administration also increased, from approximately 2000 agencies in 1974 to 3196 agencies in 1979 to 5053 in 1984.

Several activities influenced the development of computers in community and home health. First, many projects were initiated to develop out-of-institution computerized information systems to manage community health agencies (see Chap. 1). Second, many large community health agencies began to develop their own computerized information systems. Finally, some service bureaus and vendors started offering computerized information services in the community health field.

Forty of these early systems, described in a book published by the National League for Nursing (NLN), operated in a variety of visiting nurse associations (nonofficial) and in state and local official health departments. They included financial, billing, and statistical reporting systems. The book provided an analysis of each of these systems, with a flowchart depicting the computer processing configuration along with other pertinent information (NLN, 1978) (Fig. 11-1).

As community health programs expanded, the advantages of computerization became evident, and several models emerged. A community health nursing assessment tool (Taylor and Johnson, 1974) and a patient problem classification scheme (Simmons, 1980) for community health nursing also were developed for computerization. The special statistical studies, screening programs such as monitoring immunization status and audiovisual screening of children, epidemiological projects, and other prevention projects and programs that emerged also required computer systems.

Models

The community health nursing models have been developed as frameworks for community health information systems. They identified necessary database content to make the systems operable.

NLN Statistical Reporting Model

The most widely used model in community health nursing is the NLN statistical reporting model. It identifies the content needed for a computerized management information system (MIS) for community health nursing agencies (National League for Nursing, 1977).

This document contains the procedures for collecting, using, and analyzing statistical information for community health and home care. Also included are samples of agencies' data collection forms. The NLN recommends that the statistical information needed be divided into five areas (Fig. 11-2):

Legal requirements
Patients' rights

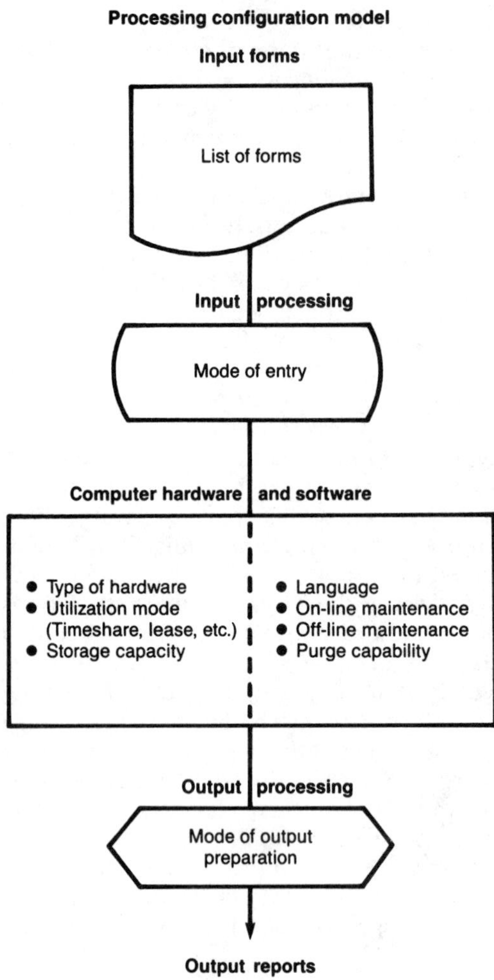

FIG. 11-1. Processing configuration of a management information system. Selected management information systems for public health/community health agencies. New York (Courtesy National League for Nursing, 1978)

Fiscal accountability
Program planning and evaluation
Community planning

Client Management Information System Model

Another community health nursing model is one that illustrates a management information system for community health nursing clients (Simmons, 1980) (Fig. 11-3). This model illustrates how the patient problem classification scheme, developed by the Visiting Nurse Association of Omaha, can be adapted to a computer system. Coded client problem data can be entered separately as input into a computerized MIS and integrated with other data to provide management reports, which can be used to assist in supervising patients and administering agency programs.

Visits to individuals
Basic data set

Case record data	Statistical reporting			
	On admission and revisit		On discharge	
	Minimum	Supplementary	Minimum	Supplementary
Demographic data and related information				
Name and unique ID number	X		X	
Residence address				
Living arrangements		X		X
Date of birth	X		X	
Sex	X			X
Race/ethnicity	X		X	
Marital status				
Usual occupation				
Place of birth				
Education				
Employment status				
Total family income				
Individual attributes				
Primary diagnosis or problem	X		X	
Additional diagnoses/problems		X		X
Functional status (physical, mental, social, etc.)		X		X
Service and administrative elements				
Source of referral and date		X		X
Source of medical (physician) care		X		X
Date of admission	X		X	
Type of visit (first, revisit, last)	X		X	
Site where service is rendered		X		X
Discipline of person providing service	X		X	
Date of service	X		X	
Primary diagnosis (care related)	X		X	
Category of program (as appropriate to agency)		X		X
Time spent (when appropriate)	X		X	
Reimbursement source(s) (when appropriate)	X		X	
Date of discharge from service (last visit)			X	
Reason for discharge				X
Disposition (when appropriate)				X

FIG. 11-2. National League of Nursing statistical reporting model. Indented items represent information in addition to usual minimum requirements. Statistical reporting of Home and Community Health Services. New York (Courtesy National League of Nursing, 1977)

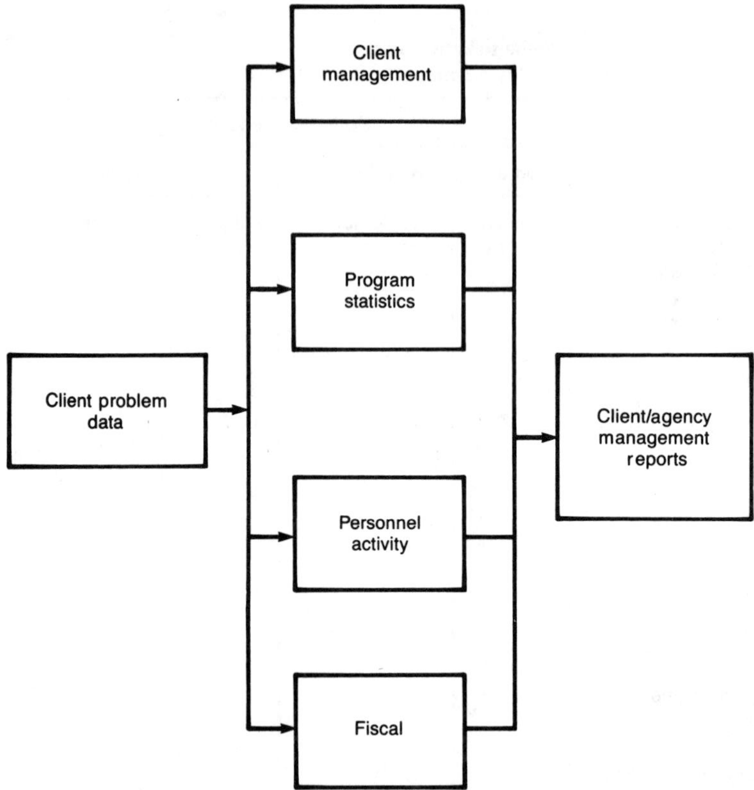

FIG. 11-3. A client management information system model. (Simmons DA: A classification scheme for client problems in community health nursing [nurse planning information series, vol 14] [NTIS no. HRP-0501501]. Springfield, VA, National Technical Information Series, 1980)

The four basic modules in this system model are as follows:

Client management
Personnel activity
Fiscal statistics
Program statistics

Data can be integrated in all the modules. The modules contain the following:

1. Client management module: Client demographic characteristics, problems, and information such as health status
2. Personnel activity module: Activities of personnel providing client care, time cards, payroll history, and other information
3. Fiscal module: Client invoices, agency chart of accounts, agency expenditures, and funding sources
4. Program statistics module: Client management, demographics, personnel activity, and fiscal data

Ambulatory Care Nursing Model

The ambulatory care nursing model, developed by Verran (1981), provides a classification system for nursing care in ambulatory care settings. Ambulatory care is considered to contain the full range of nursing practice in out-of-institution settings. The model contains and defines the content for seven areas of responsibility in ambulatory care nursing:

Patient counseling
Health care maintenance
Preventive care
Primary care
Patient education
Therapeutic care
Normative care

Each of these areas is delineated in Figure 11-4. This model, developed from a research study, has been tested by the Delphi method with a panel of experts. It provides not only a framework for a computerized MIS but also the structure for evaluating ambulatory nursing care.

Scope of Computer Applications

Computer applications in community health focus not only on community health nursing services but also on the programs administered by various types of community health agencies, including home health. They are aided by computerized MISs used to administer the different types of community health agencies as well as to document the delivery of patient care.

Other computer systems, developed especially to collect, store, and process statistics applicable to community health nursing programs, include the following:

- Community health MISs
- Ambulatory care systems
- Special-purpose applications

COMMUNITY HEALTH MANAGEMENT INFORMATION SYSTEMS

Definition

A MIS has been described as an organized system that manages the flow of information in the proper time frame and thus assists in the decision-making process (Kennevan, 1974; Saba, 1974).

A computerized MIS in a community health setting serves to satisfy growing demands for information. The specific benefits of such a system in community health include the following:

Increased statistical information required by local, state, and federal governments
Reports to facilitate management of agency resources
Precise information on billing patients, which in turn improves agency cash flow
Information essential to program planning and budgeting

Such a system also helps identify community needs and evaluate the impact of out-of-hospital nursing on community health conditions (Saba, 1982a, 1982b).

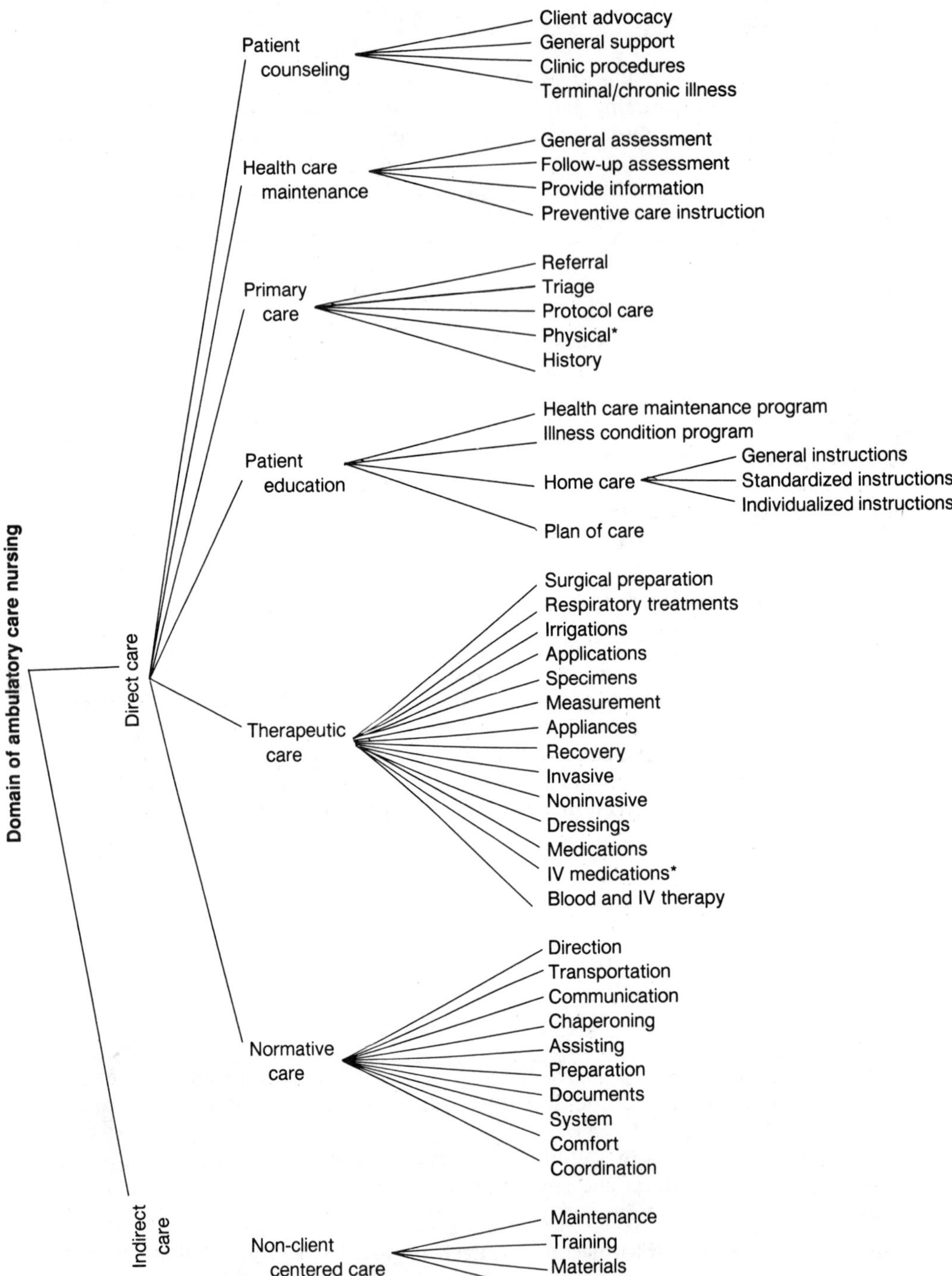

FIG. 11-4. An ambulatory care model for taxonomy of domain of ambulatory care nursing. Consensus not achieved. (Verran J: Delineation of ambulatory care nursing practice. J Ambul Care Nurs 4(2): 7, 1981)

According to the 1979 Survey of Community Health Nursing, approximately 26 state departments of health reported having a computerized information system for processing information on nursing personnel, community health nursing programs, or nursing services. Furthermore, the majority of community health nursing agencies with more than 50 nurses reported having some type of computerized information system (U.S. Department of Health and Human Services, 1982).

Three types of community health MISs are usually found in community health agencies. Used to provide the various applications unique to community health nursing services, they include the following:

- Financial and billing systems
- Statistical reporting systems
- Patient care systems

Financial and Billing Systems

Financial and billing systems are found mainly in large visiting nurse associations and other voluntary agencies that administer programs of home care. These systems are designed to furnish information essential for payment by Medicare and Medicaid and other third-party payers.

These systems use data collected from a variety of forms — an admission form, a plan of treatment, an activity form, and a patient encounter form completed by providers. Further, providers generally collect and record eligibility data for the Medicare form as required by the Health Care Finance Administration. However, when microcomputers are used, "menus" and "templates" are designed and formatted for data entry. Such screens are essentially used to enter the same data as collected on the paper forms (Figs. 11-5 to 11-8).

The financial and billing systems provide such applications as general ledger, accounts receivable, accounts payable, and payroll and billing and, in some cases, actually prepare patient bills. Such systems also generate financial reports such as costs per visit and personnel costs. Some of these systems may offer statistical information and management statistics on patient visits and services received.

Statistical Reporting Systems

Statistical reporting systems are mainly found in large local or state health departments and other official agencies that administer programs of health promotion and disease prevention. Designed to furnish statistics needed to manage patient services, these systems provide such applications as visit reports and patient services statistics. They collect and summarize management data on nursing visits and services in the clinic, school, and home, and they provide statistics needed to obtain block grant monies or federal, state, or local funds. Family planning, immunization, early periodic screening and testing, maternal and infant care, care of children and youth, crippled children, tuberculosis, and drug abuse programs, all of which have reporting requirements, may benefit from the systems.

Further, statistical reporting systems provide other applications needed to manage nursing services, including patient registration, caseload registries, census, and home, clinic, and school visit summaries. They may schedule patients for appointments, and they may even offer software packages that prepare the agency payroll and manage personnel data.

ADMISSION AND START OF CARE NOTICE

1. PATIENT'S LAST NAME | FIRST NAME | MI | 2. HEALTH INSURANCE CLAIM NUMBER

3. PATIENT'S ADDRESS (Street number, City, State, Zip Code) | 4. DATE OF BIRTH | 5. SEX ☐ M ☐ F

6. HOME HEALTH AGENCY NAME AND ADDRESS | 7. PROVIDER NO. | 8. MEDICAL RECORD NO. | 9. NAME AND ADDRESS OF ATTENDING PHYSICIAN

10. DATE CARE STARTED | 11. NAME AND ADDRESS OF INSTITUTION, IF ANY, CARING FOR CONDITION LATER REQUIRING HOME HEALTH FROM TO PRIOR: LAST: | 12. VERIFIED DATES OF STAY IN ITEM 11 FROM TO | 13. DATE HOME HEALTH PLAN ESTABLISHED

14. PAYMENT SOURCE FOR CHARGES TO PATIENT
A. ☐ SELF OR FAMILY
B. ☐ PRIVATE INSURANCE
C. ☐ BLUE CROSS BLUE SHIELD
D. ☐ EMPLOYER OR UNION
E. ☐ PUBLIC AGENCY (Give name)
F. ☐ OTHER (Explain) [ ]

[ ] *

15. PATIENT'S CERTIFICATION: AUTHORIZATION TO RELEASE INFORMATION AND PAYMENT REQUEST: I certify that the information given by me in applying for payment under Title XVIII of the Social Security Act is correct. I authorize release of all records required to act on this request. I request that payment of authorized benefits be made in my behalf.

SIGNATURE: (Patient or authorized representative) (Signature by mark must be witnessed) | DATE

SIGNATURE ON FILE

16. PRIMARY DIAGNOSES | EMPLOYMENT RELATED A. ☐ YES B. ☐ NO (If yes, give name and address of employer) | LEAVE BLANK

PRIMARY:
SECONDARY:
SECONDARY:

ADDITIONAL REQUIRED INFORMATION

SOURCES OF PAYMENT

	MEDICARE Part A	MEDICARE Part B	MEDICAID
Is Entitled	1○	1○	1○ *
Not Eligible	2○	2○	2○

19○ Private Full Pay
20○ Part Pay (See special rates)
21○ No Fee
Other Payor (Code) ☐☐

STATISTICAL DATA

New Admission ○1
Readmission
Same Diagnosis ○2
New Diagnosis ○3

Diagnosis Code ☐☐
Referral Source ☐
Ethnic ☐
(California) Medi-Cal Reason Code ☐
Area ☐☐☐
Location ☐☐

BILL TO NAME, ADDRESS

OTHER THIRD PARTY NUMBER

SPECIAL RATES (part pay patients)

Discipline | Rate | H/V | Mode

EFFECTIVE DATE OF THIS ADMISSION: Mo. Day Yr.

NOTE: If patient born before 1900, mark here ○1

FIG. 11-5. An example of an "admission and start of care" form. (Courtesy IMI Heath Systems, 1985)

```
SOC01                              START OF CARE                          mm-dd-yy
PGM VER NBR                                                           PAGE 1 OF 2
 ---------------------------------- MESSAGES ------------------------------------
|                                                                                |
|                                                                                |
 --------------------------------------------------------------------------------

    CYCLE DATE   BATCH #   TRANS COUNT

    COMPUTER BATCH TOTALS:

RECORD #:                                                        ERRORS:

  PATIENT DATA                                   DATES & INSTITUTIONS
 Medical Rec #:                               Eff Admit Date:
                                             Care Start Date:
          Name:                                    Plan Date:
       Address:                                Pat Sign Date:
City State ZIP:
                                               Hospital Name:
     Birthdate:           Century:             Hospital Stay Dates
           Sex:                                   From:              Thru:

         HIC #:                               Prior Hospital:
     Medicaid #:                               Prior Stay Dates
      Co-Payor:                                   From:              Thru:

SOURC OF PYMNT           STATISTICAL DATA            SPECIAL RATES
Medicare A:                   Admit Code:            DISC  RATE   H/V MD
Medicare B:               Diagnosis Code:
  Medicaid:              Referral Source:
     Other:                       Ethnic:
                          Medical Reason:
OTHER THIRD PARTY                   Area:
                                Location:

                BILL-TO                              PHYSICIAN DATA

        Name:                        Name:
     Address:                     Address:
        City:                        City:
```

FIG. 11-6. An example of a "start of care" microcomputer template screen. (Courtesy IMI Health Systems, 1985)

Patient Care Systems

Patient care systems, found primarily in large community health agencies and ambulatory care facilities, focus on patient–nurse encounter information and document the patient care process. Such systems, which generally contain a patient database of demographic data, patient history, nursing assessment, and care data, can usually be programmed to track and audit information on care provided.

These systems provide patient profiles, medical orders, care surveillance, problem lists, medication profiles, time-oriented flowcharts, care plans, patient visit reports, and treatment plans (Figs. 11-9 to 11-11).

The administrative advantages of patient care record systems, sometimes called ambulatory record systems, are numerous. They generally provide not only patient care information but also financial, billing, and statistical information. Such record

Is Client Aware of Referral? ______

THE VISITING NURSE ASSOCIATION OF OMAHA

Date ______

FOR VNA USE ONLY

Household No. ______ C. T. ______

District ______ Notified ______ Dictated ______

Source ______ Phone ______

Payment Discussed ______ Prev. VNA Record ______ Date ______

VNA Acct. No. ______ Medicare No. ______ Medicaid No. ______ Insurance No. ______

Patient Name ______ Birthdate ______ Sex ______ Marital Status ______

Spouse/Other ______ Birthdate ______ Sex ______ Marital Status ______

Phone ______ Street ______ City ______ Zip ______

Emergency Contact Name ______ Relationship ______ Phone ______

Hospital ______ Dates __/__/__ to __/__/__ SNF ______ Dates __/__/__ to __/__/__

Physician ______ Address ______ Phone ______

Physician ______ Address ______ Phone ______

Primary Diagnosis ______

Secondary Diagnosis ______

Mental Status ______ Safety ______ Diet ______ Rehab Potential ______ Prognosis ______

Functional Limitations ______

Reason for Referral ______

Suggested Frequency of Visit: Nursing ______ Physical Therapy ______ Speech Therapy ______ Home Health Aide ______ Companion Aide ______

Explanation of Care Requested: Treatments, Dressings, Injections, Teaching, Observation, Evaluation, Other. ______

Medication and Dosage: ______

Supplies: ______

R.N. Signature ______

M.D. Signature ______

RF-1 (8-83)

FIG. 11-7. An example of a "patient admission" paper form. (Courtesy Visiting Nurse Association of Omaha)

```
1/04/85                PATIENT  INFORMATION  RECORD                         PAGE   1
-------------------------------------------------------------------------------------

Household #:    25226                                   Station: NORTH DISTRICT
Address 1:   23 GREEN STREET                              Phone: 402 874-1629
Address 2:                                        Census Tract:  13.01
City/St/Zip: OMAHA              NE 68111        Monthly Income:    520
Directions:

                                ACCOUNTS IN HOUSEHOLD
Patient's Name:                     Account #:   Birth Date:      Rel. to HH:
EWING, GEORGE                           25226     2/16/1906       HEAD OF HOUSEHOLD
EWING, MARTHA                           25227    10/17/1908 -NA   WIFE
-------------------------------------------------------------------------------------
-------------------------------------------------------------------------------------
Patient's Name:                     Account #:
EWING, GEORGE                           25226

** EMERGENCY INFORMATION            Relation:  Address:                   Phone:
   EWING, GEORGE JR.                SON        896 SEQUOIA ST             402 926-1478

** ADMISSION INFORMATION
   Soc Sec #:     205-27-3289           Rel. to HH: HH- HEAD OF HOUSEHOLD
   Birth Date:      2/16/1906             Religion:  2- PROTESTANT
   Admit Date:      9/17/84          Referral Code: UNIV. OF NEBRASKA MEDICAL CNTR
   Refer Date:      9/16/84                Program: 202 - HOME HEALTH CARE
   1st Contact:     9/17/84                   Race: 01- CAUCASIAN
   Care Started:    9/17/84                    Sex: MALE
   Plan Establ.:    9/16/84            Marital Sts: MARRIED
   Discharged:      0/00/00        Discharge Reason:
   Special Instructions:
   ICDA Diagnosis:           DIABETES MELLITUS WITHOUT COMPLICATIONS
                             EMPHYSEMA

** DIAGNOSIS INFORMATION
   21       DIABETES
   140      RESPIRATORY SYS DISORDERS

** FUNDING SOURCES                 Billing #:          Comment:            Effect Date:
   01- MEDICARE                    205-27-3289

** EMPLOYER  -     /

** OTHER AGENCIES                  Contact:                         Phone:

                                                        Orders Cover
** PHYSICIAN INFORMATION                              From Date:   To Date:
   BROWN, JAMES R.                       12441        9/17/84     11/15/84
```

FIG. 11-8. An example of a "computer-generated admission." (Courtesy Visiting Nurse Association of Omaha)

systems are generally on-line, real-time integrated systems that allow for interaction between users and patients' files. They can also be used to classify and schedule patients, determine staffing requirements, and cost nursing care.

These systems can be used by all members of the health care team of a community health agency to assist in delivery of patient care. They can be used by the following:

- Policymakers to assist in planning and evaluating community health status
- Administrators to assist in establishing more efficient and effective management practices
- Staff nurses to assist in managing and auditing patients care
- Patients themselves to help understand their care

```
                                                        10/07/82 4:30 PM
BORDON, LIZZIE L                        B805-8022-4     F
000 HATCHETT LANE                                       COMP. ID:116      W
APT #201                                                PHONE:000-00000
HATCHET, NOWHERE                                        NONE
000000                                                  000-00-0000
13K               BIRTHDATE: 01/21/1879                 (103 YRS)
BROWARD COUNTY
STATUS: ADMITTED/ACTIVE
. . . . . . . . . . . . . . . . . . . CARE PLAN . . . . . . . . . . . . . . . . .
----------------------------VISIT SCHEDULE FOR RN----------------------------
CURRENT SCHEDULE : QD - EVERY DAY
VISIT UNITS: 1

COMMENTS: Prob# 1 Urinary Elimination, Impairment of: Retention
                  *inserted cath 4/28; next change approx 5/28
          Prob# 2 Thought Process, Impaired
                  *impaired attention span, distractibility

----------------------------VISIT SCHEDULE FOR HHA---------------------------
CURRENT SCHEDULE : Q2D - EVERY OTHER DAY
VISIT UNITS: 1

COMMENTS: Prob# 3 Self-Care Deficit, Bathing, Grooming
                  *inability to obtain or get to water source
                  *intolerance to activity

----------------------------VISIT SCHEDULE FOR PT----------------------------
CURRENT SCHEDULE : 2XW - 2 TIMES A WEEK
SCHEDULE:      MON  TUE  WED  THU  FRI  SAT  SUN
VISIT UNITS:    1              1

COMMENTS: PROB #4  Mobility, Impaired Physical
                   *limited active joint range of motion

------------------------------------MEDICATIONS------------------------------------
05/05/82 : DIGOXIN .5MG QOD
           RX: 000000  ORDERED BY HELP, DR GOOD  Hold if pulse goes below 60
05/05/82 : LASIX 40MQD
           RX: 22202  ORDERED BY HELP, DR GOOD
05/05/82 : Dilantin 1 cap qhs
           RX: 22222  ORDERED BY HELP, DR GOOD
05/05/82 : Insulin U100  25 units qam
           RX:    ORDERED BY WACKS, DR FORTY
PHAR: Medi-co  123-4567
PHAR: Village Drugs  345-2345
------------------------------------TREATMENTS------------------------------------
05/03/82 : (ORDERED BY HELP, DR GOOD)
           Clean wounds with sterile H20
05/22/82 : (ORDERED BY HELP, DR GOOD)
           Apply DSD during day, leave to air at HS (left ankle)
05/22/82 : (ORDERED BY HELP, DR GOOD)
           Change foley q month
05/22/82 : (ORDERED BY HELP, DR GOOD)
           Irrigation /c N/S prn- teach family
05/22/82 : (ORDERED BY HELP, DR GOOD)
           Foley # 20 with 30cc
05/22/82 : (ORDERED BY WACKS, DR FORTY)
           Draw FBS on 5-23-82
```

FIG. 11-9. An example of a computer-generated "care plan." (Computer Resources Inc. STAT: The Complete Home Health Information System. Fort Lauderdale, FL, Computer Resources, Inc., 1984)

Integrated patient care information systems can measure and evaluate the quality of patient care as well as improve and standardize the documentation of community health nursing. They can be used to network the documentation of patient care in and out of institutions, including the patient's use of other health care resources, thus reflecting a totality of care by tracking the patient throughout the care process (Saba, 1982b, 1983a).

VISITING NURSE ASSOCIATION OF HOUSTON, INC.
3100 TIMMONS LANE, SUITE 200 • HOUSTON, TEXAS 77027 • (713) 840-7744
PHYSICIAN'S PLAN OF TREATMENT

DATE MAILED TO DR. 12/19/1984
PHONE
PHONE
REC'D

PATIENT NO.	MEDICARE NO.	MEDICAID NO.	CT	TEAM	D.O.B.	SEX	PHONE
000034803-7	454053973D	500692135	0317	SCBT	09/02/1910	F	713-7473928

PATIENT NAME (L)	(F)	(M)
BUTLER	ERMA	

ADDRESS	CITY	COUNTY	STATE	ZIP
3906 DAPHNE	HOUSTON	HARRIS	TX	000077021

RELATIVE'S NAME	RELATIVE PHONE	RELATIONSHIP

SOURCE OF REFERRAL #	NAME	PHONE
0100005	BTGH 1502 TAUB LOOP, HOUSTON, TX.	(713) 791-7000

CLINIC NO.	PHYSICIAN NO.	PHYSICIAN'S NAME	PHONE
0012046057	0300092	BEN TAUB STAFF PHYSICIAN	(713) 791-7000

ADDRESS	CITY	COUNTY	STATE	ZIP
1502 TAUB LOOP	HOUSTON,		TX	000077030

DOES PATIENT KNOW DIAGNOSIS? YES
CAN PATIENT OR FAMILY BE TAUGHT TO GIVE: TREATMENT? YES INJECTION? NO

MENTAL STATUS	PROGNOSIS	PHYSICAL/FUNCTIONAL LIMITATIONS
ALERT	FAIR	INCONTINENT BLADDER & BOWEL

DIAGNOSIS
428.0 CONGESTIVE HEART FAILURE

HOSPITAL DISCHARGE DIAGNOSIS (Including surgical procedure)

HOSPITAL	ADDRESS	ADMITTED	DISCHARGED
BEN TAUB GENERAL	1502 TAUB LOOP	11/23/1984	12/07/1984

CLINIC APPOINTMENTS	PLANS FOR DISCHARGE OR REFERRAL
SEE SLIP	HOME CARE

ACTIVITIES PERMITTED	SUGGESTED VISIT FREQUENCY
AS TOL	SEE MEDS

TREATMENT & INSTRUCTIONS	MEDICATIONS
VS & BP Q VISIT. S\I DSG CHG TO FOOT ULCER WET-DRY BID. OBS FOR SIDE EFFECTS MEDS., HEALING OF ULCER. CHG IN MENTAL STATUS & ANY VAG BLEEDING. ENC. TO SET UP IN CHAIR & AMB AS TOL. ASSIST WITH TRANSP. PRN TO CLINIC.	NITROPASTE 1INCH Q6H, COLACE 100MG PO TID DUCOLAX TABS 2 PO QHS PRN CONSTIPATION. MYLANTA 30CC PO Q3H P RN INDG. TYLENOL 2 PO Q4H PRN PAIN DIGOXIN 0.125MG Q AM, LASIX 40MG Q AM, HYDRALAZINE 50MG BID SLOWK 2QAM NURSING DAILY X 10 INCLUDING WKENDS THEN 3 X WK UNTIL ULCER HEALS

DIET	ALLERGIES
2GM NA	NKA

PT. SPECIFY: Amount/Frequency/Duration
OT SPECIFY: Amount/Frequency/Duration
MSW SPECIFY: Amount/Frequency/Duration
SPEECH/LANGUAGE SPECIFY: Amount/Frequency/Duration
NUTR SPECIFY: Amount/Frequency/Duration

REHABILITATION POTENTIAL: FAIR SAFETY MEASURES: PREVENT INFECTION
EQUIPMENT NEEDED HOW LONG?
HOME HEALTH AIDE 2 X WK times per week for personal care and other duties as directed by the Registered Nurse or Therapist

ORDERS REC'D BY: T. MOORE, RN S PHONE ☐ MAIL ☐ STAFF #

DATE CARE ESTABLISHED	VISITED BY	DATE OF FIRST VISIT
12/12/1984		

NOTE: The above orders are effective for 60 days. If services are needed for a longer period, it will be necessary for the physician to review the treatment plan and sign a new TREATMENT Plan Form. SERVICE COVERAGE DATES: FROM 12/12/1984 **TO** 02/09/1985

THE PATIENT, WHO IS UNDER MY CARE, IS ESSENTIALLY HOMEBOUND FOR HEALTH REASONS AND IS IN NEED OF INTERMITTENT HOME VISITS ACCORDING TO THE ABOVE TREATMENT PLAN.

PHYSICIAN'S SIGNATURE ____________________ DATE: __________

DOCTOR, PLEASE SIGN & RETURN TO V.N.A.

FIG. 11-10. An example of a "plan of treatment" paper form. (Courtesy Visiting Nurse Association of Houston, Inc.)

System Options

Most of the community health MISs, regardless of type, are obtained in similar ways. The agency can design its own system, including obtaining its own hardware and software, purchase a complete stand-alone system, or contract to timeshare or purchase system services from a service bureau or vendor. Many of the service bureaus or vendors offer several different options, including the following:

PHYSICIAN'S PLAN OF TREATMENT
MODIFICATION TO PLAN

CRI HOME HEALTH AGENCY
6289 W SUNRISE BLVD, STE 117 FORT LAUDERDALE, FL. 33313
(305) 791-6080

PATIENT BORDON, LIZZIE L
000 HATCHETT LANE
HATCHET, NOWHERE 000000
PHONE 000-00000
D.O.B. 01/21/1879
HIC# 000-00-0000A
MR# B805-8022-4
PAT ID# 116
ADMIT 05/05/82
EXPECTED SERVICE: 3 Months
SPECIAL SUPPLIES: Bed; 4x4 sterile gauze

PHYSICIAN DR FORTY WACKS
00A HATCHET STREET
SUITE 201
HATCHET, NOWHERE 000000
000-0000
POST INSTITUTIONAL CARE?
PROGNOSIS: fair
REHAB POTENTIAL: fair
TEACH FAMILY AND/OR SIGNIFICANT OTHER : Yes
VITAL SIGNS: B/P: 100/60; T-99.9; P-80-100; R-24

DIAGNOSES
INJ INNOMIN/SUBCLAV VEIN (9013); ANEMIA NEC (2858); DRUG MENTAL DISORDER NEC (29289);

SURGICAL PROCEDURES
09/02/81 SKIN TRANSPLANTS
09/02/81 SUTURING

ACTIVITIES PERMITTED: PRN WALK

ONSET OF ILLNESS: 3-23-81
DIET: Hold- start beet juice in 2 wks-100cc/hour
ALLERGIES: METAL

- -

Nursing Services (QD)
MONITOR: vital signs and symptoms; ASSESS: cardiopulomonary status.
EDUCATE: patient in proper use of axe. TEACH: aiming techniques; potential side effects of improper administration.

------MEDICATIONS-----
05/05/82 Insulin U100 25 units qam

I hereby certify that the above services are required for my patient who is primarily confined to his home for health reasons.

____
Physician's signature

FIG. 11-11. An example of a computer-generated "plan of treatment." (Computer Resources Inc. STAT: The Complete Home Health Information System. Fort Lauderdale, FL, Computer Resources, Inc., 1984)

- Batch processing
- Remote entry
- Complete package

Batch Processing

Many service bureaus still offer automated batch processing, whereby the service bureau uses its own computerized MIS to store and process the agency's data. In this option the agency sends patient and visit data forms (paper) to the service bureau. The service bureau edits the forms, enters the data into its system, and then batch processes them. The service bureau is also responsible for preparing patients' bills and producing financial, statistical, and other reports for the agency.

Remote Entry

Another option offered by service bureaus or vendors is remote entry, whereby the service bureau also uses its own computerized MIS to store and process a community or home health agency's data. In this instance, however, the service bureau receives the patient and visit data through an on-line terminal or a microcomputer. A computer terminal or microcomputer, installed in the community or home health agency, transmits data over telephone lines to the service bureau's computer facility. The service bureau generally trains agency personnel to edit and enter data for transmission. The service bureau is responsible for processing data, preparing patients' bills, and producing financial, statistical, and other reports for the agency. If the service bureau installs a microcomputer in the agency, the agency can use it for other applications, such as word processing. The service bureau may even offer the agency special stand-alone software packages, such as a personnel system, to run on the microcomputer.

Complete Package

The complete package option, also called a *turnkey* system, is generally a stand-alone computerized MIS installed by the service bureau or vendor in the community or home health agency. With this option, the agency stores, processes, and controls its own patient and visit data. The service bureau provides the agency with all the necessary hardware—a mainframe, minicomputer, or microcomputer—and any other required peripheral equipment. The service bureau also provides the software needed to run the MIS, including all computer programs or software packages prepared for that particular agency. The service bureau or vendor generally trains agency users on how to run the system and maintains and updates the software. In some cases it even services the hardware for the agency. The agency can use the computer system for other applications.

Service Bureau/Vendor Systems

Many service bureaus or vendors offer an MIS for community and home health care agencies. These systems, primarily designed for management and administration of community and home health nursing services, provide financial, billing, and statistical applications and, sometimes, patient care applications. The more common ones are described below and listed in Table 11-1:

- Computer Resources, Inc.
- Delta Computer Systems, Inc.
- Fleet Information Systems, Inc.
- IMI Health Systems, Inc.

TABLE 11-1 *List of Selected Service Bureaus and Vendors of Community Health Information Systems*

Accounting Corporation of America
1505 Commonwealth Ave.
Boston, MA 02135
Home Health Care

Allen Associates, Inc.
968 Main Street, Box G122
Wakefield, MA 01880
VMIS Home Health Care Management Information System

Comprehensive Management Health Care System
555 Metro Place North, Suite 200
Dublin, OH 43017
Comprehensive Management Health Care System

Computer Resources, Inc.
Suite 117, 6289 W. Sunrise Blvd.
Ft. Lauderdale, FL 33313
STAT

Creative Socio-Medics Corp.
16 E. 32nd St.
New York, NY 10016
Comprehensive Systems for the Health Field

Delta Computer Systems Inc.
P.O. Box 1824
Altoona, PA 16603
Home Health Management System

Fleet Information Systems, Inc. (Formerly Information Sciences Inc.)
125 Dupont Drive
Providence, RI 02906
Home Health Systems

Information Management International Inc. (Formerly Diversified Computer Applications)
1101 S. Winchester Blvd.
San Jose, CA 95128
and
151 Lavan St.
Warwick, RI 02888
IMI Health Systems

InfoMed
1101 State Road, Building J
Princeton, NJ 08540
Home Health Care Information Systems

Minicomputer Consultants Data Services, Inc.
Two Glenhardie Corporate Center
Suite 100, 1285 Drummers Lane
Wayne, PA 19087
Automation for Health Care Providers

New York Information Systems
1653 E. Main St.
Rochester, New York 14609
Home Health Care Management Information System

Omaha Health Resources'
10828 Harney Circle
Omaha, NB 68154
Management Information System for Home and Community Health Care

Picker Business Systems
2321 Cromwell Hills Dr.
Cromwell, CT 06416
Microcomputer Software

Pierson, Miller & Young
310 N. Hammes St.
Joliet, IL 60435
Management System for Home Health Agencies

Q.S., Inc. Systems Group
P.O. Box 847
Greenville, SC 20602
Health Management Information Software

Visiting Nurse Association of Houston, Inc.
3100 Timmons Lane, Suite 200
Houston, TX 77027
and
Benchmark Computer Systems, Inc.
3715 Dacoma
Houston, TX 77092
Casalud

- InfoMed
- Q.S., Inc.

Computer Resources, Inc.

Computer Resources, Inc. (CRI) offers a complete on-line integrated home health management information system called STAT, which is designed to provide financial/billing applications for home health visits. It also provides patient and personnel statistics and clinical applications including medical orders, treatments plans, and discharge summaries. CRI only offers STAT as a complete package or turnkey system, including hardware (an on-line minicomputer or hard disk microcomputer system). All necessary software, written in the high-language MUMPS, is also included (Computer Resources, 1984).

Delta Computer Systems, Inc.

Delta Computer Systems offers an in-house home health management system (HHMS) to community health nursing agencies that provides financial billing, and statistical reporting applications primarily for home visiting nursing services. Delta uses its own minicomputer system to process patient and visit data from its customers. It offers two options—batch processing and remote entry. Delta either obtains agency data from forms, sent weekly by agencies through a courier service, or receives the data through a remote entry microcomputer (Delta Computer Systems, 1984).

Fleet Information Systems, Inc.

Fleet Information Systems, formerly known as Information Sciences, Inc. (ISI), offers an in-house home health system for community and home health agencies with two options—batch processing or on-line remote entry to timeshare the Fleet computer system. In this case, the Fleet system is used not only to store and process the agency data but is accessed directly by the agency to interact with its own database. The agency thus uses the on-line terminal to edit and transmit data to the system and to query and communicate with its own database (Fleet Information Systems, 1984).

IMI Health Systems, Inc.

IMI Health Systems (IMI), formerly known as Diversified Computer Applications, offers its in-house MEDI-VISIT computer systems for home care providers. This system provides financial, billing, and statistical applications and some patient care treatment plans. IMI offers three processing options (IMI Health Systems, 1984):

1. MEDI-VISIT, the first option and the oldest, is batch processing.
2. MEDI-VISITplus, the next level, is the on-line remote entry option, consisting of a microcomputer installed in the agency to edit and transmit data to the IMI facilities.
3. MEDI-VISIT/TOPS, a stand-alone complete package system, enables IMI to install, service, and update a complete home care system using a minicomputer.

InfoMed

InfoMed also offers its home health care information systems to home health agencies. It provides financial, billing, and statistical applications for home visiting services, using its in-house system to process an agency's patient and visit data. InfoMed offers its customers either batch processing or on-line remote entry. The remote entry consists of a microcomputer installed in the agency to edit and transmit data for processing to the InfoMed central facility. Several other stand-alone software packages, such as payroll, personnel, and word processing, are also offered.

Q.S., Inc.

Q.S., Inc. (QSI) offers an integrated, on-line, patient-oriented medical information system, primarily with statistical and administrative applications, for community health agencies providing clinic services. Some of its uses include patient registration, patient scheduling, immunization and patient tracking. Each of these applications are stand-alone modules that can perform a specific function or that can be combined to form a multifunction information system. QSI offers a complete package consisting of a minicomputer with specific software applications (Q.S., Inc., 1982; Saba, 1982a).

Local Management Information Systems

Many local community health management information systems have also been developed and designed by local community health nursing agencies, primarily to focus on agency reporting requirements. These systems vary depending on whether the agency is official or nonofficial. Official agency systems generally consist of management statistics, whereas nonofficial ones have financial, billing, and statistical reports produced from patient and visit data. Some of these local agencies are marketing their own systems; examples include the "MIS for Home and Community Health Care" developed by the Visiting Nurse Association of Omaha, "Casalud" by the Visiting Nurse Association of Houston, and the "Computerized Record System" by the Ramsey County Public Health Nursing Service.

MIS for Home and Community Health Care

The MIS for Home and Community Health Care, developed by the Visiting Nurse Association of Omaha, is an integrated on-line computerized patient management system that generates a patient or client and family problem-oriented record. The system analyzes community health problems in relation to outcome criteria for the assessment of patient care and generates patient and visit statistics and billing and payroll information (Simmons, 1981, 1984; Saba, 1982a, 1982b, 1983b).

The system includes both patient and personnel data. The patient data includes patient/family characteristics, a narrative assessment database, a list of the patient's health care problems, the expected outcomes for the problems, the patient's care plans or progress notes. The problems and expected outcomes are selected from a community health problem classification scheme and expected outcome scheme developed by the association. The personnel activity data includes the patient and visit data collected from a personnel activity sheet.

Data are entered into the system by nurses dictating, by telephone, into recording devices (tapes). The tapes are transcribed by staff into CRT terminals with word processing capability. As a result, the system produces not only a hard copy (paper) of the dictated data for the patient record but also numerous management reports that reflect the data processing and analysis. This system uses an IBM minicomputer with on-line CRTs located in the branch offices of the agency.

This MIS is being offered to other local community health agencies by the Omaha Health Resources, a subsidiary of the Visiting Nurse Association of Omaha, as a complete or partial package–turnkey system (Omaha Health Resources, 1984).

Casalud

Casalud was developed by the Visiting Nurse Association of Houston. A MIS for the home health care industry, Casalud addresses the reporting requirements of home health care agencies. Providing financial, billing, and management applications, it is an on-line, interactive system that uses a minicomputer and is written in COBOL. The association offers Casalud as a complete package to other home health agencies (Visiting Nurse Association of Houston, 1984).

Computerized Record System

The computerized record system developed by the Ramsey County Public Health Nursing Service of St. Paul is another example of a local community health information system. The computerized system, developed by the State of Minnesota, incorporates a measurement of patient and family functioning and is unique in the design of its database. It provides information in three areas: services to individuals, services to families, and nursing activities. All patient/family files contain the functional status of the patient or family; that is, the nurse assesses the health status of each patient on admission and discharge using three functional instruments (O'Grady, 1984; Saba, 1983a):

A psychosocial assessment based on a social dysfunction rating scale (Linn, 1969)
A functional assessment of the activities of daily living adapted from Katz's ADL scale (Katz and colleagues, 1963)
A family assessment based on a family coping scale (Freeman, 1961)

The functional assessment scores are used by nursing personnel to help establish assignment priorities by identifying which clients or patients are functioning poorly. These persons are then targeted to be seen first. Evaluation of services, program decisions, and financial allocations are made based on information derived from this system.

State Management Information Systems

Many states have developed statewide management information systems to collect and process information from local health agencies, including Arizona, Colorado, Florida, Hawaii, Michigan, Minnesota, North Carolina, and Washington (Saba, 1982a). Two such systems follow:

Florida Client Information System

The client information system (CIS) developed by the State of Florida Department of Health and Rehabilitative Services is the only on-line statewide computerized system in the nation. Consisting of an on-line communication network, with terminals located in each of the local health departments statewide and connected to the state computer facility, this system collects, stores, and processes data.

The CIS health management component consists primarily of census and patient encounter data on all eligible Florida residents receiving services from official health departments. Census data include demographic data; the patient encounter data include service and program data on all patients treated (State of Florida, 1983; Saba 1982b; Saba 1983b).

The census is obtained from the client registration form, called Client Service Record—Personal Health Form (Fig. 11-12). It provides base line statistical information for managing the local public health service. The encounter data are obtained from the "Employee Activity Record" form (Fig. 11-13). The form collects encounter data on all clients receiving care directly or from contract health providers, including public health nurses. The encounter data are used to produce statistical reports outlining services provided statewide and to manage and plan the health care services.

Michigan State System

The Michigan State Department of Health is currently designing an on-line information state system that will aid in the statistical management of the agency. This

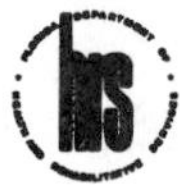

STATE OF FLORIDA
DEPARTMENT OF HEALTH & REHABILITATIVE SERVICES
CLIENT INFORMATION SYSTEM
HEALTH MANAGEMENT COMPONENT
CLIENT SERVICE RECORD
PERSONAL HEALTH

A. CLIENT DEMOGRAPHIC INFORMATION

1. TRANSACTION CONTROL: CI0011. Add Client; CI0012. Update Demo. Inf.; CI0013. Change Client I.D.

2. HRS Client I.D. — Input For All CIF Transactions

3. SSN

4. Medicaid I.D. No.

5. Last Name — Suffix — First — MI

6. Mailing Address, Number & Street — 7. Zip — 8. County

9. Date of Birth (mo da yr) — 10. Sex — 11. Race — 12. Ethnicity — 13. Employment Status — Income: 14. Amount — 15. Freq. — 16. Source

17. Language — 18. Education — 19. Client Type — 20. Family I.D. — 21. Member No. — 22. Living Arrangement — 23. Marital Status — 24. Head of Household

B TRANSACTION CONTROL NO.: CI0181.

25. Servicing Unit (a. Dist, b. Net, C. Unit) — 26. Service Location — 27. Date (mo da yr)

Use ONLY if Instructed: 28. Special Group — 29. Family Income — 30. Family Size

LOCAL USE ONLY

C	31. Prog. Comp.	32. Service	33. FTTY	34. Results	35. Outcome	36. Employee Position No.	Notes
1							
2							
3							
4							
5							
6							
7							
8							

HRS Form 50-9, Oct 81 (obsoletes previous editions and HRS-H Form 3034) Original—DATA ENTRY Yellow—FILE Pink—BILLING

FIG. 11-12. (Courtesy Division of Nursing, State of Florida Department of Health and Rehabilitative Services)

system, which will allow for easy generation of reports, is being developed by Comprehensive Management Health Care Systems (CMHCS). The software being developed will define the files, format the screens, and develop the output reports. The system reports will be designed to meet the statistical reporting requirements of the state (CHMC System, 1984). Once developed, the software will be made available to the local health departments. For a modest fee, the local health departments will be able to obtain duplicates of the system's software, which they then can adapt to meet both their own and the state's reporting requirements.

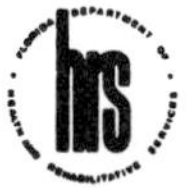

STATE OF FLORIDA
DEPARTMENT OF HEALTH & REHABILITATIVE SERVICES
CLIENT INFORMATION SYSTEM
HEALTH MANAGEMENT COMPONENT
EMPLOYEE ACTIVITY RECORD

TRANSACTION CONTROL NO.: C10201.

A 1. Employee Name (Please Print) | 2. Position Number | 3. Servicing Unit a. Dist b. Net c. Unit | 4. Date mo da yr

B	5. Services Provided to	6 Age	7 Sex	8 Race	9 Ethnic	10 Prog Comp	11. Service	12. No of Services	13 FTTY	14. Results	15. Outcome	16 Service Location	17. Service Time (min)	18. Travel Time (min)	19. Travel Miles
1															
2															
3															
4															
5															
6															
7															
8															
9															
10															
11															
12															

HRS Form 50-8, Oct. 81 (Obsoletes previous editions) Original—DATA ENTRY Yellow—FILE

FIG. 11-13. (Courtesy Division of Nursing, State of Florida Department of Health and Rehabilitative Services)

AMBULATORY CARE SYSTEMS

Ambulatory care is a part of community health. Although ambulatory care settings vary greatly, the one that involves community health nursing is the HMO, the health care plan that delivers comprehensive, coordinated, prepaid medical care services to voluntarily enrolled members. Many HMOs have emerged because of legislation —HMO Act of 1973 (PL 93-222)—that promoted their development. Many

HMOs also offer preventive health care and community health nursing services (Pollack, 1979).

Many ambulatory care computerized information systems have been developed for HMOs. These are primarily medical record systems designed to handle financial and administrative needs. The most widely used ambulatory care system is the computer-stored ambulatory record system (COSTAR).

Computer-Stored Ambulatory Record System (COSTAR)

This system is used in various ambulatory care settings, including HMOs and clinical and community health settings. Developed by the Laboratory of Computer Science at the Massachusetts General Hospital in collaboration with the Harvard Community Health Plan, an HMO in Boston, COSTAR was funded by grants from the National Center for Health Services Research (see Chap. 1) (Barnett, 1976; Reno, 1981).

A comprehensive system that documents the entire medical record, including nursing care, COSTAR is an integrated system designed to meet the medical, administrative, financial and billing, and other needs of diverse ambulatory care agencies (Saba, 1982a, 1982b, 1983b). It contains five functionally independent but interrelated modules based on sets of terms, words, or phrases for documenting all possible activities. A directory contains the system vocabulary for the entire system, which is organized into coded categories. The major ones include administrative items, diagnostic terms, medical procedures, laboratory tests, medications, therapies, and accounting terms. The five modules are as follows (Barnett, 1976):

Registration
Security and integrity
Scheduling
Medical record
Accounts receivable

The registration module consists of all patient identification data, and the security and integrity module includes measures to protect data from loss. The scheduling module schedules patient visits with providers. The accounts receivable module handles all data related to patient billing, and the medical record module documents the total medical record by collecting coded data elements structured to generate output reports to highlight the medical care. The output reports from this module consist of three standard reports — an encounter report, a status report or patient summary, and a flowchart (Figs. 11-14 and 11-15).

COSTAR also uses a medical query language (MQL) to allow users without programming knowledge to interact and search the structured database. This language, written in MUMPS, a high-level programming language designed to meet the needs of medical computing, uses a hierarchical database system to allow for dynamic storage. It runs on several types of minicomputers; it is available from the Massachusetts General Hospital and is marketed by several vendors (Table 11-2) (COSTAR User's Group, 1984).

COSTAR is being adapted by many community health agencies, including the North County Health Services of San Diego, California, where all health providers, including public health nurses, use it (Reno, 1981; Saba, 1983a). COSTAR is also being used abroad, since it is considered the most advanced system for managing primary care. The Finland National Board of Health and the Fund for Research and Development adapted COSTAR and renamed it FINSTAR. FINSTAR took 15 man-

```
ENCOUNTER REPORT
PATIENT,TEST (F) 36 YRS  (12/25/47)


7/16/84    SITE EVERNIA 826   TYPE OF VISIT WALK IN   REPEAT VISIT PRIMARY CARE
           MEDICARE  REYNOLDS,BEVERLY,RN

                                 DIAGNOSES/PROBLEMS

MHAB1       HYPERTENSION

                                   PHYSICAL EXAM

CAEF1 *     BLOOD PRESSURE             130/95 LEFT ARM
CAKH1       WEIGHT                     125

                                     THERAPIES

YSFE1-1     DIAZEPAM (VALIUM)
              5 MG ORAL USE WITH DISCRETION
              QTY: 50 REFILL: 2

                                     PROCEDURES

BTSP3       INTERMEDIATE PPD TUBERCULIN TEST ADMINISTERED
QYFD4       PROCTOSIGMOIDOSCOPY INDEPEN
JYPZ6-A     UNILATERAL REMOVAL OF IMPACTED CERUMEN,

                                       TESTS

CNAT7       DIGOXIN LEVEL [ORDERED]
CNEC2       GLUCOSE FASTING [ORDERED]
MNAA2       CBC WITH DIFFERENTIAL [ORDERED]
MNAF6       GLYCOHEMOGLOBIN [ORDERED]
MNHF1       SEDIMENTATION RATE WESTERGREN ESR [ORDERED]

RNGJ1       STS VDRL [ORDERED]
WNAY6       GLUCOSE DEXTROSTIX [ORDERED]
WNBQ1       URINALYSIS COMPLETE W MICRO [ORDERED]
WRCT6       SMAC 25 [ORDERED]
WRCR9       THYROID PROFILE [ORDERED]
WRQD2       SMITH KLINE HANDLING [ORDERED]
WRQB5       STATE LAB HANDLING [ORDERED]
```

FIG. 11-14. An example of a COSTAR "encounter report." (Courtesy Mitre Corp)

years to develop and is now used to document primary health care in Finland. An interactive system using video terminals connected to a minicomputer, it has clearly reduced the time staff spend on data processing. Less time is spent searching for information since all client data can be viewed or obtained from the computer terminals (Hynninen, 1983).

Patient Care Information System

The patient care information system (PCIS) is another ambulatory care system used by the Indian Health Service. An on-line system designed to support the direct delivery of health services to Indians and the Alaska natives and developed on the Papago Indian Reservation in Tuscon, the PCIS is used to promote comprehensive

```
PATIENT SUMMARY

PATIENT,TEST (F) 36 YRS   (12/25/47)
     1804 CAPISTRANO ST SAN DIEGO,CA 92106
                                                       SSN:  555646810

                                      PROBLEMS

MAJOR
     10/2/84              WIEWORA,R       FAMILY PLANNING
                                            SERVICE
MINOR
     10/2/84              WIEWORA,R       MENSTRUAL DISORDER
     5/3/84-7/21/84       WIEWORA,R       HYPERTENSION
     7/15/84              WIEWORA,R       DIABETES MELLITUS
     7/5/84               DUMBAUGH,R      CLUSTER HEADACHES
     7/2/84               SALK,J          WELL BABY
     4/12/84              HYDE,D          IMPETIGO
     4/9/84-4/11/84       TEUFEN,N        CHRONIC OBSTRUCTIVE
                                            LUNG DISEASE
     4/11/84              TEUFEN,N        PNEUMONIA
     4/9/84               SALK,J          ANEMIA
     4/9/84               SALK,J          FATIGUE
     6/6/75               SALK,J          SYPHILIS

                                       TESTS

CHEMISTRY
     5/3/84-7/16/84       REYNOLDS,B    * GLUCOSE FASTING
                                            [57-110]
     5/3/84               SALK,J        * GLUCOSE FASTING      200
                                            [57-110]
     4/13/84              SALK,J          GLUCOSE TOLERANCE    FBS 110, 1HR 185,
                                            TEST 3 HOUR          2HR 200, 3HR 100,
                                                                 FAST UR NEG, 1HR
                                                                 UR NEG, 2HR UR
                                                                 NEG, 3HR UR NEG,
                                                                 4HR U NEG, 5HR U
                                                                 NEG
     8/3/84               SALK,J          SODIUM URINE TEST
                                            [ORD]
     8/3/84               SALK,J          LEUCINE AMINO
                                            PEPTIDASE BLOOD [12-33] [ORD]
     7/16/84              REYNOLDS,B      DIGOXIN LEVEL
                                            [.5-2.5] [ORD]
     4/30/84              STAEFE,J        PREGNANCY TEST
                                            URINE HCG [ORD]
HEMATOLOGY
     4/13/84              SALK,J          HEMOGLOBIN [12-16]  13.5
     4/12/84-7/16/84      REYNOLDS,B      SEDIMENTATION RATE
                                            WESTERGREN ESR [0-20] [ORD]
     5/30/84-7/16/84      REYNOLDS,B      CBC WITH
                                            DIFFERENTIAL [ORD]
     7/16/84              REYNOLDS,B      GLYCOHEMOGLOBIN
                                            [ORD]
```

FIG. 11-15. An example of a COSTAR "patient summary." (Courtesy Mitre Corp)

TABLE 11-2 *List of COSTAR Vendors*

Colorado
Computer Systems, Inc.
1375 Walnut #222
Boulder, CO 80302

Innovative Computer Systems
1660 S. Albion St.
Suite 902
Denver, CO 80222

Connecticut
Professional Service Bureau
5 Town Street
Norwich, CT 06360

Illinois
GLS, Inc.
3525 W. Petersen, Suite 306
Chicago, IL 60659

Maryland
Global Health Foundation, Inc.
1300 Piccard Dr.
Rockville, MD 20850

Micronetics Design Corporation
932 Hungerford Dr., Suite 11
Rockville, MD 20850

Massachusetts
Laboratory of Computer Sciences
Massachusetts General Hospital
55 Fruit St.
Boston, MA 02114

Pennsylvania
Med Design, Inc.
1409 Penn Ave.
Scranton, PA 18509

Virginia
CTS, Inc. of Virginia
6728 Rosewood St.
Annadale, VA 22003

Medical Information Management, Inc.
107 Park Washington Ct.
Falls Church, VA 22046

(COSTAR User's Group: Vendor/Consultant List. San Marcos, CA, COSTAR User's Group, 1984)

care to address all known health problems and preventive health needs of patients (Brown and colleagues, 1971; IHS, 1982; Saba, 1982a, 1983b).

Currently all Papago Indian Reservation residents and Alaska natives receiving care at an Indian Health Service hospital or clinic are a part of the system, which contains complete medical care data on all care provided. Community health nurses also enter encounter data of clients seen in the home, clinic, school, or hospital. The PCIS is the only system that integrates patient information from the home to the hospital and back home again.

The PCIS provides summary reports of all health care encounters at the reservation health care facilities. A copy of a sample health summary is shown in Figure 11-16. The PCIS provides microfiche printouts for all medical and nursing health care centers on the reservation for use in providing health care. The community health nurses can obtain information from this system by querying the on-line computer system, by telephone, from any location on the reservation, that is, from car, clinic, or home.

SPECIAL-PURPOSE APPLICATIONS

Many activities conducted in the field of community health nursing require special purpose applications, including studies conducted to obtain statistics necessary to plan, administer, budget, and evaluate nursing care. Data gathering for screening programs for early detection of diseases, epidemiological activities, and other projects that use the computer for health promotion and prevention of disease are still other activities. Many such studies, programs, and projects have been described in the literature; each of these required a special computer system or application designed to process them.

```
HEALTH SUMMARY
  (10/13/81)

NAME:  DOE,      JANE       LOUISE
RESIDENCE:    PRYOR, MT
SEX:  FEMALE
BENEFICIARY:  01 INDIAN
BIRTH:  09/20/1979
MOTHER:   DOE,        MARY
PCIS ID NO:  DCA-123456
SOCIAL SECURITY NO:  999-88-7777

REGISTER NOS:  AR-SU-TY REG NO
  HNDCP.  CH.  40-42-HC 111111

H.R. NOS:      AR-SU-FY REC NO
  CROW HOSP    40-42-01 123456
  PRYOR HS     40-42-30 222222

ACTIVE PROBLEMS
        YR     DATE
NO.     ENT    MOD        FACILITY     DIS       PROBLEM
005     79   12/23/79     PRYOR HS     MD     R PARIETAL TEMPORAL SKULL FRACTURE
008     80   09/04/81     CROW HOSP    MD     RECURRENT PNEUMONIA
             09/04/81     N003         MD      PLAN BRONCHOSCOPY AFTER NEXT EPISODE
009     81   09/04/81     CROW HOSP    MD     ANEMIA
             09/04/81     N004         MD      ON FE SUPPLEMENT FOR ONE YEAR

INACTIVE PROBLEMS
        YR     DATE
NO.     ENT    MOD        FACILITY     DIS       PROBLEM
004     79   12/17/79     PRYOR HS     CHM    R HILAR PNEUMONITIS
006     79   09/04/81     PRYOR HS     MD     MENINGITIS
007     00   04/13/80     CROW HOSP    MD     ACUTE SUPPURATIVE OTITIS MEDIA

ACTIVE MEDICATIONS
 09/04/81  ASPIRIN                  2 TAB 60MG          6 TIMES/DAY
 09/04/81  FERROUS SULFATE          1 TAB 300MG         3 TIMES/DAY   000
 08/16/81  BACITRACIN               OINT 500U/GM        3 TIMES/DAY   015
 08/16/81  PENICILLIN V K           5 SOLN 4CMU/5ML     4 TIMES/DAY   200

INPATIENT ENCOUNTERS (MAX 9 OR 5 YRS)
 04/10  04/13/80  CROW HOSP    ACUTE SUPPURATIVE OTITIS MEDIA
                               RECURRENT PNEUMONIA
 12/23  12/30/79  CROW HOSP    SEPTIC H INFLUENZA
                               MENINGITIS H INFLUENZA
                               PNEUMONIA
                               LINEAR SKULL FRACTURE R PARIETAL

OUTPATIENT AND FIELD ACTIVITIES (MAX 18 OR 2 YRS)
 09/04/81  MD   CROW HOSP     ANEMIA
                              URI, PROBABLY VIRAL
 08/16/81  CHM  PRYOR HS      IMPETIGO
 03/20/81  MD   PRYOR HS      WELL CHILD CARE
 10/24/80  CHN  HOME          HEALTH SURVEILLANCE
 10/19/80  MD   PRYOR HS      S P MENINGITIS X2
                              RECURRENT LEFT OTITIS MEDIA
 04/21/80  MD   HOME          RIGHT SEROUS OTITIS MEDIA
 12/23/79  MD   PRYOR HS      ANEMIA
                              MENINGITIS
                              R HILAR PNEUMONITIS
                              R PARIETAL TEMPORAL SKULL FRAC
 12/17/79  CHM  PRYOR HS      R HILAR PNEUMONIA
                              R PARIETAL SKULL FRACTURE, ND

MEASUREMENTS (MAX 5 OR 2 YRS)
   DATE       WT     PCT    HT     PCT     BLD PRS     HD CIRC
 09/04/81   030-04    80    31      36     060/040       19.5
 08/16/81   029-08    81
 10/24/80   024-00    78    30      61                   19.0

IMMUNIZATIONS (MAX 5 FOR EACH TYPE)
 DPT         3  03/20/81  PRYOR HS
 DPT         2  10/24/80  HOME
 DPT         1  04/21/80  HOME
 SABIN TRI   3  03/20/81  PRYOR HS
 SABIN TRI   2  10/24/80  HOME
 SABIN TRI   1  04/21/80  HOME
 MMR            03/20/81  PRYOR HS

SKIN TESTS (MAX 3 FOR EACH TYPE)
 PPD            03/20/81  PRYOR HS    N 00
 PPD            10/24/80  CROW HOSP   N 00

LAB/X-RAY RESULTS (MAX 7 OR 2 YRS)
             09/04/81  06/20/81  03/20/81  01/06/80  12/16/79
 SKUL X-RAY                                              P
 CHST X-RAY                                    9         9
 WBC                                        10.5      23.6
 HEMOGLOBN                12        12      10.7       8.8
 HEMATOCRT     32.0                         31.8      27.4

REGULAR SURVEILLANCE
              LAST         NEXT
 DPT        03/20/81     03/20/82
 SABIN TR   03/20/81     03/20/82
 HEARING                 DUE NOW
 VISION                  DUE NOW

               **END**
```

FIG. 11-16. An example of a PCIS "health summary." (Courtesy Indian Health Service, United States Public Health Service)

The following examples illustrate the computer applications developed for special studies, programs, and projects:

- Special statistical studies
- Screening programs
- Epidemiologic projects
- Prevention projects

Special Statistical Studies

Military Ambulatory Care Study

One special statistical study that required a specially designed computer application is the military ambulatory care study. Conducted in a military clinical area seeing 13,000 outpatients a month, the 6-month project was done to ascertain if outpatient encounter data could be used to develop an outpatient information system. Such a system is needed to assist the U.S. Army in the management and planning of its outpatient services (Misener, 1983).

Even though the U.S. Army serves as one of the largest HMOs in the world, it did not have reliable outpatient data that could be used to plan services. Thus, the need for an ambulatory database system mandated the project to examine the feasibility of developing such a system.

The pilot study consisted of data collected on a one-page optical mark-sense readable encounter form. The mark-sense form was processed by a desktop mark-sense reader that could be off loaded onto a host computer for processing. The form collected data on client demographics, diagnosis using the international classification of health problems in primary care, and provider of services.

The forms, once computer processed, generated several reports that were prepared for providers. They included a list of the primary diagnosis, the frequency of each diagnosis, and secondary diagnoses. Other reports provided information on procedures, and still others reflected demographic information such as age, beneficiary status, and average time per client. It was determined that these monthly reports were useful enough to be used as management tools.

Once completed, the study was considered a success because it met study objectives. It proved that this method of collecting outpatient data on mark-sense forms, and then using a computer system to process them was valuable, even though only limited data were collected. The computer application developed for this feasibility study could be used as a prototype for developing a U.S. Army outpatient information system.

1979 Survey of Community Health Nursing

Another special statistical study is the 1979 Survey of Community Health Nursing. All the study data collected from a multipage form were completely processed by computer, making it possible to analyze the hundreds of data elements collected from all federal, state, and local community health agencies. Providing a statistical description and an analysis of community health nursing in the United States and territories, the study was used to plan community health nursing requirements for the nation (U.S. Department of Health and Human Services, DN, 1982; Saba, 1983b).

This survey is just one of the many studies in the field of community health nursing conducted by the Division of Nursing, U.S. Department of Health and Human Resources. The division's periodic census of nurses, begun in 1937, is taken to support Federal legislation for improving national health care. The early counts, needless to say, were not processed by computer. These censuses are considered the forerunner of public health nursing classification schemes and database structures used in community health information systems of today.

Screening Programs

California Neonatal Screening Program

A screening program in California illustrates a special project computer application. It uses a minicomputer to collect important public health information mandated by state regulations. The California State Department of Health Services, Genetic Disease Branch, initiated a neonatal screening program to detect infants affected with Phenylketonuria (PKU), a hereditary metabolic disease. If treated, patients do not become mentally retarded (Gordon and colleagues, 1982).

This program uses a minicomputer system to monitor and evaluate the laboratory results of the newborn's screening tests. The data on all the screened newborns are captured on disk. From these data, all laboratory runs are monitored. Once the results are printed, the record is deleted from the dedicated system and transferred to a large computer facility for program analysis. This application allows for retrospective analysis of a large database that can be used to measure the effectiveness of the screening program.

North Carolina Neonatal Screening Program

Another screening program is found in North Carolina, where microcomputers are used to process a similar neonatal screening program (Guthrie, 1980). In both states the primary purpose of the screening program is to monitor large numbers of newborns. The microcomputer system processing is so efficient that the results of the tests are transmitted to the health care providers within 10 dayas after the test is conducted.

Epidemiologic Projects

CASS

Computer-Assisted disease Surveillance System (CASS) illustrates a computer application for an epidemiologic project. The State of Wisconsin Division of Health, Section of Acute and Communicable Disease Epidemiology, has developed one of the few on-line interactive computer systems for disease surveillance. CASS provides communicable disease surveillance as an approach to controlling and preventing communicable diseases (LaVenture and colleagues, 1982).

CASS is a user-oriented system with conventional hardware; its software allows users to access records on demand. The system keeps records of each reported case of communicable disease and produces on-line routine case reports and statistical summaries of diseases. By channelling communications on communicable diseases to the appropriate clinicians, it can assist in controlling these diseases.

Preschool Health Assessment Project

Nursing health assessment of preschool children is done in an urban-rural health unit in Ontario, Canada. The unit has a computer-assisted school health program that computerizes the school health record. The results of each child's assessments—audiovisual testing, immunization profile, health appraisal by a public health nurse, and dental checkup—are computerized. The system, which demonstrates that this type of standardized assessment assists in detecting health care needs, was found to be less expensive than fees charged by a private physician (Robertson and colleagues, 1976).

Prevention Projects

Teletriage Program

The teletriage program, a prevention project that illustrates the use of a computer system, was developed by a group of nurses in Minneapolis. Designed to provide standardized interviewing, by telephone, of clients who call a health care facility for assistance or information, it collects client data using a set of standardized triage questions and protocols. An Apple II microcomputer system systematizes the interviewing. The system, which generates summaries of the interviews and selected care plans, demonstrates how a microcomputer system helps assess clients' problems (Moreland and colleagues, 1982).

Total Child Health Data System

The total child health data system in Japan, developed by a team of health professionals in the Osaka PL Hospital, Osaka, Japan, is an on-line system that provides early detection and prevention of children's diseases and follow-up consultation services. The system was designed for health care, education, and research. Data on clients are entered into the system at birth; clients are tracked until school age. The system attempts to devise a method that uses information to detect high-risk infants so that they can receive more nursing care and their parents more advice (Ohata, 1983).

Caseload/Workload Planner Project

A caseload/workload planner project is being conducted at the University of Michigan School of Nursing. Developed to provide a low-cost system using a microcomputer to plan nurses' caseloads and workloads in community health nursing agencies, the system will contain two modules—a caseload and a workload planner. They are used to assess staff caseloads based on time requirements and level of services. The time requirements are based on four categories, and the level of service is based on six dimensions: clinical judgment, physical care, psychosocial care, teaching needs, multiagency involvement, and number and severity of problems. This system will generate the number of cases required per month and expected workload and will provide the workload for each staff member (Schultz, 1983).

SUMMARY

This chapter describes the various computer applications found in community health nursing. Community health nursing, also called public health nursing, is discussed, and computer applications for this specialty are reviewed, including community health management information systems, ambulatory care systems, and special purpose applications.

The community health management information systems found in community and public health agencies are primarily financial and billing, statistical reporting, and patient care systems. Applications for each type are described and examples are given.

Ambulatory care systems are described, and two systems—COSTAR and the PCIS—discussed. Finally, special purpose applications are presented, including those computer applications developed for special statistical studies, screening programs, epidemiological projects, and prevention projects. Examples are given.

ISSUES

1. Some community health agencies implemented computerized management information systems in the early 1970s that were discontinued by the early 1980s. Objections to such systems included (1) length of time to complete forms, (2) frequent system breakdowns, (3) slow turnaround time for producing reports, and (4) incomplete documentation of patient care.
2. Confidentiality of patient records is a concern for community health and ambulatory care information systems. Today, nursing personnel can access these systems from their homes and other sites outside the agency, making these systems open to outside manipulation and intrusion.
3. Few evaluations of community health and ambulatory care systems have been conducted to assess the changes in the quantity and quality of nursing documentation of patient care, the scope of information for billing and statistics, and the referral of patients from home to hospital and home again.
4. The data used in hospital information systems can also be used to format community health and ambulatory care information systems.
5. Community health management systems can identify regional health problems, predict high-risk groups of clients, and determine needs for personnel education and research.
6. Few schemes exist to classify patients receiving services from community health nursing agencies.
7. A comprehensive record for a community health nursing system can be used by both community health nurses and community health nurse practitioners.
8. The quality of patient care can be determined from a community health information system. This includes the use of what variables?
9. Databases from other non-health-related sources such as census and labor should be integrated into community health management information systems.
10. State and local community health management information systems should be networked together inside and outside a state.
11. A standardized community health nursing database(s) is needed. What should it encompass? Who should develop it?

SUGGESTIONS FOR HANDS-ON EXPERIENCES

Explanation

Very few computer-assisted instruction software packages are available for community health nursing. The following exercises can help a student become familiar with community health nursing information systems.

1. Visit a local community health nurse agency with a community health nursing or ambulatory care information system. Use the following format to collect the information needed to review the system being observed:
    1. Name of agency
    2. Name of system
    3. Who developed system
       If service bureau/vendor
       (1) Name
    4. Purpose of system
    5. System information

a. Hardware
   (1) Type computer
   (2) Size computer
b. Software
   (1) Programs
   (2) Packages
   (3) Programming language
c. Applications provided
   (1) Financial billing
   (2) Statistical reporting
   (3) Patient care
d. Costs

6. Who enters data into system
   a. Clerk
   b. Nurses
   c. Other
7. List reports produced by systems and indicate for whom

2. Design an input form with codes and instructions for a community health nursing client management information system.
   a. Use basic data set for a visit to patients developed by the National League for Nursing in the publication *Statistical Report for Home and Community Health Services* (NLN Pub. No. 21-1652). New York, National League for Nursing, 1977.
3. Design several output reports produced from the community health nursing client management information system.
   a. Determine use and user of each report.
4. Prepare a flowchart of a community health nursing program (*e.g.*, a school eye testing program or well-child immunization program).
5. Solicit a vendor or service bureau offering a community health information system to demonstrate its microcomputer system.
6. Outline an on-line community health nursing client management information system that tracks a patient discharged from a hospital, referred to the community health nursing agency for home visiting, and referred back into the hospital again.

STUDY QUESTIONS

1. What major piece of legislation influenced the expansion of community health nursing services in this country?
2. Computer applications in community health centers around what three major areas?
3. Name the three types of community health management information systems.
4. Name at least three applications provided by financial and billing systems.
5. Name at least three applications provided by statistical reporting systems.
6. List the three system options that community and home health agencies can select from service bureau or vendors.
7. In what state is the only on-line statewide client information system found?
8. Name three local community health agencies that offer a management information system.
9. Name the three instruments that can be used to assess community health patients.

10. Name the most widely used ambulatory care system.
11. In what two states is the Indian health service system (patient care information system) found?
12. List the four types of community health special applications.

REFERENCES

Barnett GO: Computer-stored Ambulatory Record (COSTAR) (NCHSR Research Digest Series) (DHEW pub. no. HRA 76-3145). Rockville, MD, National Center for Health Services Research, 1976

Brown VB, Mason WT, Kaczmarski M: A computerized health information service. Nurs Outlook 19(3):158–161, 1971

CHMC System: Comprehensive Management Health Care (CMHC) System. Dublin, OH, CHMC System, 1984

Computer Resources: STAT: The Complete Home Health Information System. Ft. Lauderdale, FL, Computer Resources, 1984

COSTAR User's Group: Vendor/Consultant List. San Marcos, CA, COSTAR User's Group, 1984

DELTA Computer Systems: Home Health Management System. Altoona, PA, DELTA Computer Systems, 1984

Fleet Information Systems: Home Health Systems. Providence, RI, Fleet Information Systems, 1984

Freeman R: Measuring the effectiveness of public health nursing. Nurs Outlook 9:605–607, 1961

Gordon E, Kan K, Mordaunt, V, et al: Computer applications for California's newborn screening program. In Blum B (ed): Proceedings: The Sixth Annual Symposium on Computer Applications in Medical Care, pp 151–155. New York, IEEE Computer Society Press, 1982

Guthrie R: Organization of a regional newborn screening laboratory. In Bickel H, Guthrie R, Hammersen G (eds): Neonatal Screening for Inborn Errors of Metabolism. New York, Springer, 1980

Hynninen P: A comprehensive computer-based system for patient information in primary health care. In Scholes M, Bryant Y, Barber B (eds): The Impact of Computers on Nursing, pp 207–214. Amsterdam, North-Holland, 1983

IHS Data Advisory Committee, Study Design Team: Patient Care Information System (PCIS): PCIS Operations Manual, vol 3.2, Health Care Providers Reference Manual. Tuscon, AZ, Indian Health Service, Department of Health and Human Services, 1982

IMI Health Systems: MEDI-VISIT: Computer Systems for Home Care Providers. San Jose, CA, IMI Health Systems, 1984

InfoMed: Home Health Care Information System Highlights. Princeton, NJ, Infomed, 1984

Katz S, Ford AB, Moskowitz RW, et al: Studies in illness in the aged: The index of ADL, a standardized measure of biological and psychosocial function. JAMA 185:914–919, 1963

Kennevan WJ: General systems theory—a logical transition. In National League for Nursing: Management Information Systems for Public Health/Community Health Agencies: A Report of a Conference. New York, National League for Nursing, 1974

LaVenture M, Davis J, Faulkner J, et al: Wisconsin epidemiology disease surveillance system: User control of data base management technology. In Blum B (ed): Proceedings: The Sixth Annual Symposium on Computer Applications in Medical Care, p 156. New York, IEEE Press, 1982

Linn M, Scalthorpe WB, Evje M, et al: A social dysfunction rating scale. J Psychiatr Res 6:299–306, 1969

Misener TR: Ambulatory care database. In Dayhoff R (ed): Proceedings: The Seventh Annual Symposium on Computer Applications in Medical Care, pp 533–536. New York, IEEE Computer Society Press, 1983

Moreland H, Johnston M, Sharp D: Demonstration of the Tele-Triage system (C): A microcomputer-based telephone triage program for use by R.N.'s in ambulatory care settings or physician's offices. In Blum B (ed): Proceedings: The Sixth Annual Symposium on Computer Applications in Medical Care, p 637. New York, IEEE Computer Society Press, 1982

National League for Nursing: Selected Management Information Systems for Public Health/Community Health Agencies. New York, National League for Nursing, 1978

National League for Nursing: Statistical Reporting in Home and Community Health Services (Pub. no. 21-1652). New York, National League for Nursing, 1977

O'Grady BV: Computerized documentation of community health nursing — what shall it be? Comp Nursing 2(3):98–101, 1984

Ohata F: PL child health care systems. In Scholes M, Bryant Y, Berber B (eds): The Impact of Computers on Nursing, pp 222–229. Amsterdam, North-Holland, 1983

Omaha Health Resources: Management Information System for Home and Community Health Care. Omaha, Omaha Health Resources, 1984

Pollack B: The evolution of an HMO. Med Group Manage 26(6):3–5, 1979

Q.S. Inc, Systems Group: Health Management Information Software. Greenville, SC, Q.S. Systems Group, 1982

Reno DM: COSTAR V computer system: North county health services. In Heffernon H (ed): Proceedings: The Fifth Annual Symposium on Computer Applications in Medical Care, pp 722–724. New York, IEEE Computer Society Press, 1981

Robertson LH, McDonnell K, Scott J: Nursing health assessment of preschool children in Perth County. Can J Public Health 67:300–304, 1976

Saba VK: Computers in nursing administration: Information systems for community health nursing. Comp Nursing 1(2):1–3, 1983a

Saba VK: How computers influence nursing activities in community health. First National Conference: Computer Technology and Nursing (NIH pub. no. 83-2142). Bethesda, MD, National Institutes of Health, 1983b

Saba VK: Computerized management information system in community health nursing. In Blum B (ed): Proceedings: The Sixth Annual Symposium on Computer Applications in Medical Care, pp 148–149. New York, IEEE Computer Society Press, 1982a

Saba VK: The computer in public health: Today and tomorrow. Nurs Outlook 30(9):510–514, 1982b

Saba VK: Basic considerations in management information systems for public health/community health agencies. In National League for Nursing: Management Information Systems for Public Health/Community Health Agencies: A Report of a Conference, pp 3–13. New York, National League for Nursing, 1974

Schultz S: A microcomputer based community health nursing database management system. In Dayhoff R (ed): Proceedings: The Seventh Annual Symposium on Computer Applications in Medical Care, pp 531–532. New York, IEEE Computer Society Press, 1983

Simmons DA: Computer implementation in ambulatory care: A community health model. Second National Conference: Computer Technology and Nursing (NIH pub. no. 84-2623). Bethesda, MD, National Institutes of Health, 1984

Simmons DA: Computerized management information system in a community health nursing agency. In Heffernon H (ed): Proceedings: The Fifth Annual Symposium on Computer Applications in Medical Care, pp. 753–754. New York, IEEE Computer Society Press, 1981

Simmons DA: A Classification Scheme for Client Problems in Community Health Nursing (Nurse Planning Information Series, vol. 14, (NTIS no. HRP-0501501). Springfield, VA, National Technical Information Series, 1980

State of Florida Department of Health and Rehabilitative Services: HRS Manual: System Management: Client Information System: Personal Health. Tallahassee, FL, State of Florida Department of Health and Rehabilitative Services, 1983

Taylor DB, Johnson OH: Systematic Nursing Assessment: A Step Toward Automation (DHEW pub. no. HRA 74-17). Bethesda, MD, Department of Health, Education and Welfare, 1974

U.S. Department of Health, Education and Welfare, Public Health Service, Office of Assistant Secretary for Health and Surgeon General: Healthy People: The Surgeon's General Report on Health Promotion and Disease Prevention (PHS pub. no. 79-55071). Washington, DC, U.S. Government Printing Office, 1979

U.S. Department of Health and Human Services, Division of Nursing: Survey of Community Health Nursing 1979 (NTIS no. HRP-0904449). Hyattsville, MD, Department of Health and Human Services, 1982

Verran JA: Delineation of ambulatory care nursing practice. J Ambul Care Manage 4(2):1–13, 1981

Visiting Nurse Association of Houston: VNA Home Health Services: An Introduction to "CASALUD". A Management Information System for the Home Health Care Industry. Houston, Visiting Nurse Association of Houston, 1984

BIBLIOGRAPHY

Accounting Corporation of America: Home Health Care Management Information System. Boston, Accounting Corporation of America, 1980

Allen Associates: An Overview of VMIS Home Health Care Management Information System. Wakefield, MA, Allen Associates, 1984

American Nurses' Association: Concepts of Community Health Nursing Practice. Kansas City, MO, American Nurses' Association, 1975

American Public Health Association, Public Health Nursing Section: The Definition and Role of Public Health Nursing in the Delivery of Health Care. Washington, DC, American Public Health Association, 1980

Barnett GO, Justice ME, Somand J, et al: COSTAR system. In Blum B (ed): Information Systems for Patient Care pp 270–293. New York, Springer-Verlag, 1984

Brown VB, Mason WT, Millman S: The health information system—an example of a total health system. In National League for Nursing: Management Information Systems for Public Health/Community Health Agencies: Report of the Conference, pp 159–161. New York, National League for Nursing, 1974

Creative Socio-Medics Corp: Computer Systems for the Health Field. New York, Creative Socio-Medics Corp, 1984

Fiddleman RH: Proliferation of COSTAR—a status report. In Blum B (ed.): Proceedings: The Sixth Annual Symposium on Computer Applications in Medical Care, pp 175–178. New York, IEEE Computer Society Press, 1982

Fiddleman RH: Survey of COSTAR Installations and Vendors. McLean, VA, MITRE Corp, 1981

Fiddleman RH, Kerlin BD: Preliminary Assessment of COSTAR at the North (San Diego) County Health Services Project (con. no.: grant no. CS-D-000001-03-0). McLean, VA, MITRE Corp, 1980

Freeman R, Heinrick J: Community Health Nursing Practice, 2nd ed. Philadelphia, WB Saunders, 1981

Global Health Foundation: COSTAR: Summary of Functions. Rockville, MD, Global Health Foundations, 1982

Kerlin B, Greene P: COSTAR: An Overview and Annotated Bibliography (con. no. 233-79-3021). McLean, VA, MITRE Corp, 1981

Minicomputers Consultant Data Services: Total Office Automation for Health Care Services. Wayne, PA, Minicomputers Consultant Data Services, 1984

National Center for Health Services Research: Computer-stored Ambulatory Record. (NCHSR research digest series, DHEW pub. no. 77-3160). Rockville, MD, National Center for Health Services Research, 1977

New York Information Systems: Home Health Management Information System. Rochester, NY, New York Information Systems, 1983

Picker Business Systems: VNA Computer Software System. Cromwell, CT, Picker Business Systems, 1984

Pierson, Miller, Young: Management System for Home Health Agencies. Joliet, IL, Pierson, Miller & Young, 1984

State of Florida Department of Health and Rehabilitative Services: Management Information Systems for Community/Public Health Nursing Services (con. no. No1-NU-34036). Washington, DC, Department of Health, Education and Welfare, 1973

U.S. Department of Health and Human Services: Prospectus on Health Maintenance Organizations (DHHS pub. no. PHS 82-50180). Rockville, MD, Department of Health and Human Services, 1981

U.S. Department of Health and Human Services, Division of Nursing: Nurse Supply, Distribution and Requirements: Third Report to the Congress: Nurse Training Act of 1975 (DHHS pub. no. HRA 82-7). Hyattsville, MD, Department of Health and Human Services, 1982

U.S. Department of Health and Human Services, Bureau of Health Professions: Public health practice and program management: Public health nursing. In Public Health Personnel in the United States (DHHS pub. no. HRA 82-6). Hyattsville, MD, Department of Health and Human Services, 1982

U.S. Department of Health and Human Services, Office of Disease Prevention and Health Promotion: Prevention 1982 (DHHS pub. no. 82-50157). Hyattsville, MD, Department of Health and Human Services, 1982

Waxman BD: Implementation of the COSTAR System in San Diego and Other California Health Departments (NCHSR 83-90). Rockville, MD, National Center for Health Services Research, 1983

12 Nursing Practice Applications

Objectives

- Understand the current standards governing documentation of nursing practice.
- Describe the basic categories and potential components of documentation systems on mainframes, minicomputers, and microcomputers.
- Identify documentation applications available from vendors.
- Identify nursing documentation capabilities from admission to discharge.
- Understand the issues related to computerized documentation.

Is a pocket computer terminal at the bedside a reality in the future of nursing? Whether this concept is myth or reality, computers are being used more frequently to document nursing practice in both U.S. and foreign hospitals. The applications on mainframes, minicomputers, and microcomputers available to document direct patient care, the issues related to computerized nursing documentation, current standards, and possible future uses are discussed in this chapter.

The computer provides accurate and accessible information that is perhaps as important to nursing as knowledge and practical skills in determining the quality and cost of nursing care. In order to appreciate the magnitude of information available on the computer for documentation and retrieval, this chapter presents a hypothetical patient's computerized nursing documentation from admission to discharge. A composite of available computer products is used. (Chap. 13 describes documentation applications in the intensive care unit and specialty areas.)

MANUAL TO COMPUTER NURSING DOCUMENTATION: HISTORICAL PERSPECTIVE

Historically, nursing documentation has been consistent with hospital standards, nurse practice acts, and legal definitions of nursing (see Chap. 1). As these controls grew, the amount and quality of nursing documentation also increased. Nursing documentation in the medical record has become more complex as nursing practice has expanded to encompass care to critically ill and specialty patients. However, nursing documentation, whether manual or computerized, must adhere to certain professional standards and state laws. Nurses should refer to the current standards governing computerized documentation before its applications.

STANDARDS GOVERNING COMPUTERIZED DOCUMENTATION

Table 12-1 summarizes standards governing nursing documentation in the medical record that must be adhered to when computerized documentation is considered. Practice acts establish regulatory and statutory rules, The Joint Commission on Accreditation of Hospitals (JCAH) and The American Nurses' Association (ANA) set standards required for hospital accreditation and professional practice, and hospitals establish policies on which malpractice negligence rules are supported. The computer only automates what other forces mandate; it cannot improve nursing practice or patient care. The computer should only facilitate documentation of nurses' actions, patients' conditions, and outcomes of care planning.

Legally, an undisputed independent area of professional nursing is the recording and reporting of a nursing note. Legal definitions of nursing include necessary documentation requirements. Documentation is also clearly a nursing function recognized equally by judicial decisions (Lesnik and Anderson, 1955). Nurses can be found negligent in a malpractice case with supporting evidence from a nursing note. In a legal defense, if the hospital or staff are not legally responsible for a negligent act, conclusions may be drawn from the records. A court faced with a conflict between the record of an event made at the time and evidence of a witness relying on several years' memory is hard pressed to accept the witness's evidence. A witness is preferable only when the records are "inaccurate, illegible, or obviously unreliable" (Rozovsky, 1978).

Despite legal arguments, nursing research studies have shown that nurses have not always recorded in the nursing note. As early as the 1950s standards of recording and reporting were found wanting (Lesnik and Anderson, 1955). A study of the nature and uses of nurses' notes stated that frequently phrases used to describe patients were stereotyped and meaningless (Walker, 1964). Although inaccuracies were infrequent, significant omissions were common. In 1966 a study on the effectiveness and acceptance of nurses' notes revealed that nurses' notes often lacked detail, that some gave no information, and that many were incomplete or repetitive and usually reported what procedure was performed rather than observations on the patient (Healy and McGurk, 1966). Internal hospital audits and JCAH accreditation reports continually chide nurses for deficiencies in documentation, even though after medical orders are written, nurses' notes hold the only clue on whether orders were carried out and what the results were (Kerr, 1975).

The discrepancy between what is required by law, standards, the profession, nurse practice acts, and actual documentation is great. Documentation should reflect an expanding profession's numerous independent and interdependent functions, particularly when evidence of assessment, planning, implementation, and evaluations is required by JCAH and ANA standards.

AUTOMATED NURSING NOTES

Because nurses are requested to assess patient-centered problems on which patient care decisions are based, the methods employed in collecting and recording data have changed. As early as the 1950s health care agencies began using computers to facilitate handling patient data. By the 1960s nurses began to recognize computers' potential for improving documentation of nursing practice and its impact on the quality of patient care (Hannah, 1976).

TABLE 12-1 *Standards of Nursing Documentation in the Medical Record*

PRACTICE ACT (Example: Maryland)	JCAH STANDARDS	ANA STANDARDS	MALPRACTICE NEGLIGENCE DEFENSE	HOSPITAL POLICIES
STATUTORY AND REGULATORY	*REQUIRED INFORMATION*	*SUGGESTED RECORDING*	*SUGGESTED RULES*	*REQUIRED*
Licensing may be withheld, denied, revoked or suspended for 1. Failing to file or record health records 2. Willfully and knowingly filing false reports	Hospital accreditation may be denied for failure to record 1. Nursing process 2. Care plan including: Physiological factors Psychosocial factors Environmental factors Patient/family teaching Patient discharge planning 3. Patient's health status: problems, needs, capabilities, limitations 4. Nursing interventions, patients' responses, patient/family understanding, counselling 5. Routine elements of care: hygiene, medication administration, physiological parameters	Record 1. Patient's health status 2. Nursing process	Record 1. Accurately 2. Concisely 3. Legibly 4. Timely 5. Right person 6. Chronologically ordered 7. Fully signed 8. Uniformity—format 9. Uniformity—terminology 10. Errors corrected by a. Stroking out b. Dated c. Signed	Establish policies for 1. Frequency 2. What/content 3. Who 4. Where 5. Uniformity in format 6. Distribution outside hospital 7. Uniformity in terminology 8. Signature 9. Error correction procedures

DOCUMENTING PRACTICE WITH MAINFRAMES AND MINICOMPUTERS

Basic Categories of Nursing Documentation Systems

The documentation of patient care falls within the capability of computers to document the following two categories:

Direct patient care
Nursing unit management reports

In direct patient care, the computer documents nursing care activities. In nursing unit management reports the computer documents administrative applications. Nursing unit management is described in Chapter 9. This chapter describes the use of computers to document direct patient care.

Potential Components of a Direct Patient Care System

The potential components of the direct patient care system for documenting nursing practice, listed below, are based on the nursing process as defined by Yura and Walsh (1973). Both in the United States and abroad, nursing documentation organization has been committed to nursing process designs (Ashton, 1983).

No one system currently contains all the following components, which were derived from several nursing evaluation studies (McCormick, 1983; Rieder and Norton, 1984; Edmunds, 1984; Lombard and Light, 1983; Scholes and colleagues, 1983).

I. Nursing Process
- **A.** Assessment
  - **1.** Admission assessment
    - **(a)** Defining characteristics
    - **(b)** Nursing physical examination
    - **(c)** Vital signs, height and weight, and other flowsheets.
  - **2.** Reassessments
    - **(a)** New defining characteristics
- **B.** Planning
  - **1.** Patient problem list (*e.g.*, allergies, medical diagnosis, behavioral problems)
  - **2.** Potential nursing diagnosis
  - **3.** Nursing diagnosis
  - **4.** Replanning
    - **(a)** New nursing diagnosis or new patient problems
- **C.** Implementation
  - **1.** Nursing actions responsive to nursing diagnosis and risk management
    - **(a)** Nursing order entry and transmission
  - **2.** Nursing actions responsive to physicians' orders and risk management
    - **(a)** Medication administration, intravenous medications, and blood
    - **(b)** Vital signs and graphic flowsheets
    - **(c)** Intake and output
    - **(d)** Diet
  - **3.** Nursing actions responsive to procedures and unit tests and risk management
    - **(a)** Automatic schedule reminders

4. Patients' actions
5. New actions

D. Evaluations
1. Patients' response and expected outcomes resulting from nursing actions
2. Patients' response and expected outcomes resulting from physicians' orders
3. Patients' response and expected outcomes resulting from procedures and tests
4. Patients' response and expected outcomes resulting from patients' expectations
5. Daily progress note

II. Transfer note

III. Discharge care plan and summary

The following reports could result from a direct patient care system:

Admission assessment
Nursing care plan, including nursing diagnosis or KARDEX
Daily nursing progress note, including documentation of every problem or potential problem identified in the initial admission assessment and a reassessment, analysis of new nursing diagnosis, nursing actions, and evaluations
Medication administration sheets, including regularly scheduled medications, intravenous medications, and blood administration
Vital signs and other flowsheets, including intake and output, height and weight, and diet
Nursing order summary sheets
Automatic schedule summaries for special procedures and unit tests
Transfer note and care plan
Discharge care plan and summary

Examples of an Ideal Direct Patient Care System

An ideal computer system could operate as follows to document nurses' notes, care plans, and other traditional documentation requirements.

1. *Assessment.* On admission the nurse could complete a nursing assessment covering the patient's history; this includes physical characteristics, signs, and symptoms. The assessment is made 24 to 72 hours after admission depending on the hospital's policy. The nurse would enter the information into the computer through a terminal at the nursing station.
2. *Plan.* Either potential or confirmed nursing diagnosis and other patient problems are then listed. The nurse could select from predefined screens or enter these nursing and other patient problems into the computer through a terminal.
3. *Interventions.* The computer could prompt the nurse to describe interventions (actions), observations, further assessments, or teaching that the nurse determines necessary for patient care. Included in these interventions are actions that the nurse accomplishes because the patient has nursing care problems and actions taken in response to a physician's order. From the list of nursing actions, the computer could print automatic schedule reminders as needed. Included in these interventions are the patient's actions.
4. *Evaluation.* The nurse could enter evaluation information into the computer,

including the patient's response to actions, expected outcomes, and dates of expected outcomes. An expected outcome can be established for every patient, every nursing or medical problem, or every action. The nurse signs his or her name and the date.

If the computer can accept order entry from the physician, other patient problems (*e.g.*, allergies) could be added to the nursing assessment. Those orders for special procedures and medications may also become a part of the nursing implementation profile (nursing actions responsive to physicians' orders and procedures and unit tests). The system could then prompt nurses to identify nursing care problems resulting from physicians' orders. The computer output generated from physicians' orders that nurses would need include medication administration sheets, vital signs and other flowsheets, and additional physician-ordered actions on the nursing order summary sheet.

Later, the nursing progress note could contain

1. New observations, signs, and symptoms
2. Current nursing or other problems; the computer then could prompt the nurse to comment if problems have changed or new problems have occurred.
3. Previously ordered actions are documented as done/not done and given/not given, and new orders are prompted or summarized.
4. The patient's response to all actions is documented (*e.g.*, ability to learn a certain principle of hygiene).

The transfer note could summarize most of the above information when the patient is transferred. The nurse determines what information will be processed. The discharge care plan and summary are similar; the nurse determines the content from the patient's hospitalization—current problems, procedures, and nursing actions.

Major Vendors and Nursing Documentation Capabilities

Although almost 1.5 million JCAH-accredited hospital beds exist in the United States, only about 2500 have some form of computerized medical records (Downey and colleagues, 1983). The first hospitals to be automated totally usually had over 300 beds. It is not known how many of these hospitals have computerized nursing documentation. These systems were developed by approximately 30 major companies or suppliers; some suppliers have produced more than one kind of system. Each system was developed by the supplier and set up in a prototype hospital. Table 12-2 lists the major suppliers.

Several hospitals are set up to share the same computer. Today, many systems are being adapted for new facilities with software developed by a prototype hospital. Each system has its own capabilities, which are described as the standards for those systems.

The existing systems have been predominantly developed by commercial vendors, are marketed as prototype systems, and are adapted as required for a specific facility. The Burroughs Hospital Information System (HIS) (Burroughs Corporation), Patient Care Information System (Datacare Incorporated), Health Care Support Patient Care System (IBM), SMS HIS (Shared Medical Systems), Spectra 1000 HIS (Spectra Medical Systems), and MATRIX MIS (Technicon Medical Information Systems) are some of the systems with nursing documentation available. Such vendors generally timeshare the hardware or provide dedicated equipment and have standard software packages that can be adapted to the needs of a specific hospital with minimal effort, time, and expense.

TABLE 12-2 *List of Major HIS Suppliers*

SUPPLIER	SYSTEM NAME
Burroughs Corporation	BHIS
Compucare, Inc.	Compucare HIS
Computer Sciences Corporation	Not identified
Datacare, Inc.	Patient care information system
Dynamic Control Corporation	Not identified
Electronic Data Systems Corporation	PCIS
General Computer Corporation	Not identified
Global Health Systems	OE/RR
HBO and Company	IFAS/MEDPRO
Healthcare Data Systems	Not identified
Health Care Information Systems, Inc.	PAIRS
Honeywell Information Systems, Inc.	Not identified
Hospital Computer Systems, Inc.	HDC/financial system
Hospital Data Center of Virginia	HDCV
IBM Corporation—Data Processing Division	Not identified
IBM Corporation—General Systems Division	System/3 model 15D
International Data Systems, Inc.	Not identified
Jones Health Systems Management, Inc.	HOSPLEX
Martin Marietta Data Systems	H.I.S.
McAuto Hospital Services Division	HDC/HFC
McAuto Health Services Division	HFC/PCS
Medical Information Technology, Inc.	Hospital information system
M.J.S. Systems, Inc.	S/80 MIS
NCR Corporation	NCR MEDNET
National Data Communications, Inc.	NADACOM data base
Pentamation Enterprises, Inc.	PLUS/7
Shared Medical Systems	COMMAND
Space Age Computer Systems, Inc.	Mini-Master
Spectra Medical Systems	Spectra 1000 HIS
Spectra Medical Systems	Spectra 2000 FIS/MIS
Sperry Univac Corporation	WHIS-1100
Technicon Medical Information Systems	MATRIX MIS
Tymshare Medical Systems	TYMCARE/TYMMED

(After Young E, Brian E, Hardy D: Automated Hospital Information Systems Workbook, vol 1, Guide to Planning, Selecting, Acquiring, Implementing, and Managing an AHIS. Los Angeles, Center Publications, 1981)

Nursing Documentation Capabilities

Specific nursing documentation applications are related to the type of system used, and in order to understand the applications of a particular system, it is helpful to know the specifications for which suppliers designed the system. For example, system types and how nursing staff use systems can be compared (Young and colleagues, 1981). Ten major areas of nursing-related content have been developed for the computer by vendors and are listed below. (Of the ten applications, only nos. 1 and 4 relate to nursing practice documentation. The others were discussed in Chap. 9).

1. Assign/update a nursing care plan
2. Charge compilations on patients' bills that includes billing for stock items used from the inventory of a nursing unit
3. Inpatient census and census reporting

4. Recording of nurses' notes and vital signs
5. Nurse staffing management that includes rosters of available statistical reports
6. Automatic nursing reminders that include staffing schedule reports or the availability of continuing education classes
7. Nursing staff rosters that include the maintenance of personnel files, qualifications of nurses, and assignments
8. Order formatting or order entry for medical orders as well as supplies
9. Order transmission (*e.g.,* ordering supplies from the nursing station through a terminal)
10. Pharmacy floor stock inventories in order to charge patients for medications used

Table 12-3 identifies actual nursing capabilities for the major systems. It is expected that by 1990 each system will have all the above functions (Young and colleagues, 1981).

Examples of Nursing Documentation with Mainframes and Minicomputers

Many major hospital facilities document nursing practice with a computerized system. As mentioned previously, a theoretical framework reflecting nursing practice is essential to the organization of a nursing database. If data organization is understood, a computer can be more effectively used to communicate information on the nursing note. A model developed for the Technicon system that includes data organization and reflects nursing practice, JCAH standards, and legal protection for nurses is discussed below.

Many descriptions exist in the nursing literature on how nurses have used computers to document their practice. Some systems use large mainframe computers for hospital and medical information systems.

Each nurse must know the type of computer system in the hospital. The publication *Software in Healthcare* lists and describes the latest software for the health care profession. Nurses who seek to be information specialists must know what hardware and software are available to document patient care. Examples of the nursing documentation components of HIS mainframes follow.

IBM Patient Care System. IBM has nursing care plans on the computer. The patient care system developed at the State University of New York at Stony Brook incorporates many applications essential for documenting patient care, including medical and nursing order entry, patient assessment protocols, and discharge planning guides. It also contains reference data for nursing such as pharmacy and dietary guides (Edmunds, 1984).

At Crouse-Irving Memorial Hospital, Syracuse, New York, the nursing content on the PCS contains nursing care plans, and the system includes a nursing problem list based on nursing diagnosis. The care plans are based on the nursing process: assessment, planning, intervention, and evaluation. Each plan is divided into six parts, leading the nurse through a series of displays on the terminal screen at the nurses' stations. The displays help the nurse to develop the patient's care plan. Once completed, the plans become part of patients' medical records. The system also contains a miscellaneous diagnosis category that allows freeform entry into the care plans in several content areas (Lombard and Light, 1983). These care plans are being marketed as the nursing care plan installed user program (IUP), part of the IBM PCS.

The basic framework of the IBM PCS at the Brigham and Women's Hospital in Boston includes individualized patient care records that integrate medical and

TABLE 12-3 *Major Nursing Capabilities on HIS*

HIS SUPPLIER	NURSING APPLICATIONS 1	2	3	4	5	6	7	8	9	10
Burroughs Corporation	X	X	X						X	X
Compucare, Inc.			X					X	X	X
Computer Sciences Corporation	Not identified									
Datacare, Inc.	X		X		X	X	X	X	X	
Dynamic Control Corporation	Not identified									
Electronic Data Systems Corporation	X	X	X	X	X	X	X	X	X	X
General Computer Corporation		X	X							X
Global Health Systems	Not identified									
HBO and Company	X	X	X	X				X	X	
Healthcare Data Systems	Not identified									
Health Information Systems, Inc.	Not identified									
Honeywell Information Systems, Inc.	X	X	X	X			X		X	X
Hospital Computer Systems, Inc.	Not identified									
Hospital Data Center of Virginia		X	X					X	X	
IBM Corporation — Data Processing Division	X	X	X	X	X	X	X	X	X	X
IBM Corporation — General Systems Division		X	X					X	X	X
International Data Systems, Inc.	Not identified									

CORRESPONDING CODES

1. Assign/update nursing care plan
2. Charge compilation
3. Inpatient census/reports
4. Nurses' notes/vital signs update chart
5. Nurse staffing management
6. Nurse scheduling automatic reminders
7. Staff rosters
8. Order format tailoring to type of order
9. Order transmission
10. Pharmacy floor stocks inventory

Jones Health Systems Management, Inc.	Not identified									
Martin Marietta Data Systems	X									
McAuto Hospital Services Division		X	X		X				X	
McAuto Health Services Division	Not specified which McAuto									
Medical Information Technology, Inc.		X	X					X	X	
M.J.S. Systems, Inc.	Not identified									
NCR Corporation	X	X	X		X			X	X	X
National Data Communications, Inc.	X	X	X	X	X	X	X	X	X	X
Pentamation Enterprises, Inc.		X	X		X		X	X	X	
Shared Medical Systems	X	X	X					X	X	X
Space Age Computer Systems, Inc.	Not identified									
Spectra Medical Systems 1000 HIS	X	X	X		X		X		X	X
Spectra Medical Systems 2000 FIS/MIS	Not specified which spectra									
Sperry Univac Corporation	Not identified									
Technicon Medical Information System	X	X	X	X		X		X	X	
Tymshare Medical Systems	Not identified									

(After Young E, Brian E, Hardy D: Automated Hospital Information Systems Workbook, vol 1, Guide to Planning, Selecting, Acquiring, Implementing, and Managing an AHIS. Los Angeles, Center Publications, 1981) nursing problem lists, physicians' orders, care plans, medication and nutrition plans, the charting of vital signs, and nursing notes. This design produces a nursing care plan and nursing notes that become a part of the patient's medical record (Fig. 12-1) (Gebhardt, 1983).

Martin Marietta. The Martin Marietta HIS provides several components for on-line charting and nurses' notes. Nurses can chart vital signs and medications. Nurses' notes are typed in using a terminal keyboard or lightpen selections. Menu-selected observations and notes are categorized into the following sets of observations: gastrointestinal, musculoskeletal, -ostomy, stool, skin, neuro-, cardiovascular, urology, intravenous site, labor, postpartum, intravenous administration, and blood administration. Nursing care plans can be entered using the nursing diagnosis format. Nursing documents normally printed by the computer include vital sign flowsheets, care orders by shift, medication record, nurses' notes and observations by shifts, and care plans. Other HIS components used by nurses are also available, such as order entry (Martin Marietta, 1983).

Shared Medical Systems. The Shared Medical Systems (SMS) HIS offers documentation advantages as well as administrative applications. In the documentation components, the SMS facilitates care plan development with hospital-defined care plans for "various diagnoses" (Shared Medical Systems, 1983). These care plans can serve as standards on which individualized care plans can be developed.

```
ROOM 14A111 DOE, JANE        MRN 000-000-0        AGE 082Y       DR. ALAN JOSEPH
  RES =                      H.O. = J. GREEN                     NURSE = S. SNUTA
                       DIET->  7/8 REGULAR PUREED FOODS

  P R O B L E M   L I S T
                A         FRACTURED LEFT HIP
                B         PRE-OP LEFT HIP SURGERY
                C         POST-OP LEFT HIP SURGERY
                D         IMMOBILITY
                E         CONFUSION

  D O C T O R S   O R D E R S
                XXX       07/16/82   ALLERGIES: N.K.
                DG        FRACTURED LEFT HIP
                XXX       06/24/82   ADM TO 14A - COND. SATISFACTORY
                XXX       07/08/82   NUTRITION: PUREE REGULAR DIET
  18    22      Q4H       07/16/82   ROUTINE VITAL SIGNS
                XXX       07/16/82 - PRE/OP HIP SURG.

  C A R E   P L A N
                A         FRACTURED LEFT HIP
                          1.   POSITION PT. IN PROPER BODY ALIGNMENT
                          2.   ASSIST AS NEEDED
                B         PRE-OP LEFT HIP SURGERY
                          1.   PRE-OP TEACHING
                          2.   PHISOHEX SCRUBS AS TOLERATED
                          3.   EXPLAIN USE OF IV THERAPY AFTER SURGERY
                          4.   EXPLAIN THE IMPORTANCE OF PROPER BODY ALIGNMENT
                          5.   NPO AFTER MN 6/24
```

FIG. 12-1. Sample printout of care plan. (Gebhardt AN: Developing a patient care program. In Scholes M, Bryant Y, Barber B [eds]: The Impact of Computers on Nursing: An International Review, p 102. Amsterdam, North-Holland, 1983)

SMS has a unique system that integrates the patient's clinical data with financial data, nurse staffing data, and patient acuity information. Based on nursing assessments, the system accumulates information on what nursing actions have affected nursing time for patient care.

Integrated with physicians' orders, this system provides the automated medication administration record so that nurses can document medications given. In addition to drug name, route of administration, dose, and start and stop dates, auxiliary drug-specific information is given while the nurse administers the medication. An order history (summary) can be retrieved from the system at any time during a patient's hospitalization.

The system keeps track of special procedures and physicians' orders. It identifies medications for which physicians' orders will expire and automatically notifies the dietary department to restrict a patient's diet when a barium enema is ordered for the next day.

In view of its retrieval capabilities, the system can be used in quality assurance audits if nursing personnel document patients' problems, actions taken, patients' response, and whether outcomes were met. Improvements in care can be monitored, and thus the effectiveness of specific nursing actions are documented.

National Cash Register. The National Cash Register (NCR)/MEDNET system can include nursing documentation linked to the patient accounting system in the financial office. This system also has a portable nursing unit terminal called the P-NUT, designed to accompany the nurse to the bedside. Consisting of a keyboard and an integrated digital temperature probe and blood pressure cuff, the P-NUT is used in conjunction with the NCR Decision Mate V, a terminal linked to the NCR/MEDNET communication network. The P-NUT receives information from the main computer and can hold the nursing information on 8 to 12 patients. The design is based on the primary nurse model (Buthker, 1983).

P-NUT allows nursing documentation in the following areas: vital signs, recall and documentation of medications, and nursing process documentation. The nursing process documentation includes assessment, care plan, interventions, and patients' responses. Nurses' notes are integrated with the care plan. After the information is collected at bedside, the P-NUT is returned to a terminal that communicates with the main computer. The vital sign flowsheets, the medical record, and nursing notes are generated (Buthker, 1983).

Burroughs. The Burroughs Corporation HIS is an integrated system developed by the Medi-Data Corporation at the Charlotte Memorial Hospital, Charlotte North Carolina. One of the early systems developed for hospitals, its major goal is to communicate the care given to a patient to all hospital units and care providers (Somers, 1971). The system has been upgraded and changed as computer technology has progressed.

This system is available to hospitals in this country and abroad. Allowing documentation of patient care orders using on-line display terminals integrated throughout the hospital, the system includes a patient care database containing profiles of all patients. It allows patient care plans to be produced for each shift change, and it also provides a care plan summary on discharge. The system includes a nursing component, and patient care plans can be documented using nursing diagnoses, standard care plans, or problem-oriented care plans. The system also offers administrative applications, including patient classification, quality monitoring, staffing framework, and management reporting (Burroughs Hospital Information System, 1978).

Technicon MATRIX MIS. An early nursing system that used computers for nursing care planning is in use at El Camino Hospital, in Mountain View, California. Designed by Technicon, this system allowed nurses to develop standard care plans in matrix format (Mayers, 1974). One of the first systems to include nursing documentation, it has been described extensively in the nursing literature. Since it was a prototype system, it has also undergone in-depth evaluations.

The content for documenting nursing care plans is also available on the Technicon MIS (Howe, 1980). Six categories were described for this system in 1970; each category has additional problems identified and desired outcomes listed. Over 200 assessment factors were organized under the six basic categories. An example of this type of documentation is shown in Table 9-7. The structured format was intended to guide nurses in assessing patients' needs. Because the problems were identified with specific patient outcomes intended, the model was designed to use actual nursing documentation with quality assurance audit criteria.

The NIH Experience. Another model developed for the Technicon MIS was a system to document nursing care at the Clinical Center, National Institutes of Health, Bethesda, Maryland. Initially the content included admission notes, care plans, observational status reports, suicidal assessment, and interim information (Gearhart, 1981). In general, in the NIH computer system, all patients are admitted to the facility through the computer system. The physician enters all orders for the patient into the computer. A lightpen is used to make selections from a display

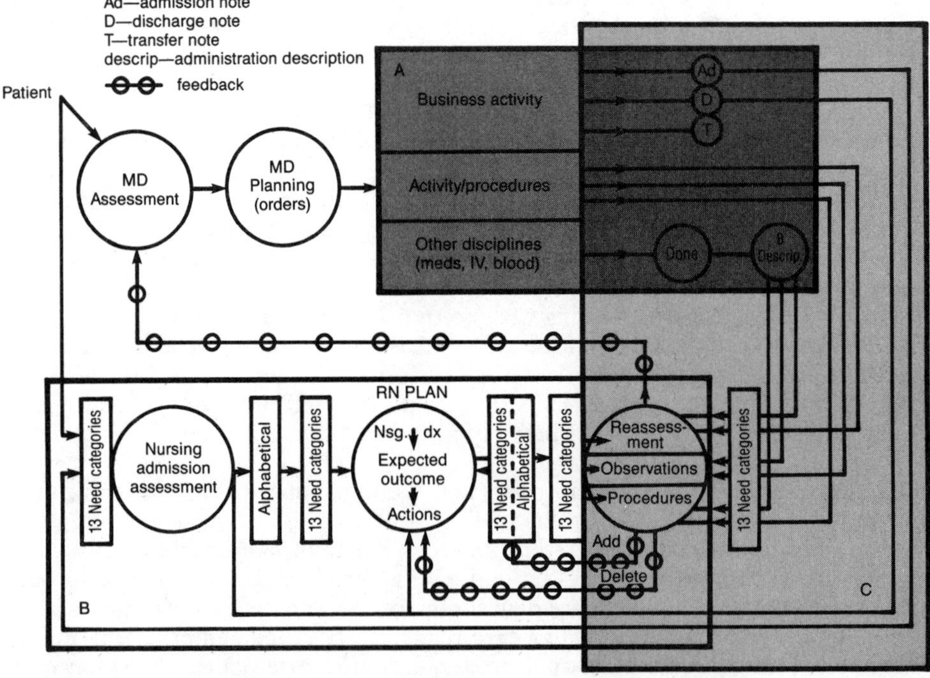

FIG. 12-2. Three modules of documentation in the Technicon MATRIX MIS system. (Romano C, McCormick K, McNeely L: Nursing documentation: A model for a computerized data base. Adv Nurs Sc 4:43–56, 1982)

terminal. Nurses can record patient observations, vital signs, medications and intravenous administration, and other activities on the terminal. Nurses access the computer through a code given to them after an orientation. Other health professionals also have access codes. Printers are available in the nursing areas to provide copies of the forms that become the nurses shift reports, summary reports, worksheets, and patients' medical records. Both nursing notes and nursing care plans are printed from data entered by nursing personnel through the lightpen selection items or typed in through a keyboard. One terminal in a nursing station can serve 10 patients (Romano and colleagues, 1982).

Basic Areas of Documentation. Three modules of nursing documentation were identified on the Technicon System (Fig. 12-2).

Interdependent nursing, documentation of nursing actions that require a medical order
Independent nursing, which includes care plans and nursing notes
A combination of the above (Romano and colleagues, 1982)

In Module A physicians write orders for nurses, including vital signs, respiratory therapy, suctioning, tracheostomy care, positioning, cardiac monitors, pacemakers, compresses and soaks, hyperalimentation catheters, enemas, irrigation and instillations, restraints, supports and binders, dressings, hygiene, seclusion, activity, sedation, wet sheet packs, and unit tests.

In Module B, when nursing enters nursing process content in the computer, the essential components are assess, plan, implement, and evaluate. The format for the Technicon system accommodates the nursing process in the form shown in Figure 12-3.

Cluster	Category	Subcategory	Pathway	Data Point
Nursing Admission Assessment	Air Circulation Comfort/Pain Elimination- bowel bladder Food/Fluid Hygiene/Skin Mobility Neuro Sensory Physical Safety Sexuality Sleep/Rest Socio-Psychological Teaching/Learning		Pattern/Impairment/Aid Neuro Sensory Neuro Sensory Specialty Socio-Psychological 11 pathways Teaching/Learning Home Management Learning	Infinite
Nursing Care Plan		Nursing Diagnosis	Expected Outcome Nursing Actions	Current Revised Complete Content Chart Point Deadlines
Nursing Reassessment/ Observations		Reassessment Observations Procedures	Pattern/Impairment/Aid Specific Type Specific Type	Infinite

FIG. 12-3. Format of nursing process content (Technicon MATRIX MIS). (Romano C, McCormick K, McNeely L: Nursing documentation: A model for a computerized data base. Adv Nurs Sc 4:43–56, 1982)

In Module C, the nursing part of the note responding to medical orders is in the form given/not given and to be done/not done. A description of the procedure can be entered through the nursing observation content (Romano and colleagues, 1982).

File Structure MATRIX MIS. The file structure MATRIX MIS uses data trees to describe nursing content (Fig. 12-4). After being assessed, data are divided into pattern, impairment, and aid. For instance, if a patient has trouble breathing, *air*

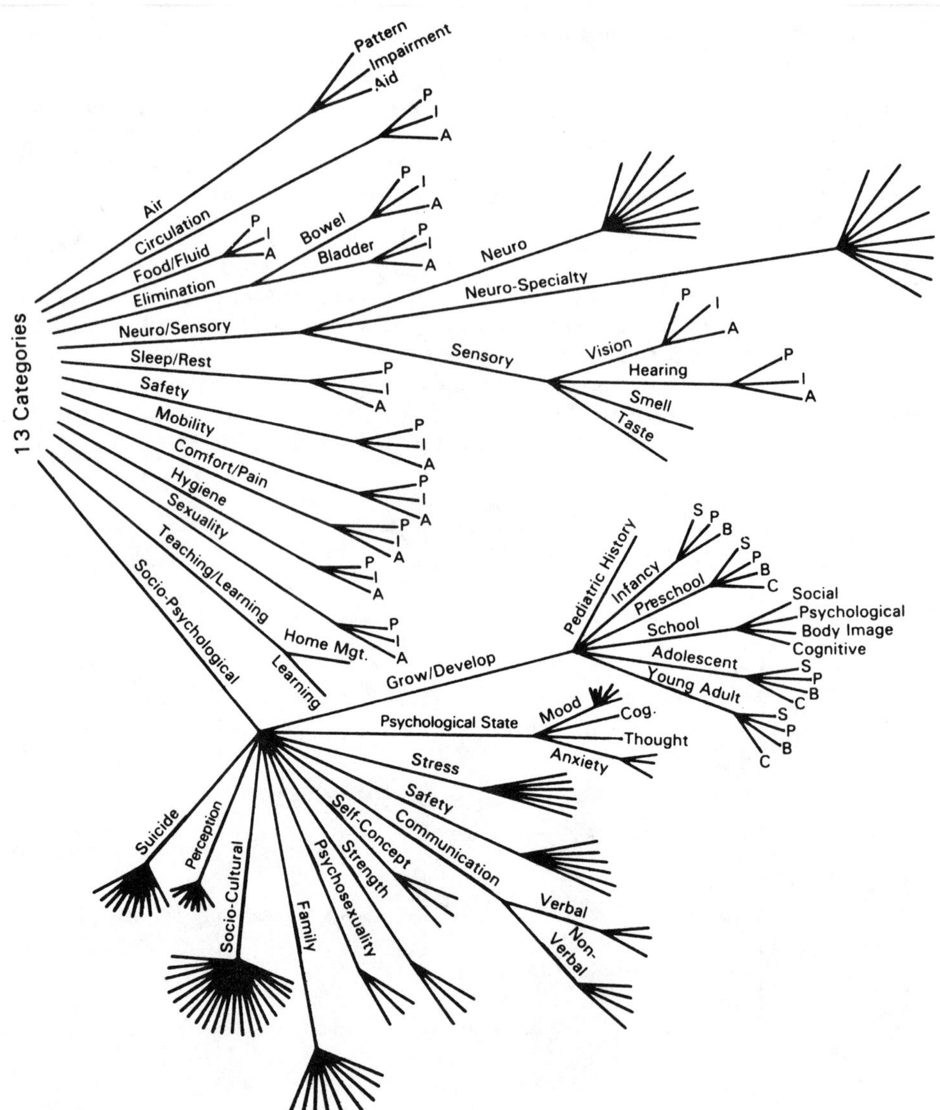

FIG. 12-4. Nursing assessment data tree (Technicon MATRIX MIS). (Romano C, McCormick K, McNeely L: Nursing documentation: A model for a computerized data base. Adv Nurs Sc 4:43–56, 1982)

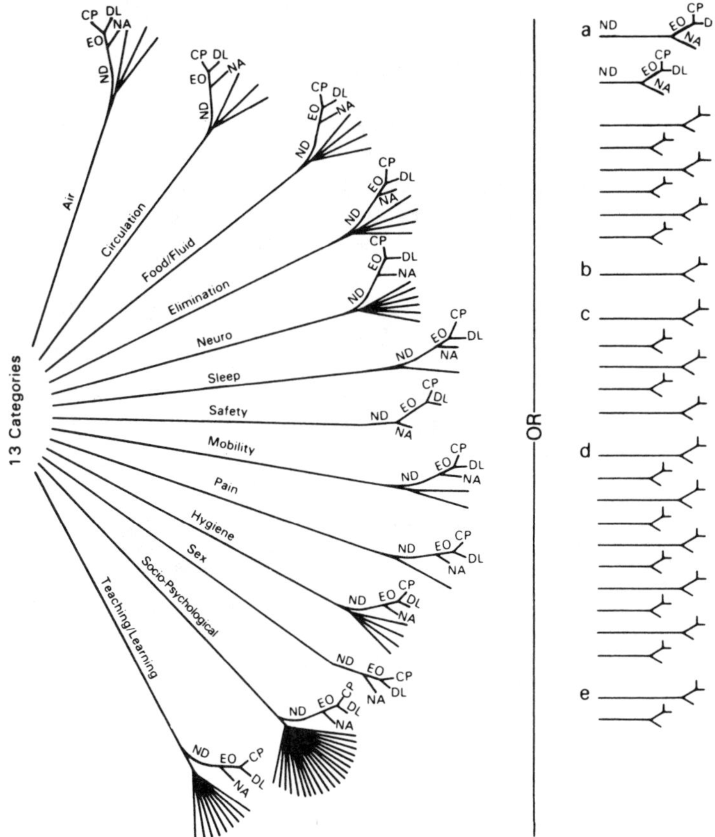

FIG. 12-5. Nursing care plan data tree. *ND*, nursing diagnosis; *EO*, expected outcomes; *CP*, check progress; *DL*, deadline; *NA*, nursing action (Technicon MATRIX MIS). (Romano C, McCormick K, McNeely L: Nursing documentation: A model for a computerized data base. Adv Nurs Sc 4:43–56, 1982)

would be selected as a category. The pattern of breathing (rate, depth, rhythm) would then be assessed, and the impairment would be selected as the observable deficiency that interferes with meeting a basic need. The aid describes the device or activity used to take care of the problem — in this example, oxygen (Romano and colleagues, 1982). An assessment tree of improvement, stabilization, or deterioration could also be chosen.

The data tree for the nursing care plan component of this system is shown in Figure 12-5. The Technicon system accommodates the use of nursing diagnosis after a category is chosen. The nurse can then chart an expected outcome, a nursing action, a progress point, or a deadline. Care plans designed on admission can be checked periodically, and outcomes can be charted as met or not (Romano and colleagues, 1982).

The data tree components of the nursing observation component resembles the assessment component except that observation and procedure sections were added to contain additional descriptions.

This system has approximately 4000 screens and data organized into data trees with data points into infinity, allowing for endless opportunities for documentation. An evaluation of the impact of this type of system has been described (Anser, 1982).

The New York University Medical Center Experience. Figure 12-6 shows another style of nursing documentation available on IBM hardware with Technicon software and peripheral hardware in a 727-bed tertiary care teaching hospital. In this system, medical orders are entered into the computer directly by physicians.

Nursing has developed the content within the computer to perform assessments, which are described by physical assessment needs; a patient who had suffered a cerebrovascular accident, for instance, would receive an in-depth assessment of neurological status (Kelly, 1983).

In addition, nursing care planning is possible after assessment and nursing diagnosis have been made. After the severity of a disease is staged, the nurse can select treatment from a menu (Fig. 12-7). (Kelly, 1983).

This system integrates nursing with risk management. The nursing orders

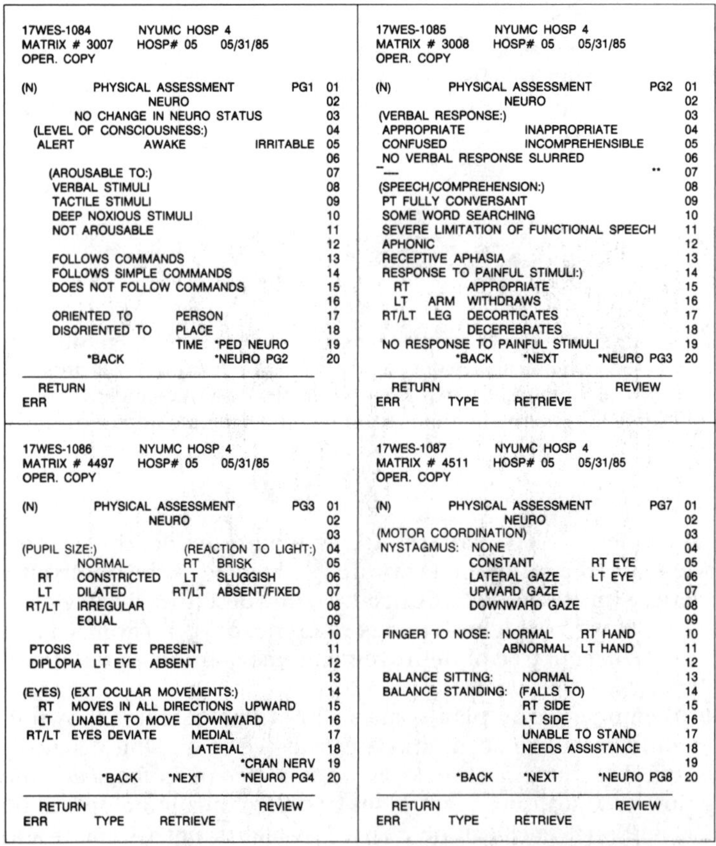

17WES-1084 NYUMC HOSP 4
MATRIX # 3007 HOSP# 05 05/31/85
OPER. COPY

(N) PHYSICAL ASSESSMENT PG1
NEURO
NO CHANGE IN NEURO STATUS
(LEVEL OF CONSCIOUSNESS:)
ALERT AWAKE IRRITABLE

(AROUSABLE TO:)
VERBAL STIMULI
TACTILE STIMULI
DEEP NOXIOUS STIMULI
NOT AROUSABLE

FOLLOWS COMMANDS
FOLLOWS SIMPLE COMMANDS
DOES NOT FOLLOW COMMANDS

ORIENTED TO PERSON
DISORIENTED TO PLACE
TIME *PED NEURO
*BACK *NEURO PG2

RETURN
ERR

17WES-1085 NYUMC HOSP 4
MATRIX # 3008 HOSP# 05 05/31/85
OPER. COPY

(N) PHYSICAL ASSESSMENT PG2
NEURO
(VERBAL RESPONSE:)
APPROPRIATE INAPPROPRIATE
CONFUSED INCOMPREHENSIBLE
NO VERBAL RESPONSE SLURRED

(SPEECH/COMPREHENSION:)
PT FULLY CONVERSANT
SOME WORD SEARCHING
SEVERE LIMITATION OF FUNCTIONAL SPEECH
APHONIC
RECEPTIVE APHASIA
RESPONSE TO PAINFUL STIMULI:)
RT APPROPRIATE
LT ARM WITHDRAWS
RT/LT LEG DECORTICATES
DECEREBRATES
NO RESPONSE TO PAINFUL STIMULI
*BACK *NEXT *NEURO PG3

RETURN REVIEW
ERR TYPE RETRIEVE

17WES-1086 NYUMC HOSP 4
MATRIX # 4497 HOSP# 05 05/31/85
OPER. COPY

(N) PHYSICAL ASSESSMENT PG3
NEURO

(PUPIL SIZE:) (REACTION TO LIGHT:)
NORMAL RT BRISK
RT CONSTRICTED LT SLUGGISH
LT DILATED RT/LT ABSENT/FIXED
RT/LT IRREGULAR
EQUAL

PTOSIS RT EYE PRESENT
DIPLOPIA LT EYE ABSENT

(EYES) (EXT OCULAR MOVEMENTS:)
RT MOVES IN ALL DIRECTIONS UPWARD
LT UNABLE TO MOVE DOWNWARD
RT/LT EYES DEVIATE MEDIAL
LATERAL
*CRAN NERV
*BACK *NEXT *NEURO PG4

RETURN REVIEW
ERR TYPE RETRIEVE

17WES-1087 NYUMC HOSP 4
MATRIX # 4511 HOSP# 05 05/31/85
OPER. COPY

(N) PHYSICAL ASSESSMENT PG7
NEURO
(MOTOR COORDINATION)
NYSTAGMUS: NONE
CONSTANT RT EYE
LATERAL GAZE LT EYE
UPWARD GAZE
DOWNWARD GAZE

FINGER TO NOSE: NORMAL RT HAND
ABNORMAL LT HAND

BALANCE SITTING: NORMAL
BALANCE STANDING: (FALLS TO)
RT SIDE
LT SIDE
UNABLE TO STAND
NEEDS ASSISTANCE

*BACK *NEXT *NEURO PG8

RETURN REVIEW
ERR TYPE RETRIEVE

FIG. 12-6. Nursing assessment using IBM hardware and Technicon software. (Kelly J: Computers in hospitals: Nursing practice defined and validated. In Dayhoff R [ed]: Proceedings from the Seventh Annual Symposium on Computer Applications in Medical Care. Silver Spring, MD, IEEE Computer Society Press, 1983)

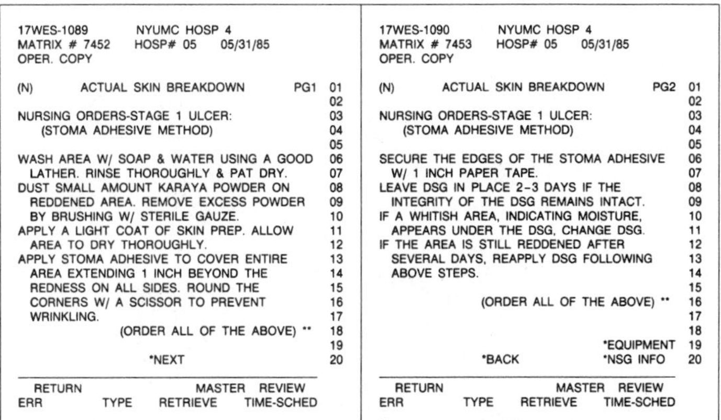

17WES-1089 NYUMC HOSP 4
MATRIX # 7452 HOSP# 05 05/31/85
OPER. COPY

(N) ACTUAL SKIN BREAKDOWN PG1

NURSING ORDERS-STAGE 1 ULCER:
(STOMA ADHESIVE METHOD)

WASH AREA W/ SOAP & WATER USING A GOOD LATHER. RINSE THOROUGHLY & PAT DRY.
DUST SMALL AMOUNT KARAYA POWDER ON REDDENED AREA. REMOVE EXCESS POWDER BY BRUSHING W/ STERILE GAUZE.
APPLY A LIGHT COAT OF SKIN PREP. ALLOW AREA TO DRY THOROUGHLY.
APPLY STOMA ADHESIVE TO COVER ENTIRE AREA EXTENDING 1 INCH BEYOND THE REDNESS ON ALL SIDES. ROUND THE CORNERS W/ A SCISSOR TO PREVENT WRINKLING.
(ORDER ALL OF THE ABOVE) **

*NEXT

RETURN MASTER REVIEW
ERR TYPE RETRIEVE TIME-SCHED

17WES-1090 NYUMC HOSP 4
MATRIX # 7453 HOSP# 05 05/31/85
OPER. COPY

(N) ACTUAL SKIN BREAKDOWN PG2

NURSING ORDERS-STAGE 1 ULCER:
(STOMA ADHESIVE METHOD)

SECURE THE EDGES OF THE STOMA ADHESIVE W/ 1 INCH PAPER TAPE.
LEAVE DSG IN PLACE 2-3 DAYS IF THE INTEGRITY OF THE DSG REMAINS INTACT.
IF A WHITISH AREA, INDICATING MOISTURE, APPEARS UNDER THE DSG, CHANGE DSG.
IF THE AREA IS STILL REDDENED AFTER SEVERAL DAYS, REAPPLY DSG FOLLOWING ABOVE STEPS.

(ORDER ALL OF THE ABOVE) **

*EQUIPMENT
*BACK *NSG INFO

RETURN MASTER REVIEW
ERR TYPE RETRIEVE TIME-SCHED

FIG. 12-7. Examples of nursing orders (IBM hardware, Technicon software). (Kelly J: Computers in hospitals: Nursing practice defined and validated. In Dayhoff R [ed]: Proceedings from the Seventh Annual Symposium on Computer Applications in Medical Care. Silver Spring, MD, IEEE Computer Society Press, 1983)

shown in Figure 12-8 would be the screens that follow the nurse's diagnostic selection. In addition, if the nurse selected "one siderail only" the policy regarding this would be shown on the next screen. This would remind the nurse that the policy is limiting and warrants a nursing justification. In this way the computer interrelates nursing decision making with risk management. Issues that present specific risk management problems to a hospital can be interrelated with nursing documentation by simple policy reminders. Nursing personnel are thus kept aware of nursing orders that may not be appropriate (Kelly, 1983).

If the content within the nursing system contains risk management data, policies can be added to the screens. If certain patient care problems are uncommon, standard care plans can be added to the system so that nurses can learn appropriate assessments and actions. For example, if patients are admitted only rarely for outpatient elective surgery, standard postoperative nursing actions can be added to the content screens.

POMR. Many descriptions of nursing content have used the problem-oriented medical record (POMR) (Weed 1969). The problem-oriented MIS (PROMIS), the information system technologically supported by two Control Data Corporation 1700 Series computers, was initiated with terminals located on a ward and in the radiology, surgery, pharmacy, laboratory, library, and maintenance and development sections of the Medical Center Hospital of Vermont (Weed and Hertzberg, 1976).

POMR is used to document direct patient care in four parts: database, problem list, initial plans for each problem, and progress notes. In PROMIS the care plan format included subjective symptoms, objective signs, assessment, and plans (SOAP). The SOAP note includes patient problems, needs, nursing actions, and patient responses. Many mainframes and microcomputers still use the POMR and SOAP formats.

International Systems. The Department of Health and Social Security in the United Kingdom established an experimental program to develop computerized nursing documentation. Since 1974, a computer project nurses' group has met to

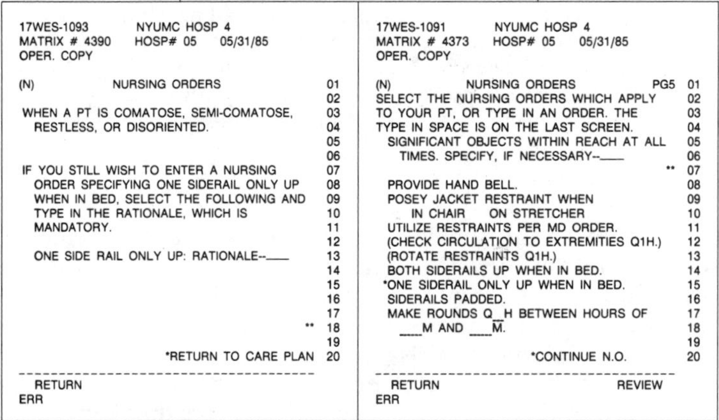

17WES-1092 NYUMC HOSP 4
MATRIX # 4389 HOSP# 05 05/31/85
OPER. COPY

(N) NURSING ORDERS
VIEW ONLY
EXCEPT WHEN A STAFF MEMBER IS GIVING DIRECT CARE, BOTH SIDERAILS MUST BE UP IN THE FOLLOWING CIRCUMSTANCES:

AFTER PT HAS RECEIVED PRE-ANESTHETIC MEDICATION.
AFTER PT HAS BEEN HEAVILY SEDATED PRIOR TO TESTS, TREATMENTS OR EXAMS.
POST-OPERATIVELY UNTIL PT HAS FULLY REACTED & IS ORIENTED TO PERSON, PLACE & TIME.
WHEN A PT HAS SEVERE VISUAL LIMITATIONS IS BLIND, OR HAS BOTH EYES COVERED.
WHEN A PT HAS NEURO-MUSCULAR IMPAIRMENT &/OR OTHER PHYSICAL LIMITATIONS, & HAS NOT ACHIEVED CONTROL OF BALANCE & MOVEMENT WHILE IN BED.
*CONTINUE

RETURN
ERR

17WES-1093 NYUMC HOSP 4
MATRIX # 4390 HOSP# 05 05/31/85
OPER. COPY

(N) NURSING ORDERS

WHEN A PT IS COMATOSE, SEMI-COMATOSE, RESTLESS, OR DISORIENTED.

IF YOU STILL WISH TO ENTER A NURSING ORDER SPECIFYING ONE SIDERAIL ONLY UP WHEN IN BED, SELECT THE FOLLOWING AND TYPE IN THE RATIONALE, WHICH IS MANDATORY.

ONE SIDE RAIL ONLY UP: RATIONALE--____

**

*RETURN TO CARE PLAN

RETURN
ERR

17WES-1091 NYUMC HOSP 4
MATRIX # 4373 HOSP# 05 05/31/85
OPER. COPY

(N) NURSING ORDERS PG5
SELECT THE NURSING ORDERS WHICH APPLY TO YOUR PT, OR TYPE IN AN ORDER. THE TYPE IN SPACE IS ON THE LAST SCREEN.
SIGNIFICANT OBJECTS WITHIN REACH AT ALL TIMES. SPECIFY, IF NECESSARY--____
**
PROVIDE HAND BELL.
POSEY JACKET RESTRAINT WHEN
IN CHAIR ON STRETCHER
UTILIZE RESTRAINTS PER MD ORDER.
(CHECK CIRCULATION TO EXTREMITIES Q1H.)
(ROTATE RESTRAINTS Q1H.)
BOTH SIDERAILS UP WHEN IN BED.
*ONE SIDERAIL ONLY UP WHEN IN BED.
SIDERAILS PADDED.
MAKE ROUNDS Q_H BETWEEN HOURS OF ___M AND ___M.

*CONTINUE N.O.

RETURN REVIEW
ERR

FIG. 12-8. Nursing documentation integrated with nursing policies and risk management (IBM hardware, Technicon software). (Kelly J: Computers in hospitals: Nursing practice defined and validated. In Dayhoff R [ed]: Proceedings from the Seventh Annual Symposium on Computer Applications in Medical Care. Silver Spring, MD, IEEE Computer Society Press, 1983)

network about computer development and other applications. Two hospitals were the site of the computer program development: the Royal Devon and Exeter Hospital and the Queen Elizabeth Hospital, Birmingham. A similar development project was undertaken in Ninewells Hospital, Dundee, Scotland. The hospitals developed their computer systems for patient care planning and were committed to the nursing process. Each hospital organized its nursing record according to nursing unit needs and special patient care problems. An example of a care plan from the Exeter Hospital is shown in Figure 12-9 (Ashton, 1983; Astbury, 1983).

Discharge Care Planning

The documentation of patient care usually begins with the admission assessment and ends with the discharge care plan. Discharge care planning provides for continuity of care from the home to the hospital and back to the community, another care facility, an outpatient department, or the home. The computer facilitates this communication network and can provide for this continuity when computer systems within hospitals and other care facilities can communicate with each other.

Components. Computers within a single hospital are being used to generate a discharge care plan for each patient. In such automated systems, the discharge care plan includes five components (Romano, 1982):

A summary of the admission assessment
A summary of learning needs that the patient had at discharge
A multidisciplinary plan including problems still unresolved and outcomes not met during hospitalization
Medications and procedures that the patient must continue
A summary of selected patient outcomes that a multidisciplinary team desired as minimal criteria for the patient to have achieved during hospitalization

Computerized discharge care plans have the potential to be used for quality assurance, audit, research data, and information necessary for categorizing persons at discharge for prospective payment.

Patients can be sent home with printed discharge plans if the content of the computerized nursing interventions or those outcomes not met while the patient was hospitalized are used. The problem list can also be sent with patients who are transferred to different institutions or to different wards within the same hospital (Wessling, 1972). An example of content that might appear on a display terminal documenting a discharge care plan through an MIS is shown in Figure 12-10.

International Experiences. In countries with health care access to all citizens, interrelated communication networks and continuity of care through discharge care plans are vital. In Sweden, for example, Stockholm County has had an interactive regional health information system in use at all 74 hospitals for over 15 years. The documentation on each patient contained in this system is administrative information and recent examinations and tests. The information can be accessed by medical and nursing staff working at any of the hospitals.

The vital information on each patient that must be communicated to all health professionals has been identified as follows (Jelger and Regid, 1983):

Summary of all previous admissions, diagnoses, or symptoms of those admissions, physicians and nurses who treated the patient, and what hospital or clinic the patient was admitted to
Information on transfers or referrals to other health care facilities
Most common medical diagnoses and treatment protocols
Overview of previous and planned consultations
Summary of previous and planned special procedures and tests
Common medications taken
Sick leave taken from the person's place of employment

United Kingdom Experience. The discharge care plan, called the discharge print in the United Kingdom, has been used to include the nursing care plan, hospital record number, patient name, consultants attending the patient, bed number on a ward, date, and time. It also includes all patient information still current on the day of discharge, nursing orders administered during hospitalization, and current orders that the patient must continue. Using the computer for the discharge care plan facilitates communication among nurses (Astbury, 1983).

-1149-HOURS- SINGLE ROOMS WARD OKEMENT

A.N. OTHER 123456 WHO ________________1149-HOURS-02.11.82 — Tuesday

Special Needs & Precautions

PROTECTIVE ISOLATION (BLUE CARD).
WEARS GLASSES.
WEARS DENTURES, UPPER.
SOAK DENTURES IN NYSTATIN FOUR TIMES DAILY.

More Information on VDU

Basic Care

WASH AT WASH BASIN, OR SHOWER, WITH HELP. (—)
MOUTHCARE, 2-HOURLY. (chart)
TREAT PRESSURE AREA 4-HOURLY WITH SOAP AND WATER. (R1, R2, R3, R4, R5, R6
PATIENT LIKES 3 PILLOWS AT NIGHT. (—)

Mobility

UP AS ABLE.

Diet & Fluids	
DIET: NORMAL.	
FREE FLUIDS.	(chart)
Observations & Recordings	
RECORD TEMPERATURE, PULSE 4 × DAILY.	(SF'10, 14, 21)
RECORD BLOOD PRESSURE 2 × DAILY.	(10, 16)
RECORD WEIGHT WEEKLY ON SUNDAY.	(—)
Tests & Investigations	
ROUTINE URINE TEST, 2 × WEEKLY ON THURSDAY AND SUNDAY.	(—)
TEST URINE FOR BLOOD, DAILY.	(SF)
Technical Care	
INTRAVENOUS MEDICATION AS PRESCRIPTION SHEET.	(chart)
CARE OF VENFLON.	

FIG. 12-9. An example of a nursing care plan printout from the Exeter Hospital. (Astbury C: Nursing care plans: Aspects of computer use in nurse-to-nurse communication. In Fokkens O et al [eds]: Medinfo 83 Seminars. Amsterdam, North-Holland, 1983)

DISCHARGE CARE PLAN

PATIENT NAME: ADMISSION DATE:

IDENTIFICATION NUMBER: MEDICAL DIAGNOSIS:

DOCTOR (NAME): NURSING DIAGNOSIS:

NURSE (NAME): SPECIAL TESTS AND PROCEDURES:

SOCIAL WORKER (NAME):

PHARMACIST (NAME):

PHYSICAL THERAPIST (NAME):

MEDICAL OUTCOMES MET DURING HOSPITALIZATION:

NURSING OUTCOMES MET DURING HOSPITLIZATION:

PATIENT OUTCOMES MET DURING HOSPITALIZATION:

UNMET MEDICAL NEEDS:

UNMET MEDICATION NEEDS:

UNMET NURSING NEEDS:

UNMET SOCIAL NEEDS:

MEDICATIONS PATIENT TAKES (LIST):

SPECIAL PROCEDURES:

SPECIAL EQUIPMENT NEEDS:

DIET:

REFERRALS:

ACTIVITY:

DATE OF RETURN APPOINTMENT:

FIG. 12-10. Discharge care plan format.

A COMPUTERIZED NURSING RECORD FROM ADMISSION TO DISCHARGE—A COMPOSITE VIEW

Many different approaches to document nursing practice now exist. Some systems use nursing problem lists; others use nursing diagnosis, medical diagnosis, or frequent orders to drive the menu selections. Although specialty units are known to require particular documentation requirements, common elements in nursing assessment, planning, implementation, and evaluation have not yet been identified. Most important, however, is that the student become familiar with many existing systems (Scholes and colleagues, 1983).

A composite view of computer screens that could appear on a cathode ray tube (CRT) is shown in Figures 12-11 to 12-23. With a lightpen selector or teletypewriter, the matrix selection on a hypothetical patient will respond to the displays. These figures display screens that could be used to admit a patient (Fig. 12-11), do

```
█          P R E - A D M I S S I O N - P E R S O N A L   D A T A
 PATIENT-ID PATIENT NAME                ADDITIONAL NAME TTL  SEX AGE  ADM.DATE TIME
▶   803254◀▶MYERS MARTHA R              ◀▶GRAYSON      ◀▶MRS ◀▶F◀▶24Y◀▶07-29---◀▶1400
 PATIENT ADDRESS                                           CITY/STATE          ZIP
▶1901 SOUTH BOULEVARD              ◀▶APT 3A           ◀▶CHARLOTTE, N C      ◀▶28209◀
 HOME-PHONE    BIRTHDATE   BIRTHPLACE                  REL/CHURCH
▶704-535-4163◀ ▶8-31-53 ◀ ▶WILMINGTON N C        ◀ ▶METHODIST                  ◀
 ROOM-BD    FC    CR  RACE  M/S NOTABLE   SVC   DR-CD  DOCTOR NAME
▶        ◀ ▶02◀  ▶   ◀ ▶ ◀   ▶M◀  ▶N◀     ▶SUR◀ ▶16025◀ BROWN J C
HIST# ▶K36752     ◀  PREV-ADM ▶03-75   ◀ SS ▶241-88-3141  ◀ SG-DTS
EST-DAYS ▶    ◀ DIAGNOSIS ▶POSSIBLE CHOLECYSTOLITHIASIS                         ◀
REMARKS▶NOTIFY DR BROWN WHEN PATIENT ARRIVES                                      ◀
 POSITION       EMPLOYER NAME/ADDRESS                                    TELEPHONE
▶SECRETARY    ◀ ▶APEX BUILDING SUPPLIES                             ◀ ▶704-523-1641◀
 RESPONSIBLE PARTY              RELATION     TELEPHONE
▶MYERS MARTHA R              ◀ ▶SELF      ◀ ▶704-535-4163◀
 RESPONSIBLE PARTY ADDRESS                                  CITY/STATE          ZIP
▶1901 SOUTH BOULEVARD              ◀▶APT 3A           ◀▶CHARLOTTE, N C      ◀▶28209◀
POSTN▶SECRETARY    ◀EMP NM/ADDR▶APEX BUILDING SUPPLIES                             ◀
 EMERGENCY CONTACT NAME       RELATION     EMERG CONT CITY/STATE          TELEPHONE
▶ROBERT E MYERS              ◀ ▶HUSBAND   ◀ ▶CHARLOTTE, N C          ◀▶704-535-4163◀
 INS?
 ▶Y◀
                                                                            Page  1
```

FIG. 12-11. Patient admission screen (Burroughs HIS).

a nursing assessment (Fig. 12-12), chart a nursing care plan (Fig. 12-13), obtain medication information (Fig. 12-14), enter a medication order (Fig. 12-15), chart administration of medications (Fig. 12-16), display laboratory test results (Fig. 12-17), review current physicians' orders (Fig. 12-18), schedule a patient for surgery (Fig. 12-19), chart a patient's progress (Fig. 12-20), plan a discharge summary (Fig. 12-21), register the patient for an outpatient visit (Fig. 12-22), and look at patient cost per DRG (Fig. 12-23). The screens are from test screens produced by several vendors of mainframe HISs.

MICROCOMPUTERS IN NURSING DOCUMENTATION

Seven essential elements must be considered when the use of microcomputers to document nursing practice is discussed. Although the applications are few, the potential for microcomputers in facilitating nursing with small-scale documentation and care plans is great (Scholes, 1983; Ball, 1984; Grobe, 1984). This section highlights some basic elements to consider when evaluating microcomputer use for nursing documentation.

1. The amount of memory available. If care plans are done daily on a 20-bed ward, a potential amount of information that can be stored in a particular time must be identified.
2. Input mode. How is information entered?
3. Output features. Is a television type of screen, a paper chart or copy for the permanent medical record, or cassette tapes required?

Page Nos. for Nursing Orders

Basic Care

1. General Hygiene—excluding Facial Hygiene.
2. Facial Hygiene.
3. Pressure Area & Sore Care.
4. Aids for Relief of Pressure.
5. Position.
6. Mobility.
7. Intake—Diet.
8. Intake—Fluids.
9. Observation Charts.
10. Observations.
13. Recordings.

Tests

20. Urine Tests (Ward).
21. Urine Tests (Laboratory).
22. Tests—Execretary (except urine) & Blood.
26. Swabs & Aspirates.
28. Biopsies.
30. X-Ray Investigations.
35. Investigations—excluding X-rays.
39. Bovey Day Cases.

Treatments

40. Alimentary Canal—Upper.
41. Cardiac Therapy.
42. Dialysis.
43. Genito—Urinary Tract—Catheters.
44. Urology.
45. Genito—Urinary Tract—excluding Catheters.
47. Infusion Therapy.
48. Intestinal Tract.
50. Orthopaedic—Traction.
51. Orthopaedic—Plaster.
52. Orthopaedic—Exercise & Appliances.
53. Ear, Nose & Throat.
55. Radiotherapy—Oncology.
56. Respiratory Tract—Inhalations.
57. Respiratory Tract—excluding Inhalations.
58. Skin—Topical Applications.
59. Skin—Non Topical.
60. Bandages.
61. Clips, Sutures, Clamp & Rod.
63. Drains.
64. Dressings.
66. Packs.
67. Operation or Investigation.
69. Treatments & Applications—Hot & Cold.

Miscellaneous

70. Patient/Relative Tuition.
71. Patient/Relative Appointments, etc.
72. Therapy, Clinics, Visits & Domiciliary Services.
73. Transfer & Transport.
74. Handicaps, etc.
75. Special Precautions
76. Reminders to Nurse in Charge.
77. }Nursing Problems (Printed on Care
78. }Plans).
79. Sensitive Problems (Not printed on Care Plans).

FIG. 12-12. Nursing assessment menu. (Astbury C: Nursing care plans: Aspects of computer use in nurse-to-nurse communication. In Fokkens O et al [eds]: Medinfo 83 Seminars. Amsterdam, North-Holland, 1983)

4. Is the language easy to understand and can it communicate easily with the user?
5. Can the microcomputer communicate with the telephone modem or can the output be communicated to another computer?
6. Is software available for the computer? Have any nursing documentation systems been described for the system?
7. Is the system flexible? Could it be expanded, a voice synthesizer added, or output tabulated and graphed?

Available on the IBM PC or the Apple II is software similar to the POMR. This program facilitates the discovery of correct clinical problems and develops diagnostic and management hypotheses based on information in the literature. The system has been developed and applied in physicians' offices. The software pro-

(Text continues on p. 289.)

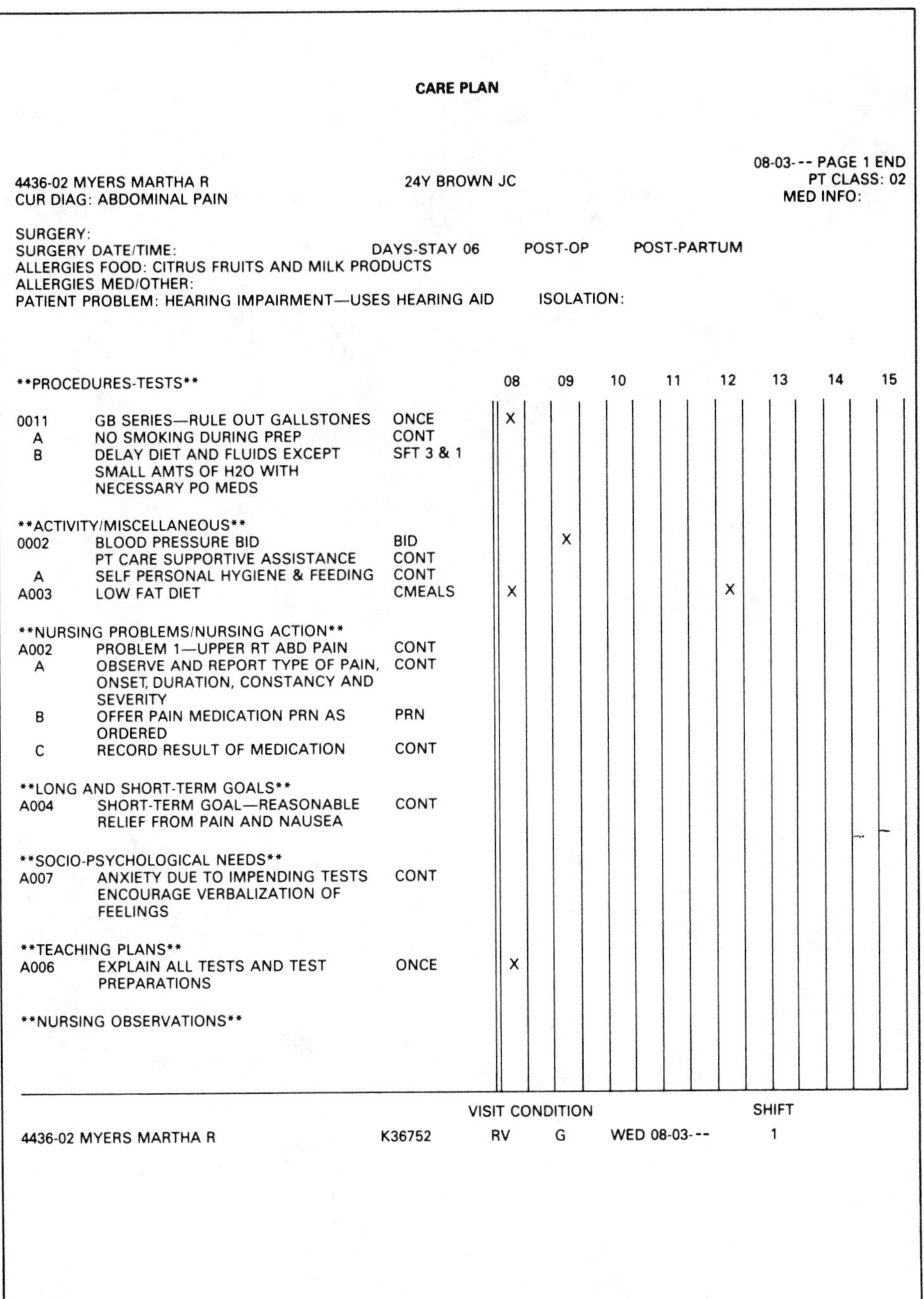

CARE PLAN

08-03--- PAGE 1 END
4436-02 MYERS MARTHA R 24Y BROWN JC PT CLASS: 02
CUR DIAG: ABDOMINAL PAIN MED INFO:

SURGERY:
SURGERY DATE/TIME: DAYS-STAY 06 POST-OP POST-PARTUM
ALLERGIES FOOD: CITRUS FRUITS AND MILK PRODUCTS
ALLERGIES MED/OTHER:
PATIENT PROBLEM: HEARING IMPAIRMENT—USES HEARING AID ISOLATION:

			08	09	10	11	12	13	14	15
PROCEDURES-TESTS										
0011	GB SERIES—RULE OUT GALLSTONES	ONCE	X							
A	NO SMOKING DURING PREP	CONT								
B	DELAY DIET AND FLUIDS EXCEPT SMALL AMTS OF H2O WITH NECESSARY PO MEDS	SFT 3 & 1								
ACTIVITY/MISCELLANEOUS										
0002	BLOOD PRESSURE BID	BID		X						
	PT CARE SUPPORTIVE ASSISTANCE	CONT								
A	SELF PERSONAL HYGIENE & FEEDING	CONT								
A003	LOW FAT DIET	CMEALS	X				X			
NURSING PROBLEMS/NURSING ACTION										
A002	PROBLEM 1—UPPER RT ABD PAIN	CONT								
A	OBSERVE AND REPORT TYPE OF PAIN, ONSET, DURATION, CONSTANCY AND SEVERITY	CONT								
B	OFFER PAIN MEDICATION PRN AS ORDERED	PRN								
C	RECORD RESULT OF MEDICATION	CONT								
LONG AND SHORT-TERM GOALS										
A004	SHORT-TERM GOAL—REASONABLE RELIEF FROM PAIN AND NAUSEA	CONT								
SOCIO-PSYCHOLOGICAL NEEDS										
A007	ANXIETY DUE TO IMPENDING TESTS ENCOURAGE VERBALIZATION OF FEELINGS	CONT								
TEACHING PLANS										
A006	EXPLAIN ALL TESTS AND TEST PREPARATIONS	ONCE	X							
NURSING OBSERVATIONS										

VISIT CONDITION SHIFT
4436-02 MYERS MARTHA R K36752 RV G WED 08-03--- 1

FIG. 12-13. Nursing care plan (Burroughs HIS).

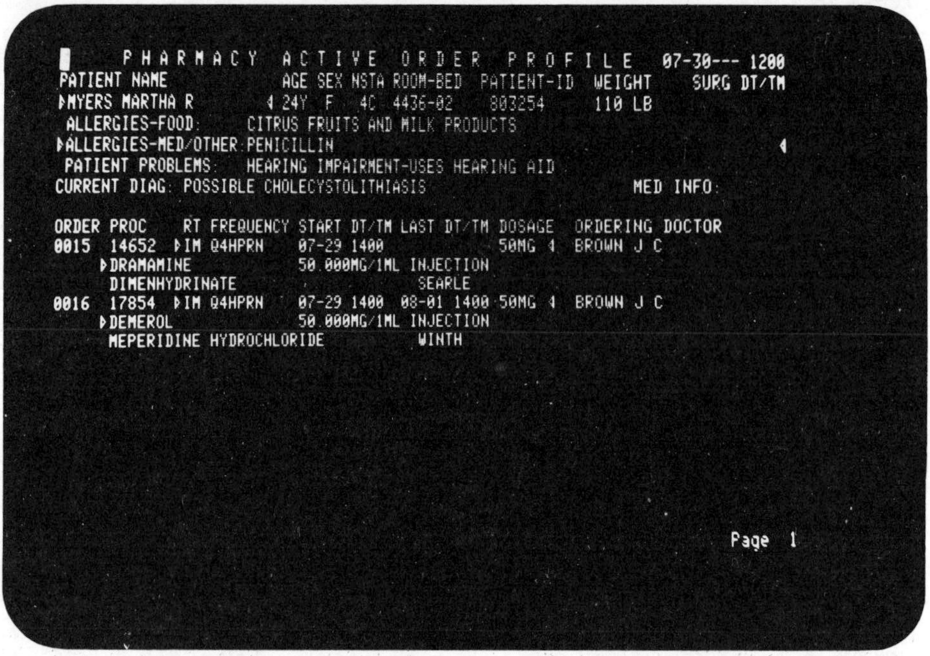

```
▌    P H A R M A C Y   A C T I V E   O R D E R   P R O F I L E   07-30--- 1200
PATIENT NAME            AGE SEX NSTA ROOM-BED  PATIENT-ID  WEIGHT     SURG DT/TM
▶MYERS MARTHA R        ◀ 24Y  F   4C  4436-02    803254     110 LB
 ALLERGIES-FOOD:       CITRUS FRUITS AND MILK PRODUCTS
▶ALLERGIES-MED/OTHER:PENICILLIN                                               ◀
 PATIENT PROBLEMS:   HEARING IMPAIRMENT-USES HEARING AID
CURRENT DIAG: POSSIBLE CHOLECYSTOLITHIASIS                           MED INFO:

ORDER PROC     RT FREQUENCY START DT/TM LAST DT/TM DOSAGE   ORDERING DOCTOR
0015  14652  ▶IM Q4HPRN    07-29 1400              50MG ◀  BROWN J C
     ▶DRAMAMINE            50.000MG/1ML INJECTION
      DIMENHYDRINATE                       SEARLE
0016  17854  ▶IM Q4HPRN    07-29 1400  08-01 1400 50MG ◀  BROWN J C
     ▶DEMEROL              50.000MG/1ML INJECTION
      MEPERIDINE HYDROCHLORIDE            WINTH

                                                                    Page  1
```

FIG. 12-14. Obtaining medication information from a pharmacy profile (Burroughs HIS).

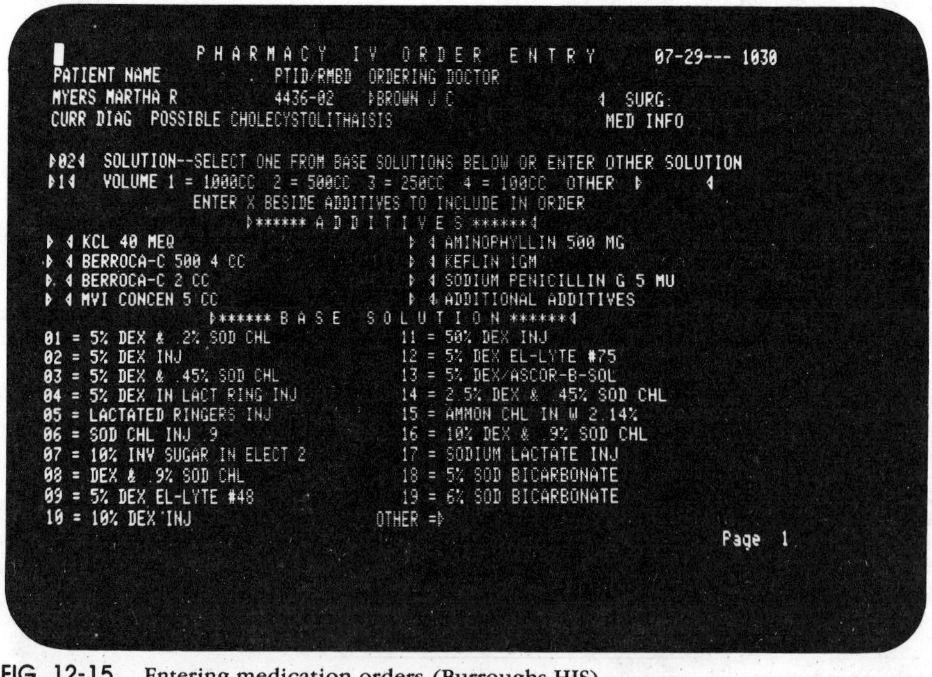

```
▌             P H A R M A C Y   I V   O R D E R   E N T R Y      07-29--- 1030
PATIENT NAME          PTID/RMBD  ORDERING DOCTOR
MYERS MARTHA R        4436-02    ▶BROWN J C                  ◀  SURG:
CURR DIAG  POSSIBLE CHOLECYSTOLITHAISIS                          MED INFO

▶02◀  SOLUTION--SELECT ONE FROM BASE SOLUTIONS BELOW OR ENTER OTHER SOLUTION
▶1◀   VOLUME 1 = 1000CC  2 = 500CC  3 = 250CC  4 = 100CC  OTHER  ▶      ◀
               ENTER X BESIDE ADDITIVES TO INCLUDE IN ORDER
                     ▶****** A D D I T I V E S ******◀
▶ ◀ KCL 40 MEQ                           ▶ ◀ AMINOPHYLLIN 500 MG
▶ ◀ BERROCA-C 500 4 CC                   ▶ ◀ KEFLIN 1GM
▶ ◀ BERROCA-C 2 CC                       ▶ ◀ SODIUM PENICILLIN G 5 MU
▶ ◀ MVI CONCEN 5 CC                      ▶ ◀ ADDITIONAL ADDITIVES
                ▶****** B A S E   S O L U T I O N ******◀
01 = 5% DEX & .2% SOD CHL                11 = 50% DEX INJ
02 = 5% DEX INJ                          12 = 5% DEX EL-LYTE #75
03 = 5% DEX & .45% SOD CHL               13 = 5% DEX/ASCOR-B-SOL
04 = 5% DEX IN LACT RING INJ             14 = 2.5% DEX & .45% SOD CHL
05 = LACTATED RINGERS INJ                15 = AMMON CHL IN W 2.14%
06 = SOD CHL INJ .9                      16 = 10% DEX & .9% SOD CHL
07 = 10% INV SUGAR IN ELECT 2            17 = SODIUM LACTATE INJ
08 = DEX & .9% SOD CHL                   18 = 5% SOD BICARBONATE
09 = 5% DEX EL-LYTE #48                  19 = 6% SOD BICARBONATE
10 = 10% DEX INJ                       OTHER =▶
                                                                  Page  1
```

FIG. 12-15. Entering medication orders (Burroughs HIS).

```
▌     D E T A I L   M E D I C A T I O N   C O N F I R M A T I O N
PATIENT-ID   ORDER #  PATIENT NAME            LOCATION       PROCEDURE #
   803254    0015    MYERS MARTHA R          4C  4436-02    14652
BRAND NAME                     DOSAGE FORM                   STRENGTH
▸DRAMAMINE                    ◂▸INJECTION  ◂             ▸     50 000MG/1ML◂
GENERIC NAME                    ORDER WORDS                  ROUTE
DIMENHYDRINATE                  GIVE FOR NAUSEA              IM
     FROM          TO
07-29--- 1000 07-29--- 1800          TO STOP CONFIRMATIONS ENTER STOP IN NEXT
DATE ADMINISTERED  ▸07-29---◂              PATIENT AND SPACE OUT THE REST OF
TIME ADMINISTERED  ▸1400◂                  THE SCREEN
QTY  ADMINISTERED  ▸50  ◂
UNITS              ▸MG◂
PROFESSIONAL ID    ▸400194◂
REASON NOT ADMINISTERED ▸ ◂
  1 = PAT REFUSED 2 = PAT NPO  3 = PAT NAUSEATED  4 = OTHER-COMMENTS REQUIRED
COMMENTS - ENTER Y ▸ ◂
SITE               ▸   ◂
NEEDLE             ▸       ◂
BAG NUMBER         ▸    ◂
OVERRIDE           ▸ ◂?

NEXT PATIENT       ▸          ◂
NEXT ORDER         ▸    ◂
                                                               Page  1
```

FIG. 12-16. Chart medication administration (Burroughs HIS).

RESULT SUMMARY FOR MYERS MARTHA R THROUGH 08-06---

ROOM BD	PATIENT ID	HISTORY NO.	ADM.	ATTENDING DR.
4436-02	803254	K36752	07-28---	BROWN JC

HEMATOLOGY

1213 DIFFERENTIAL —BLOOD **0001 08-04 0900 08-04 1200

RBC MORPHOLOGY:	PLATELETS	WBC	JUV	BAND	SEG	LYM	MONO	EO	BASG
SL ANISOCYTOSIS	ADEQ	9.6			66	37	3	4	

9508 SMA 6/60 —SERUM **0003 08-04 0900 08-04 1200

GLUCOSE MG%	BUN MG%	SODIUM MEQ/L	POTASSIUM MEG/L	CO2 MM/L	CHLORIDE MEQ/L	
107	19	130 LO	3.6	27.0	97	
						**0007 08-05 0900 08-05 1000
104	18	132 LO	4.6	25.0	102	

URINALYSIS

7248 URINALYSIS, ROUTINE —URINE **0002 08-05 0800 08-05 1000

MICROSCOPIC	APPEARANCE	SP GR	PH	ALB	GLU	KETONE	BILE	OCC BL
C: 0-2	YELLOW HAZY	1.015	5.0	0	0	0	0	0

RBC: 0
EPITH: OCC
BACT: 1+
OTHER:

RADIOLOGY

2320 GALLBLADDER SERIES **0011 08-03 0800 08-03 1000

FAINTLY OUTLINED GALLBLADDER WITH NUMEROUS SMALL STONES PRESENT.
IMP: EXTENSIVE CHOLECYSTOLITHIASIS

4436-02 MYERS MARTHA R PAGE 1

FIG. 12-17. Display of laboratory results (Burroughs HIS).

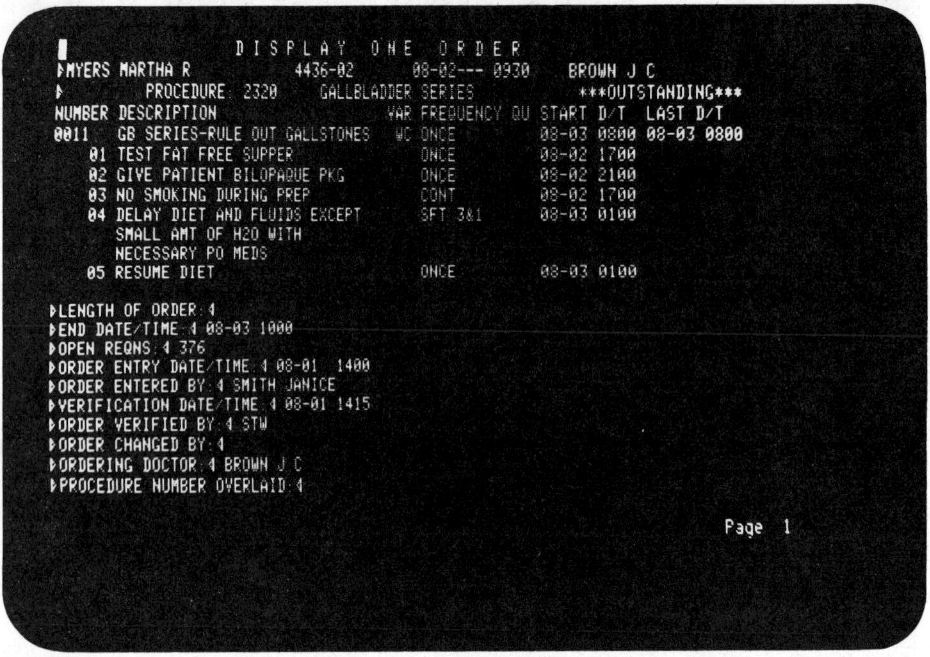

```
█                 D I S P L A Y   O N E   O R D E R
▶MYERS MARTHA R              4436-02       08-02--- 0930    BROWN J C
▶         PROCEDURE: 2320     GALLBLADDER SERIES           ***OUTSTANDING***
NUMBER DESCRIPTION                      VAR FREQUENCY QU START D/T  LAST D/T
0011   GB SERIES-RULE OUT GALLSTONES    WC ONCE          08-03 0800 08-03 0800
    01 TEST FAT FREE SUPPER                ONCE          08-02 1700
    02 GIVE PATIENT BILOPAQUE PKG          ONCE          08-02 2100
    03 NO SMOKING DURING PREP              CONT          08-02 1700
    04 DELAY DIET AND FLUIDS EXCEPT        SFT 3&1       08-03 0100
       SMALL AMT OF H2O WITH
       NECESSARY PO MEDS
    05 RESUME DIET                         ONCE          08-03 0100

▶LENGTH OF ORDER:◀
▶END DATE/TIME:◀ 08-03 1000
▶OPEN REQNS:◀ 376
▶ORDER ENTRY DATE/TIME:◀ 08-01  1400
▶ORDER ENTERED BY:◀ SMITH JANICE
▶VERIFICATION DATE/TIME:◀ 08-01 1415
▶ORDER VERIFIED BY:◀ STW
▶ORDER CHANGED BY:◀
▶ORDERING DOCTOR:◀ BROWN J C
▶PROCEDURE NUMBER OVERLAID:◀

                                                       Page  1
```

FIG. 12-18. An overview of current physicians' orders (Burroughs HIS).

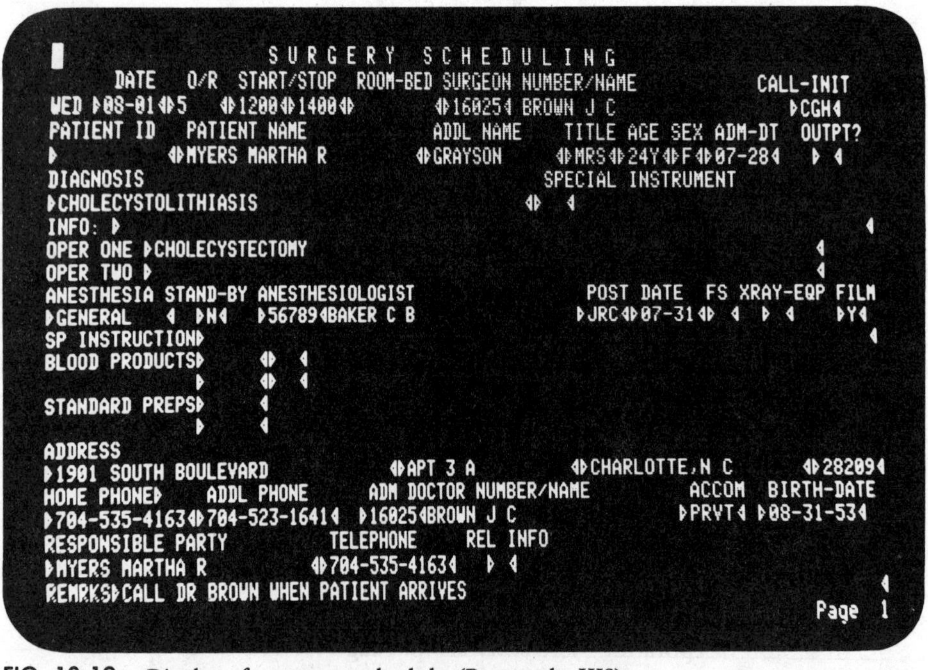

```
█                    S U R G E R Y   S C H E D U L I N G
      DATE   O/R  START/STOP  ROOM-BED SURGEON NUMBER/NAME            CALL-INIT
WED ▶08-01◀▶5   ◀▶1200◀▶1400◀▶         ◀▶16025◀ BROWN J C              ▶CGH◀
PATIENT ID   PATIENT NAME            ADDL NAME    TITLE AGE SEX ADM-DT  OUTPT?
▶          ◀▶MYERS MARTHA R        ◀▶GRAYSON     ◀▶MRS◀▶24Y◀▶F◀▶07-28◀   ▶ ◀
DIAGNOSIS                                         SPECIAL INSTRUMENT
▶CHOLECYSTOLITHIASIS                            ◀▶ ◀
INFO: ▶                                                                    ◀
OPER ONE ▶CHOLECYSTECTOMY                                               ◀
OPER TWO ▶                                                              ◀
ANESTHESIA STAND-BY ANESTHESIOLOGIST                 POST DATE   FS XRAY-EQP FILM
▶GENERAL    ◀ ▶N◀   ▶56789◀BAKER C B                  ▶JRC◀▶07-31◀▶ ◀  ▶ ◀    ▶Y◀
SP INSTRUCTION▶                                                            ◀
BLOOD PRODUCTS▶      ◀▶ ◀
              ▶      ◀▶ ◀
STANDARD PREPS▶      ◀
              ▶      ◀
ADDRESS
▶1901 SOUTH BOULEVARD           ◀▶APT 3 A         ◀▶CHARLOTTE,N C        ◀▶28209◀
HOME PHONE▶     ADDL PHONE       ADM DOCTOR NUMBER/NAME           ACCOM  BIRTH-DATE
▶704-535-4163◀▶704-523-1641◀ ▶16025◀BROWN J C                   ▶PRVT◀ ▶08-31-53◀
RESPONSIBLE PARTY            TELEPHONE      REL INFO
▶MYERS MARTHA R            ◀▶704-535-4163◀  ▶ ◀
REMRKS▶CALL DR BROWN WHEN PATIENT ARRIVES                                  ◀
                                                                     Page  1
```

FIG. 12-19. Display of a surgery schedule (Burroughs HIS).

```
                             PATIENT CARE PROFILE
PIEDMONT HOSPITAL                       12/06/83  4:29PM          PAGE   1  SHIFT:A

ACTIVITIES OF DAILY LIVING                |610-01            000192983 7691819   6C
  VITAL SIGNS      RT                     |   BAXTER FREDRICK ALLEN          SEX:M
  BATH             SELF                   |   ADM:11/29/83           SRV:ORT  SMK:N
  ELIMINATION      FRACTURE PAN           |   DOB:10/26/16 67    COND:G   LEVEL:2
  TRANSPORT BY     STRETCHER              |   HT :5/08  F/I       WT :185/000 P/O
  CIRC/SENS/MOTIO  RT LEG                 |   26100 MORRISON JACK L      200
  B/P              QID                    |   ALG:PCN, SULFA
  B/P              L ARM ONLY             |   DX :OSTEOTOMY R KNEE 12/1 - UTI
                                          |
.LL          SURGICAL OR CLEAR LIQUID     |NURSING GOALS
                                          | D/G:PT. WILL DEMONSTRATE KNOWLEDGE TO
PRC:SEIZURE PRECAUTIONS                   |     COMPLY WITH PRESCRIBED REGIMEN
                                          | GL :PT. WILL RECEIVE PRE-OP TEACHING AS
ACTIVE ORDERS                             |     PER PROTOCOL __________
    WALKER W/2 FOREARM 12/02              |
    PHYSICAL THERAPY-O 12/05              |NURSING INTERVENTIONS
    INCENT.SPIR.TREATM 12/06              |   1:REVIEW INFORMATION IN PRE-OP BOOKLET
    PYELOGRAM INTRAVEN 12/06 IH           |     W PT. INCLUDING PRE-OP PROGRAMS ON
  1:PYELOGRAM INTRAVENOUS (IVP)(400)      |     CHANNEL 13.______________
    MAY HAVE LIQUIDS ON THE DAY OF EXAM   |   2:ASSIST PT. TO PERFORM POST-OP
    UNLESS UPPER G.I. SERIES,GALLBLADDER  |     BREATHING EXERCISES (RESPRIX,___ETC)
    SERIES OR SONOGRAM IS ORDERED         |
                                          |   3:EXPLAIN WHAT PT.SHOULD EXPECT PRE-OP
TREATMENTS                                |     (PREPS,MEDS,DRESSING,ETC)__________
  1:ELEVATE RIGHT LEG ON _____PILLOW (S)  |
  2:FOLEY CATHETER TO BSB                 |
    CATH CARE BID.  D/E:______________    |
  3:HEAD OF BED FLAT EXCEPT FOR MEALS     |
    AND BEDPAN                            |
  4:CHANGE DRESSING TID. D/E:_______      |

DATE:               NURSING NOTES

 INT   SIGNATURE            INT  SIGNATURE            INT  SIGNATURE
|   |                      |   |                     |   |
|---| ____________________ |---| ___________________ |---| ___________________
|   |                      |   |                     |   |
```

FIG. 12-20. An example of a patient progress format (HBO, Medpro System).

vides a framework for nurses to use nursing diagnosis problem lists (Weed and Hertzberg, 1983).

Already available for nursing care plans is the framework established for the IBM-PC by Roton Corporation. The software package is entitled RNact. The program aims to facilitate creating and documenting the nursing care plan. It is flexible in that the nurse can edit, substitute, or design nursing problem lists, patient goals,

```
08/23/82   **  NURSING SERVICE - PROBLEMS/ORDERS/CAREPLAN  **        19.33.47
DOE, JANE                MRN = 000-000-0    ROOM 10B391          DIVISION = N5
POR NO    FREQ    CARE PLAN
 21    XXX

  08/23/82:     DISCHARGE PLANNING          EXPECTED DATE OF DISCHARGE:__/__/__
 ______________________________            DESTINATION:
  HOME-                                     NURSING HOME I-
  NURSING HOME II-                          NURSING HOME III-
  NURSING HOME IV-                          OTHER:______________________
  TRANSPORTATION:                           FAMILY -
  AMBULANCE-                                CHAIR CAR -
  TIME ORDERED:________  -                  PT./FAMILY INSTRUCTION:
  CONFERENCE NEEDED ___ DATE _____ -        MEDICATION SCHEDULE: __________
  ACTIVITIES ___________________ -          TREATMENTS: ___________________
  COMMUNITY HEALTH:                         SERVICES NEEDED:
  NURSING-                                  PT-
  HHA-                                      HOMEMAKER-
  MEALS ON WHEELS-                          OTHER __________________________

  ______________________________

  NEXT PAGE          REMOVE WORD            READY                  GO BACK
```

FIG. 12-21. An example of a discharge summary plan. (Gebhardt A: Developing a patient care program. In Scholes M, Bryant Y, Barber B [eds]: The Impact of Computers on Nursing: An International Review. Amsterdam, North-Holland, 1983)

```
                 O U T P A T I E N T   R E G I S T R A T I O N
PATIENT ID  PATIENT NAME               ADDL NAME   TITLE SEX AGE  REGSTRN.DT/TM▶
   ◀03254◀▶MYERS MARTHA R            ◀▶GRAYSON    ◀▶MRS ◀▶F◀▶24Y◀▶07-29---◀▶1200
◀PATIENT CLASSIFICATION        DOCTOR NUMBER/NAME               SVC  FC  CR REGBY
▶01◀PRIVATE REFERRED          ▶16025◀BROWN J C                ▶SUR◀▶02◀▶  ◀▶CGH◀
 HISTORY NO  SOC-SEC-NO  CLINIC REFERRING DOCTOR NAME/ADDRESS
▶K26752    ◀▶241-88-3141◀▶SUR ◀▶
◀PLACE OF ACCIDENT                DATE ONSET CASH RCVD RCP NO PROF FEE  DC CHART?
▶                                ◀▶07-15---◀ ▶10.00  ◀ ▶248  ◀▶        ◀▶ ◀  ▶Y◀
CUR DIAG▶POSSSIBLE CHOLE                                     ◀
INFO ▶                                                                         ◀
 INFORMANT   METHOD OF ARRIVAL     ALLERGY
▶PATIENT   ◀▶                     ◀▶CITRUS FRUITS AND PENICILLIN               ◀
RMARKS▶                                                                        ◀
ORD SET ORD SEL ORDERING DOCTOR             ENTER Y BESIDE SCHEDULED PROCEDURES
▶     ◀   ▶ ◀  ▶BROWN J C                ◀  TO BE VERIFIED
SEL PROC NO/DESCRIPTION                     SCH DATE/TIME
▶Y◀▶12011  ◀▶CBC                           ◀  07-29---  1200
▶ ◀▶       ◀▶                              ◀
▶ ◀▶       ◀▶                              ◀
▶ ◀▶       ◀▶                              ◀
▶ ◀▶       ◀▶                              ◀
▶ ◀▶       ◀▶                              ◀
▶ ◀▶       ◀▶                              ◀                 MORE SCH ORD ▶N◀
                                                                       Page  1
```

FIG. 12-22. Registering patients for outpatient appointments (Burroughs HIS).

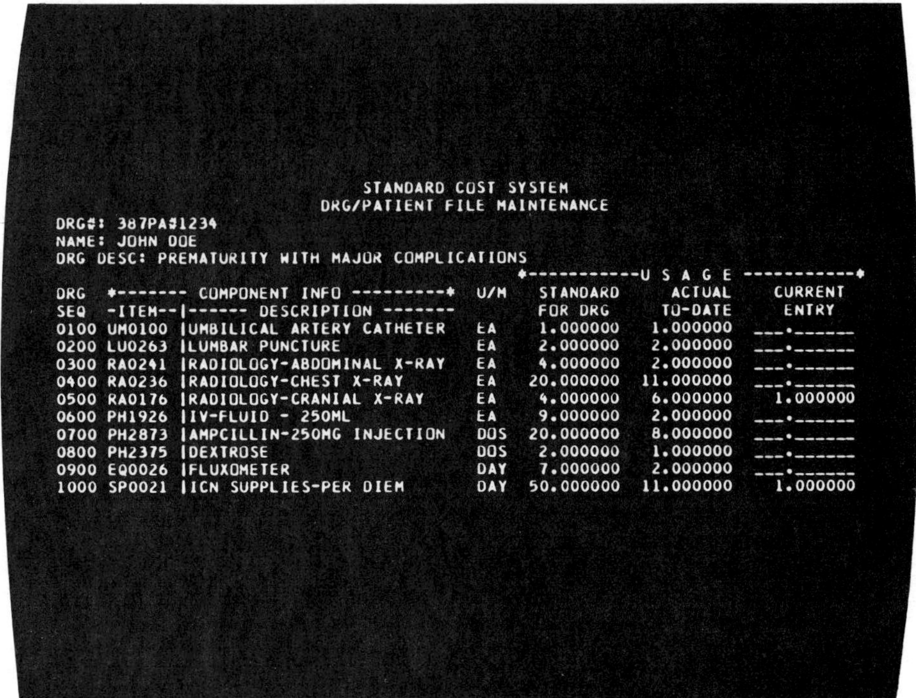

STANDARD COST SYSTEM
DRG/PATIENT FILE MAINTENANCE

DRG#: 387PA#1234
NAME: JOHN DOE
DRG DESC: PREMATURITY WITH MAJOR COMPLICATIONS

DRG SEQ	COMPONENT INFO -ITEM--	DESCRIPTION	U/M	USAGE STANDARD FOR DRG	ACTUAL TO-DATE	CURRENT ENTRY
0100	UM0100	UMBILICAL ARTERY CATHETER	EA	1.000000	1.000000	___.______
0200	LU0263	LUMBAR PUNCTURE	EA	2.000000	2.000000	___.______
0300	RA0241	RADIOLOGY-ABDOMINAL X-RAY	EA	4.000000	2.000000	___.______
0400	RA0236	RADIOLOGY-CHEST X-RAY	EA	20.000000	11.000000	___.______
0500	RA0176	RADIOLOGY-CRANIAL X-RAY	EA	4.000000	6.000000	1.000000
0600	PH1926	IV-FLUID - 250ML	EA	9.000000	2.000000	___.______
0700	PH2873	AMPCILLIN-250MG INJECTION	DOS	20.000000	8.000000	___.______
0800	PH2375	DEXTROSE	DOS	2.000000	1.000000	___.______
0900	EQ0026	FLUXOMETER	DAY	7.000000	2.000000	___.______
1000	SP0021	ICN SUPPLIES-PER DIEM	DAY	50.000000	11.000000	1.000000

FIG. 12-23. An example of patient costs per DRG (Global software, HCCS software).

nursing approaches, and discharge objectives. The second part of the program allows the nurse to use a reference library that includes pretyped care plans. An example of a microcomputer-based nursing care plan that fits into an $8\frac{1}{2} \times 11$ care plan book is shown in Figure 12-24 (RNact, 1984).

An example of a microcomputer used in a specialty area such as hemodialysis has also been described. A desktop Hewlett-Packard was used to record the daily nursing documentation in a hemodialysis unit. The software package is called DIALAZA. The dialysis data was organized into the permanent patient data and orders, the medication profile, and dialysis data. Figures 12-25 and 12-26 are copies of the worksheet and summary form that resulted. This system has been positively evaluated for facilitating recordkeeping to improve patient care, save time, and facilitate clinical research (DePooter and colleagues, 1983).

SUMMARY

Nurses seem to approve of using computers to document nursing practice. However, content format and hardware must be developed with the same amount of precision and effort as the microchip has been.

The computer is a clinical tool that nurses can use daily, just as they use a blood pressure cuff, and, like other tools, the computer will never replace the nurse's knowledge and skills of patient assessment. The computer assessments serve as general "blueprints" against which the nurse makes clinical judgments; the nurse must also make nursing judgments when available data are inadequate. The com-

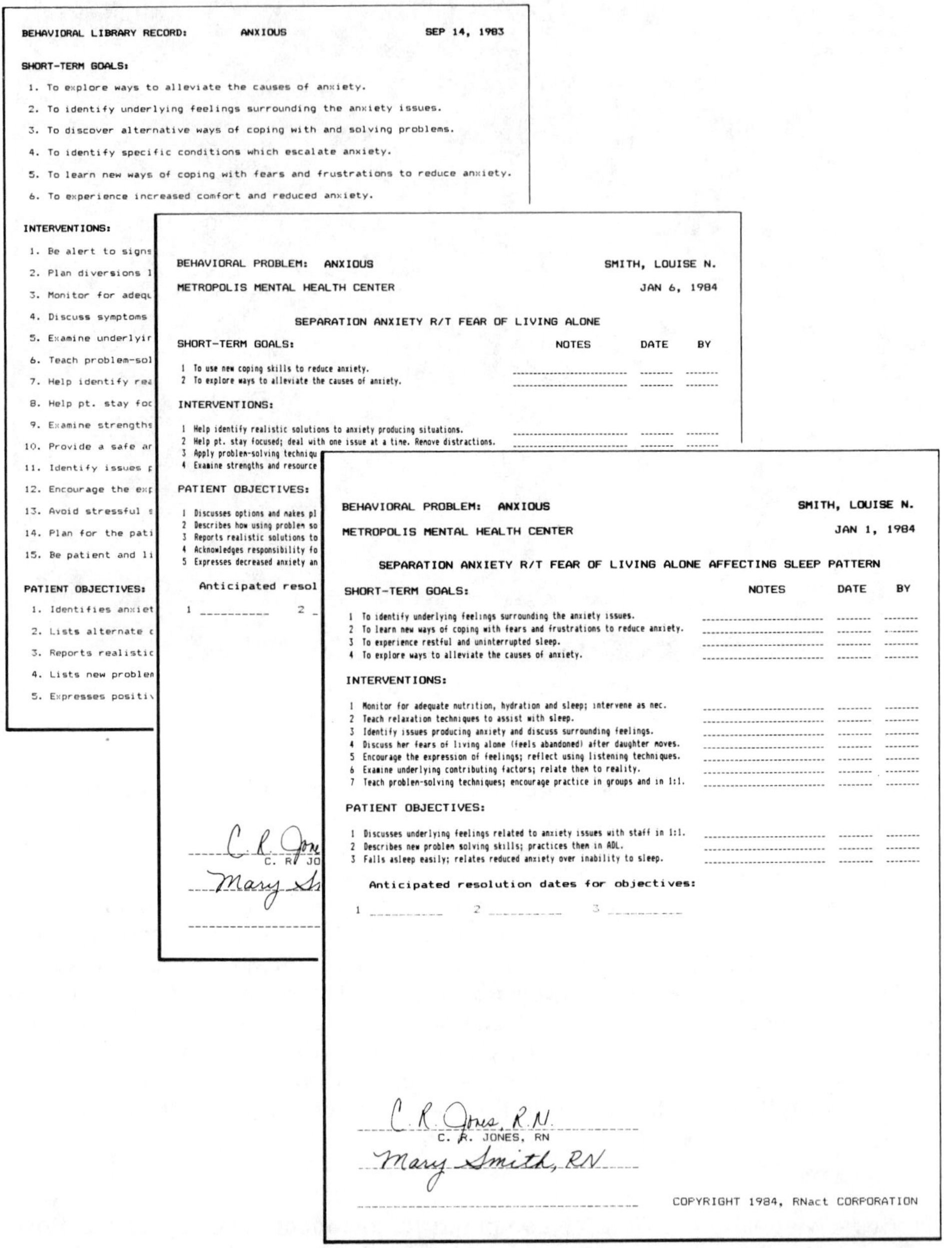

BEHAVIORAL LIBRARY RECORD: ANXIOUS SEP 14, 1983

SHORT-TERM GOALS:

1. To explore ways to alleviate the causes of anxiety.
2. To identify underlying feelings surrounding the anxiety issues.
3. To discover alternative ways of coping with and solving problems.
4. To identify specific conditions which escalate anxiety.
5. To learn new ways of coping with fears and frustrations to reduce anxiety.
6. To experience increased comfort and reduced anxiety.

INTERVENTIONS:

1. Be alert to signs
2. Plan diversions 1
3. Monitor for adequ
4. Discuss symptoms
5. Examine underlyir
6. Teach problem-sol
7. Help identify rea
8. Help pt. stay foc
9. Examine strengths
10. Provide a safe ar
11. Identify issues p
12. Encourage the exp
13. Avoid stressful s
14. Plan for the pati
15. Be patient and li

PATIENT OBJECTIVES:

1. Identifies anxiet
2. Lists alternate c
3. Reports realistic
4. Lists new problem
5. Expresses positiv

BEHAVIORAL PROBLEM: ANXIOUS SMITH, LOUISE N.

METROPOLIS MENTAL HEALTH CENTER JAN 6, 1984

SEPARATION ANXIETY R/T FEAR OF LIVING ALONE

SHORT-TERM GOALS:	NOTES	DATE	BY
1 To use new coping skills to reduce anxiety.			
2 To explore ways to alleviate the causes of anxiety.			

INTERVENTIONS:

1 Help identify realistic solutions to anxiety producing situations.
2 Help pt. stay focused; deal with one issue at a time. Remove distractions.
3 Apply problem-solving techniqu
4 Examine strengths and resource

PATIENT OBJECTIVES:

1 Discusses options and makes pl
2 Describes how using problem so
3 Reports realistic solutions to
4 Acknowledges responsibility fo
5 Expresses decreased anxiety an

Anticipated resol

1 ________ 2 _

C. R. Jones
C. R. JO
Mary Sm

BEHAVIORAL PROBLEM: ANXIOUS SMITH, LOUISE N.

METROPOLIS MENTAL HEALTH CENTER JAN 1, 1984

SEPARATION ANXIETY R/T FEAR OF LIVING ALONE AFFECTING SLEEP PATTERN

SHORT-TERM GOALS:	NOTES	DATE	BY
1 To identify underlying feelings surrounding the anxiety issues.			
2 To learn new ways of coping with fears and frustrations to reduce anxiety.			
3 To experience restful and uninterrupted sleep.			
4 To explore ways to alleviate the causes of anxiety.			

INTERVENTIONS:

1 Monitor for adequate nutrition, hydration and sleep; intervene as nec.
2 Teach relaxation techniques to assist with sleep.
3 Identify issues producing anxiety and discuss surrounding feelings.
4 Discuss her fears of living alone (feels abandoned) after daughter moves.
5 Encourage the expression of feelings; reflect using listening techniques.
6 Examine underlying contributing factors; relate them to reality.
7 Teach problem-solving techniques; encourage practice in groups and in 1:1.

PATIENT OBJECTIVES:

1 Discusses underlying feelings related to anxiety issues with staff in 1:1.
2 Describes new problem solving skills; practices them in ADL.
3 Falls asleep easily; relates reduced anxiety over inability to sleep.

Anticipated resolution dates for objectives:

1 ________ 2 ________ 3 ________

C. R. Jones, R.N.
C. R. JONES, RN
Mary Smith, RN

FIG. 12-24. An example of a microcomputer-generated nursing care plan (IBM hardware, RNact, A Division of ROTON Corporation: An untitled marketing report. Villa Park, IL, RNact, 1984)

UNIT POST: RESP. NURSE: TRANSPORT: BLOOD GROUP: ALLERGY: HEPATITIS B Ag: DIET:	TYPE OF TREATMENT: TYPE OF DIALYZER: DIALYSATE: PRIMING: BLOOD FLOW: HEPARINE (ml/h): OPTIMAL WEIGHT:	MEDICATION DURING DIALYSIS	ALARM CONTROLS: TEMPERATURE ART. PRESSURE VEN. PRESSURE BLOOD LEAK DETECT. AIR DETECTOR STROKE VOLUME
DATE HOSPITALISED (1 = NO, 2 = YES) RESP. AT START RESP. AT END	WEIGHT GAIN U.F. COEFFICIENT DATA FROM PRECEDING DIALYSIS: WEIGHT E.D.: BLOOD VOLUME:	VASCULAR ACCESS: NUMBER OF PUNCTURES COMPLICATIONS 1 = NONE — 2 = HEMATOMA — 3 = BLEEDING (PRE-DIAL.) 4 = BLEEDING (POST-DIAL.) — 5 = THROMBOSIS	

HOUR	B.P.		WEIGHT		PRESSURES		Q.B.	VOLUME		HEPARIN	REMARKS	
	SYST.	DIAST.	PROGRAMM.	EFFECT.	V.D.	D.D.		PROGRAMM.	EFFECT.			
												SALISE (ml): HEMACEL (ml): BLOOD/PACKED CELLS (ml): COMPL. M2 1: 2: 3: 4:
												1 = SOME 2 = HYPOTENSION SYMPT. 3 = HYPOTENSION A-SYMPT. 4 = HYPERTENSION 5 = CRAMPS 6 = HEADACHE 7 = VOMITING 8 = NAUSEA 9 = ANGINA 10 = HYPOGLYCEMIA

PROBLEMS	PLANNED FOR TODAY	FURTHER PLANNING

FIG. 12-25. Worksheet from the microcomputer program called DIALAZA. (DePooter G, Elseviers M, Verpooten G, et al: Nurses' experience with a computer in a nephrology-hypertension department. In Scholes M, Bryant Y, Barber B [eds]: The Impact of Computers on Nursing: An International Review. Amsterdam, North-Holland, 1983)

NAME OF THE PATIENT	26/07	28/07	30/07	02/08	05/08	06/08	09/08	MEAN	
BP SYST. PRE D. BP DIAST. PRE D. BP SYST. POST D. BP DIAST. POST D. WEIGHT PRE D. WEIGHT POST D. TOTAL BLOOD VOLUME HEPARINE SALINE HEMACEL BLOOD/PACKED CELLS NUMBER OF PUNCTURES FISTULA RELATED COMPL. OTHER COMPLICATIONS									

VASCULAR ACCESS RELATED COMPLICATIONS	DIALYSIS RELATED COMPLICATIONS	REMARKS

LABORATORY RESULTS	PLANNING
MEDICATION SURVEY	**GENERAL DATA**
	DIET: LONGTERM GOAL: HEPARINE: OPTIMAL WEIGHT:

FIG. 12-26. Summary form from the microcomputer program called DIALAZA. (DePooter G, Elseviers M, Verpooten G, et al: Nurses' experience with a computer in nephrology-hypertension department. In Scholes M, Bryant Y, Barber B [ed]: The Impact of Computers on Nursing: An International Review. Amsterdam, North-Holland, 1983)

puter data must fit patients' needs, and it is the nurse who envisions modifications in computer content to facilitate better documentation of patient care (Tamarisk, 1982).

This chapter has described the current standards governing documentation, whether manual or computerized; computers do not change nursing accountability, but merely facilitate documentation of patient care. The potential components of a direct patient care system were described within a nursing process framework, since nursing practice in the United States and abroad is committed to this standard. Major vendors and documentation capabilities were described, and mainframe documentation systems were presented. The ease of using documentation systems for providing discharge care plans was summarized. Screens available for documenting practice from admission to discharge on a composite of mainframes were illustrated. Finally, although few applications of nursing documentation related to microcomputers exist to date, the essential components of a microcomputer system can be defined; a few examples of microcomputer documentation capabilities were described.

ISSUES

1. Most nurses are pleased with computerized documentation, even though the development of content has been tedious.
2. The amount of data, storage capabilities, and content formats that can be obtained from mainframes versus microcomputers have not been compared.
3. A universal nursing database has not been developed to provide high-quality and timely documentation that is valid for quality assurance or research retrieval.
4. The costs of implementing a nursing documentation system have not been thoroughly evaluated to determine if they also decrease the costs of nursing care.
5. Time-consuming clerical duties seem to be lessened after computerized direct order entry systems are integrated with the nursing process.
6. No one system hardware or software design contains all the potential elements of a direct patient care system.
7. Nursing records generated from computerized documentation add to the bulk of medical records, which may indicate that duplication and overlap exist in the current models.
8. Guidelines must determine who gains access to which parts of the nursing record.
9. Hospital policies related to security, confidentiality of information, and backup policies for "downtime" have not been adequately described.
10. Many nurses who have developed systems have not evaluated them or described them in the literature.
11. If nursing does not integrate nursing process with patients' medical diagnosis, documentation may be fragmented, and patient care for which nurses are accountable may be overlooked.
12. Should patients communicate with the computer to enter their own assessments and goals?
13. Computer documentation produces more legible medication orders, notes, and care plans.
14. The automated care plans have not eliminated the need for administration to chide nurses for not updating care plans.

15. It is the nursing professional's responsibility to ensure that future nursing systems benefit nurses.
16. One way to become comfortable with computers is to know how they have been applied to real nursing problems, for example, documentation.
17. The next generation of computer applications in nursing documentation will include artificial intelligence expert systems on mainframes or microcomputers in sequence.
18. A nursing documentation integrated with the nursing unit management reports and the hospital's financial system can provide information needed to document practice, evaluate personnel, validate the costs of nursing care, and provide valid information for clinical nursing research and quality assurance.
19. Computers have been programmed to automate what nurses did manually, but they have the potential to do more.
20. It is unclear what knowledge is needed to use these systems.
21. New legal issues are arising because of computerized nurses' notes.

SUGGESTIONS FOR HANDS-ON EXPERIENCES

1. Few areas in the country have schools of nursing with a mainframe with nursing documentation content, but schools located near hospital centers that have mainframes or minicomputers may have a teaching database used when new nursing personnel are oriented to the hospital. Negotiations to provide access to those systems with terminals on line or through telephone modems is possible. The current hospital mock databases include most aspects of documentation that a nurse encounters in hospital practice.
2. In schools of nursing with computer laboratories, software is now available for doing nursing care plans with microcomputers. If the school purchases such systems, students can have hands-on experience with using and authoring nursing content.
3. At most nursing conferences and conferences related to computers in nursing, vendors exhibit on-line communications to computer resources. The personnel from these companies provide walk-through demonstrations of their nursing documentation components and written literature about their new updates.
4. Query a major company near you and ask its educational representatives to provide classroom access to the computer system and nursing content on a contract basis with rental of computer time by the week, month, or year. This could be accomplished with terminals and telephone modems.
5. Consider a link with the major hospital in the area that has computerized nursing documentation. Negotiate a contract for student rotations through the computer and nursing department as a senior or leadership course for a semester. A model for this exists in medicine; medical students nationwide come to the National Institutes of Health Clinical Center for a clinical electives program that includes access and hands-on experience with computers in administration, practice, research, and education.

STUDY QUESTIONS

1. What major standards govern nursing documentation?
2. Define the two basic categories of documentation of patient care.

3. How are the potential components of documenting direct patient care universally organized in mainframe systems?
4. Name five records that could be produced from a direct patient care system.
5. Name five vendors of mainframe computers with nursing documentation capabilities.
6. Nursing content can be integrated with risk management information. True or false?
7. If so, where has this been done and on what system?
8. What three areas of documentation are found within the Technicon system?
9. The Technicon system uses pattern, impairment, and aid as one example of content flow. From the other examples provided, what is another content flow?
10. What are the five components of a discharge care plan?
11. Describe the seven essential elements to consider in a microcomputer for documenting nursing practice.
12. Are any documentation systems available on microcomputers?

REFERENCES

Anser Analytical Services: Evaluation of the Medical Information System at the NIH Clinical Center, vols 1–6, (report no. NIH-79-302, National Technical Information Service accession number PB 82-1900TS). Springfield, VA, NTIS, 1982

Ashton C: Caring for patients within a computer environment. In Scholes M, Bryant Y, Barber B (eds): The Impact of Computers on Nursing: An International Review pp 105–114. Amsterdam, North-Holland, 1983

Astbury C: Nursing care plans: Aspects of computer use in nurse-to-nurse communication. In Fokkens O, et al (eds): Medinfo 83 Seminars, pp 332–336. Amsterdam, North-Holland, 1983

Ball M, Hannah K: Using Computers in Nursing. Reston, VA, Reston Publishing, 1984

Buthker J: Computers and nursing a likely combination. Comp Health Care, 4:44–45, 1983

Burroughs Hospital Information System: An untitled marketing handout. Charlotte, NC, Burroughs Hospital Information System, October 1978

DePooter G, Elseviers M, Verpooten G, et al: Nurses' experience with a computer in a nephrology-hypertension department. In Scholes M, Bryant Y, Barber B (eds): The Impact of Computers on Nursing: An International Review, pp 163–168. Amsterdam, North-Holland, 1983

Downey J, Walczak R, Hohri W: Evaluating hospital compliance with JCAH quality assurance standards. In Dayhoff R (ed): Proceedings of the Seventh Annual Symposium on Computer Applications in Medical Care, pp 94–97. Silver Spring, MD, IEEE Computer Society Press, 1983

Edmunds L: Computers for inpatient nursing care. Comp Nursing 2:102–108, 1984

Gearhart M: Nursing input: Patient outcomes? In Werley H, Grier M (eds): Nursing Information Systems, pp 91–96. New York, Springer, 1981

Gebhardt A: Developing a patient care program. In Scholes M, Bryant Y, Barber B (eds): The Impact of Computers on Nursing: An International Review, pp 95–104. Amsterdam, North-Holland, 1983

Griffith M: The computer as an aid to improving patient care. In Scholes M, Bryant Y, Barber B (eds): The Impact of Computers on Nursing: An International Review, pp 120–125. Amsterdam, North-Holland, 1983

Grobe S: Computer Primer and Resource Guide for Nurses. Philadelphia, JB Lippincott, 1984

Hannah K: The computer and nursing practice. Nurs Outlook, 24:555–558, 1976

Healy E, McGurk W: Effectiveness and acceptance of nurses' notes. Nurs Outlook 14:32–34, 1966

Howe M: Developing instruments for measurement of criteria: A clinical nursing practice perspective. Nurs Res 29:100–103, 1980

Jelger U, Regid K: Coordinating nursing systems with other medical and health care systems. In Fokkens O, et al (eds): Medinfo 83 Seminars, pp 364–366. Amsterdam, North-Holland, 1983

Kelly J: Computers in hospitals: Nursing practice defined and validated. In Dayhoff R (ed): Proceedings from the Seventh Annual Symposium on Computer Applications in Medical Care, pp 545–550. Silver Spring, MD, IEEE Computer Society Press, 1983

Kerr A: Nurses' notes—that's where the goodies are. Nursing 75 5:34–41, 1975

Lesnik M, Anderson B: Nursing Practice and the Law, 2nd ed. Philadelphia, JB Lippincott, 1955

Lombard N, Light N: On-line nursing care plans by nursing diagnosis. Comp Healthcare 4:22–23, 1983

Martin Marietta: An untitled marketing handout. Greenbelt, MD, Martin Marietta, 1983

Mayers M: Standard Nursing Care Plans. Palo Alto, CA, K. P. Co Medical System, 1974

McCormick K: Nursing research using computerized data bases. In Heffernan H (ed): Proceedings of the Fifth Annual Symposium on Computer Applications in Medical Care, pp 738–743. Silver Spring, MD, IEEE Computer Society Press, 1981

Rieder K, Norton D: An integrated nursing information system—a planning model. Comp Nursing 2:73–79, 1984

RNact, A Division of ROTON Corporation: An untitled marketing handout. Villa Park, IL, RNact, 1984

Romano C: Computerized multidisciplinary discharge care planning. In Blum B (ed): Proceedings of the Sixth Annual Symposium on Computer Applications in Medical Care, pp 587–589. Silver Spring, MD, IEEE Computer Society Press, 1982

Romano C, McCormick K, McNeely L: Nursing documentation: A model for a computerized data base. Adv Nurs Sc 4:43–56, 1982

Rozovsky L: Medical records as evidence. Dimen Health Serv 55:16–17, 1978

Scholes M, Bryant Y, Barber B: The Impact of Computers on Nursing: An International Review. Amsterdam, North-Holland, 1983

Shared Medical Systems: An untitled marketing handout. King of Prussia, PA, Shared Medical Systems, 1983

Somers J: A computerized nursing care system. Hospitals 45:96–100, 1971

Tamarisk N: The computer as a clinical tool. Nurs Manage, 13:46–49, 1982

Walker S: A study of the nature and uses of nurses' notes. Nurs Res 13:113–121, 1964

Weed L: Medical Records, Medical Education, and Patient Care: The Problem-Oriented Record as a Basic Tool. Cleveland, Case Western Reserve University Press, 1969

Weed L: Automation of a Problem-Oriented Medical Record. (National Technical Information Service order no. PB-263-578/7). Springfield, VA, U.S. Department of Commerce, 1976

Weed L, Hertzberg R: The use and construction of problem-knowledge couplers. The knowledge coupler editor knowledge networks and the problem-oriented medical record for the microcomputer. In Dayhoff R (ed): Proceedings from the Seventh Annual Symposium on Computer Applications in Medical Care, pp 831–836. Silver Spring, MD, IEEE Computer Society Press, 1983

Wessling E: Automating the nursing history and care plan. J Nurs Admin 2:34–38, 1972

Young E, Brian E, Hardy D: Automated Hospital Information Systems Workbook, vol 1, Guide to Planning, Selecting, Acquiring, Implementing, and Managing an AHIS. Los Angeles, Center Publications, 1981

Yura H, Walsh M: The Nursing Process: Assessing, Planning, Implementing, Evaluating, 2nd ed. New York, Appleton-Century-Crofts, 1973

BIBLIOGRAPHY

Abdellah F, Beland I, Martin A, Matheney R.: Patient-Centered Approaches to Nursing. New York, Macmillan, 1960

American Nurses' Association: Statement of function. Am J Nurs 54:686, 1954

Brimm J, O'Hara M, Peters R: An adaptable system for keeping intake and output records for fluid management of the critically ill. In Proceedings of the Second Annual Symposium on Computer Applications in Medical Care, pp 620–624. Silver Spring, MD, 1978

Bronzino J: Computer Applications for Paient Care. Reading, MA, Addison-Wesley, 1982

Butler E: An automated hospital information system. Nurs Times 245–247, 1978

Carriker D: Automated nurses' notes. J Pract Nurs 20–26, 1970

Cook M: Using computers to enhance professional practice. Nurs Times 78:1542–1544, 1982

Cornell S, Brush F: Systems approach to nursing care plans. Am J Nurs 71:1376–1378, 1971

Davis K: Give nurses the chance to explore these twelve routes to better care. Mod Hosp 82–85, 1968

Dietz L: History and Modern Nursing. Philadelphia, FA Davis, 1963

Dehlinger M: Nurses' utilization of the computerized records at NIH Clinical Center. In Heffernan H (eds): Proceedings of the Fifth Annual Symposium on Computer Applications in Medical Care, pp 744–747. Silver Spring, MD, IEEE Computer Society Press, 1981

Dynamic Control Corporation: An untitled marketing handout. Coral Gables, FL, Dynamic Control Corp, 1983

Edmunds L: Computer-assisted nursing care. Am J Nurs 82:1076–1079, 1982

Eggland E: Charting: How and why to document your care daily and fully. Nursing 80 10:38–43, 1980

Gane D: The computer in nursing. In Hursh J, Walker H (eds): The Problem-Oriented System, pp 251–257. New York, Medcom Press, 1982

Goodwin J, Edwards B: Developing a computer program to assist the nursing process. I. From system analysis to an expandable program. Nurs Res 24:29–305, 1975

Greene R, Kerr H, Likely N, Stephenson P: Computers and patients: The user system. Can Nurse 78:24–26, 1978

HBO & Company: An untitled marketing handout. Atlanta, GA, HBO & Co, 1983

Head A: Planning and controlling patient care with the Exeter system. In Scholes M, Bryant Y, Barber B (eds): The Impact of Computers on Nursing: An International Review, pp 115–119. Amsterdam, North-Holland, 1983

Henderson, V: The Nature of Nursing. New York, Macmillan, 1961

Hughes S: Computers in support of patient care. In Scholes M, Bryant Y, Barber B (eds): The Impact of Computers on Nursing: An International Review, pp 91–94. Amsterdam, North-Holland, 1983

Joint Commission on Accreditation of Hospitals: Standards for Hospital Accreditation. Chicago, Joint Commission on Accreditation of Hospitals, 1953, 1956, 1960, 1965, 1979, 1980.

Lesnik M: Nursing functions and legal control. Am J Nurs 53:1210–1211, 1953

MacEachern M: How hospital standardization can improve the professional work and the service to the patient in the hospital. Surg Gynecol Obstet 34:149–160, 1922

McCormick K: Monitoring and evaluating implemented HIS. In Dayhoff R (ed): Proceedings of the Seventh Annual Symposium on Computer Applications in Medical Care, pp 507–510. Silver Spring, MD, IEEE Computer Society Press, 1983

Muirhead R: Happening now. The decline and fall of paperwork. RN 45:34–40, 1982

NCR: MEDNET. Dayton, OH, NCR, 1983

Nightingale F: Notes on Nursing: What It Is and What It Is Not (facsimile of 1859 edition). Philadelphia, Edward Stern, 1946

Olsson D: Automating nurses' notes—first step in a computerized record system. Hospitals 41:64–78, 1967

Prendergast J: Implementing problem-oriented records in a primary nursing system. Nurs Clin North Am 12:235–246, 1977

Rosenberg M, Carriker D: Automating nurses; notes. Am J Nurs 66:1021–1023, 1966

Rosenberg M, Glueck B, Stroebel C, et al: Comparison of automated nurses' notes as recorded by psychiatric and nursing service personnel. Nurs Res 18:350–356, 1969

Sherman L: Nursing and computers: The present and implications for the future. Virginia Nurse 51:211–216, 1983

Simborg D: The development of a ward information management system. Meth Inform Med 12:17, 1973

Toy M: The observation study: A method of teaching in nursing arts. Am J Nurs 47:120–122, 1947

Watkins B: A pocket computer in the ward. Nurs Times 78:1468–1471, 1982

When AHA discussed records for the first time. Hosp Manag, 1932

Wilson G: A clinical chart for the records of patients in small hospitals. JAMA 45:920–921, 1905

Zielstorff R: Computers in Nursing. Wakefield, MA, Nursing Resources, 1980

Zielstorff R: The planning and evaluation of an automated system: A nurse's point of view. J Nurs Admin 5:22–25, 1975

13 Intensive Care Unit, Emergency Room, and Operating Room Applications

Objectives

- Identify computer applications in the intensive care unit, emergency room, and operating room.
- Understand the basic elements of arrhythmia monitors and physiologic monitors.
- Understand the basic types of computers in intensive care units.
- Identify dedicated, distributed, and integrated systems.
- Identify special-purpose applications available.
- Discuss the issues related to computers in the intensive care unit, emergency room, and operating room.

Nurses in critical care, including the intensive care unit (ICU), the emergency room (ER), and the operating room (OR), are exposed to different computer resources than nurses who work with hospital information systems (HISs) alone. This chapter describes several computer systems available for ICUs, ERs, and ORs that are designed for intensive patient and equipment management in sites where time and information are critical. The chapter includes a description of special-purpose systems in specialty areas where nurses may also work that provide accurate information, analysis, and reporting.

BACKGROUND

The average patient in an ICU may have from 1000 to 1500 nursing observations within a 24-hour period, which must be recorded and correlated. In the ER and the OR a patient may have up to 20 physiologic variables needing assessment each minute. Since a patient's condition is almost always serious in these intensive care areas, information is generally needed immediately. Documentation requires little time for planning, and long-term outcome goals are often inappropriate. Because the trajectory of hospitalization is short, documentation requirements are not the same as for chronically ill patients.

The developers of automated approaches for intensive care environments have thus computerized complex physiologic formulas; stored large volumes of data that would otherwise be disorganized, lost, inaccurate, or illegible; rapidly analyzed small samples of gas or fluids, and maintained near-normal physiologic ranges with life-supporting equipment. In addition, they automated alarm systems so that nurses make use of each vital second.

The advantages of these systems seem to resemble the advantages of computerizing nursing documentation: better control of nursing observations to promote better assessment of immediate patient needs. However, these systems do not provide all components of the nursing process; there are usually no outcome objectives, implementation strategies, or evaluation mechanisms.

Probably the most widespread use of computers in ICU, ER, and OR nursing has been in arrhythmia detection. Computerized arrhythmia monitors have been demonstrated to increase the detection of fatal arrhythmias and have even been linked to decreased mortality in coronary care patients (Badura, 1980). In these areas computers have been used to detect arrhythmias, generate alarms for heart rates that go out of a predetermined range, store data, provide graphic trends of heart rates, and correlate heart rates with medication administration and special procedures. The computer has also been used as an advanced calculator to calculate physiologic variables such as total peripheral resistance, cardiac output, and oxygen consumption.

Many of the applications described below refer to a microprocessor, which is another name for the central processing unit (CPU), or silicon chip. The CPU is composed of memory, the arithmetic and logic unit, and the control unit. A microprocessor installed into a monitor or other equipment is described as microprocessed equipment; it allows the equipment to behave like a computer, since the microprocessor allows the equipment to store and process information.

COMPUTERS' CAPABILITIES IN INTENSIVE CARE ENVIRONMENTS

Computers in ICUs, ERs, and ORs have seven major capabilities:

Microprocess physiologic data
File documentation of patient care
Graph trend data
Regulate physiologic equipment through microprocessors
Microprocess diagnostic equipment
Recognize deviations from preset ranges by an alarm
Comparatively evaluate patients with similar diagnoses

Nurses not involved in these intensive environments of computer technology may be surprised at the simplicity of these systems.

COMPUTER APPLICATIONS IN THE INTENSIVE CARE UNIT

Although many of the applications described in this chapter are also used in the ER and OR, they were often developed for the ICU and will thus be described within the ICU framework. Specifically, three types of computer applications will be described:

- Arrhythmia monitors
- Physiologic monitors
- Special-purpose systems

Arrhythmia monitoring systems and special-purpose systems are usually dedicated systems; that is, the computer processes information that is used for a special purpose. Physiologic monitoring systems are distributed or integrated. Distributed systems provide system-to-system communication; for example, these systems link the arrhythmia monitoring system with the blood pressure monitoring system. A new design is the modular system, in which microcomputer networks that include support modules are used. Integrated systems integrate all bedside recordkeeping and may include a nursing note. They are often called patient data management systems (PDMSs).

Arrhythmia Monitors

The electrocardiogram (ECG) and arrhythmia monitors led computerization into the ICUs, ERs, and ORs. The computerized patient care arrhythmia monitoring systems are generally used to collect data on electrical activity of the heart, blood pressure, and heart rate. They provide continuous telemetric measurements of a patient's cardiopulmonary function. Books have been written about the use of computers for arrhythmia monitoring (Bronzino, 1982).

Basic Elements

An arrhythmia system is composed of seven basic elements (Table 13-1):

A sensor (electrodes)
A signal conditioner
The cardiograph
Pattern recognition
Rhythm analysis
Diagnosis of the results
A subsequent written report

System Types

The two types of arrhythmia systems are detection surveillance and diagnostic or interpretive. In a detection system the criteria for a normal ECG are programmed into the computer. The computer might survey the ECG for wave amplitude and duration and the intervals between waves. The program may even include an alarm response if either the R-R interval is less than or equal to two thirds of the average R-R interval. Each signal may then be analyzed to determine whether the QRS duration is greater than normal.

The next programmed search may be for the presence of a compensatory pause, that is, a prolonged R-R interval after a premature ventricular contraction (PVC). The computer may then be programmed to store the number of PVCs per minute and sound an alarm or alert the nurse visually (flashing red light) and audibly (loud

TABLE 13-1 *Basic Components of Arrhythmia Monitors*

Sensor
Signal conditioner
Cardiograph
Pattern Recognition
Rhythm analysis
Diagnosis
Written report

sound) when more than five PVCs occur within a minute. Detection systems can even store in memory the type of arrhythmia and time of occurrence so that the patient's arrhythmia history can be plotted and compared to medication administration and cardiopulmonary pressures (Sorkin and Bloomfield, 1982).

Arrhythmia systems can also be diagnostic; after the analog signals are interfaced to digital information for processing, the program analyzes and diagnoses the ECG. The computer, after processing the ECG, generates an analysis report that is confirmed by a cardiologist at another site. The computers that support these types of ECGs are usually dedicated systems; that is, main memory is used only for ECG acquisition, analysis, and report generation. These systems are usually communicated by telephone.

Interpretive systems are beneficial because they do the following (Bronzino, 1982):

Reduce nursing time
Standardize terminology
Can be used as teaching aids
Rapidly transmit information for diagnosis
Reduce clerical duties
Eliminate potential errors of interpretation

Interpretive systems search the ECG complex for five parameters:

Location of QRS complex
Time from the beginning to end of the QRS
Comparison of amplitude, duration, and rate of QRS complex with all limb leads
P and T waves
Comparison of P and T waves with all limb leads

The findings are then compared to predetermined diagnostic specifications.

Examples of Arrhythmia Computer Systems

The following three systems are examples of arrhythmia computer systems:

- Hewlett-Packard arrhythmia monitoring system
- Phone-A-Gram-System
- CAPOC

The IBM/Bonner, which requires only 20 seconds of ECG data to perform its analysis, and TELEMED are two additional systems.

Hewlett-Packard Arrhythmia Monitoring System. The Hewlett-Packard Management System, an automatic ECG analysis, detection, and diagnostic system, monitors the ECG, blood pressure, and pulmonary artery pressure. It has software routines that provide analysis and diagnosis. Bedside carts with telephones transmit the ECG to an interpretive computer, and the diagnosis is recorded. This system can be used in the ICU, ER, or OR. Emergency rooms throughout the country can rely on on-line ECG arrhythmia recognition and diagnosis systems or can use telephone lines connected to emergency rescue squads within regional and national ECG service centers. Figure 13-1 shows a final ECG report from the Hewlett-Packard system.

Phone-A-Gram-System. National service centers make economic sense for the small hospital that has no more than 50 to 200 ECGs per day. National centers such as Phone-a-Gram-System in San Francisco (and TELEMED in Chicago) record and process ECGs, which are transmitted by telephone within minutes or the

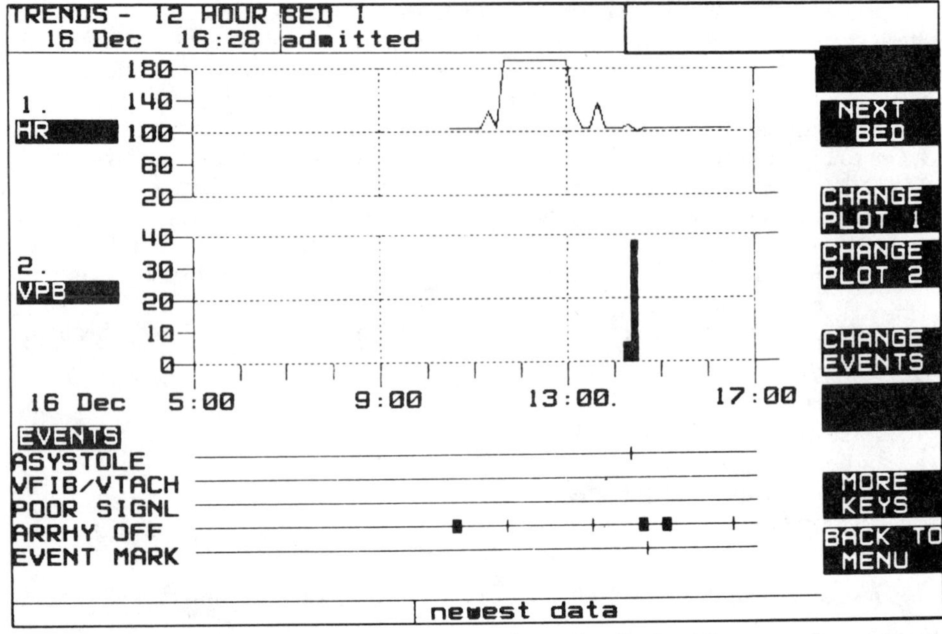

FIG. 13-1. A typical trend plot. (Copyright 1984, Hewlett-Packard Company. Reproduced with permission)

results mailed to hospitals within 1 day (Phone-A-Gram-System, Inc., 1983; TELEMED, 1983).

CAPOC. CAPOC (computer-assisted practice of cardiology) provides computer-assisted interpretation of ECGs. These systems accept simultaneous 12-lead ECGs, process and analyze information, read ECGs, print an analysis report, provide for short- and long-term ECG storage and retrieval, acquire system statistics and administrative reports, and provide for automated backup in the event of a system failure (TRIMIS Fact Sheet, 1983).

Physiologic Monitors

In 1975 the essential computers at the bedside of a critically ill patient consisted of an $800 Hewlett-Packard programmable calculator and a $3000 cardiac output computer. The remaining equipment included ECG leads, pressure transducers, oxygen and carbon dioxide analyzers, an oscilloscope, and a chart recorder. What facilitated the patient's records were worksheets, formulae, and glossaries of terms. About 10 parameters of physiologic data could be collected on line; approximately 12 additional parameters had to be calculated. The entire patient profile could take as long as 1 hour to assess, and then data had to be collected again. On-line continuous monitoring was restricted to heart rate, respiratory rate, blood pressure, and pulmonary artery pressure.

Today, computers facilitate the processing of large amounts of physiologic data, including bedside physiologic monitoring and PDMSs.

Bedside Physiologic Monitoring Systems

Most physiologic monitoring equipment consists of five basic parts (Table 13-2):

The sensor, which is the instrument that provides information (*e.g.*, the thermometer, the arterial pressure transducer)
The signal conditioner, which amplifies or filters the display device (*e.g.*, the signals, amplifier, oscilloscope, or paper record)
The file, which holds the information (*e.g.*, the storage file, signals, or alarms)
The computer processor, which analyzes information, stores pertinent information in specific places, and controls the direction of reporting (*e.g.*, a paper report, storage for graphic files, shift summary reports)
The evaluation or controlling component, which either regulates the infusion pumps electromechanically or alerts the nursing personnel through a report, an alarm, or a visual notice (*e.g.*, a notice on the display screen: "increase patient's oxygen or check for leaks")

The three basic types of physiologic monitoring systems are as follows:

Detection or surveillance systems
Diagnostic or interpretive systems
Treatment intervention system

The principles of detection and diagnostic systems are similar to those described for arrhythmia monitoring systems but also include treatment interventions. When the microprocessing includes changing an administered gas (*e.g.*, oxygen or carbon dioxide) or changing tidal volume or pressure after lung functions are diagnosed as being out of range, then microprocessing has been extended to treatment interventions.

Computers and their software provide dedicated systems with practical use for special care areas. One step beyond the dedicated system is the distributed system, where one computer communicates with another, such as the hospital information system or the clinical laboratory system. Two examples of bedside physiologic monitoring systems are as follows:

- Burdick: A modular system
- Trinity modules

Burdick: A Modular System. A relatively new design is the modular system available from Burdick. The Burdick color-trend patient bedside monitor is a multiparameter monitor for ICUs and coronary care units. It consists of compact plug-in modules that receive signals from the ECG, respiration, blood pressure, cardiac output, peripheral pulse, or temperature. In addition, this equipment stores infor-

TABLE 13-2 *Basic Components of Physiologic Monitoring Equipment*

1. Sensor (*e.g.*, thermometers, arterial pressure transducer)
2. Signal conditioners to amplify or filter the display device (*e.g.*, amplifier, oscilloscope, paper recorder)
3. File to rank and order information (*e.g.*, storage file, alarm signal)
4. Computer processor to analyze data and direct reports (*e.g.*, paper reports, storage for graphic files, summary reports)
5. Evaluation or controlling component to regulate the equipment or alert the nurse (*e.g.*, a notice on the display screen, alarm signal)

mation and allows 27-hour color graphic displays for three different parameters. After values are entered into the system, additional physiologic information can be calculated and graphed. Examples of this system are shown in Figures 13-2 and 13-3 (The Burdick Corporation, 1983).

Trinity Modules. The intensive care support system from Trinity computer systems is part of a microcomputer network that includes support modules for monitoring cardiovascular, respiratory, renal, and fluid balance in critically ill patients. The system's special feature is to use the monitored and laboratory data to provide a condensed evaluation of a patient's condition within seconds. The system analyzes and stores data, then reports trends of the patient's profile during the intensive care stay. It operates on various microcomputers. Output reports from this system are shown in Figures 13-4 and 13-5 (Trinity Computing Systems, 1983).

Integrated Patient Data Management Systems

An integrated system is one that combines physiologic monitoring systems and patient data management systems. Included in this description are the three major integrated systems described in the literature:

- HELP
- Hewlett-Packard PDMS
- Quantitative Medicine QS-2

HELP. The computers in intensive care environments also create files to document patient care. A system called HELP (Health Evaluation through Logical Processing) at the Latter Day Saints Hospital in Salt Lake City is used for decision making. It establishes quality instrumentation and standardized procedures for test performance and standardizes measurements. HELP is a hospitalwide computer system that integrates patient information from physiologic monitors and many other sources. Using a communication network to integrate clinical laboratory data with the ICU, including all pulmonary function testing, the system allows decision making in the form of interpretations, warning alerts, or treatment protocols. Figure 13-6 shows an example of an alert printout (Johnson and colleagues, 1980).

When such large volumes of data are being recorded in the intensive environment, a "data cemetery" is possible; that is, continuous monitoring of data occurs, summary reports are composed of all data stored, and the nurse does not use the information to evaluate the patient's status clinically. When a computer has the potential to file continuous physiologic data on patients, nursing personnel may study the retrieved information when the patient is discharged or dies to determine patterns of actions that most appropriately facilitated or inhibited patients' outcomes.

When the output of computerized intensive care systems is designed appropriately, the continuous data can be formatted so that the output record serves as the unit report. Critical conditions in the day of an intensive care patient could be integrated from the continuous monitoring and nursing interventions to prepare unit reports. With the HELP system, nurses have designed a nursing care plan that includes plans for critical care patients. The unique problems of critical care patients are listed in Table 13-3. An example of a care plan that could be printed at discharge from the ICU is shown in Figure 13-7 (Cengiz and colleagues, 1983).

Hewlett-Packard PDMS. The Hewlett-Packard patient data management system integrates physiologic data with other patient information such as fluid management (intake and output), clinical observations (nurses' notes), and diagnostic studies (laboratory data). The system is composed of a "soft key" key pad and video

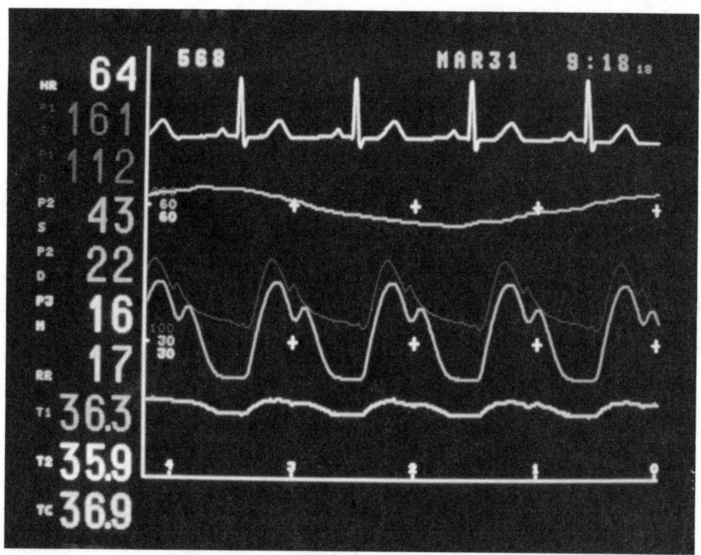

FIG. 13-2. An example of the Burdick Color-Trend screen with data related to hemodynamic function.

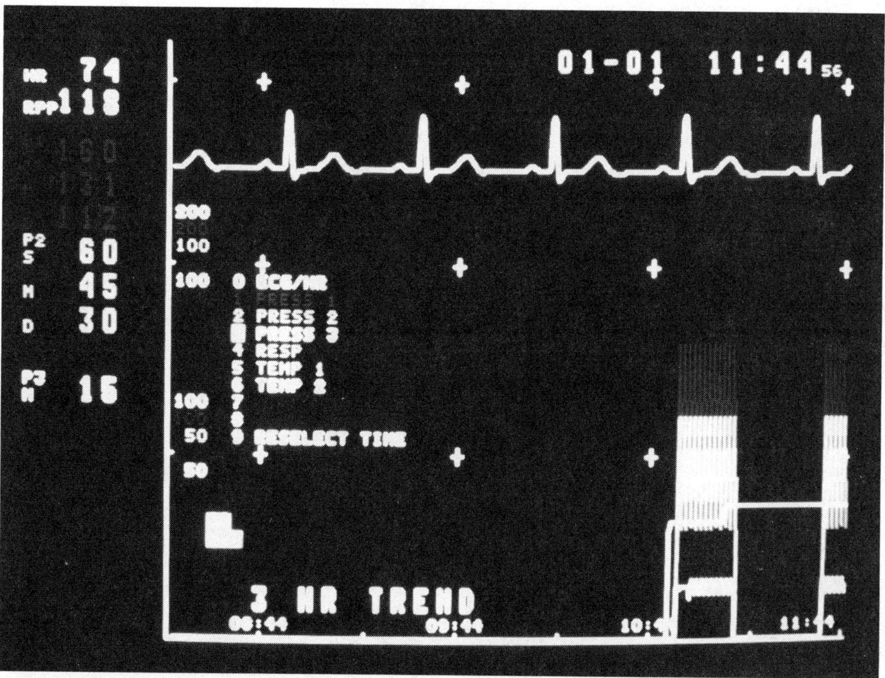

FIG. 13-3. An example of a Burdick Color-Trend display of 3-, 9-, 27-hour trend data of hemodynamic function.

FIG. 13-4. Trinity respiratory and cardiovascular output reports.

Hemodynamic Tracking Profile

Pulmonary Edema Trends

CV Respiratory Data

((CU RESPIRATORY DATA)) DATE 01/24/83

PATIENT NO. TC12345678 TIME OF READINGS 1400 HOURS DATE 01/24/83

PATIENT'S NAME: JAMES PRITCHETT AGE: 30 SEX: MALE
INTITIAL DIAGNOSIS WAS: MULTIPLE STAB WOUNDS

HEIGHT (CM) 103.0 (IN) 72.0 WEIGHT (KG) 00.0 (LB) 194.0
BODY SURFACE AREA 2.1 TEMP (C) 37.5 (F) 99.5

CARDIOVASCULAR

	NORMAL VALUES	CALCULATED VALUES		INPUT VALUES
MEAN ART PRESS	(82 - 102)	101.3	SYSTOLIC B/P	134.0
STROKE VOLUME	(60 - 70)	28.4	DIASTOLIC B/P	85.0
CARDIAC INDEX	(2.8 - 3.6)	1.2	CARDIAC OUTPUT	2.5
STROKE INDEX	(30 - 50)	13.5	HEART RATE	88.0
SUR	(900 - 1200)	2858.1	CUP	12.0
SURI	(1760 - 2600)	6013.6	PCWP	22.0
PUR	(150 - 250)	−149.5	PUL ARTERY SYS	28.0
PURI	(45 - 225)	−314.6	PUL ARTERY DIA	12.0
LUSW	(VARIES)	30.6	MEAN PAP	17.3
LUSWI	(44 - 68)	14.6		
RUSW	(VARIES)	2.1		
RUSWI	(4 - 8)	1.0		
LUMWI	(3 - 4.6)	1.6		
RUMWI	(0.4 - 0.6)	0.3		
TRIPLE INDEX	(150,000)	259424.0		

RESPIRATORY

	NORMAL VALUES	CALCULATED VALUES		INPUT VALUES
CAO2	(18 - 20)	15.9	PH(A)	7.38
CUO2	(13 - 16)	13.6	PAO2	99.0
A-UDO2	(4 - 5.5)	2.3	PACO2	44.0
A-ADO2	(0 - 20)RM AIR	452.1	SAO2	97.2
SHUNT QS/QT (%)	(0 - 8)	44.1	PH(U)	7.42
02 (AVAILABLE)	(520 - 720)	189.4	PUO2	48.0
02 (EXTRACTION)	(22% - 30%)	14.7	PUCO2	42.0
RQ (RESP QUOT)	(.8)	−0.9	SUO2	83.6
CO2 (PROD INDEX)	(VARIES)	−23.8	%IO2	85.0
02 (CONSUMP IND)	([illegible] - [illegible])	27.8	HB	12.0
RME (RES META EX)	(VARIES)	75.9	COHGB	1.5

TEMP CORRECTED VALUES

PH(A)	7.37
PAO2	101.88
PACO2	44.95
PH(U)	7.41
PU02	49.70
PUCO2	42.90

Cardiogenic Parameter Trends

Oxygen Delivery Trends

Acid — Base Chart Graph

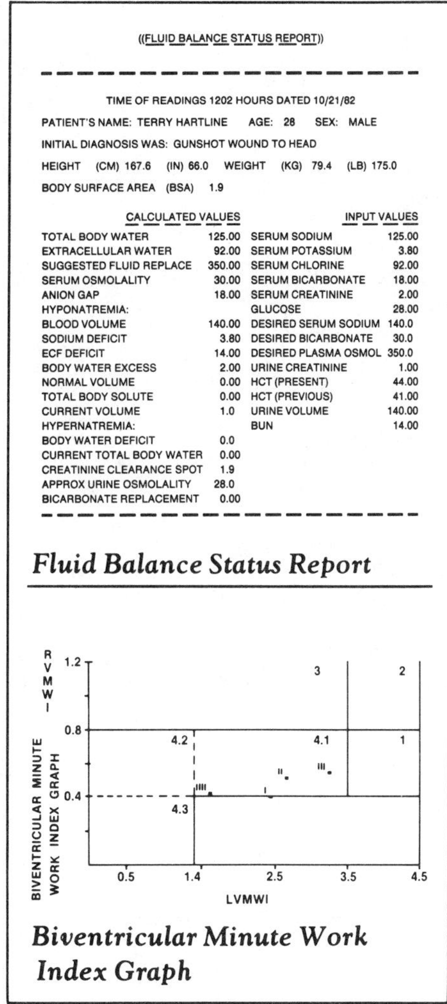

((FLUID BALANCE STATUS REPORT))

TIME OF READINGS 1202 HOURS DATED 10/21/82

PATIENT'S NAME: TERRY HARTLINE AGE: 28 SEX: MALE

INITIAL DIAGNOSIS WAS: GUNSHOT WOUND TO HEAD

HEIGHT (CM) 167.6 (IN) 66.0 WEIGHT (KG) 79.4 (LB) 175.0

BODY SURFACE AREA (BSA) 1.9

CALCULATED VALUES		INPUT VALUES	
TOTAL BODY WATER	125.00	SERUM SODIUM	125.00
EXTRACELLULAR WATER	92.00	SERUM POTASSIUM	3.80
SUGGESTED FLUID REPLACE	350.00	SERUM CHLORINE	92.00
SERUM OSMOLALITY	30.00	SERUM BICARBONATE	18.00
ANION GAP	18.00	SERUM CREATININE	2.00
HYPONATREMIA:		GLUCOSE	28.00
BLOOD VOLUME	140.00	DESIRED SERUM SODIUM	140.0
SODIUM DEFICIT	3.80	DESIRED BICARBONATE	30.0
ECF DEFICIT	14.00	DESIRED PLASMA OSMOL	350.0
BODY WATER EXCESS	2.00	URINE CREATININE	1.00
NORMAL VOLUME	0.00	HCT (PRESENT)	44.00
TOTAL BODY SOLUTE	0.00	HCT (PREVIOUS)	41.00
CURRENT VOLUME	1.0	URINE VOLUME	140.00
HYPERNATREMIA:		BUN	14.00
BODY WATER DEFICIT	0.0		
CURRENT TOTAL BODY WATER	0.00		
CREATININE CLEARANCE SPOT	1.9		
APPROX URINE OSMOLALITY	28.0		
BICARBONATE REPLACEMENT	0.00		

Fluid Balance Status Report

Biventricular Minute Work Index Graph

FIG. 13-5. An example of a Trinity fluid balance output report.

display unit. The programs or software are structured around six soft keys used to view data and read from the monitor equipment, including the arrhythmia monitoring system. It aids the nurse by providing rapid access to physiologic information.

The following information may be entered into the computer:

Heart rate	Blood pressure
Central venous pressure	Intracranial pressure
Temperature	Urine output
Respiratory rate	Pulmonary artery pressure medications
Intravenous rate	Intake and output
Weight	Nurses' notes

The nurses' notes allow systematic assessment of patients. The computer is

PRINTOUT OF ALERTS FOR ONE TIME PERIOD

AS OF 16:23 ON 2/18/78

```
288144  NAME                          76  4E61   DR. UNKNOWN
POSTED: 2/18/78  16:11  DATA: 2/18/78  15:5
RENAL FAILURE (BUN IS 108)

290066  NAME                          60  5N79   DR. DOCTOR NOT ASSIGNED
POSTED: 2/18/78  14:49  DATA: 2/18/78  14:33
SEVERE HYPOXEMIA ON OXYGEN

29006  NAME                           60  5N79   DR. DOCTOR NOT ASSIGNED
POSTED: 2/18/78  14:49  DATA: 2/18/78  14:33
SEVERE CHRONIC RESPIRATORY ACIDOSIS—

287199  NAME                          70  3W03   DR. UNKNOWN
POSTED: 2/18/78  14:48  DATA: 2/18/78  14:30
CONSIDER METABOLIC ACIDOSIS

327865  NAME                          58  2E61   DR. WARNER, HOMER R.
POSTED: 2/18/78  14:35  DATA: 2/18/78  07:05
HEMATOCRIT FALLING (HCT 26.1)
```

FIG. 13-6. An example of an alert printout available on the HELP system. (Johnson D, Ranzenberger J, Herbert R, et al: A computerized alert program for acutely ill patients. J Nurs Admin 10:26–35, 1980)

TABLE 13-3 *Unique Problems of Critical Patients Using the HELP System*

1. Altered ventilation/oxygenation
2. Hemodynamic instability
3. Fluid/electrolyte imbalance
4. Altered level of consciousness/impaired neurological state
5. Cardiac rhythm disturbance
6. Pain
7. Altered gastrointestinal function
8. Infection/compromised defense mechanisms
9. Immobility/Impaired musculoskeletal function
10. Patient/family anxiety
11. Inadequate nutrition
12. Altered hematologic status

(Cengiz M, Ranzenberger J, Johnson D, et al: Design and implementation of computerized nursing care plans. In Dayhoff R [ed]: Proceedings of the Seventh Annual Symposium on Computer Applications in Medical Care. Silver Spring, MD, IEEE Computer Society Press, 1983) used to track patients' physiologic responses correlated with pharmacologic treatments. In addition to nursing input, a clerk may enter the patient's name, diagnosis, physician record number, and laboratory results. The blood gas technician enters the results of arterial and venous blood gases, the monitoring technician enters cardiac output data and the respiratory therapist enters ventilatory parameters and results from pulmonary function tests. Entry into the computer is controlled by an identification number, so that the output is recorded by the name of the person entering the information. In order to orchestrate this interdisciplinary access to the system, a 12-bed unit may have a keyboard at a nurses' station, a portable terminal, keyboards at each bedside, screens at each bedside, and terminals in the blood gas laboratory and nursing office (Beckmann and colleagues, 1981).

During 2 years' experience with this system, one ICU has entered nursing records for 2000 patients. The main advantages of the system are reported in terms of time; more time was left for nurses to do nursing care. Also, nursing notes are more legible and accurate. In addition, the retrieval of patient information has been facilitated (Beckmann, 1981).

These computers are also in use in the intensive care nursery. Nurses' progress notes are recorded with a computer-assisted PDMS. A modified menu selection of problem-oriented notes has been described as expediting recordkeeping and providing well-organized, precise notes. This system allows selection from 13 categories of problems frequently occurring in the intensive care nursery (Table 13-4). The second level of selection are objectives, evaluations, assessments, and care plans. The last segment is the ability to incorporate phrases that describe the problem. It is estimated that the new nurse working with this system is comfortable within 5 working days of orientation (McCarthy and colleagues, 1982).

Hewlett-Packard to IBM Link. A Hewlett-Packard minicomputer with PDMS software links an IBM PCS to an IBM clinical laboratory system. It is a distributed system where peripheral computers exchange information with a large host computer and thereby greatly reduce redundant data entry. The system allows a progress note for respiratory care, statistical information for unit management, computation of cardiac and pulmonary parameters, intravenous schedules for vasoactive drugs, data collection for retrospective audits, and daily compilation of TISS (therapeutic intervention scoring system) and APACHE (acute physiology and chronic health evaluation: a physiologically based classification system). The advantage for nursing is the reduction in redundant information. The functions of such a system are listed in Table 13-5 (Shinozaki and colleagues, 1982).

Quantitative Medicine. The Quantitative Sentinel (QS) is an interactive computer database system designed for use in a 54-bed facility of the Maryland Institute for Emergency Medical Services System. It includes critical care areas such as a hyperbaric oxygen unit, ICU, intermediate care, a neurotrauma center, a critical care recovery unit, an admitting area, and an OR. Its primary goals are to assist clinical staff in patient care by offering the best computer technology without increasing staff work time and to incorporate the entire clinical patient record into the computer system. It is only when the patient is discharged from the trauma unit that a paper record is printed.

The information that the QS system allows is from many sources: either directly from the physiologic monitors or manually by the clinical nursing staff. The major functions of the system include database definition, database management, data entry, real-time monitoring of physiological variables, data display, and fluid balance calculation. The system consists of two types of calculators, one that computes

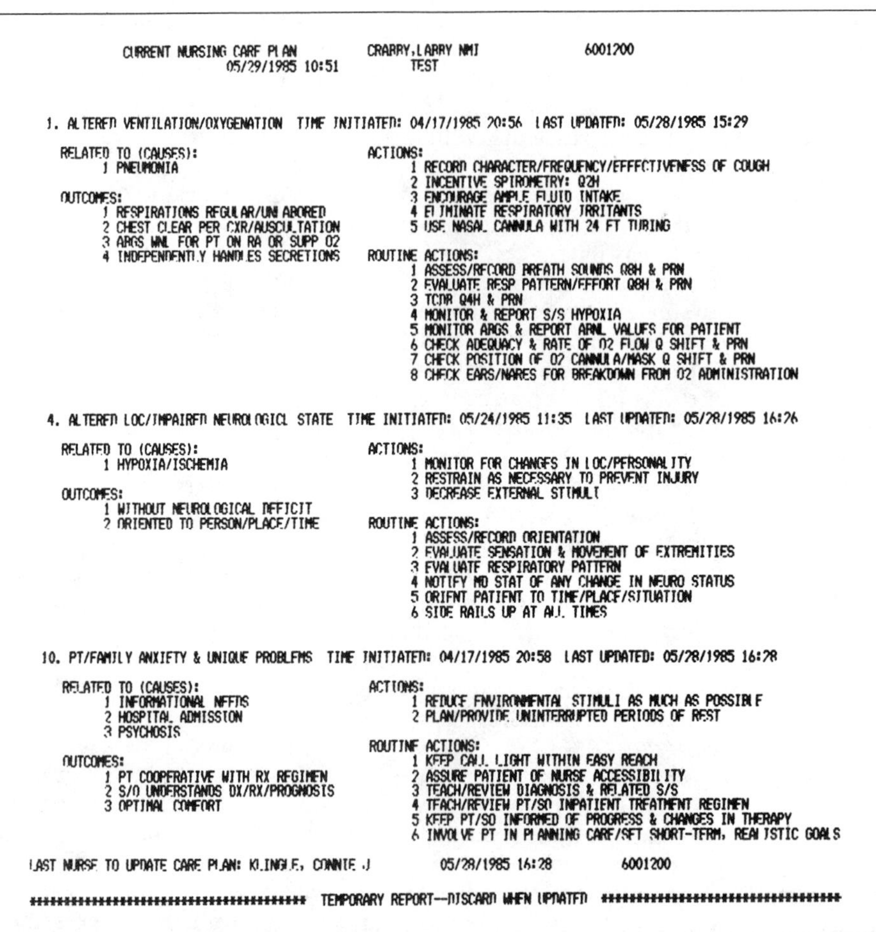

```
          CURRENT NURSING CARE PLAN         CRABBY,LARRY NMI              6001200
                      05/29/1985 10:51           TEST


 1. ALTERED VENTILATION/OXYGENATION  TIME INITIATED: 04/17/1985 20:56  LAST UPDATED: 05/28/1985 15:29

   RELATED TO (CAUSES):                     ACTIONS:
         1 PNEUMONIA                              1 RECORD CHARACTER/FREQUENCY/EFFECTIVENESS OF COUGH
                                                  2 INCENTIVE SPIROMETRY: Q2H
   OUTCOMES:                                      3 ENCOURAGE AMPLE FLUID INTAKE
         1 RESPIRATIONS REGULAR/UNLABORED         4 ELIMINATE RESPIRATORY IRRITANTS
         2 CHEST CLEAR PER CXR/AUSCULTATION       5 USE NASAL CANNULA WITH 24 FT TUBING
         3 ABGS WNL FOR PT ON RA OR SUPP O2
         4 INDEPENDENTLY HANDLES SECRETIONS  ROUTINE ACTIONS:
                                                  1 ASSESS/RECORD BREATH SOUNDS Q8H & PRN
                                                  2 EVALUATE RESP PATTERN/EFFORT Q8H & PRN
                                                  3 TCDB Q4H & PRN
                                                  4 MONITOR & REPORT S/S HYPOXIA
                                                  5 MONITOR ABGS & REPORT ABNL VALUES FOR PATIENT
                                                  6 CHECK ADEQUACY & RATE OF O2 FLOW Q SHIFT & PRN
                                                  7 CHECK POSITION OF O2 CANNULA/MASK Q SHIFT & PRN
                                                  8 CHECK EARS/NARES FOR BREAKDOWN FROM O2 ADMINISTRATION

 4. ALTERED LOC/IMPAIRED NEUROLOGICL STATE  TIME INITIATED: 05/24/1985 11:35  LAST UPDATED: 05/28/1985 16:26

   RELATED TO (CAUSES):                     ACTIONS:
         1 HYPOXIA/ISCHEMIA                       1 MONITOR FOR CHANGES IN LOC/PERSONALITY
                                                  2 RESTRAIN AS NECESSARY TO PREVENT INJURY
   OUTCOMES:                                      3 DECREASE EXTERNAL STIMULI
         1 WITHOUT NEUROLOGICAL DEFICIT
         2 ORIENTED TO PERSON/PLACE/TIME     ROUTINE ACTIONS:
                                                  1 ASSESS/RECORD ORIENTATION
                                                  2 EVALUATE SENSATION & MOVEMENT OF EXTREMITIES
                                                  3 EVALUATE RESPIRATORY PATTERN
                                                  4 NOTIFY MD STAT OF ANY CHANGE IN NEURO STATUS
                                                  5 ORIENT PATIENT TO TIME/PLACE/SITUATION
                                                  6 SIDE RAILS UP AT ALL TIMES

 10. PT/FAMILY ANXIETY & UNIQUE PROBLEMS  TIME INITIATED: 04/17/1985 20:58  LAST UPDATED: 05/28/1985 16:28

   RELATED TO (CAUSES):                     ACTIONS:
         1 INFORMATIONAL NEEDS                    1 REDUCE ENVIRONMENTAL STIMULI AS MUCH AS POSSIBLE
         2 HOSPITAL ADMISSION                     2 PLAN/PROVIDE UNINTERRUPTED PERIODS OF REST
         3 PSYCHOSIS
                                             ROUTINE ACTIONS:
   OUTCOMES:                                      1 KEEP CALL LIGHT WITHIN EASY REACH
         1 PT COOPERATIVE WITH RX REGIMEN         2 ASSURE PATIENT OF NURSE ACCESSIBILITY
         2 S/O UNDERSTANDS DX/RX/PROGNOSIS        3 TEACH/REVIEW DIAGNOSIS & RELATED S/S
         3 OPTIMAL COMFORT                        4 TEACH/REVIEW PT/SO INPATIENT TREATMENT REGIMEN
                                                  5 KEEP PT/SO INFORMED OF PROGRESS & CHANGES IN THERAPY
                                                  6 INVOLVE PT IN PLANNING CARE/SET SHORT-TERM, REALISTIC GOALS

 LAST NURSE TO UPDATE CARE PLAN: KLINGLE, CONNIE J        05/28/1985 16:28        6001200

 ###################################### TEMPORARY REPORT--DISCARD WHEN UPDATED ##################################
```

FIG. 13-7. An example of a care plan summary when a patient is discharged from an ICU equipped with a HELP System. (Cengiz M, Ranzenberger J, Johnson D, et al: Design and implementation of computerized nursing care plans. In Dayhoff R [ed]: Proceedings of the Seventh Annual Symposium on Computer Applications in Medical Care. Silver Spring, MD, IEEE Computer Society Press, 1983)

and stores physiologic data and a clinical calculator for which results are not stored. Graphic displays are available for trend analysis. Figure 13-8 is an example of a nursing note from this system. A survey of use, including nursing use and satisfaction with this type of system, showed nurse satisfaction to be above average, but software and hardware changes were deemed necessary (Milholland and Cardona, 1983).

A Microcomputer Integrated System

A computerized notation system (CNS) has been introduced to ICUs in the United States. This system relies on a portable microprocessor and was designed for use in outpatient departments, hospital wards, and the ICU. It automates the previous bedside daily note or patient summaries produced by nurses and physicians. The

```
NURSING CARE PLAN HISTORY   MCC    , HE    RRO              369     W5     05/29/1985 10:49

  9. IMMOBILITY/IMPAIRED MUSCULO-SKELETAL FUNCTION        TIME INITIATED: 05/25/1985 20:49  TIME RESOLVED: 05/29/1985 10:48

   A. RELATED TO (CAUSE) (BT - ET *) :
    1. FRACTURES       (05/25  -  05/29)
    2. PROLONGED BEDREST       (05/25  -  05/29)
    3. COMMENT:DVT RIGHT LEG       (05/25  -  05/29)

   B. ACTIONS (BT - ET *):
    1. POSITIONING:ELEVATE RIGHT LEG ON PILLOWS       (05/25  -  05/29)
    2. TEACH/REVIEW S/S WHICH REQUIRE MEDICAL ATTENTION       (05/25  -  05/29)

   C. ROUTINE ACTIONS (BT - ET *):
    1. CHECK/RECORD MOVEMENT/STRENGTH/SENSATION OF EXTREMITIES       (05/25  -  05/25)
    2. EVALUATE/RECORD RANGE OF MOTION Q SHIFT & PRN       (05/25  -  05/25)
    3. CHECK FOR/RECORD SKIN DISCOLORATION/BREAKDOWN/IRRITATION       (05/25  -  05/29)
    4. EVALUATE/RECORD ADEQUACY OF PERIPHERAL CIRCULATION Q SHIFT       (05/25  -  05/29)
    5. MONITOR FOR S/S THROMBOPHLEBITIS       (05/25  -  05/25)
    6. MASSAGE BONY PROMINENCES/PRESSURE AREAS PRN       (05/25  -  05/29)
    7. TURN & REPOSITION Q2H & PRN       (05/25  -  05/25)
    8. MAINTAIN PROPER BODY ALIGNMENT       (05/25  -  05/29)
    9. ASSIST WITH ADLS PRN       (05/25  -  05/29)
   10. EVALUATE & RECORD ACTIVITY TOLERANCE       (05/25  -  05/29)
   11. TEACH/REVIEW PT/SO INPATIENT TREATMENT REGIMEN       (05/25  -  05/29)

   D. EXPECTED OUTCOMES (BT - ET *):
    1. SKIN INTACT/NO BREAKDOWN       (05/25  -  05/29)
    2. BOWEL FUNCTION WNL FOR PATIENT       (05/25  -  05/29)
    3. OPTIMAL COMFORT       (05/25  -  05/29)

 12. ALTERED HEMATOLOGIC/COAGULATION STATUS              TIME INITIATED: 05/25/1985 20:44  TIME RESOLVED: 05/29/1985 10:48

   A. RELATED TO (CAUSE) (BT - ET *) :
    1. ANTICOAGULANT THERAPY       (05/25  -  05/29)

   B. ACTIONS (BT - ET *):
    1. USE INFUSION PUMP FOR CONTINUOUS HEPARIN DRIP       (05/25  -  05/29)
    2. TEACH/REVIEW ANTICOAGULANT REGIMEN/PRECAUTIONS       (05/25  -  05/29)
    3. TEACH/REVIEW S/S REQUIRING MEDICAL ATTENTION       (05/25  -  05/29)

   C. ROUTINE ACTIONS (BT - ET *):
    1. HANDLE PT GENTLY AT ALL TIMES       (05/25  -  05/25)
    2. CONTINUOUSLY MONITOR FOR S/S BLEEDING       (05/25  -  05/25)
    3. ASSESS/RECORD TEMP,COLOR,SENSATION OF FINGERS & TOES       (05/25  -  05/29)
    4. HEMATEST ALL URINE & EMESIS/GUAIAC ALL STOOLS       (05/25  -  05/29)
    5. OBSERVE FOR PETECHIAE/CONTUSIONS       (05/25  -  05/25)
    6. OBSERVE FOR BLEEDING GUMS OR MUCOUS MEMBRANES       (05/25  -  05/25)
    7. MONITOR ARTIERAL/VENIPUNCTURE & INJECTION SITES FOR BLEEDING       (05/25  -  05/29)
    8. CAUTIOUS MOUTH CARE WITH SOFT BRUSH OR SWABS       (05/25  -  05/25)
    9. SHAVING WITH ELECTRIC RAZOR ONLY       (05/25  -  05/25)
   10. MONITOR PERTINENT LAB: ..............................       (05/25  -  05/29)
   11. TEACH/REVIEW PT/SO INPATIENT TREATMENT REGIMEN       (05/25  -  05/25)

   D. EXPECTED OUTCOMES (BT - ET *):
    1. PT WITHIN THERAPEUTIC RANGE       (05/25  -  05/29)
    2. PT/SO UNDERSTAND HOSPITAL ROUTINE       (05/25  -  05/29)

XX. RN'S INITIATING/CHANGING CARE PLAN FOR THIS PATIENT
     1. KLINGLE, CONNIE J                  05/25
     2. PED     , SHE    J                 05/25
```

FIG. 13-7. *(Continued)*

report is a legible printout comparable and compatible with the manually prepared documentation. The system encourages but does not mandate a forced use of problem-oriented identification. The CNS uses a portable Hewlett-Packard microprocessor.

The program consists of three basic portions directed by five key functions: notation/problem identification, medications/therapies, numerical/laboratory selection. Figure 13-9 is an example of the output from this system. The notes are "type-in problems" and "actions taken." Compression of the numerical section allows 11 or more numbers to be placed on a 45-degree slant underneath the titles displayed. Current medications and therapies such as ventilator settings, diet, or intravenous rate can be recorded. It takes approximately half an hour to train a user (Ash and colleagues, 1981).

TABLE 13-4 *Thirteen Components Categorized for Intensive Care Nursery Problems*

1. Cardiac status
2. Respiratory status
3. Thermoregulation
4. Hematologic status
5. Hyperbilirubinemia
6. Infection
7. Nutrition
8. Gastrointestinal status
9. Renal status
10. Neurologic status
11. Congential anomalies
12. Social/family care
13. Routine care

(McCarthy M, Townsend M, Thorp J: Computer assistance to record problem oriented notes for intensive care nursery patients. In Blum B [ed]: Proceedings of the Sixth Annual Symposium on Computer Applications in Medical Care. Silver Spring, MD, IEEE Computer Society Press, 1982)

Special-Purpose Systems

The following seven types of special-purpose systems are described in this chapter:

- Ventilators
- Blood gas analyzers
- Pulmonary function systems
- Intracranial pressure monitors
- Cardiac and other diagnostic systems
- Drug administration system
- Newborn nursery system

Nurses today might work in the ICU, ER, and OR, or they use these systems because they work in the cardiac catheterization laboratory, the pulmonary function department, or another specialty area.

Ventilators

An advantage of computer facilities in intensive environments has been the regulation of equipment through microprocessors. Ventilators are used to deliver an adequate volume of gas to the patients' lungs and to control the pressure, volume, flow rate, inspiratory: expiratory time ratio, and oxygen concentration. The two types of ventilators, pressure cycled and volume cycled, have time-cycled devices that are regulated by microprocessors.

Ventilators have relied on surveillance systems by providing alarms when pulmonary function appears out of a present range or by communicating the integrity of the ventilator to the nurses' station when the patient in question is not in the intensive care environment. Computer-assisted ventilators have been developed and frequently use a microprocessor chip. Electromechanically controlled by a

TABLE 13-5 ***Functions of a Distributed Minicomputer System Used in an Intensive Care Environment***

1. Admission/discharge entry
   Most of the demographic data are obtained from the host computer. Problem lists pertinent to the admission to the unit, are entered to facilitate coding at discharge.
2. Presentation of laboratory data on screen or by printout in special format.
3. Interface between blood gas and respiratory parameters for intelligent interpretation.
4. Entry of chest radiographic findings by a standardized numeric system.
5. Daily printout for progress note in flowchart form and uniform narrative form.
6. Periodic printout of respiratory parameters for all patients in unit which enhances the smooth transfer of respiratory care from daytime to nighttime coverage.
7. Data entry and subsequent display of TISS and APACHE scores.
8. Aid to nursing and medical auditing.
9. Use as a computation aid for cardiac parameters. All additional data (age, sex, surface area, blood gases, hemoglobin concentration) are obtained from the computer memory and are interfaced with manually entered cardiac output and pressure data. Results are retained for graphic display.
10. Computation of IV schedule for vasoactive drugs. These are calculated specifically for a patient in terms of weight, surface area or caloric need.
11. Narrative information.
    This section is used to keep an updated list of problems which necessitate the intensive care unit stay of the patient.
12. Monthly log of patients, audit results, cumulative TISS and APACHE scores by admitting service.
13. Statistics to manage the unit. The statistics include length of various active respiratory interventions, average TISS and APACHE scores per patient day.
14. Collection of physiologic data for the group of patients who are under various clinical protocols. Barbiturate coma for head injury, high frequency ventilation trial, and long-term endotracheal intubation are examples.

(Shinozaki T, Deane R, Mazuzan J: A devoted mini-computer system for the management of clinical and laboratory data in an intensive care unit. In Blum B [ed]: Proceedings of the Sixth Annual Symposium on Computer Applications in Medical Care. Silver Spring, MD, IEEE Computer Society Press, 1982)

closed-loop feedback system, they analyze and control ventilation, blood volumes, and alveolar gases, which change as the patient's metabolic rate changes.

Processing signals by breath analysis of flow and volume has been done with various forms of microprocessors for years. The signals from respiratory pneumotachographs in association with differential pressure transducers allows on-line data collection of inspiration and expiration phases of the respiratory cycle. Such systems have been thoroughly described (McCormick, 1978; Dolcourt and Harris, 1982).

For: Kathy Milholland, R.N.

Quantitative Medicine, Inc
3806 Baker Avenue
Abingdon, Maryland
21009

Patient: Sample, Demo

ID: 101 Location: ICU 1

Nursing Notes

For the time: 4/29/85 14:00:00 EDT

Authored by Kathy Milholland, R.N.

Awake, alert, and oriented. Pupils equal and reactive to light. Corneals brisk. Follows commands and moves spontaneously - all extremities.
Intubated and on ventilator; breath sounds equal and clear; suctioned for clear secretions. R chest tube draining moderate amounts of blood; no air leak; Breathing in-phase with ventilator.
Peripheral pulses all present; skin warm and dry; vital signs stable; Arterial line (R wrist) - patent & has good wave form; normal sinus rhythm by monitor; p-a line patent and wedges well.
Abdomen soft and flat; bowel sounds active; n/g tube draining small amounts of green fluid; no stools.
foley catheter draining clear amber urine in moderate amounts.
Long-leg cast on R - dry; neurovascular checks o.k.
Medicated q2h with mso4 for pain with good effect.

FIG. 13-8. An example of a nursing note capability (Quantitative Sentinel, QS-2).

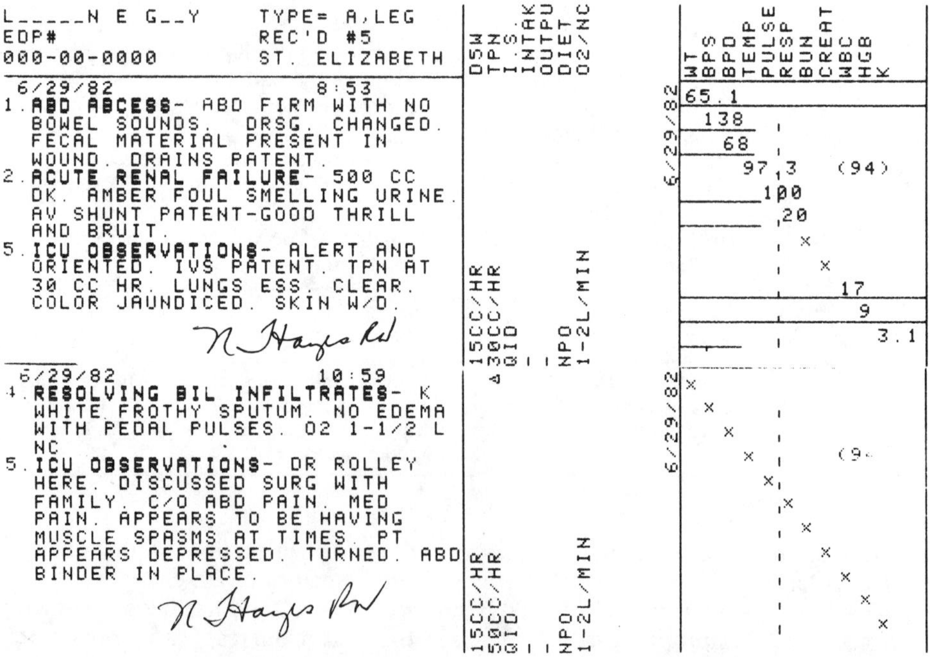

L______N E G__Y TYPE= A,LEG
EDP# REC'D #5
000-00-0000 ST. ELIZABETH

D5W TPN I.S. INTAK OUTPU DIET O2/NC

WT BPPS BPPD TEMP PULSE RESP BUN CREAT WBC HGB K

6/29/82 8:53
1. **ABD ABCESS**- ABD FIRM WITH NO BOWEL SOUNDS. DRSG. CHANGED. FECAL MATERIAL PRESENT IN WOUND. DRAINS PATENT.
2. **ACUTE RENAL FAILURE**- 500 CC DK. AMBER FOUL SMELLING URINE. AV SHUNT PATENT-GOOD THRILL AND BRUIT.
5. **ICU OBSERVATIONS**- ALERT AND ORIENTED. IVS PATENT. TPN AT 30 CC HR. LUNGS ESS. CLEAR. COLOR JAUNDICED. SKIN W/D.

N Hayes RN

15CC/HR 30CC/HR QID - - NPO 1-2L/MIN

6/29/82 65.1 138 68 97.3 (94) 100 20 17 9 3.1

6/29/82 10:59
4. **RESOLVING BIL INFILTRATES**- K WHITE FROTHY SPUTUM. NO EDEMA WITH PEDAL PULSES. O2 1-1/2 L NC
5. **ICU OBSERVATIONS**- DR ROLLEY HERE. DISCUSSED SURG WITH FAMILY. C/O ABD PAIN. MED PAIN. APPEARS TO BE HAVING MUSCLE SPASMS AT TIMES. PT APPEARS DEPRESSED. TURNED. ABD BINDER IN PLACE.

N Hayes RN

15CC/HR 50CC/HR QID - - NPO 1-2L/MIN

6/29/82 (9

FIG. 13-9. An example of output from a portable microprocessor (HP-85) computerized notation system. (Ash S, Mertz S, Ulrich D: The computerized notation system: A portable, self-contained system for entry of physicians' and nurses' notes. In Heffernan H [ed]: Proceedings of the Fifth Annual Symposium on Computer Applications in Medical Care. Silver Spring, MD, IEEE Computer Society Press, 1981)

SensorMedics MMC Horizon System. In the spontaneously breathing patient, a new concept in critical care monitoring is the SensorMedics Metabolic Measurement Cart (MMC), which integrates the metabolic and respiratory measurement systems. Through a mobile bedside unit with a built-in microprocessor, the unit combines breath-by-breath monitoring of volume, alveolar ventilation, and flow rates with the continuous assessment of cellular metabolism. It saves information on two floppy disks and graphically plots basic and comparison information on paper plots or graphically on a cathode ray terminal (CRT). This system combines physiologic microprocessing, file documentation, graph and trend capabilities, physiologic equipment regulated with automated recalibration, and automated diagnostics. Approximately 54 patient variables can be entered, calculated, stored, and analyzed with this one piece of equipment. Figure 13-10 shows a copy of a MMC report (Norton, 1983).

Respitrace. A semiquantitative method of evaluating breath-by-breath tidal volume, minute volume, and respiratory rate that noninvasively separates rib cage from abdominal contributions of breathing has been described by many authors. The device can either be electromagnetic or inductive plethysmography. The output may be displayed digitally or on an analog recorder and stored for archival purposes (Ackerman, 1981; Watson, 1979). A computer can be used. The following information is displayed: tidal volume, minute ventilation, rate, inspiratory time, fractional inspiratory time, and mean inspiratory flow. An analysis program can calculate the frequency distributions and plots histograms. Since this system can separate chest from abdominal breathing, nurses can use the output to assess the rate and pattern of ventilation. Figure 13-11 shows an example of Respitrace output.

Blood Gas Analyzers

Other diagnostic or interpretive types of equipment found in critical care environments are blood gas analyzers. They are also available with microprocessor chips that are used to maintain and assist with the calibration of electrodes. As an analyzer system, the microprocessor automatically senses and calculates arterial blood gases, saturation curves, and buffer curves from normal data. These analyzers may also store data and graphically present trend analysis (Corning, 1983).

Microprocessing techniques have been used for almost 10 years in calculations related to blood gas analysis. Recently, the use of a Hewlett-Packard computer in a hospital that decided to automate as much of the processing of calculations and reports as possible was described (Hercz and Coates, 1981). In blood gas testing the computer facilitates the following:

Calculating variables
Entering primary results as they are available
Communicating results quickly to medical personnel
Generating trend analysis results for patients from admission to discharge

This exceeds the usual computer adjuncts to blood gas analysis, since the standard equipment calculates variables and prints a readable report. Blood gas reports must then be fed into a larger system, such as a HIS.

Pulmonary Function Systems

Computer-assisted pulmonary diagnostic systems enhance spirometric testing by increasing test accuracy while decreasing test time. They automate and simplify routine lung mechanics, lung volume, diffusion capacity, and other pulmonary function tests.

REAL-TIME REPORT

Page 1

Name: | Date: Aug 13, 1984
ID Number: | Time: 11:25
Preset Name: Classic#1

Time	VE BTPS	VT	f	VO2 STPD	VCO2 STPD	RER	PETO2	PETCO2	Vd/Vt anat	VO2/KG	CO2VE	O2VE	FEO2	FECO2
min	L/min	L/br	br/min	L/min	L/min		mmHg	mmHg		ml/min /kg	L/L	L/L		
0:17	8.7	0.504	17.2				126.	19.						
0:33	7.9	0.413	19.0	0.142	0.104	0.73	126.	19.	0.15	1.7	75.4	55.3	0.1885	0.0164
0:46	6.6	0.348	18.9	0.124	0.092	0.74	126.	19.	0.05	1.5	71.6	52.9	0.1875	0.0173
1:01	9.4	0.595	15.9	0.180	0.137	0.76				2.2	69.0	52.6	0.1873	0.0179
1:17	10.1	0.672	15.1	0.180	0.142	0.79				2.2	71.6	56.2	0.1886	0.0173
1:33	8.4	0.720	11.7	0.157	0.120	0.76				1.9	70.2	53.5	0.1877	0.0176
1:49	7.2	0.481	15.0	0.142	0.107	0.76				1.7	67.4	50.9	0.1866	0.0184
2:03	7.7	0.628	12.2	0.151	0.116	0.77				1.8	66.4	51.1	0.1866	0.0186
2:17	14.3	0.826	17.3	0.275	0.216	0.79				3.4	66.0	51.8	0.1869	0.0188
2:32	20.4	1.200	17.0											
2:46	16.3	1.000	16.3	0.246	0.224	0.91	129.	18.	0.22	3.0	72.9	66.5	0.1913	0.0170
3:03	9.3	0.515	18.1	0.148	0.115	0.78				1.8	80.9	62.8	0.1908	0.0153
3:17	7.0	0.412	17.0	0.122	0.086	0.71				1.5	81.5	57.5	0.1894	0.0152
3:31	5.9	0.349	17.0	0.106	0.073	0.68				1.3	81.8	55.9	0.1890	0.0152
3:47	7.6	0.333	22.8	0.142	0.096	0.68				1.7	79.0	53.5	0.1881	0.0157
4:02	6.8	0.339	20.1	0.130	0.087	0.67				1.6	78.7	52.7	0.1878	0.0158
+++++	EVENT1 # 1 occurred at 5:12 +++++													
4:19	7.8	0.442	17.8	0.153	0.098	0.64				1.9	80.1	51.1	0.1873	0.0155
4:32	6.6	0.355	18.6	0.139	0.087	0.63				1.7	75.6	47.5	0.1857	0.0164
4:49	5.3	0.306	17.2											
5:01	5.3	0.339	15.7											
5:17	9.5	0.615	15.4											
5:32	23.4	1.550	15.1											
5:46	17.8	1.037	17.1	0.261	0.266	1.02	133.	17.	0.15	3.2	66.9	68.0	0.1913	0.0185
6:04	19.7	1.407	14.0	0.274	0.303	1.11				3.4	65.1	72.0	0.1920	0.0190
6:16	19.3	1.375	14.1	0.250	0.293	1.13				3.2	66.0	74.5	0.1925	0.0187
6:33	22.5	1.500	15.0	0.301	0.342	1.14				3.7	65.8	74.7	0.1926	0.0188
6:45	20.7	1.460	14.2	0.293	0.320	1.09				3.6	64.7	70.5	0.1917	0.0191
7:04	18.8	1.450	13.0	0.274	0.289	1.05				3.4	65.1	68.6	0.1914	0.0190
7:19	19.3	1.573	12.2	0.279	0.297	1.06				3.4	64.7	68.9	0.1914	0.0191
7:33	18.9	1.483	12.8											
7:45	23.4	1.552	14.2											
8:03	18.4	1.366	13.5	0.265	0.273	1.03	133.	16.	0.13	3.2	67.5	69.6	0.1917	0.0183
8:17	16.9	1.297	13.0	0.248	0.248	1.00				3.0	68.1	68.2	0.1914	0.0182
8:33	19.4	0.989	19.6	0.279	0.279	1.00				3.4	69.5	69.4	0.1918	0.0178
8:47	15.0	1.187	12.7	0.224	0.221	0.99				2.7	68.1	67.2	0.1912	0.0182
9:02	19.1	1.552	12.3	0.270	0.275	1.02				3.3	69.5	70.8	0.1920	0.0178
9:15	21.2	1.592	13.3	0.273	0.290	1.06				3.3	73.2	77.8	0.1935	0.0169
9:32	21.7	1.517	14.3	0.283	0.301	1.06				3.5	72.0	76.5	0.1932	0.0172
9:49	21.7	1.491	14.5	0.273	0.288	1.06				3.3	75.2	79.4	0.1938	0.0165
10:01	23.5	1.568	15.0											
10:16	20.0	1.310	15.3											
+++++	EVENT1 # 2 occurred at 10:45 +++++													
10:31	18.5	1.153	16.1	0.264	0.255	0.96	133.	15.	0.13	3.2	73.0	70.4	0.1921	0.0170

FIG. 13-10. A copy of an MMC report (SensorMedics, Metabolic Measurement Cart).

Specifically, a spirometric system quantifies breath-by-breath measurements of lung volume, calibrates a series of data points from the spirometer, and transmits them to the computer memory. The input represents instantaneous flow of gas volumes at each discrete interval of time, after the point recognized as the beginning of a breath or until the end of a breath. The volume input is collected with a

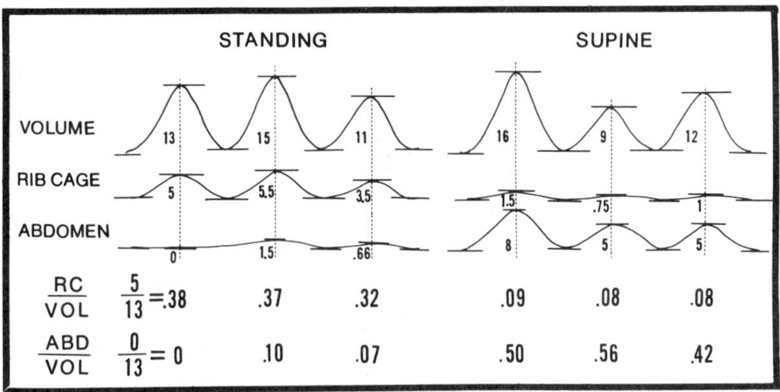

FIG. 13-11. An example of Respitrace output.

recording device and converted to digital measurements. These measurements of the various spirometric indexes are compared with normal values, and the output is generated. Such a system can also be programmed to sequence the test procedures, store all data points during the test, calculate the results, and generate a report numerically, and graphically display volume with time and flow volumes. It can also generate trend tables and graphics. The system depicts the presence and severity of expiratory and inspiratory obstructions that restrict the patients' vital capacity and is used to detect pulmonary diseases. An example of a computerized pulmonary function report is shown in Figure 13-12.

Spirometric systems are availabe as small stand-alone systems using microprocessors with dedicated software or as larger integrated systems using either a minicomputer or a mainframe. Microcomputer and minicomputer systems are usually dedicated systems with preprogrammed software packages like those made by Hewlett-Packard. They are available for all sizes of health care facilities; a Collins Eagle II is available for physicians' offices. This microcomputer system stores and interprets patient information (Collins W. Eagle II, 1984).

Panasonic or Quasar. Nurses can use a hand-held computer made by Panasonic or Quasar to simplify lung function assessment. This equipment analyzes spirometric variables and tests and prints a report that includes the predicted normal values with correction factors applied. The input is BTPS, sex, age, height, race, FVC, and FEVI, FEF 25 – 75%, MVV, and postbronchodilator comparisons. The output data is percentage predicted and categorized by type of obstruction: mild, moderate, or severe according to American Lung Association/American Thoracic Society standards (Enright, 1982).

Intracranial Pressure Monitoring

Neurosurgical nurses may use computer microprocessing in assessing intracranial pressure in patients with head injuries. The use of theoretical models for predicting the control of pressure and volume in the cerebrospinal fluid and intracranial space of head-injured patients has been tested using microprocessing techniques. A minicomputer programmed with a combination of predicted pressure curves simulating intracranial pressure volume increases or decreases has been described. Further applications of this theoretical model with computer applications could allow intracranial pressure to be assessed and therapy introduced earlier in the course of treatment (Marmarou and colleagues, 1981).

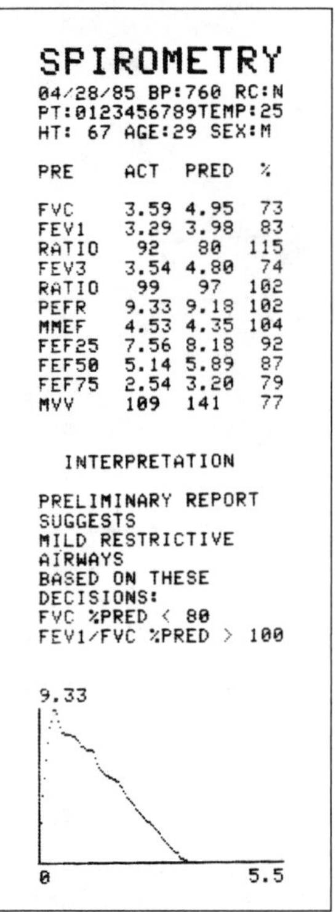

SPIROMETRY

04/28/85 BP:760 RC:N
PT:0123456789TEMP:25
HT: 67 AGE:29 SEX:M

PRE	ACT	PRED	%
FVC	3.59	4.95	73
FEV1	3.29	3.98	83
RATIO	92	80	115
FEV3	3.54	4.80	74
RATIO	99	97	102
PEFR	9.33	9.18	102
MMEF	4.53	4.35	104
FEF25	7.56	8.18	92
FEF50	5.14	5.89	87
FEF75	2.54	3.20	79
MVV	109	141	77

INTERPRETATION

PRELIMINARY REPORT
SUGGESTS
MILD RESTRICTIVE
AIRWAYS
BASED ON THESE
DECISIONS:
FVC %PRED < 80
FEV1/FVC %PRED > 100

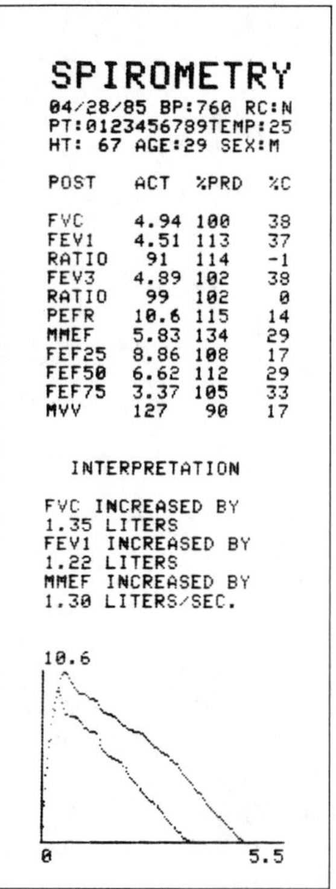

SPIROMETRY

04/28/85 BP:760 RC:N
PT:0123456789TEMP:25
HT: 67 AGE:29 SEX:M

POST	ACT	%PRD	%C
FVC	4.94	100	38
FEV1	4.51	113	37
RATIO	91	114	-1
FEV3	4.89	102	38
RATIO	99	102	0
PEFR	10.6	115	14
MMEF	5.83	134	29
FEF25	8.86	108	17
FEF50	6.62	112	29
FEF75	3.37	105	33
MVV	127	90	17

INTERPRETATION

FVC INCREASED BY
1.35 LITERS
FEV1 INCREASED BY
1.22 LITERS
MMEF INCREASED BY
1.30 LITERS/SEC.

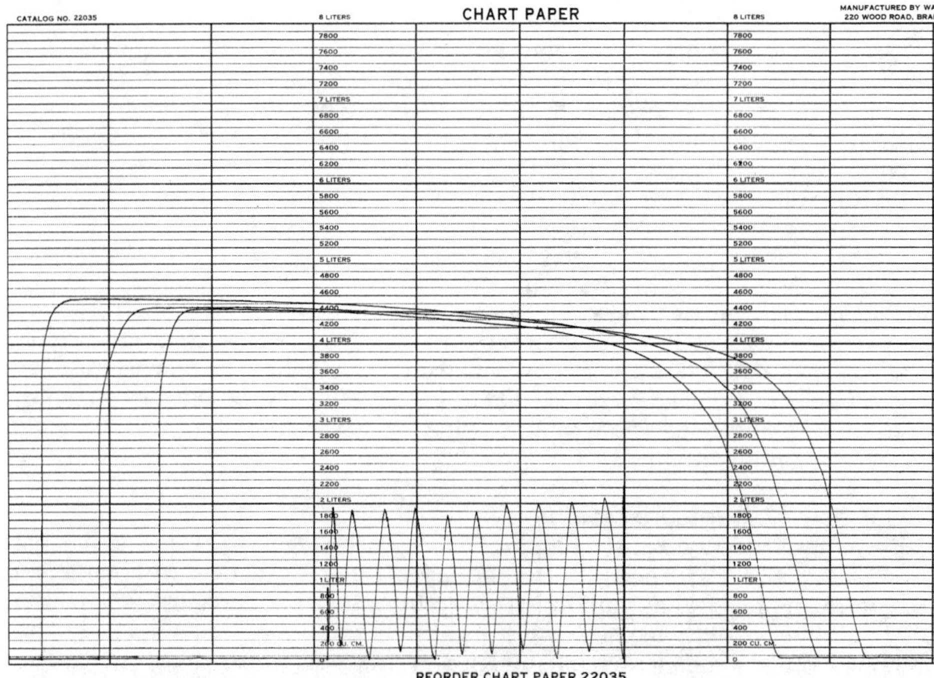

FIG. 13-12. Computerized pulmonary function report (Collins Eagle II: Pulmonary function testing system. Braintree, MA, Collins W. Eagle II, 1984)

Cardiac and Other Diagnostic Systems

Echocardiography, diagnostic radionuclides, and the cardiac catheterization functions are becoming more closely linked to critical care environments. Each of these equipment technologies with diagnostic capabilities uses microprocessing for integrating sensors, analyzing information, and reporting. One such system is described below.

CARDIONET. CARDIONET is a special-purpose system that uses microcomputer hardware to network several areas in a cardiology department, including the cardiac catheterization laboratory, the coronary care unit, and the echocardiography laboratory. Individual modules available include the following:

- Catheterization Laboratory support system
- Pacemaker follow-up system
- Echocardiography support system
- Coronary care unit support system

1. In the Catheterization Laboratory system, blood pressure levels and laboratory results are entered into the system and cardiac output, flow resistances, valvular areas, pressure gradients, congenital shunts, blood gases, and oxygen content and consumption can be calculated. This module also includes a quality control component that tracks equipment problems.
2. The pacemaker follow-up system was designed to provide continuity of care for patients with pacemakers and includes maintenance information on pacemakers.
3. The echocardiography support system analyzes the echocardiograph tracing and calculates the distance between the points selected, projections on the X axis, and projections on the Y axis and compares values obtained as low, normal, or elevated.
4. The coronary care unit support system includes a cardiovascular support module, a respiratory module, and a renal and fluid balance module (Trinity Computing Systems, 1983).

Drug Administration Systems

Infusion Pumps. Implantable infusion pumps are also regulated by microprocessors. The most developed system administers medication and stores information pertaining to equipment operation. The equipment can be programmed to deliver medication on an established, regular basis for a 24-hour period. Up to six different programs, or variations in medication schedules, can be stored. The equipment is currently used experimentally in patients with diabetes; however, these microprocessors are being tested in the laboratory for applications to hormone regulation and hormone delivery for human fertility, treatment of hypertension, cancer, chronic intractable pain, thrombosis, and delivery of growth hormone (Sanders and Radford, 1982).

Pharmacy Systems

Because nursing personnel interact with several types of pharmacy systems, they may be considered a special application for nursing. Three types of pharmacy systems are relevant to nurses:

- Unit dose order entry and supply system
- Drug interaction programs
- Intravenous systems

Unit Dose Order Entry. Whether they stand alone or are apart of larger HISs, pharmacy modules are important for nursing. In one type of system, after the physician orders medication, a pharmacy computer company picks up copies of the hand-written medication order form. Within 24 hours, the standard orders are entered into a computer, the medications are noted, and a unit-dose cart is filled with the medication. A computerized sheet is delivered with the medications for nursing personnel to document whether medications were given. Medications to be given immediately are held in stock supplies on nursing units and charted manually. A sample copy of this type of system is shown in Figure 13-13.

When pharmacy modules are a part of larger HIS, the physician writes medication orders directly at a terminal and the order is received in the pharmacy department. The computer establishes the timeframes for each medication order and dispenses approved orders. Carts are filled with lists, and medication envelopes are prepared for unit-dose dispensing. Medication administration records are made available on line and are printed on a nursing unit at specified times. These records are used by nursing personnel to document medications given. Notification to administer a medication immediately will automatically generate a refill request. All medications about to expire are listed at a nursing unit.

Drug Interaction Programs. Hospital formulary information is available on several HISs. Nurse may access these files to determine the usual purpose of a medication, maximum doses, side-effects, and drug interactions. One problem with the number of drug interaction problems occurring in hospitals is the complexity of drug information available, the lack of time for nursing personnel to look up references, and the difficulty finding needed references. Computerized systems facilitate access to drug interaction information (Hansten, 1983).

The drug interaction capabilities are also available from COMSHARE, an international network. Through a terminal in a hospital, a nurse can communicate with a centralized computer. This computer service provides clinical evaluation of the administration of digitalis, glycosides, procainamide, lidocaine, antibiotics, and six inhalation anesthetics. Individualized pharmacokinetic models are plotted for each patient's response to a drug dose regimen. COMSHARE also has a service for analyzing cardiology information and pulmonary function laboratory data (COMSHARE, 1984).

Intake and Output Systems. In intake systems, computers are linked to infusion pumps that control arterial pressure, drug therapy, fluid resuscitation, anesthesia, and serum glucose levels. They can include just the infusion system and the computer or the infusion system, the computer, and the physiologic monitors.

One of the most useful advantages of these systems for nursing is the use of intravenous drip rate calculation and regulation. The microprocessed infusion systems can calculate the following (Jelliffe and colleagues, 1983):

Intravenous concentrations in milligrams per milliliter or microns per milliliter
Dose rate with body weight index
Intravenous rate
Required medication administration to intravenous preparations
Required intravenous volume for intravenous preparations

Most of these capabilities are available from IVAC. These systems have been integrated with Hewlett-Packard computers and are also available from Hewlett-Packard and IMED alone or in combination. The IMED 929 pump has been interfaced with IBM, HP, DEC, Motorola, and Apple computers (IMED Corporation, 1984).

MONTH JUN YEAR 1985 | 1 2 3 4 5 6 7 8 9 10 11 12 13 14 15 16 17 18 19 20 21 22 23 24 25 26 27 28 29 30 31

INSULIN NPH U-100

10 UNITS SQ EACH MORNING

START DATE RENEW DATE STOP DATE | REFRIGERATE;

NITRODISC 5 MG

APPLY ONE PATCH TO SKIN 2 X DAILY (HOLD ONE DOSE IF DIASTOLIC BP <50)

START DATE RENEW DATE STOP DATE | TRANSDERMAL NITROGLYCERIN; REMOVE PREVIOUS APPLICATION !;

PRAMILET FA

1 TAB BY MOUTH DAILY

START DATE RENEW DATE STOP DATE

PROCARDIA (NIFEDIPINE) 10 MG

1 CAP BY MOUTH EVERY 6 HRS (HOLD ONE DOSE IF DIASTOLIC BP <60)

START DATE RENEW DATE STOP DATE

TENORMIN (ATENOLOL) 50 MG

1/2 TAB (25 MG) BY MOUTH DAILY

START DATE RENEW DATE STOP DATE | CHECK APICAL PULSE RATE & RHYTHM DAILY; CHECK BLOOD PRESSURE WEEKLY;

START DATE RENEW DATE STOP DATE

MONTH JUN YEAR 1985 | 1 2 3 4 5 6 7 8 9 10 11 12 13 14 15 16 17 18 19 20 21 22 23 24 25 26 27 28 29 30 31

DIET:
3GM NA, 2.4GM K, NO PROT. REST, 1000ML/24H FLUID RESTR.

DIAGNOSIS:
DIABETES/S/P CVA/S/P (R) AKA/CRF /

PATIENT | ROOM | I.D. NO. | PHYSICIAN | ALLERGIES NO KNOWN ALLERGY | REVIEWED BY: DATE

FIG. 13-13. Example of a pharmacy system report. (© Copyright, Hessler Enterprises, 1984. Reproduced by permission)

Even urine output has been microprocessed in the intensive care environment with the UROTRACK PLUS system supplied by Vitalmetrics. This system monitors core body temperature from urinary output. The total volume in the container and the urine volume within a given timeframe is stored, recorded, and shown on a digital readout. A continuous internal bladder temperature is recorded (Vitalmetrics, 1984).

Newborn Nursery Systems

In the newborn intensive care setting, computers are routinely used to microprocess information relative to an infants' heart and respiratory rates. In addition, a system regulates the isolette temperature by sensing the infant's temperature and the air of the isolette. Called Alcyon, it was designed in 1971 and described in the literature in 1977. Under normal circumstances the computer automatically controls the temperature of the isolette to maintain a 36 C to 36.5 C environment. Because Alcyon also has been modified to store respiratory and heart rate data, the nurse has graphic data available to interpret changes in neonates' vital signs caused by environmental controls or physiologic function (Endo, 1981).

The nurse's role with this type of equipment in the neonatal intensive care unit has also been described. Equipment must be maintained so that the system can alert nurses by an alarm if a malfunction exists or an abnormal physiologic range is recorded. In addition, information that the computer generates must be interpreted (Endo, 1981).

A microprocessor may be used to measure the stiffness of the lung (compliance) and lung volumes in the premature infant with respiratory distress syndrome. Information on breath-by-breath regulation of lung volume in premature infants can help prevent the development of bronchopulmonary dysplasia and potential ventilator dependence (Dolcourt and Harris, 1982).

COMPUTER APPLICATIONS IN THE EMERGENCY ROOM

Emergency Medical Systems

The basic elements of an emergency medical system are threefold:

Continuous patient monitoring
Communication with interpretive and diagnostic centers
Consultation using immediate access to large databases

By 1977 emergency medical services in many parts of the country were using computers. By 1981 a comprehensive emergency room service system patient-related database (PRDB) used a minicomputer and a microcomputer. The main features of this system were to enter rescue squad reports, patient symptoms, laboratory data, treatment, outcomes, and demographic data. The system interacted with a poison differential diagnosis system; a pharmacokinetic system also was maintained. Output information provided frequency distributions to assess quality control.

Database content was ordered as follows (Anne and colleagues, 1981):

Complaints and history, which lists 50 symptoms, 23 sites, and 15 causes of injuries
Diagnosis in terms of illness (48 categories) or injuries (28 categories)
Status classification in the emergency room (urgent or nonurgent)

Length of stay reports
Linking emergency data with prehospital evaluations from the rescue squad
Concise and complete emergency room records
A database for disaster planning in a small community
Evaluation mechanisms to track persons who use an emergency facility as a primary care facility

The cost of such a service is estimated to be less than $1.50 per patient visit.

Poison Indexes

A poison index is an information system that contains nearly 200,000 listings and differential diagnosis related to acute poisoning from 476 agents. A toxicology pharmacokinetics reference system also offers individualized patient information sheets, pharmacokinetic calculations, and graphic plots (Attinger and colleagues, 1977). These systems are used in many major hospitals throughout the country.

COMPUTER APPLICATIONS IN THE OPERATING ROOM

Operating Room Management Systems

Basic Elements

Microcomputers, minicomputers, and HISs also have practical nursing applications for OR nurses. The basic elements of an operating room management system include managing records for the following:

OR schedules
Nursing personnel schedules
Budgeting supplies used in the OR during procedures
Infection control mapping
Documenting medications
Intake and output
Retrospective chart audit for quality control

Examples

The OR-MS, developed by Perimeter Systems, has subroutines for operating room scheduling, instrument preparation, operating room reports, and status information on equipment and patients before transfer. Inventory control is a projected option (Paquet, 1982).

Computers in ORs may eventually reduce nursing time. One option is the development of the universal bar code for controlling operating room supplies. During procedures, the nurse could use a portable device to record supplies used. This device would be similar to the light coding system used in grocery and department stores (Paquet, 1982).

Surgical Procedure Systems

Computers are being used more frequently for actual surgical procedures. Computers assist in arteriography and angiography and participate in autotransfusion during open heart, vascular, and orthopedic surgery. One computer has functioned to maintain intraocular pressure during eye surgery (Paquet, 1982).

With computer graphics, the computer could be used on line during diagnostic procedures or reconstructive surgery or to prepare graphic simulations or holography during procedures. Each surgical incision would be microprocessed to display the potential result of the surgical procedure (Paquet, 1982).

Computer communications, computer-facilitated surgical procedures, and computer monitoring systems should increase the incidence of 1-day surgery in outpatient clinics. Operating room procedures and personnel requirements may also be reduced as computer use grows (Paquet, 1982).

SUMMARY

The numbers of observations that nursing is accountable for in the ICU, ER, and OR have necessitated the development of computer adjuncts to nursing care. This chapter has described the seven major capabilities of computers in these highly technological areas. Three specific types of computer applications were described: the arrhythmia monitoring system, physiologic monitors, and special-purpose systems. These three types of applications may be used in the ICU, ER, or OR. The basic elements of arrhythmia monitoring systems and physiologic monitors were also described. Common to both systems are sensors, signal conditioners, the computer as a processor, and display elements. Arrhythmia systems were categorized as detection or surveillance and diagnostic or interpretive systems; they are usually dedicated systems. Physiologic monitoring systems, which include these types and treatment intervention systems, have expanded to integrate patient data management systems. Physiologic monitoring systems tend to be distributed and modular or integrated. Examples of these designs were provided.

Seven special-purpose systems were described. Because nurses work in new specialty areas such as echocardiography and cardiac stress test laboratories, some computer systems in these areas were also described. Pharmacy systems were categorized, and the basic elements of computer applications in the ER and OR were included. Examples of ER computers and computer applications for OR management and surgical procedures were presented.

Computers have been present in these high-technology areas since arrhythmia monitors were introduced. The use of computers in intensive care areas is predicted to expand more rapidly than in any other area of nursing practice. The "burnout" problem in ICUs, ERs, and ORs may be a result of technology being introduced so rapidly into these areas. Five years after nurses are graduated from nursing school, 50% of the skills they have learned about specialty equipment are obsolete. This chapter should provide students with the basic elements of many technologies; the principles will not change during the next decade. The new equipment introduced will merely include an application of what already exists.

ISSUES

1. Patients in the ICU, ER, and OR are in critical condition. Most computer systems used by nurses in these areas include physiologic variables and nursing process documentation but have not been thoroughly exploited by nursing for other uses.
2. Graphic reports could provide information for nursing personnel to evaluate patients' conditions and nursing actions.
3. The use of computers for physiologic monitoring and special-purpose systems has extensive implications for nursing, yet less has been written in the nursing literature about these systems than in the biomedical literature.

4. If nurses want to expand nursing applications of these systems, all nurses will need a beginning level of understanding of the system capabilities, types of basic elements, applications, and projected use.
5. Patients who rely on these computerized devices, equipment, and procedures require unique nursing care.
6. In the future, nursing must be more responsive to these types of computers by predicting the types of nursing care that patients will require, by using the equipment to its fullest, and by expanding the use of these technologies to improve quality of nursing care in critical care environments.
7. Do critical care nurses feel like they are nurse machines?
8. Can increased knowledge about these machines help nurses to provide quality care for patients needing these technologies?

STUDY QUESTIONS

1. What are the seven major capabilities of computers in the ICU, ER, and OR?
2. What are the three types of computer applications in the ICU?
3. Name the basic elements of an arrhythmia monitor.
4. Identify the types of arrhythmia system.
5. Name a vendor of an arrhythmia monitoring system.
6. List the five basic parts of physiologic monitoring systems.
7. What are the three basic types of physiologic monitoring systems?
8. Name a distributed physiologic monitoring system.
9. Describe two modular systems that extend the concept of distributed systems.
10. Define an integrated physiologic monitoring system.
11. Name the seven special-purpose systems that nurses may use in hospital practice today.
12. What are the basic elements of an emergency medical system?
13. What are the basic elements of an OR management system?
14. What surgical procedure may be facilitated by computers?

REFERENCES

Ackerman M: Non-invasive continuous monitoring of pulmonary performance. In Heffernan H (ed): Proceedings of the Fifth Annual Symposium of Computer Applications in Medical Care, pp 433–434. Silver Spring, MD, IEEE Computer Society Press, 1981

Anne A, Spyker D, Edlich R, Attinger E: A comprehensive information system for emergency medical services. In Heffernan H (ed): Proceedings of the Fifth Annual Symposium on Computer Applications in Medical Care, pp 979–983. Silver Spring, MD, IEEE Computer Society Press, 1981

Ash S, Mertz S, Ulrich D: The computerized notation system: A portable, self-contained system for entry of physicians' and nurses' notes. In Heffernan H (ed): Proceedings of the Fifth Annual Symposium on Computer Applications in Medical Care, pp 129–135. Silver Spring, MD, IEEE Computer Society Press, 1981

Attinger E, Anne A, Edlich R: Preliminary results with a computerized information system for emergency medical services. Proceedings of the First Annual Symposium on Computer Applications in Medical Care, pp 190–199. Silver Spring, MD, IEEE Computer Society Press, 1977

Badura F: Nurse acceptance of a computerized arrhythmia monitoring system. Heart Lung 9:1046, 1980

Beckmann E, Cammack B, Harris B: Observation on computers in an intensive care unit. Heart Lung 10:1055–1057, 1981

Brozino J: Computer Applications for Patient Care. Reading, MA, Addison-Wesley, 1982

The Burdick Corporation: Burdick Color Trend. Milton, WI, The Burdick Corp, 1983
Cengiz M, Ranzenberger J, Johnson D, et al: Design and implementation of computerized nursing care plans. In Dayhoff R (ed): Proceedings of the Seventh Annual Symposium on Computer Applications in Medical Care, pp 561–564. Silver Spring, MD, IEEE Computer Society Press, 1983
Collins W. Eagle II: Pulmonary function testing system. Braintree, MA, Collins W. Eagle II, 1984
COMSHARE: The USC Pack. Los Angeles and Ann Arbor, MI, COMSHARE, 1984
Corning Medical: An untitled marketing handout. Medfield, MA, Corning Medical, 1983
Dolcourt J, Harris T: Pulmonary function in critically-ill newborn infants: Measurement by microprocessor. In Blum B (ed): Proceedings of the Sixth Annual Symposium on Computer Applications in Medical Care, pp 686–689. Silver Spring, MD, IEEE Computer Society Press, 1982
Endo A: Using computers in newborn intensive care settings. Am J Nurs 81:1336–1337, 1981
Enright P: A hand held computer simplifies lung testing. In Blum B (ed): Proceedings of the Sixth Annual Symposium on Computer Applications in Medical Care, p 649. Silver Spring, MD, IEEE Computer Society Press, 1982
Hansten P: Utilization of drug information in pharmacy systems. In Fokkens, O et al (eds): Medinfo 83 Seminars, pp 123–125. Amsterdam, North-Holland, 1983
Hercz L, Coates A: Blood gas system for result acquisition, calculation and reporting in the Montreal children's hospital. In Heffernan H (ed): Proceedings of the Fifth Annual Symposium on Computer Applications in Medical Care, pp 435–439. Silver Spring, MD, IEEE Computer Society Press, 1981
IMED Corporation: An untitled marketing handout. San Diego, IMED Corp, 1984
Jelliffe R, Shumitzky A, D'Argenio D, et al: Improved 2-compartment time-shared programs for adaptive control of digitoxin and digoxin therapy. In Dayhoff R (ed): Proceedings of the Seventh Annual Symposium on Computer Applications in Medical Care, pp 231–234. Silver Spring, MD, IEEE Computer Society Press, 1983
Johnson D, Ranzenberger J, Herbert R, et al: A computerized alert program for acutely ill patients. J Nurs Admin 10:26–35, 1980
Marmarou A, Shapiro K, Kosteljanetz M, Pasternack D: A microprocessor based analysis of raised intracranial pressure in head injured patients. In Heffernan H (ed): Proceedings of the Fifth Annual Symposium on Computer Applications in Medical Care, pp 644–646. Silver Spring, MD, IEEE Computer Society Press, 1982
McCarthy M, Townsend M, Thorp J: Computer assistance to record problem-oriented notes for intensive care nursery patients. In Blum B (ed): Proceedings of the Sixth Annual Symposium on Computer Applications in Medical Care, p 675. Silver Spring, MD, IEEE Computer Society Press, 1982
McCormick K: An animal model for the adult respiratory distress syndrome: Pathophysiologic mechanism. Doctoral dissertation, University of Wisconsin–Madison, WI, 1978
Milholland DK, Cardona V: Computers at the bedside. Am J Nurs 83:1304–1307, 1983
Milholland DK: Clinical staff satisfaction with a computerized critical-care database system. In Dayhoff R (ed): Proceedings of the Seventh Annual Symposium on Computer Applications in Medical Care, pp 516–518. Silver Spring, MD, IEEE Computer Society Press, 1983
Norton A: Development and testing of a microprocessor-controlled system for measurement of gas exchange and related variables in man during rest and exercise. Anaheim, CA, SensorMedics, Beckman reprint no. 025, 1983
Paquet J: OR computers: The future is today. Today's OR Nurse 4:10–15, 1982
Phone-A-Gram-System, Inc: An untitled marketing handout. San Francisco, Phone-A-Gram-System, 1983
Sanders K, Radford W: The computer in a programmable implantable medication system (PIMS). In Blum B (ed): Proceedings of the Sixth Annual Symposium on Computer Applications in Medical Care, pp 682–685. Silver Spring, MD, IEEE Computer Society Press, 1982
Shinozaki T, Deane R, Mazuzan J: A devoted mini-computer system for the management of

clinical and laboratory data in an intensive care unit. In Blum B (ed): Proceedings of the Sixth Annual Symposium on Computer Applications in Medical Care, pp 267–269. Silver Spring, MD, IEEE Computer Society Press, 1982

Sorkin J, Bloomfield D: Computers of critical care. Heart Lung. 11:287–293, 1982

TELEMED: An untitled marketing handout. Chicago, TELEMED, 1983

TRIMIS Fact Sheet. Bethesda, MD, Computer Assisted Practice of Cardiology (CAPOC), 1983

Trinity Computing Systems: CARDIONET: The Intensive Care Support System. Houston, Trinity Computing Systems, 1983

Vitalmetrics, Inc.: An untitled marketing handout. San Diego, Vitalmetrics, 1984

Watson H: The technology of respiratory inductive plethysmography. In Third International Symposium on Ambulatory Monitoring. Clinical Research Center. Harrow, Middlesex, United Kingdom, 1979

BIBLIOGRAPHY

Brown A: Computer management of operating room time information with proposed standard definitions for the measurement of utilization. In Blum B (ed): Proceedings of the Sixth Annual Symposium on Computer Applications in Medical Care, pp 246–250. Silver Spring, MD, IEEE Computer Society Press, 1982

Dawson A, Mohler J: Microprocessor-assisted spirometry. In Clausen J, Zarins L (eds): Pulmonary Function Testing Guidelines and Controversies. New York, Academic Press, 1982

Duraiswamy N, Welton R, Reisman A: Using computer simulation to predict ICU staffing needs. J Nurs Admin 11:39–44, 1981

EPIC Systems Corporation: Madison, WI, 1983

Gardner R, Crapo R, Morris AL, Beus M: Computerized decision-making in the pulmonary function laboratory. Resp Care. 27:799–808, 1982

Hanson K: Four years of computer assisted operating room scheduling. In Blum B (ed): Proceedings of the Sixth Annual Symposium on Computer Applications in Medical Care, p 252. Silver Spring, MD, IEEE Computer Society Press, 1982

Hewlett-Packard: Waltham, MA, 1983

Joshi M: The computer in coronary care. Nurs Times 78:358–360, 1982

Kane F: Operating room status monitoring system. In Blum B (ed): Proceedings of the Sixth Annual Symposium on Computer Applications in Medical Care, pp 244–245. Silver Spring, MD, IEEE Computer Society Press, 1982

Kiely M: Utilization of computers in the management of critically ill patients. Focus 9:4–5, 1983

Litton Medical Electronics: Dallas, 1984

McAuto Health Service, McDonnell Douglas Automation Company: Hazelwood, MO, 1983

McColligan E: Operating room scheduling and utilization. In Blum B (ed): Proceedings of the Sixth Annual Symposium on Computer Applications in Medical Care, p 243. Silver Spring, MD, IEEE Computer Society Press, 1982

McCormick K: Nursing in the computer revolution. Comp Nursing 4:30, 1984

Mertz S, Ash S, Farrell J: The CNS in the ICU: A bedside notation system for nurses. In Blum B (ed): Proceedings of the Sixth Annual Symposium on Computer Applications in Medical Care, pp 577–582. Silver Spring, MD, IEEE Computer Society Press, 1982

Miller J, Preston T, Dann P, et al: Charting via computers in a post-operative cardio-thoracic ICU. Nurs Times 74:1423–1425, 1978

Muirhead R: Nursing evaluation of monitoring methods in CCU. Superv Nurse 11:13, 1980

Respitrace. Ardsley, NY, Ambulatory Monitoring, 1983

Quantitative Medicine, Inc.: Quantitative Sentinel. Abingdon, MD, Quantitative Medicine, 1984

SensorMedics (formerly Beckman), MMC Horizon Systems: Systemetrics. Physiology Measurements Operations. Anaheim, CA, 1983

Siegel J, Cerra F, Moody E: The effects on survival of critically ill and injured patients of an ICU teaching service organized about a computer-based physiologic care system. J Trauma 209:558–579, 1982

14 Research Applications

Objectives

- Describe two major research applications in nursing.
- Describe computer capabilities to assist nursing research from document retrieval to manuscript preparation.
- Understand statistical packages relevant to nursing available on mainframes, minicomputers, and microcomputers.
- Describe the use of computers for data related to nursing practice.
- Discuss the issues confronting nursing related to the use of computers for nursing research.

Two main applications of computers in nursing research exist:

- Computers in the nursing research process
- Computers in clinical nursing research

For many years, computers have supported the entire research process. Computer applications have included ways to facilitate research. More recently, because of the advancement and implementation of computerized information systems in health care facilities and the introduction of microcomputers to collect patient care data, computers have increasingly been used to provide data needed for clinical nursing research.

COMPUTERS IN THE NURSING RESEARCH PROCESS

The six major uses of computers in the nursing research process are as follows:

- Information retrieval
- Data processing
- Statistical analysis
- Graphic displays
- Database management systems
- Text editing

Most significant is the retrieval of information, since the amount of information is so extensive that computerized document retrieval systems can facilitate a literature search for an essay, a thesis, or a research project. Data processing allows the user to enter, store, and process large amounts of information. Computer software packages for statistical analysis are available, as are graphic displays of that data to make slides for presentations or graphs and charts for publication. Database management systems are used to manage the data that is collected, analyzed, and represented. Text editing is the final step; text editing software packages make information dissemination easier.

These uses of computers in the nursing research process are discussed in detail below.

Information Retrieval Systems

A great advantage of computers in nursing research is their use in searching the literature. Between 6000 and 7000 scientific papers are written each day, and knowledge is expected to double every 20 months in the 1990s. Therefore, 5 years after a person is graduated from college, about 50% of the knowledge he or she has acquired will be obsolete (Naisbitt, 1982). This massive information database must rely on computers for literature organization and retrieval. The amount of knowledge a nurse needs exceeds the time available to read and synthesize the literature. The computer can synthesize and search specific literature. Nursing now needs information specialists who can search the literature by computers.

Several computerized document retrieval systems that yield bibliographic references are available:

- MEDLARS
- MEDLINE
- Excerpta Medica
- Special List Nursing/INI
- ERIC
- SOCIAL SCISEARCH

MEDLARS

Searches for the research literature have been carried out in the United States since the early 1960s in the United States Public Health Service, National Library of Medicine's (NLM) MEDLARS (Medical Literature Analysis and Retrieval Systems) (see Chap. 1).

There are 20 MEDLAR system databases on line (Table 14-1). Individual categories of MEDLAR databases should be searched when the subject of a proposed nursing study is within a specialty category. For example, if a proposed study involves informed consent or related bioethics issues, the BIOETHICSLINE should be searched.

The 20 MEDLAR on-line databases are described below (National Library of Medicine Fact Sheet, 1983):

1. AVLINE (audiovisuals online) is a catalog of audiovisual teaching materials.
2. BIOETHICSLINE references law, religion, and philosophy.
3. CANCEREXPRESS contains bibliographic records identifying articles covering aspects of the therapy, etiology, and biology of cancer as well as studies of mutagenic agents that stimulate cell division.
4. CANCERLIT (cancer literature) is an index of journals.
5. CANCERPROJ (cancer research projects) is a summary of ongoing cancer research projects.
6. CATLINE (catalog on line) includes references to books and serials in the NLM.
7. CHEMLINE (chemical dictionary) is a chemical dictionary.
8. CLINPROT (clinical cancer protocols) describes all cancer research.
9. DIRLINE (directory of information resources on line) is an experimental file that includes the National Referral Center (NRC) database developed and maintained by the Library of Congress.
10. HEALTH PLANNING AND ADMIN contains references and abstracts from nursing literature related to health planning, organizing, financing, management, personnel, and related subjects of medical and hospital literature.
11. HISTLINE (history of medicine on line) provides historical facts.

TABLE 14-1 *Available MEDLARS*

1. AVLINE	12. MESHVOCABULARY
2. BIOETHICSLINE	13. NAME AUTHORITY
3. CANCEREXPRESS	14. PDQ
4. CANCERLIT	15. PDQ/DIRECTORY
5. CATLINE	16. POPLINE
6. CHEMLINE	17. RTECS
7. CLINPORT	18. SERLINE
8. DIRLINE	19. TDB
9. HEALTH PLANNING AND ADMIN	20. TOXLINE
10. HISTLINE	
11. MEDLINE	
MED 77	
MED 75	
MED 71	
MED 66	
SDILINE	

12. MEDLINE (Medical Literature Analysis and Retrieval System On Line) contains approximately 6 million references to biomedical journal articles.
13. MESHVOCABULARY contains information on 14,000 medical subject headings and 28,000 chemical substances used for indexing and retrieving references.
14. NAME AUTHORITY lists 130,000 personal and corporate names and decisions on how monographs series are classified.
15. PDQ (protocol data query) lists 700 research protocols active with the National Cancer Institute, institutions, and contact persons.
16. POPLINE (population information on line) contains population indexes and research.
17. RTECS (registry of toxic effects of chemical substance) contains basic acute and chronic toxicity data for 57,000 toxic chemicals.
18. SERLINE (serials on line) gives bibliographic information on journals and other serials catalogued or on order for the NLM collections.
19. TDB is a toxicology data bank.
20. TOXLINE (toxicology information on line) contains data on 2000 chemical, pharmacologic, and toxicologic facts and references, adverse drug reactions, human and animal toxicity studies, environmental chemicals, pollutants, and other pharmacologic and toxicologic subjects.

Besides being available from the NLM, MEDLARS is also available internationally (Table 14-2). The NLM enters into an international MEDLARS bilateral agreement with a non–United States institution designated to serve as a national biomedical information resource center. The international centers may access MEDLARS through tapes, software, or directly from on-line access to NLM computers. Access to TOXLINE and CHEMLINE requires an additional fee, since these are proprietary information files from organizations external to the NLM.

MEDLINE

MEDLINE (Medical Literature Analysis and Retrieval System On Line) is probably the largest document retrieval system in the world. In 1983 it contained approximately 6 million references to biomedical journal articles and books (NLM Fact

TABLE 14-2 *International MEDLARS Centers*

COUNTRY	ORGANIZATION
Australia	The National Library of Australia
Canada	Canada Institute for Scientific and Technical Information National Research Council of Canada
Colombia	Fundacion OFA and Fondo Colombiano de Investigaciones Científicas (Colciencias)
France	Institut National de la Santé et de la Recherche Medicale (INSERM) Ministère de la Santé Publique et de la Sécurité Sociale
Italy	Instituto superiore di Sanita Ministero della Sanita
Japan	Japan Information Center of Science and Technology (JICST) Science and Technology Agency
Mexico	Centro Nacional de Información y Documentación en Salud Ministerio de Salud
South Africa	Institute for Medical Literature South African Medical Research Council
Sweden	Karolinska Institut
Switzerland	Schweizerische Akademie der Medizinischen Wissenschaften
United Kingdom	The British Library
West Germany	Deutsches Institut für Medizinische Dokumentation und Information (DIMDI) Der Bundesminister für Jugend, Familie und Gesundheit
Intergovernmental Health Organization	Biblioteca Regional de Medicina (BIREME) Pan American Health Organization

Sheet, 1983). It is used to produce three major health indexes: *Index Medicus,* the *International Nursing Index* (INI), and the *Index to Dental Literature* (Lancaster, 1978). It also contains references to 23 of the most widely used nursing journals (International Nursing Index, 1983).

MEDLINE computer searches are available for a fee from most libraries that have approved access to the MEDLINE databases. A MEDLINE search usually requires a search strategy in accordance with the requestor's interest. A search request for literature on a particular topic is matched against the file of citations. The match to retrieve a reference is usually done on terms that describe the contents of an article. Search results consist of a list of references from each file that has been searched. Files usually contain all references for a 2- or 3-year period.

The indexing terminology (thesaurus) of the journal literature is selected from a controlled list of terms of medical subject headings (MeSH) description of contents (Principles of MEDLARS, 1970). The MEDLINE database uses MeSH, which is a controlled vocabulary; it contains approximately 14,000 subject headings classified by both major broad subject categories and subcategories. It contains cross-references to other headings, using related terms arranged in hierarchies (Strauch and Brundage, 1980). It also contains a separate listing for the nursing literature.

Special List Nursing/INI

MEDLINE also contains the special list nursing file, which produces the *INI* and can be specially searched. The *INI* is published in cooperation with the American Journal of Nursing Company and the NLM.

The *INI* cites references to approximately 200 nursing journals throughout the world. Approximately half of these journals are sponsored by national and state nurses' associations; foreign countries account for the other half. Also included in the *INI* are approximately 3000 non-nursing journals that contain nursing articles.

The *INI* lists the indexed journals, a thesaurus of the subject categories, an alphabetical listing of articles and authors, a list of corporate authors or organizational names of reports, documents, and a list by country of nursing journals published during the year. The *INI* indexes all published articles according to its own nursing thesaurus, a classification method developed particularly for this system. Most articles are indexed under three or more subject categories and therefore can be found in several sections of the subject index. In addition, references are identified by the original language of the document. The nursing thesaurus has approximately 750 subject categories as well as numerous subheadings that provide a breakdown of the major categories (International Nursing Index, 1975, 1976, 1977). The MeSH contain broad nursing subject headings, which are not the same as those found in the *INI* nursing thesaurus, the latter being specific for nursing. Each indexed article in MEDLINE has its full bibliographic description, as well as 10 to 20 keywords that describe the contents of the articles. All descriptors used to index an article are searchable in MEDLINE.

Excerpta Medica

Another internationally known database system is Excerpta Medica, which includes articles referenced from 43 abstract journals and two drug-related literature indexes. Although this service does not include nursing, it does include several sections important to nursing research (Table 14-3). For example, a section on health economics and hospital management and one on arthritis and rheumatism are contained in this system (Excerpta Medica, 1983).

Cumulative Index To Nursing Literature

Also important to nursing is the Cumulative Index to Nursing and Allied Health Literature (CINAHL), which duplicates information available in the *INI*. This index, covering over 260 journals and popular-type magazine articles, includes 100 or so journals not listed in the on-line MEDLINE nursing search; it therefore should be used for extensive nursing literature searches. CINAHL is now on line to its subscribers.

Other Databases Relevant To Nursing

Additional computerized document retrieval systems are relevant to nursing, two of which are ERIC (Educational Resources Information Center) and SOCIAL SCISEARCH (Social Science Search), produced by the Institute for Scientific Information from the Social Sciences Citation Index (SSCI).

ERIC. The ERIC database, developed by the National Institute of Education, Educational Resources Information Center, contains references to journal articles on education in general, including nursing education. ERIC was developed because of the "literature explosion" in the field of education that evolved after Sputnik in 1957. Following the passage of the Elementary and Secondary Education Act of 1965, ERIC was designed to contain literature on the educationally disadvantaged. Later it was mandated to provide comprehensive coverage of the educational materials from the Education Resources Information Center (Mathies and Watson, 1973). The ERIC database is composed of two files: resources in education, which contains research reports and other such documents, and the periodical literature catalogued in the current index to journals in education. The index contains references to approximately 700 journal publications with an educational focus for every aspect and segment of the educational profession.

The vocabulary, or indexing language, of ERIC is a controlled vocabulary of educational terms. It uses a subject focus thesaurus, or dictionary of ERIC descriptors, which contains a core of terms for indexing ERIC documents. Acquired documents are processed for input systematically. Each document must meet standard requirements and is catalogued, analyzed, indexed through use of the thesaurus, and finally abstracted with a 20- to 50-word summary or descriptive annotation. Each ERIC bibliographic reference that is retrieved from searches contains the complete bibliographic citation, descriptors from the thesaurus of ERIC descriptors, and the annotation (Mathies, and Watson, 1973). The ERIC database can best be searched by using its dictionary. Since it is an on-line interactive system, searches can be conducted at a computer terminal. Users can obtain access to ERIC through several commercial vendors that conduct searches of document retrieval systems.

SOCIAL SCISEARCH. SOCIAL SCISEARCH, a database prepared by the Institute for Scientific Information from the Social Sciences Citation Index (SSCI), was established by Eugene Garfield in 1963. The first edition was published in 1963 (Weinstock, 1971). SOCIAL SCISEARCH is a unique system because the indexed journals are selected to provide wide coverage of the social sciences. Cited references are indexed to allow access to newly published articles through subject comparisons established by an author's reference to earlier publications (DIALOG, 1977).

Although its main focus is on social science, SOCIAL SCISEARCH accounts for a large percentage of relevant articles for many scientific fields. By taking a selected few journals and indexing them by computer, SOCIAL SCISEARCH offers a representation of the literature. Moreover, by achieving multidisciplinary searching capability, the SOCIAL SCISEARCH takes into account the linkages between documents that the authors themselves found. In principle, citation indexing can serve as a tool to evaluate scientific literature. By using citation analysis and networks, scientific topics can be analyzed, traced historically, and used as a predictor for scientific topics (Weinstock, 1971). The SOCIAL SCISEARCH is a multidisciplinary database that indexes all significant items from approximately 1400 social science journals throughout the world, including nursing, and selectively indexes items from 2400 other journals in the natural, physical, and biomedical fields.

The SOCIAL SCISEARCH index contains all natural language words of subject importance that are meaningful and found in the title of the cited article. The information retrieval techniques are unique in this system because the citations are also indexed. It processes articles not only by the traditional title words, author, and corporate source but can also be searched through authors' cited references.

The SOCIAL SCISEARCH computer-readable bibliographic database is used to

TABLE 14-3 *Excerpta Medica Abstract Journals*

Adverse Reaction Titles
(1 volume in 12 issues)

Anatomy, Anthropology, Embryology and Histology
(1 volume in 10 issues)

Anesthesiology
(1 volume in 10 issues)

Arthritis and Rheumatism
(1 volume in 10 issues)

Biophysics, Bio-engineering and Medical Instrumentation
(1 volume in 10 issues)

Cancer
(4 volumes in 32 issues)

Cardiovascular Disease and Cardiovascular Surgery
(3 volumes in 30 issues)

Chest Diseases, Thoracic Surgery and Tuberculosis
(2 volumes in 20 issues)

Clinical Biochemistry
(4 volumes in 32 issues)

Dermatology and Venereology
(1 volume in 10 issues)

Developmental Biology and Teratology
(1 volume in 8 issues)

Drug Dependence
(1 volume in 6 issues)

Drug Literature Index
(1 volume in 24 issues)

Endocrinology
(3 volumes in 30 issues)

Environmental Health and Pollution Control
(1 volume in 10 issues)

Epilepsy
(1 volume in 6 issues)

Forensic Science
(1 volume in 6 issues)

Gastroenterology
(2 volumes in 20 issues)

General Pathology and Pathological Anatomy
(2 volumes in 20 issues)

Gerontology and Geriatrics
(1 volume in 10 issues)

Health Economics and Hospital Management
(1 volume in 8 issues)

Hematology
(2 volumes in 20 issues)

Human Genetics
(3 volumes in 30 issues)

Immunology, Serology and Transplantation
(3 volumes in 30 issues)

Internal Medicine
(3 volumes in 30 issues)

Mycobacterial Diseases: Leprosy, Tuberculosis and Related Subjects
(1 volume in 10 issues)

Microbiology: Bacteriology, Mycology and Parasitology
(3 volumes in 30 issues)

Neurology and Neurosurgery
(4 volumes in 32 issues)

Nuclear Medicine
(2 volumes in 20 issues)

Obstetrics and Gynecology
(2 volumes in 20 issues)

Occupational Health and Industrial Medicine
(1 volume in 10 issues)

Ophthalmology
(1 volume in 10 issues)

Orthopedic Surgery
(1 volume in 10 issues)

Otorhinolaryngology
(1 volume in 10 issues)

Pediatrics and Pediatric Surgery
(2 volumes in 20 issues)

Pharmacology
(2 volumes in 20 issues)

TABLE 14-3 *(Continued)*

Physiology (4 volumes in 32 issues)	**Rehabilitation and Physical Medicine** (1 volume in 10 issues)
Plastic Surgery (1 volume in 6 issues)	**Surgery** (2 volumes in 20 issues)
Psychiatry (2 volumes in 20 issues)	**Toxicology** (2 volumes in 20 issues)
Public Health, Social Medicine and Hygiene (2 volumes in 20 issues)	**Urology and Nephrology** (2 volumes in 20 issues)
Radiology (2 volumes in 20 issues)	**Virology** (1 volume in 10 issues)

access the citation in the computerized database. It is a good source of references to journal articles and monographs in every area of the social and behavioral sciences. It differs from other computerized databases in that it offers two different means of searching the database: source searching of references to journal literature and citation searching. Source searching is the traditional method of accessing document retrieval systems; it provides for searches by using words in the title (DIALOG, 1977). The SOCIAL SCISEARCH database is usually retrievable through commercial vendors that search on-line services of document retrieval systems.

• • •

The characteristics of the four principal information retrieval systems of significance to nursing are listed in Table 14-4.

Vendors of Bibliographic Searches

The major vendors of bibliographic searches are listed in Table 14-5. DIALOG is an extensive on-line commercial information service. Research institutions, academic centers, libraries, and other large organizations may subscribe to DIALOG for searches of several databases. Besides MEDLINE, Excerpta Medica, and ERIC, DIALOG also contains access to the FEDERAL INDEX, NEWSEARCH, and National Technical Information Service (NTIS). The FEDERAL INDEX includes federal actions usually found in the *Congressional Record* and the *Federal Register;* NEWSEARCH is an index of newspaper resources; NTIS is the government-sponsored clearinghouse of technical information. The DIALOG information retrieval service offers more than 100 databases containing over 40 million records that provide references to technical reports, conference papers, newspapers, journal and magazine articles, patents, and statistical data. The system enables the user to search title and abstract works, names of authors or corporations, dates, codes, patent numbers, and other specified portions of the machine-readable record.

Systems Development Corporation (ORBIT) offers access to approximately 80 files in health sciences, science and technology, scientific research, public affairs, business, and social sciences. Users are able to retrieve citations to technical reports, magazine and journal articles, patents, monographs, and government documents.

TABLE 14-4 *Characteristics of Four Information Retrieval Databases by Coverage, Vocabulary, and Search Result*

INFORMATION RETRIEVAL SYSTEM	SYSTEM COVERAGE	VOCABULARY	SEARCH RESULT
	TYPE OF DOCUMENT	*INDEXING METHOD*	*TYPE OF REFERENCE*
ERIC	Education research reports and 700 journals from *Current Index to Journals of Education*	Controlled with a dictionary	Citation with 20- to 50-word annotated abstract and several descriptors
Special List Nursing/INI	Approximately 200 nursing journals produced by MEDLINE for the *INI*	Controlled with a thesaurus by subject	Citation by journal source
MEDLINE	Approximately 3000 biomedical journals published in *Index Medicus*	Controlled with a dictionary of medical subject	Citation by journal source and descriptors
SOCIAL SCISEARCH	Approximately 1400 science journals and 2400 journals in natural, physical, and biomedical fields from *Social Sciences Citation Index*	Uncontrolled with free text words from title	Citation by title

TABLE 14-5 *Major Vendors of Bibliographic Searchers*

Bibliographic Retrieval Services (BRS)
1200 Route 7
Latham, NY 12110

DIALOG
3460 Hillview Ave.
Palo Alto, CA 94304

Systems Development Corporation (ORBIT)
2500 Colorado Ave.
Santa Monica, CA 90406

The National Library of Medicine (MEDLARS)
8600 Rockville Pike
Bethesda, MD 20205

Computerized Data Processing

The information explosion has led to nursing research endeavors that previously would have produced too much data and extremely cumbersome processing. However, with the computer as the central processor of information, millions of research items can be processed for an individual study. More than ever before, though, computerized data input, storage, and retrieval require that the method for data collection and analysis be described with the study design.

The way the data are stored determines how data can be retrieved for statistical analysis. In the past, nurses were taught that in large studies, where the number of variables are large, computer assistance could provide easier manipulation of data for complex mathematical computations (Abdellah and Levine, 1979).

File Components

The main steps in preparing raw data for a computer system are as follows (Abdellah and Levine, 1979):

Edit the raw data
Code, score, and scale the data
Communicate the data
Input the data

Chapter 4 describes the characteristics of FILES.

If the computer is used to analyze data for nursing research, most programs for statistical analysis require that data be stored in a particular file. Creating a file includes inputting the data into the computer.

Since a computer software package may be needed to prepare a data file for computer retrieval and statistical analysis, it is important to know the basic components of a research file (Table 14-6):

1. The problem, title, or label, which defines the output
2. The input paragraph or headnote, which describes the format, where the data are located, and whether the data are in additional files
3. The variable paragraph or stub, which identifies the names of variables
4. The group, box, or head category paragraph, which stratifies and classifies data into groups or categories

TABLE 14-6 *Basic Components of a Research File*

1. Title
2. Input paragraph/headnote
3. Variable paragraph
4. Group/box/head
5. Lines/block
6. Columns/rows
7. Cells
8. Body
9. Footnotes/legends/key
10. Source

5. Lines or blocking factors, which show the data
6. Columns, which show the data
7. Cells, which intersect categories
8. Body, which aggregates all cells
9. Footnotes, which provide reference data to the table or legends
10. Source, which describes where the data came from

A program can specify how the data file can be stored for maximum analysis.

Transformational programs now exist to change existing files stored in one program into readable files for another program. File creation programs have capabilities similar to word processors and thus can create a flexible file. For example, data editing, case selections, flagging excessive range units, adding data to existing files when additional research is completed, merging files, renaming files, specifying format length, repeating numbers in a list, handling missing data, abbreviated words, tab features, reassigning values in a list, saving data, and finding data sets and costs to retrieve information become important features for file creation. Database management concepts now include file management systems, which are discussed later in this chapter.

Statistical Analysis

Approximately 180 statistical software packages are available for use on mainframes and minicomputers. These statistical software packages have evolved, since the first programs appeared in the late 1950s, from simple descriptive statistics packages to those including exploratory and model-building methods. The earlier packages also limited the number of data sets that could be included in the data file. Today statistical packages can analyze very large and complex data sets, transform data to be read in a number of statistical packages, and communicate with users who have little experience with statistics or computers (Francis, 1981).

Statistical software packages have unique categories, characteristics and capabilities. They will be described in the following sections.

Categories

The seven major categories of statistical packages reflect their intended use and capabilities:

Large, general-purpose statistical packages
Statistical packages with more restricted applications
Database management packages

Editing packages
Tabulation packages
Survey analysis
Subroutine libraries

Characteristics

The five essential characteristics of a statistical program that determine its usefulness and overall quality are listed in Table 14-7 (Francis, 1981).

The general-purpose systems provide complex mathematical formulas to manipulate large data sets in order to test statistical hypotheses or determine population parameters. Several computer programs (software packages) are available to process data (create files for storage) and analyze data statistically.

Capabilities

The mathematical analysis of statistical data can be grouped into software packages that provide capabilities within three major categories:

Statistical analysis
Sample survey
Mathematical categories

Eighteen subroutines are available as follows:

1. Statistical analysis. Multiple regression, Analysis of Variance (ANOVA)/linear models, linear multivariate, multiway tables, other multivariates, time series, nonparametric, exploratory, robust, curve fitting, bayesian, and econometrics
2. Sample survey. Computer estimates, computer variances, and select samples
3. Mathematical. Simulations, mathematical functions, and operations research

Modeling and Forecasting. Today, data sets that are input into computers can be analyzed by other computer software packages to build univariate and bivariate spectral analysis of parametric time domain models. As with most statistical model building, models may be built in steps that include several stages:

1. Identification and selection of a tentative model
2. Estimation of model parameters
3. Testing the fit
4. Forecasting of future observations

TABLE 14-7 *Five Characteristics of a Useful Statistical Program or Package*

1. Capabilities, which include filing, editing, tabulations, sample surveys, statistical analysis, language, mathematical functions, simulation capabilities, and operations research functions
2. Portability, which involves availability, number of installations, how many makes of computers can accommodate this version, memory core required, and batch versus interactive operating modes
3. Ease of learning and using, which is evaluated by time required for statistics training, computer training, language, documentation needs, and user conveniences
4. Reliability, which is judged by maintenance requirements and tests for accuracy
5. Costs, which includes on-line storage and retrieval costs

Many classes of models exist. The data collected are analyzed for potential error and outside influences to predict future trends. Models can be classed into time series or regression (parametric) time series models. Most are used for decision making or to test theories.

Three Major Software Packages

Three general-purpose statistical software packages are routinely used in nursing research. International in scope, broad in coverage of statistical capabilities, relatively easy to use, and available mostly on mainframes and minicomputers, these packages include the following:

- Statistical Package for the Social Sciences (SPSS)
- Statistical Analysis System (SAS)
- BMDP

Statistical Package for the Social Sciences. Statistical Package for the Social Sciences (SPSS) is available in 60 countries (Hull, 1981). The debut of the program packages was 1970. Social science data lends itself well to data summaries in tables, histograms, and graphs. These data types also require statistical tests that verify a hypothesis. Some of the capabilities of SPSS include descriptive statistics, frequency distributions, crosstabulations, Student's *t* test, bivariant correlation analysis, scatter diagram plots, partial correlations, multiple regression analysis, analysis of variance, discriminant analysis, factor analysis, Guttman scaling analysis, and canonical correlations.

Statistical Analysis System. Started in 1966 and revised in 1979, Statistical Analysis System (SAS) is a computer package for data analysis that includes information storage and retrieval, data modification and programming, report writing, statistical analysis, and file handling (Helwig, 1979).Once a data file has been created for SAS, computer programs read SAS data files and perform descriptive statistics, analysis of designed experiments, regressions, multivariate analysis, econometric and time series analysis. In addition, SAS can chart and graphically display data in vertical and horizontal bar charts.

In creating a file with SAS, researchers can do their own programming using SAS statements to manipulate data and to describe data sets. In the statistical analysis part of SAS, the user selects a program by name, and the program provides the statistical analysis. The user may give the program extra information in the form of procedure statements or add options to the already simple procedure statements.

BMDP. BMDP is another package of statistical programs used in biomedical research (Dixon and colleagues, 1981). The first BMD biomedical computer programs appeared in 1961 and have been followed by many editions. New programs included more robust statistical algorithms. The number of programs has grown from 26 to 42 in the 1981 edition. The statistical programs in BMDP are designed to aid in simple descriptive statistics to advanced statistical techniques. The programs are classified into eight series: data description, frequency tables, regression analysis, analysis of variance, multivariant analysis, life and survival tables, nonparametric analysis and cluster, and time series. An advantage of BMDP is the English-based instruction.

Statistical Analysis on Microcomputers

More than 40 statistical software packages are available for microcomputers. These software packages are expanding the capabilities of microcomputers and offer opportunities to perform complex statistical analyses without a mainframe or minicomputer. In 1981 only four statistical packages were available, but now both Apple and IBM have over four programs available for statistical analysis (Platt, 1981). The statistical software packages for microcomputers have unique categories, characteristics, and capabilities.

Categories. Three major categories of statistical packages for microcomputers exist:

General-purpose applications for a wide range of statistical analyses
Restricted applications that perform specific functions such as analysis of linear models (*e.g.,* multiple regression)
Database management packages

Statistical packages for microcomputers differ from those available for mainframes and minicomputers in that most of them contain a specified amount of function. More software programs are needed to extend its capabilities. Other programs are available as a set of disks; for example, speedSTAT and Human Systems Dynamics (HSD) come in a series of statistics programs, each of which has various functions.

Characteristics. Six general characteristics of a statistical program for a microcomputer exist (Table 14-8):

1. *Operating system,* which describes the type of microcomputer that the system can run on. Most packages can run on only one type of microcomputer (*e.g.,* IBM, Apple, Atari).
2. *Hardware requirements,* which determine the need for disk drives, range of storage, and format. The capacity of different disk configurations (single versus double sided, single versus double density) varies; some software cannot be used with the disk drive configuration of specific microcomputers.
3. *Limitations* include the need for additional software to run the package. For example, some statistical packages on microcomputers require an interpreter such as BASIC to run the program. Another limitation is the amount of system flexibility; some packages do not allow the user to change the formats. Because of protected formats, most packages cannot be copied (*i.e.,* backup copies cannot be made for archives). Some programs consist of a single program with subprograms; others are a series of separate programs. The series of separate programs requires the user to remember what program does what. Different operating styles exist for statistical programs. Some are menu driven; others are command language driven. Menus have long sequences of questions requiring answers, while command language requires a correct reply from the user with-

TABLE 14-8 *General Characteristics of a Statistical Program for a Microcomputer*

1. Operating system—what does it run on?
2. Hardware requirements—range of storage and format requirements
3. Limitations—ranging from flexibility to how the system handles errors
4. Documentation—how to learn to use the system
5. Data management and processing—does the information flow within the system?
6. Statistical functions—can the system add and do more sophisticated computations?

out a prompt. Although most microcomputers have potential hookups with mainframes, the ability to use an external test file of commands to run the files on a mainframe may be an option. Escape options, help functions, and error handling are also potential limitations of microcomputer statistical packages. How the program handles missing data or data out of range or identifies variables descriptively or within maximum or minimum ranges is important.

4. *Documentation* covers what screen displays the user will see, what tutorials are included about the software package, and what documentation exists on program technical formulas.
5. *Data management and processing* refers to how the package allows entry, editing, storage, retrieval, and display of data. Processing includes how the statistical program allows data to be processed through subsetting, merging, sorting, and transforming.
6. *Statistical functions* are the ways that the statistical package performs. Some microcomputer packages do one or more of the following: summary statistics, graphics, nonparametrics, linear models, and time series.

Evaluations

Some microcomputer software packages have been evaluated for statistical analysis programs that operate on the Apple, IBM, and Atari systems. Table 14-9 lists 24 programs rated good, fair, or negligible and evaluated for some characteristics. The vendors of most microcomputer statistical packages are listed in Table 14-10 (Carpenter and colleagues, 1984).

Graphic Displays

Once a data set is created in a file, many software packages provide a graphic display. A graphic display of data is a useful way to describe data and reveal trends, unusual values, or relationships between variables. Data can be plotted as a histogram of the frequency distribution or of the cumulative distribution (histograms and univariate plots) or as a graph of the data values in a normal or half-normal probability plot (bivariate scatter plots).

Data from one variable can be plotted against the data for another variable. For example, if time is in column one and blood pressure is in column two, a graph representing that data can be plotted. Symbols can be varied to represent an analysis of many variables on one graph. The user can control the size of the graph, its scale, histogram or data point intervals, and number of observations represented by each plot symbol. The vertical or Y axis can be labeled, as can the horizontal or X axis. Time or data scales can be converted to log scales, and regression lines for data can also be plotted. If a paper copy of a graph is desired, plotter equipment is available as an adjunct to the computer.

Frequency tables summarize results from surveys, clinical studies, and experiments when data are qualitative or categorical (*e.g.,* sex, or an answer to a multiple choice question), discrete but ordered (*e.g.,* educational preparation), or continuous but grouped into intervals (*e.g.,* height and weight).

Examples of computer graphics are shown in Figures 14-1 to 14-6. These graphics can be produced from a mainframe, a minicomputer, or a microcomputer connected to a proper printer with graphics capabilities (Prime Plotter, 1983).

Database Management Systems

Database management systems (DBMS) are popular systems today for mainframe, minicomputers, and microcomputers. The concept of database management is that

TABLE 14-9 *A Comparison of Statistical Analysis Packages for Microcomputers*

	DOCUMENTATION	DATA MANAGEMENT	DATA PROCESSING	SUMMARY STATISTICS	GRAPHICS	NONPARAMETRICS AND TABLES	LINEAR MODELS	TIME SERIES
ABSTAT	G	G	G	G	F	G	G	—
AIDA	G	G	G	G	G	G	F	—
A-Stat	F	G	G	G	—	G	G	—
Dynacomp Regr 1	F	F	—	—	F	—	F	—
Dynacomp Regr 2	F	F	—	—	F	—	—	—
Dynacomp Multilin	F	F	—	—	F	—	F	—
Dynacomp ANOVA	F	F	—	—	—	—	F	—
HSD Stats Plus	G	F	F	F	G	G	F	—
HSD Regress II	G	F	F	F	F	—	F	F
HAS ANOVA II	G	—	F	—	—	—	F	—
Introstat	G	G	G	F	F	G	F	—
Microstat	G	G	G	G	F	G	G	F
Micro-TSP	G	G	F	F	F	—	F	G
Number Cruncher	F	F	F	G	F	G	G	—
NWA Statpak	G	G	G	G	F	G	G	G
SAM	F	G	F	G	F	F	G	—
SpeedSTAT Vol. I	G	F	—	G	—	G	—	—
SpeedSTAT Vol. II	G	F	F	G	—	F	F	—
SPS	F	G	F	G	G	G	G	—
STAN	G	F	F	F	F	—	G	F
Statpro	G	F	G	G	G	G	G	G
SYSTAT	G	G	G	G	F	G	G	F
TWG ELF	G	G	F	G	G	F	G	—
TWG ARIMA	G	G	F	—	F	—	—	G
Wallonick Statpac	F	G	G	G	F	F	F	—

G = good; F = fair; — = none or negligible. (Carpenter J, Deloria D, Morganstein D: Statistical software for microcomputers. BYTE 9:234–264, 1984. Reprinted with permission from the April 1984 issue of BYTE magazine.)

TABLE 14-10 *Vendors of Statistical Analysis Packages for Microcomputers*

ABSTAT
Anderson-Bell
POB 191
Canon City, CO 81212
(303) 275-1661

AIDA
Dr. David Lingwood
Action-Research Northwest
11442 Marine View Dr., SW
Seattle, WA 98146
(206) 241-1645

A-Stat 83.1
Gary Grandon
Rosen Grandon Associates
7807 Whittier St.
Tampa, FL 33617
(813) 985-4911

Dynacomp
Dynacomp Inc.
1427 Monroe Ave.
Rochester, NY 14618
(716) 442-8960

EDA (Exploratory Data Analysis)
Paul Velleman
Conduit
POB 388
Iowa City, IA 52244
(319) 353-5789

HSD Stats Plus, ANOVA II, and Regress II
Stephen Madigan
and Virginia Lawrence
Human Systems Dynamics
9249 Reseda Blvd.,
Suite 107
Northridge, CA 91324
(213) 993-8536

Introstat 2.2
Ideal Systems
POB 681
Fairfield, IA 52556
(515) 472-4507

Microstat
Jack Purdham
Ecosoft Inc.
5311 North Central
Indianapolis, IN 46220
(317) 283-8883

Micro-TSP
College Division
McGraw-Hill
Princeton Rd.
Hightstown, NJ 08520
(609) 426-5000

Number Cruncher
Jerry L. Hintze
865 East 400 North
Kaysville, UT 84037
(801) 546-0445

NWA Statpak
Northwest Analytical Inc.
1532 SW Morrison St.
Portland, OR 97205
(503) 224-7727

SAM
International Software
Box 160
Welwyn Garden City
Herts, England A18 6TQ

SpeedSTAT:Volume 1: Frequencies and Crosstabs;
Volume 2: Regression and Correlation
Dennis LaRue
Softcorp International
229 Huber Village Blvd.
Westerville, OH 43081
(614) 267-3109
(800) 543-1350

SPS Version 3A.0 (Statistical Processing System)
Data Basic Inc. 102 South Main
Mount Pleasant, MI 48858
(517) 772-5055

STAN
David M. Allen
Statistical Consultants Inc.
Park Plaza Office Bldg.
462 East High St.
Lexington, KY 40508
(606) 252-3890

Statpac
Wallonick Associates
5624 Girard Ave. South
Minneapolis, MN 55419
(612) 866-9022

TABLE 14-10 *(Continued)*

Statpro
Mark Imhof and Steve Hewett
Wadsworth Electronic Publishing Company
20 Providence
Boston, MA 02116
(617) 423-0420

SYSTAT
Systat Inc.
1127 Asbury Ave.
Evanston, IL 60202
(312) 864-5670

The Winchendon Group:
ELF and ARIMA
3907 Lakota Rd.
POB 10114
Alexandria, VA 22310
(703) 960-2587

(Carpenter J, Deloria D, Morganstein D: Statistical software for microcomputers. BYTE 9:234–264, 1984. Reprinted with permission from the April 1984 issue of BYTE magazine. Copyright © by McGraw–Hill, Inc., NY 10020. All rights reserved.)

a program or series of programs (software packages) manages everything that happens to data from defining the file through statistical analysis and graphics. Database management facilitates, in a "user-friendly" way, the process of entering, storing, and retrieving data in a form suitable for analysis. (See Chap. 4 for a description of a database management system.)

Database management systems are particularly appropriate for clinical nursing research, since they reduce the amount of programming needed by older programs, are "user-friendly," and reduce the cost of manipulating large amounts of clinical data. Several database management systems can be used for clinical research, including the file management types SAS, RS/1, PROPHET, FILE MANAGER, and dBASE II or III. Five types run principally on minicomputers but may also have microcomputer versions: CLINFO, MISAR, Clinical Data Manager (CDM), INGRES,

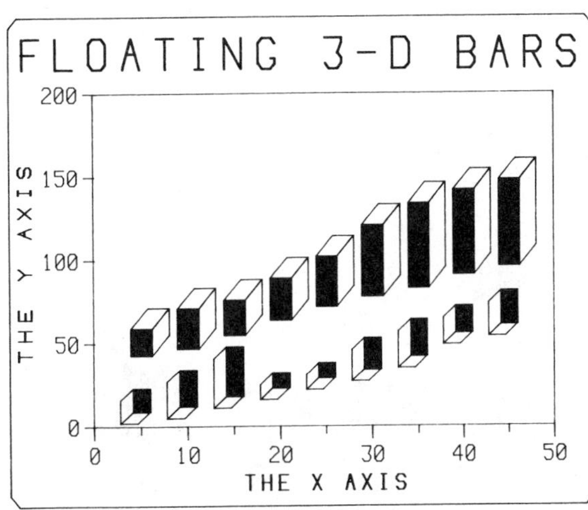

FIG. 14-1. An example of computer graphics from the Prime Plotter.

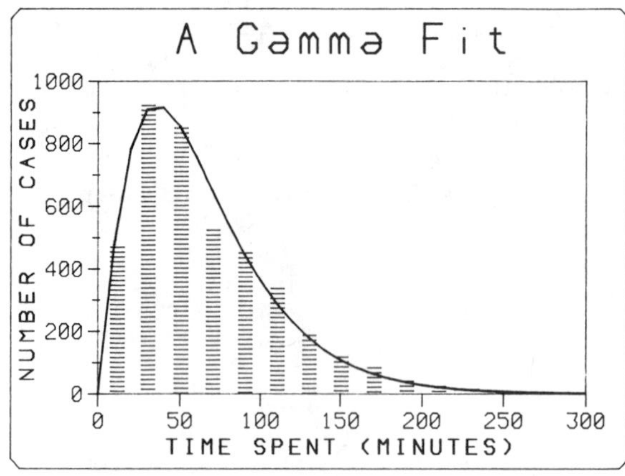

FIG. 14-2. An example of computer graphics from the Prime Plotter.

and ORACLE. Two database management systems run on mainframes: TOD and FOCUS. NPL is the microcomputer version of FOCUS. One system called SIR runs on either a mainframe or minicomputer. Table 14-11 lists the vendors of these database management systems (King and colleagues, 1983).

Text Editing

The majority of statistical software packages have an edit program to edit data in the files. These programs add new variables, replace data by corrected values, select subpopulations for specific analysis, change the data scales, record the values, and generate random numbers.

Text editing extends beyond the data points to describe the research itself. The most used text editor is the word processor, which is usually software that records type from a keyboard into magnetic memory for subsequent recall, correction, change, rearrangement, or reprinting. Some word processor equipment can be integrated with large-scale data processing computers that store research data. Word processing systems on microcomputers are usually more facile in text editing than the text editing programs available on large-scale data processing computers.

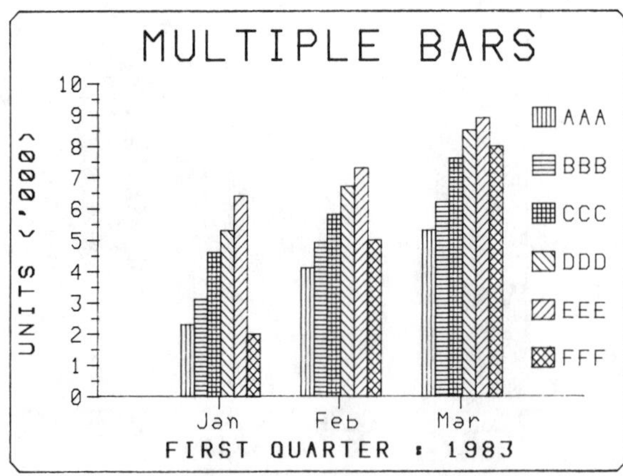

FIG. 14-3. An example of computer graphics from the Prime Plotter.

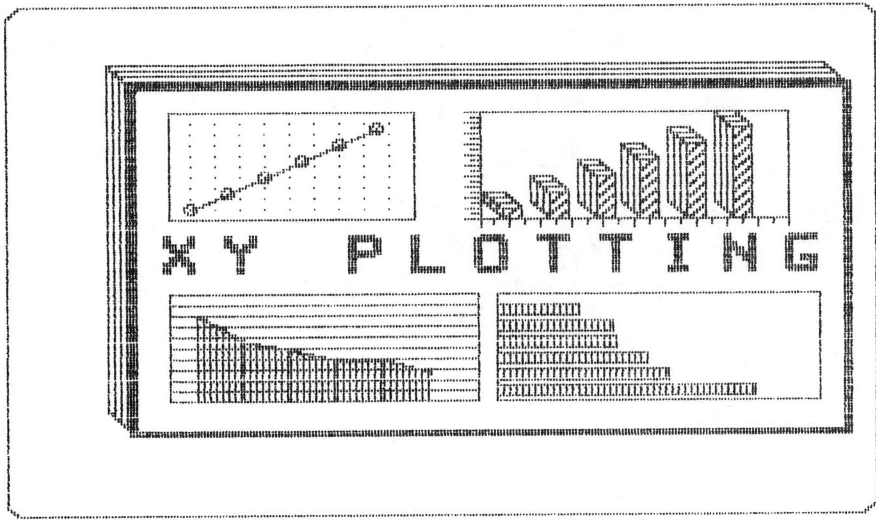

FIG. 14-4. An example of computer graphics from the Prime Plotter.

Programs available for mainframes and minicomputers usually vary from a basic editor of errors to elaborate editing and formatting (*i.e.,* right and left justification of margins and moving paragraphs). The major mainframe programs (SCRIBE, WYLBUR, TEK, and ATMS) usually have automatic indexing, checks for spelling, and footnote handling capabilities. They also allow the user to give format instructions to produce complex pages with tables in place or leave space for allocated illustrations, tables, and figures.

Additional benefits of using computerized sources for manuscript preparations are as follows:

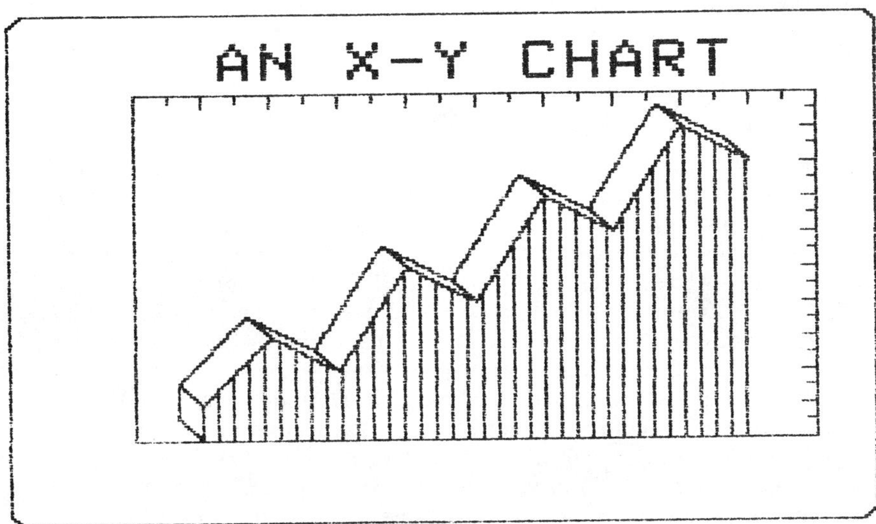

FIG. 14-5. An example of computer graphics from the Prime Plotter.

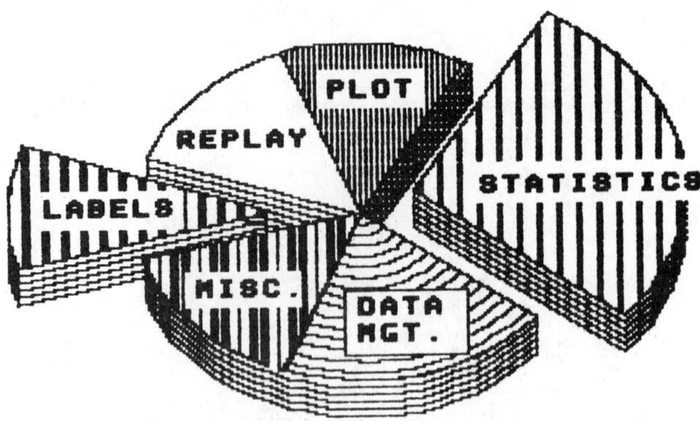

FIG. 14-6. An example of computer graphics from the Prime Plotter.

To speed up the writing and refining process
To change a manuscript from single to double or triple space with no retyping
To place footnotes at the end of a page, the end of a chapter, or the end of the manuscript
To number pages
To automate indexing
To save duplicates on disks
Print multilingual versions of texts to translate

Approximately 100 different software versions are available on microcomputers for text editing. They are usually ranked for ease of use, cost, editing capabilities, formatting potentials, interfacing capabilities, file handling, and user support documentation such as tutorials. Because new text editing disks are added to the market frequently, an interested person should consult a current software directory.

State of the Art: Computers in the Research Process

The state of the art of computer capabilities for processing data has gradually improved over the last decade. In the last 5 years there has been accelerated growth of new systems, revision of old ones, and dissemination of information regarding these programs. This growth has been enhanced by nurses' appreciation of the possibilities and new techniques now available to them through the computer. Although the computer has allowed analytic techniques, it has not reduced the need for nurses who examine their data for inaccuracies, choose appropriate statistical techniques, and analyze the results cautiously. About 20,000 microcomputers are selling each month (Naisbitt, 1982). Home computers will allow literature searches and statistical analysis of research from home, airplane, or boat. Being knowledgable about available programs will make nurses information specialists and better consumers of software for their home or office computer. The use of literature searches and statistical programs will greatly aid the research process (McCormick, 1983).

TABLE 14-11 *Vendors of Database Management Systems*

SAS
SAS Institute
SAS Circle
Box 8000
Cary, NC 27511

RS/1
Bolt, Beranek and Newman (BBN)
50 Moulton St.
Cambridge, MA 02238

PROPHET
Applied for through an NIH grant
Bolt, Beranek and Newman support and maintenance
50 Moulton St.
Cambridge, MA 02238

CLINFO
Bolt, Beranek and Newman
50 Moulton St.
Cambridge, MA 02238

MISAR (in the public domain)
Computer Medicine Laboratory
Beth Israel Hospital
330 Brookline Ave.
Boston, MA 02215

CDM
Clinical Data Manager
(formerly MEDUS/A)
Clinical Data Inc.
Box 430
Brookline, MA 02146

VA FILE MANAGER (in the public domain)
MUMPS Users' Group
P.O. Box 37247
Washington, DC 20013

INGRES
Relational Technology Inc.,
Suite 515
2855 Telegraph Ave.
Berkeley, CA 94705

ORACLE
Relational Software, Inc.
Menlo Park, CA

SIR
SIR, Inc.
P.O. Box 1404
Evanston, IL 60204

TOD
The Data Bank Network
701 Welch Rd. No. 3301
Palo Alto, CA 94306

MEDLOG (Microcomputer version of TOD)
Information Analysis Associates
490 El Capitan
Palo Alto, CA 94306

FOCUS
Information Builders, Inc.
New York, NY

NPL (Microcomputer version of FOCUS)
Desktop Software
228 Alexander Rd.
Princeton, NJ 08540

dBASE II or III
Ashton-Tate
9929 West Jefferson Blvd.
Culver City, CA 90230

COMPUTERS IN CLINICAL NURSING RESEARCH

Systems are available to provide nurse researchers with information to facilitate clinical nursing research. One such system is retrievable through DATAPAC from the University of Alberta, Canada. It provides information on current thesis and nonthesis research in Canadian institutions by telephone. Information for the system is derived from ten cooperating institutions (Canadian Nurse, 1978).

Clinical Nursing Research on Mainframes or Minicomputers

Very few descriptions in the literature exist on the actual use of mainframe or minicomputer information for nursing research purposes; more descriptions point to the potential of what nursing databases have to offer. As early as 1966 research textbooks pointed to the potential for computers to open up avenues for correlating complex physiologic data. Computers were predicted to be the sources of information for physiologic monitoring, nursing service organizational studies, and diagnostic facilitators (Abdellah and Levine, 1966).

By 1980, the technology involved in nursing research was predicted to involve computers in the future based on activities where computer applications were already in progress, that is, quality assurance programs, staffing, services and unit management, data analysis, and monitoring nursing therapies and interventions (Gortner, 1980).

By 1981 the research potential of computerized information systems was thought to lie in the areas of practice, education, administration, and health care delivery. At the June 1977 Research Conference on Nursing Information Systems, three major research directions were classified as potentials with computers (Werley and Grier, 1981):

Nursing practice content
Systematic nursing practice
System evaluation

Unfortunately, by 1983, nurse researchers were still only describing the potential for nursing databases, and few authors had described the use of computers for nursing practice research, nursing practice evaluation, or system evaluation. It has even been reiterated that if nursing objectives were established, the data on the computer could be structured so that information could be retrieved and linkages could be made between patient characteristics, nursing diagnoses, desired outcomes, nursing interventions, actual outcomes, and resource use. In fact, a list of systems that should be developed to produce more clinical nursing research has been presented again in 1983 (Kiley and colleagues, 1983).

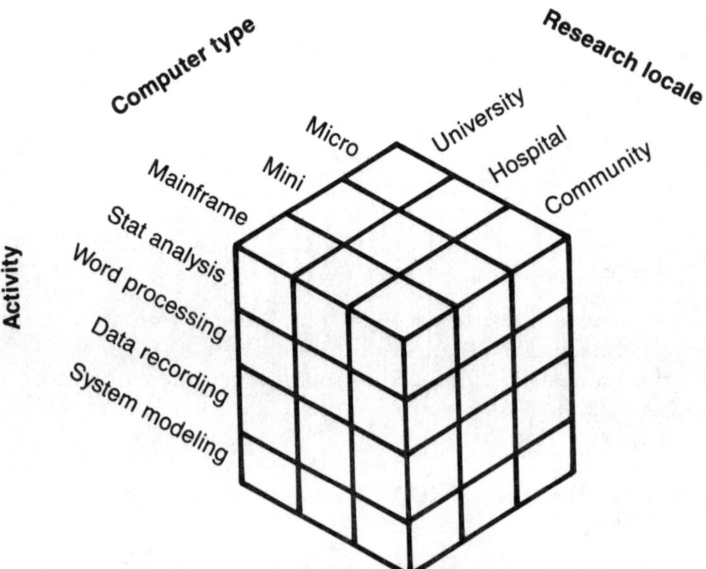

FIG. 14-7. Schwirian's cube: The research dimension.

TABLE 14-12 *Preconditions of a Nursing Information System Necessary for Research Retrieval*

1. Structure is legible, accurate, and accessible; costs are reasonable
2. Structure is theoretically logical
3. Content is standardized and brief
4. Input matches output
5. Accessory storage devices for subsequent batch processing are flexible and compatible
6. Data are appropriately coded
7. Data input and retrieval capabilities are adaptable and can interface with other equipment
8. Hardware performance is stable
9. Hardware has an appropriate response time compatible with software design
10. Data processing and printing have adequate handling speed

Schwirian's Cube: The Research Dimension

One model described to organize the potential for computers in clinical nursing research is shown in Figure 14-7. Schwirian's cube analyzes research location, computer type, and activities that enhance and support clinical nursing research. The model provides a prospective for nurses to explore what they can do with computers in a clinical research environment, what settings research takes place in, and what types of computers provide research support (Schwirian, 1983).

Preconditions of a Nursing Database

The first attempt to classify what information systems could provide for clinical nursing research was presented in 1981. Preconditions established what data available on HISs were needed for nursing research (Table 14-12) (McCormick, 1981).

Nurse researchers must first work with information and computer specialists in designing nursing information systems so that input matches potential output; that is, information systems must be designed to facilitate research retrieval. The technology must match the research needs so that output will contain valid data and retrieval costs will be reasonable.

In essence, the type of computer system and design is not only affected by standardized, logical formats, but also by processing capabilities. Processing components that must be considered include type of content being stored, amount of content needed, amount of coding involved, and degree of decision making and manipulation the coded data will be subjected to. In order to make a system available for research, it is thus important to define input, decision-making capabilities, and expected output.

If content will be useful for research retrieval, some form of reliability testing or normalization of data is necessary. (Data normalization means some information consistency.) Analysis of nonnormalized data produces databases with useless information, that is, data cemeteries (McCormick, 1981).

A Research Taxonomy for Mainframes and Minicomputers

A taxonomy of research information potentially available from HISs or minicomputers can be divided into three categories (McCormick, 1981):

- Nursing science in patient care data
- Efficacy of nursing strategies in solving patient problems
- Nursing care organization and delivery

1. *Nursing science information* is potentially available on a system, since nurses in practice usually enter data necessary to document patient care. This therefore may indicate the science of nursing. Also, if standardized valid information is input, then retrieval will provide valid information. In this way, the science of nursing will be better described.
2. *Efficacy of nursing strategies in solving patient problems* can be available from computerized information of what nurses do in practice, since computers can process large amounts of information, analyze it, and graphically present a report. A computer search of the actions that nursing personnel usually perform that result in a successful patient outcome can be printed routinely. For example, by computerizing nursing diagnosis and nursing actions, it could be determined if more patients reached their expected outcomes for pain management with more frequent tranquilizer administration, back rubs, or narcotic administration.
3. *Nursing care organization and delivery* are definite research potentials. Evaluation tools can forecast, plan, and model through computerized resources. Likewise, if computers have hospital management and unit management information capabilities, then research designs could determine if one method of delivering care was more effective than another.

   A complete taxonomy requires data sets potential within each major category. Therefore, if nursing science, efficacy, and delivery can truly be a taxonomy, seven characteristics must be met: aggregates, utility, abstractions, correlations, linear profiles, comparison, and quality. A proposed taxonomy of research is listed in Tables 14-13 to 14-15. This taxonomy includes the data sets that make the three categories a taxonomy. The examples show that the three categories include the necessary characteristics of a taxonomy.

Examples of nursing research that justifies computer data in defining nursing science, efficacy of nurses' actions, and delivery of care is limited. The majority of information about nursing's use of the computer for research comes from the summaries of professional organization meetings on computer applications. This has occurred because of the relative newness of the application and the few nurse researchers currently prepared to use computers for research.

Clinical Research on Microcomputers

Since information is the lifeline of a clinical nursing research unit, HISs and microcomputers have been used to store information necessary for clinical research. Microcomputers have specific advantages in a research unit (Schwirian and Byers, 1982):

1. They are "user friendly."
2. They are relatively inexpensive.
3. They take up little space, have minimal installation needs, and add little noise to a unit.
4. Storage of data on the diskette may be more secure than the information in a mainframe computer.
5. Supporting software packages are available to put into use within a relatively short period after purchase.

TABLE 14-13 *Research Potential of Computers to Define Nursing Science in Patient Care*

I. Nursing Science in Patient Care
   A. Aggregates
      1. Frequency distributions of nursing science data (nursing diagnosis, signs and symptoms, physiological and psychologic needs assessments, patient classifications, observations and procedures, medications administered, communication with allied departments)
   B. Utility
      1. Utilization review of nursing observation and procedures, nursing process, medication administered
      2. Use of standardized content and variable structured format
      3. Completeness of nursing data
      4. Conciseness of nursing data
      5. Appropriateness of nursing data
      6. Consistency of nursing data
   C. Abstractions
      1. Definitions of analytical methods for decision making
      2. Definitions of pathways within variable structure and standardized structure of nursing content
      3. Mathematical modeling of content data
      4. Predictions of nursing data for prevention, deterioration and stabilization of patients
   D. Correlations
      1. Correlations between nursing data and medical data
      2. Correlations between nursing data and organization and delivery data
      3. Correlations within physiologic and psychologic data in nursing data
   F. Linear profiles
      1. Linear profiles and longitudinal data reflecting nursing data from admission to discharge in inpatients and outpatients
   F. Comparisons
      1. Nursing data compared to other allied health professionals' assessments
      2. Comparisons of different theoretical frameworks for structured nursing data content
   G. Quality
      1. Reliability and validity of structured and variable content within nursing data

(McCormick K: Nursing research using computerized data bases. In Heffernan H [ed]: Proceedings of the Fifth Annual Symposium on Computer Applications in Medical Care, pp 738–743. Silver Spring, MD, IEEE Computer Society Press, 1981)

Examples of Computer Usage for Clinical Nursing Research

A computer was used to facilitate the diagnosis of anxiety in patients admitted to a hospital. The computer system was tested against nurses' ability to diagnose mild, moderate, and severe levels of anxiety in patients against an administered test (the multiple affect adjective checklist) and against the galvanic skin reaction test. The patient was interviewed with a structured format. The results of the interview were fed into an IBM computer, and the data were analyzed using a program written in Fortran IV to diagnose level of anxiety. The use of the computer was not correlated

TABLE 14-14 *Research Potential of Computers to Determine the Efficacy of Nursing Strategies in Solving Patient Problems*

II. Efficacy of Nursing Strategies in Solving Patient Problems
  A. Aggregates
    1. Frequency distributions of nursing orders (nursing actions, expected patient outcomes)
    2. Frequency distributions of nursing actions resulting from doctors' orders
    3. Frequency distributions of related nursing doctors' orders
  B. Utility
    1. Utilization review of nursing actions and expected patient outcomes
    2. Use of standardized content and variable structured format
    3. Completeness of nursing actions, patient expected outcomes
    4. Conciseness of nursing actions, expected patient outcomes
    5. Appropriateness of nursing actions, expected patient outcomes
    6. Consistency of nursing actions, expected patient outcomes
  C. Abstractions
    1. Definitions of effective nursing actions with specific medical/nursing diagnosis
    2. Definition of theoretical frameworks of nursing actions
    3. Predicting nursing actions that prevent, enhance, or deter specific patient outcomes
    4. Determination of signs and symptoms that evoke specific nursing actions
    5. Mathematical models categorizing nursing actions and patient outcomes
  D. Correlations
    1. Correlations between nursing actions and doctors' orders
    2. Correlations between nursing actions and patient expected outcomes
    3. Correlations between nursing actions and nursing science data
    4. Correlations between nursing actions and organization and delivery data
    5. Correlations between nursing actions and safety/incidents
    6. Procedures correlated with standard policies
  E. Linear profiles
    1. Nursing action profiles from admission to discharge in inpatients and outpatients
    2. Expected outcomes/patient responses to nursing actions during specific stages of illness
    3. Expected outcomes/patient response to doctors' treatment during specific stages of illness
  F. Comparisons
    1. Nursing actions compared to other allied health professionals' actions
    2. Benefits of one intervention compared to another
    3. Patient response to medical procedures compared to nursing procedures
    4. Benefits of specific treatment plans compared to patient outcomes
    5. Benefits of nursing actions on patients' physical compared to emotional outcomes
  G. Quality
    1. Reliability and validity of structured and variable content for nursing actions and patient expected outcomes
    2. Safety/incidents reported related to specific nursing actions/doctors' orders
    3. Criteria for measuring the effects of nursing actions on patient outcomes
    4. Criteria for measuring quality care given for specific nursing diagnosis standards

(McCormick K: Nursing research using computerized data bases. In Heffernan H [ed]: Proceedings of the Fifth Annual Symposium on Computer Applications in Medical Care, pp 738–743. Silver Spring, MD, IEEE Computer Society Press, 1981)

TABLE 14-15 *Research Potential of Computers to Evaluate Nursing Care Organization and Delivery*

III. Nursing Care Organization and Delivery
- A. Aggregates
  1. Frequency distributions of: error reporting, safety/incidents, patient classifications, nursing computer time, nurse entry into computer, response time/down time/nurse time, unit transfers, community resources sought in discharge care planning, admissions, communications of nurses with other allied health professionals, discharges, deaths, transfers, assignment of primary nurses
- B. Utility
  1. Utilization review of patient classification schemes
  2. Utilization review of pathways of interinstitute communication
  3. Utilization review of nurse staffing predictions
  4. Appropriateness of coding nursing data content
  5. Appropriateness of access to statistics, graphics, modeling, and data reorganization
  6. Completeness of organization and delivery data
  7. Consistency in using patient classification and nursing staffing content
  8. Conciseness of organization and delivery data
- C. Abstractions
  1. Definitions of analytical methods for decision-making processes
  2. Definition of communication channels between units and with other allied health professionals
  3. Determinations of patient loads per nursing staff personnel
  4. Predictions of professional experience needed to care for patients with certain classifications/diagnosis
  5. Definition of problems enforcing rigid structure content and variable structure format
  6. Mathematical modeling of organizational channels
- D. Correlations
  1. Staffing patterns correlated to level of difficulty/patient classifications
  2. Nurse preparation correlated with level of difficulty in assignments
  3. Assignment of primary nurses correlated with hospital stay/complications/patient satisfaction
  4. Staffing difficulties correlated with frequency, appropriateness and quality of nursing documentation
  5. Nursing diagnosis correlated with patient length of stay
- E. Linear profiles
  1. Cost analysis for patient care delivered from admission to discharge for inpatients and outpatients
- F. Comparisons
  1. Assignment of primary nurses compared to no primary nurse assignment
  2. Utilization of computerized documentation in areas of Class IV patients compared to areas of Class I patients
  3. Computerized documentation compared to manual documentation
- G. Quality
  1. Reliability and validity of organization and delivery content
  2. Safety/incident reports
  3. Criteria for measuring quality of computerized documentation

(McCormick K: Nursing research using computerized data bases. In Heffernan H [ed]: Proceedings of the Fifth Annual Symposium on Computer Applications in Medical Care, pp 738–743. Silver Spring, MD, IEEE Computer Society Press, 1981)

significantly with the other three methods for diagnosing anxiety. The researcher found that a computer program is only as valid as the information programmed into it (Lagina, 1971).

In critical care nursing, a study compared computer-recorded information available from physiologic monitors with information recorded manually by staff nurses. The computer system studied consisted of a bedside physiologic monitor, a microcomputer, and the Quantitative Sentinel, developed by Quantitative Medicine in conjunction with the Maryland Institute for Emergency Medical Service Systems. Heart rate and systolic blood pressure were the variables studied. The study was prompted by nurses' distrust of computerized information in intensive care environments.

The results demonstrated that computerized and manually recorded observations of heart rate were the same 75% of the time; the systolic blood pressure observations were the same 84% of the time. The low incidence of significant differences between the computer-averaged algorithms and the manually recorded information generally supports the use of the computer in critical care environments. More variance could result from nurses' collecting information manually than from data collected from computer programs (Milholland and Ward, 1982).

SUMMARY

The two main applications for the use of computers in nursing research, the nursing research process and clinical nursing research, were discussed. The six uses of computers in nursing research were presented.

The preconditions for a nursing database for research retrieval were described, and a taxonomy of research-related information potentially available on a nursing database was presented. Some uses of the computer for research were described.

ISSUES

1. All professional nurses must be literate as information specialists; that is, they must know where to retrieve information.
2. The nursing profession must consider its own database for retrieving information pertinent to the profession.
3. Few studies describe the use of computer information for clinical research.
4. Studies are involved in evaluating the implementation, user attitudes, the costs, and satisfaction with the equipment in nursing practice, the results of administrative applications, and educational uses of computers.
5. A few studies have monitored the content that was computerized, but as a tool that could provide information to describe the science of nursing, the efficacy of practice, and organization and delivery of nursing care, the computer potentially provides an enormous amount of information.
6. Nurses with research experience must become more involved with computer specialists in designing valid, reliable computer content that must be input in order for pertinent information to be retrieved.
7. As more nurses use computers for clinical nursing research, the issues of privacy, confidentiality, and security will heighten.
8. Because the MeSH vocabulary index of MEDLINE is a medical heading, nursing articles may be misrepresented unless journals or authors provide keywords.
9. As nurse researchers increase and as more nursing literature is written, a separate NURSELINE within MEDLARS may be required.

SUGGESTIONS FOR HANDS-ON EXPERIENCES

1. Go to a library that provides MEDLINE searches and select a topic to search.
2. Search the special-list nursing file *(INI)* for the same topic selected in the MEDLINE search.
3. Look for the *INI, Index Medicus,* and *Cumulative Index to Nursing Literature* in a library reference section.
4. Contact the National Technical Information Service (NTIS) for a search of nursing-related information for a topic selected above.
5. If your library has on-line searches, do your own on-line search.
6. If you are acquainted with someone or a company that uses microcomputer searches through specific vendors, search for a specific topic within nursing.
7. Search for specific nursing literature on ERIC.
8. Search for specific nursing literature on SOCIAL SCISEARCH.
9. Search a specific nursing literature on Excerpta Medica.
10. Ask a hospital information specialist to see nursing aggregate data obtained by computer retrieval.
11. Select one nursing manuscript published in a nursing journal and determine what keywords were used to describe the nursing article, how many places listed it, and within how many literature searches you found the article.
12. If you did not find the article listed in no. 11, discuss reasons for not finding it.

STUDY QUESTIONS

1. What are two main applications of computers for nursing research?
2. What are the six uses of computers in the research process?
3. Name the MEDLAR on-line database that is the largest information retrieval system in the world.
4. Name two databases relevant to nursing.
5. Identify the four main steps in transforming raw data into a computer file.
6. What are the main components of a file?
7. What are the seven major categories of statistics software packages?
8. Discuss the five essential characteristics of a statistical software package.
9. What are three major capabilities of a statistical software package?
10. Name the three major statistical software packages on mainframes and minicomputers.
11. List ten major statistical programs on microcomputers.
12. Name a software package for graphically displaying data.
13. Name a program for text editing on a mainframe computer.
14. Describe two essential preconditions for a nursing database.
15. Identify three categories of data available for clinical nursing information.
16. Discuss one issue confronting the nursing profession resulting from the impact of computers on nursing research.

REFERENCES

Abdellah F, Levine E: Better Patient Care Through Nursing Research. New York, Macmillan, 1979

Abdellah F, Levine E: Future directions of research in nursing. Am J Nurs 66:112–116, 1966

American Journal of Nursing: International Nursing Index (1975–1983). New York, American Journal of Nursing, 1975–1983

Canadian Nurse: The information revolution: Where does it leave nursing? Can Nurse 78:17, 1978

Carpenter J, Deloria D, Morganstein D: Statistical software for microcomputers. BYTE 9:234–264, 1984

DIALOG: The Dialog Service Has It: Pick a Subject . . . Any Subject. Palo Alto, CA, Lockheed Missiles and Space Co, 1977

Dixon W, Brown M, Engelman L, et al: BMDP Statistical Software. Berkeley, CA, University of California Press, 1981

Excerpta Medica: An untitled marketing handout. Princeton, NJ, 1983

Francis I: Statistical Software: A Comparative Review. New York, Elsevier North-Holland, 1981

Gortner S: Nursing research: Out of the past and into the future. Nurs Res 29:204–207, 1980

Helwig J, Council K: User's Guide, 1979 Edition. Raleigh, NC, SAS Institute, 1979

Hull C, Nie N: SPSS Update 7–9: New Procedures And Facilities for Releases 7–9. New York, McGraw-Hill, 1981

Kiley M et al: Computerized nursing information systems (NIS). Nurs Manage 12:26–29, 1983

King C, Manire L, Strong R: Comparing data management systems in clinical research: 1983 Survey. In Dayhoff R (ed): Proceedings of the Seventh Annual Symposium on Computer Applications in Medical Care, pp 715–719. Silver Spring, MD, IEEE Computer Society Press, 1983

Lagina S: A computer program to diagnose anxiety levels. Nurs Res 20:484–492, 1981

Lancaster F: Information Retrieval Systems: Characteristics, Testing and Evaluation, 2nd ed. New York, John Wiley & Sons, 1978

Mathies L, Watson P: Computer-Based Reference Service. Chicago, American Library Association, 1973

McCormick K: Nursing research using computerized data bases. In Heffernan H (ed): Proceedings of the Fifth Annual Symposium on Computer Applications in Medical Care, pp 738–743. Silver Spring, MD, IEEE Computer Society Press, 1981

McCormick K: Data capture: Use of statistical packages and computer literature searches. In Fokkens O, et al (eds): Medinfo 83 Seminars, pp 343–347. Amsterdam, North-Holland, 1983

Milholland K, Ward J: A comparison of computer recorded and manually recorded heart rates and systolic blood pressure. In Blum B (ed): Proceedings of the Sixth Annual Symposium on Computer Applications in Medical Care, pp 608–611. Silver Spring, MD, IEEE Computer Society Press, 1982

Naisbitt J: Megatrends: Ten Directions Transforming our Lives. New York, Warner Books, 1982

National Library of Medicine: Fact Sheet: NLM Online Databases. Bethesda, MD, U.S. Government Printing Office, 1983

National Library of Medicine: Principles of MEDLARS Bethesda, MD, U.S. Government Printing Office, 1970

Platt W, Platt C: Microcomputer statistical packages and regression performances. In American Statistical Association 1981: Proceedings of the Statistical Computer Section, pp 309–316.

The Prime Plotter. Cabin John, MD, Primesoft Corp, 1983

Schwirian P, Byers S: The microcomputer in the clinical nursing research unit. In Blum B (ed): Proceedings of the Sixth Annual Symposium on Computer Applications in Medical Care, pp 658–661. Silver Spring, MD, IEEE Computer Society Press, 1982

Schwirian P: Schwirian's cube: The research dimension. Comp Nursing 1:5, 1983

Strauch K, Brundage D: Guide to Library Resources for Nursing. New York, Appleton-Century-Crofts, 1980

Weinstock M: Citation indexes. In Encyclopedia of Library and Information Science, vol 5. New York, Marcel Dekker, 1971

Werley H, Grier M: Nursing Information Systems. New York, Springer, 1981

BIBLIOGRAPHY

Better information management policies needed: A study of scientific and technical bibliographic services. Washington, DC, U.S. Government Printing Office, 1979

Huth E: How to Write and Publish Papers in the Medical Sciences. Philadelphia: ISI Press, 1982

McCarn D: Medline: An introduction to on-line-searching. J Am Soc Inform Serv 31:181–192, 1980

MEDLARS: The computerized literature retrieval service of the National Library of Medicine. (DHEW pub. no. (NIH) 79-1286). Bethesda, MD, 1979

National Library of Medicine: Fact sheet: NLM International Medlars Bilateral Agreements. Bethesda, MD, U.S. Government Printing Office, 1983

National Library of Medicine: Nursing: A Guide to Sources of Information. Bethesda, MD, U.S. Government Printing Office, 1981

National Library of Medicine: On-line Service Reference Manual. Washington, DC: U.S. Government Printing Office, 1978

Saba V, Skapik K: Nursing information center. Am J Nurs 79:86–87, 1979

Saba V: A comparative study of document retrieval systems of nursing interest. Doct Diss Intl 42(5):8124656, 1981

Schwirian P: The comparative utility of a file cabinet program vs a general statistical program in micro-computer management and analysis of clinical nursing data. In Dayhoff R (ed): Proceedings of the Seventh Annual Symposium on Computer Applications in Medical Care, 565–567. Silver Spring, MD, IEEE Computer Science Press, 1983

Study Group Nursing Information System: Special report: Computerized nursing information systems: An urgent need. Res Nursing Health, 6:101–105, 1983

Swaine M: Can you do statistics on a microcomputer? Info/World 5:39–45, 1983

Sweeney M, Olivieri P: An Introduction to Nursing Research. Philadelphia, JB Lippincott, 1981

Werley H: Impact of computers on nursing research. In Heffernan H (ed): Proceedings of the Fifth Annual Symposium on Computer Applications in Medical Care, pp 728–729. Silver Spring, MD, IEEE Computer Society Press, 1981

Williams M: Use of machine-readable data bases. Ann Rev of Inform Sci Techno 9:221–284, 1974

Zielstorff R: Computers in Nursing. Wakefield, MA, Nursing Resources, 1980

15 Educational Applications

Objectives

- Understand the many types of education applications available.
- Describe the types of computer-assisted instruction.
- Understand computer-managed instruction applications.
- Discuss the concept of computer-assisted video instruction.
- Identify education applications encompassing expert systems, knowledge synthesizers, mainframes, and microcomputers.
- Discuss the evaluations and issues related to education applications.

Computers have been used in education for over a decade. However, only in the last few years has a definite trend occurred toward the increased use of this new technology in educational settings. The use of computers to support educational activities is commonly referred to as computer-based education (CBE) or computer-assisted learning (CAL) (Ball and Hannah, 1984). CBE encompasses two categories: computer-assisted instruction (CAI), which assists in teaching students, and computer-managed instruction (CMI), which assists managing student records, rotations, and educational resources. Other categories of educational applications may include the following:

- Computer-assisted video instruction (CAVI)
- Expert systems
- Knowledge synthesizers
- Educational applications with Hospital Information Systems (HISs) (mainframes)
- Nurse extenders for patient teaching using microcomputers
- Discharge education plans
- Potentials for home computers

Specifically, this chapter describes the following major types of computer usage in education:

- Computer-based education
- Computer-assisted instruction
- Computer-managed instruction
- Computer-assisted video instruction
- Other educational applications

COMPUTER-BASED EDUCATION

CBE encompasses all activities that involve the computer systems used in education; it also refers to computer systems that involve the instruction process, the management of records, and an evaluation of student progress.

The major CBE system available for nursing education is PLATO.

PLATO

PLATO (programmed logic for automatic teaching operations), developed at the University of Illinois, is used throughout the country through a nationwide communication network set up by Control Data Corporation (CDC). The network can be used in any setting that subscribes to the service. The method of participation is not complicated; an on-line display terminal is used to communicate by telephone with a CDC mainframe. The installation of PLATO includes the hardware communication system as well as the specific schedules, course, and profiles for subscribers (Control Data Learning Fact Sheet, 1981).

CDC also offers PLATO as a microcomputer service. PLATO Microlink offers a library of educational software to owners of the IBM PC. This service is also available through the Source Telecomputing Corporation.

PLATO can provide individualized student instruction, allowing students to progress at their own pace. At the same time it can accommodate a large number of students simultaneously. The system tracks students' progress and stores students' responses as they are made. PLATO monitors student progress, accommodates different educational and experience levels, distributes instruction nationwide, and offers relevant materials (PLATO, 1979). In 1974 approximately 1000 PLATO terminals were located in schools throughout the United States and Canada.

PLATO offers many programs available for nursing education. Each contains instructions, designs (including graphics), and feedback and reinforcement (Tymchyshyn, 1982).

COMPUTER-ASSISTED INSTRUCTION

CAI is an educational technique based on the two-way interaction between a computer and a learner. The objective is greater learning and retention than with didactic instruction, since the computer allows the learner to interact more than once in order to master content.

CAI allows a student to interact with a single computer (hardware), or terminals may interface with computers, printers, tape recorders, video players, or video discs. The information is stored on the program (software), which is the essence of CAI.

Types

Four major types of CAI exist (Hassett, 1984):

- Problem solving
- Drill and practice
- Tutorials
- Simulations

1. *Problem-solving* instruction uses programs that maximize the storage and retrieval capabilities of computers by solving specific discipline-oriented problems. For example, research problems can be analyzed through CAI problem-solving capabilities.
2. *Drill and practice* routines are self-teaching systems that usually ask students questions and indicate if the answer is correct or incorrect.
3. *Tutorials* or remedial instruction uses branching techniques that enable the student to move from easier to more advanced levels of learning. It is an extension of drill and practice but allows more feedback, since the student can

move forward to new material or backward (remedial) depending on the response.

4. *Simulation cases* and models, usually written to provide the student with individualized experiences, are designed to provide opportunities to deal with realistic clinical or administrative problems. The learner can attempt to solve problems before entering the clinical environment, thus lessening the risks of decision making while practicing clinical skills. The student can make mistakes without affecting a patient's well-being.

Some simulation programs allow students to work through assessment and nursing actions for patients with pediatric oncology and medical-surgical problems. Some college campuses even allow students to enter the HIS to learn nursing assessment and documentation of patient care through simulation programs. The training laboratories of most HISs usually have a simulated patient network to teach prospective users. Academic computer laboratories are gaining access to these hospital systems to provide learning experiences for students, which extends the capabilities of computer-assisted software for assessment and decision-making skills and shows students the actual content of nursing information systems in use to document patient care (Holzemer and colleagues, 1983).

Examples of Available Software

In the past 10 years, many educators have written software programs for the different forms of CAI instruction (Table 15-1). The section called "Software Exchange" in *Computers in Nursing* lists current software, as does CONDUIT at the University of Iowa. Several CAI program areas used in nursing are described below:

- Basic nursing skills
- Classic scientific principles
- Physical examination
- Managerial decision making
- Research process
- Practice examinations and test questions
- Authoring systems
- Inservice and staff education
- Patient education

Basic Nursing Skills

Several software programs have been designed to teach nursing students basic nursing skills. Many programs can be used on existing microcomputers, including the IBM personal computer, the TRS-80, and the Apple II Plus. One program incorporates cognitive and psychomotor skills to teach the learner to calculate and regulate intravenous flow rates on a simulated intravenous drip. Another program teaches how to measure blood pressure through computer simulation with animated graphics that the student controls. A tape recorder reproduces the sounds normally heard when blood pressure is taken.

Another program, developed for the TRS-80 model 1, teaches how to calculate and prepare a fractional medication dose. An animated graphic display of a simulated syringe appears on the screen and can be manipulated by the user. Programs available for use on the Apple II Plus include one that teaches how to test urine for sugar and ketones through color codes and another that guides the user through the appropriate steps for calculating and preparing a prescribed insulin dosage for injection (Larson, 1982).

Classic Scientific Principles

CAI programs also offer complex instruction in classic scientific principles such as the physiology and diagnosis of acid-base disorders. One program, adaptable for medical and nursing professionals, considers an approach to differential diagnosis, integrates laboratory information about a hypothetical patient, and provides a form for tabulating relative frequencies of acid-base disorders presented by the computer (Goldberg and colleagues, 1973). This program, designed for use on a PDP-6 computer from Digital Equipment Corporation (DEC), was intended to be run from remote terminals throughout an educational campus.

Physical Examination

Even physical examination skills can be learned by CAI. One program presents logical rules for teaching the approach to the physical examination (Slack and colleagues, 1967). The software for this program was developed on old equipment, the LINC computer, that needed magnetic tapes and cathode ray oscilloscopes in addition to keyboard entries to complete the physical examination results. However, the clinical portions of the program would not be limited to this particular computer.

Managerial Decision Making

Two unique educational programs that have been developed but not yet implemented were designed to assist nurses to learn decision making through instructional computer programs. One decision file has been built for each narrative file. The scenarios for simulation involve topics important to nursing management, including discipline and budgeting decisions (Brennan, 1981). Another program, similar to the HELP (which aids clinical decisions with computer-assisted programs) has been designed. (HELP was described in Chap. 13.) This prototype program is developed for a computerized information system that will not only record, transmit, and retrieve information but also aid nurses in clinical decision making. Written in PASCAL for the Apple II computer, the program facilitates the nursing process with decision-making operations at each stage when nurses record daily in the medical record. The model was also designed to increase nurses' knowledge in making everyday decisions related to patient assessment (Ozbolt, 1982).

Research Process

MESS. CAI has been used on one campus to teach the research process through simulation. This program, the Michigan experimental simulation supervisor (MESS), is a set of computer programs developed to help students design and run experiments on a variety of data-generating models. Table 15-2 shows four types of experiments that a student could perform, progressing from simple to complex. Each faculty member requires the student to state the research problem in question form, formulate a hypothesis, explain the theoretical basis for selecting independent and control variables, and visually graph the design of the raw data. The simulation program allows the student to design and experiment by specifying the number of experimental groups in the design, the values of the variables and the names of the dependent variables, and the number of subjects for each group.

(Text continues on p. 387.)

TABLE 15-1 *CAI Available*

TITLE	AUTHOR	COMPUTER	LANGUAGE	TARGET GROUP	SYNOPSIS	PRICE	AVAILABLE	SOURCE OF INFORMATION
NEMAS (Nursing Education Module Authoring System)	Susan Grobe, RN, PhD	Apple with 64K, 2 drives, coming soon for the IBM PC	Pascal	Faculty or in-service educators	An authoring system that permits the nonprogrammer to create patient simulations based on the five steps of the nursing process: nursing assessment, diagnosis, planning, intervention, and evaluation. The content is specific to your curriculum.	Upon request	January 1985	J.B. Lippincott Company East Washington Square Philadelphia, PA 19105 1-800-523-2945 In PA, call collect, (215) 238-4443
Calculation of Drug Dosages	Jame Timpke, MA; Caroline Janney, MSN	Apple IIe or Apple II+	Apple Soft, BASIC	1st- and 2nd-year nursing students, hospital nurses	The computer program consists of three diagnostic tests: basic math skills, conversions, and situations that require drug calculation. Each diagnostic test gives scores and an analysis of areas that need to be studied before the test is retaken. A workbook explains conversions, and calculations accompany the computer program. Each test contains approximately 35 questions. The computer draws from a bank of questions to give the student a different test each time the test is taken. Not a tutorial	$99.95; workbook, $6.95	Now	T.J. Designs 5905 Ironwood Ranchos Palos Verdes, CA 90274 (213) 598-1423
Case Management of Cleft Lip and Palate	MGT of America, Inc.	Apple, II+ 64K, V A1 interface card, 7820 videodisk player	Super-Pilot	Pediatric chronic care nurses/parents	Approximately 6 hours of instructional materials designed primarily as teaching tools for case management nurses to use with families of cleft lip and palate children. Lessons include general home care, feeding/weight gain, feeding techniques/devices, coordinated health care, psychosocial needs, treating the patient normally, etc. The package consists of seven diskettes, 1 videodisk, and a user's guide.	Pending	Pending	Jayne Parker, RN Children's Medical Services Florida Department of Health and Rehabilitative Services 1311 Winewood Boulevard Building 5, Room 140 Tallahassee, FL 32301 (904) 487-2690
Drug Therapy for Licensed Nurses	Lucille Pogue, RN, MSN; Virginia Marshall, RN, MSN; Phyllis Napier, RN, MSN	Apple II+, IIe with 48K, 2 drives/IBM PC/TRS-80 Model 4, 12, 16	Pascal	Nursing students at all levels and licensed nurses (RN, LPN), especially RNs returning to practice	A tutorial that reviews major drug categories	Upon request	Summer 1984	Lucille Pogue Staff Development Talmadge Hospital Medical College of Georgia Augusta, GA 30912 (404) 828-2281
'AMY'	School of Nursing, UCSF	IBM PC, 1 drive	BASIC	Nursing graduate students	A clinical simulation on postoperative care of a child with an abdominal wound	Upon request	Now	Rob Slaughter, PhD School of Nursing N 319 Y University of California at San Francisco San Francisco, CA 94143

Diabetic Patient, Patient in Pain, and Obstetric Patient	Allan Villiers, RN, MS; Cathy Michaels, PhD; Kay Brannum, MN	Apple II+, 48K, 2 drives	BASIC	Junior and senior nursing students who have completed at least one course in medical–surgical nursing	All three programs are interactive simulations for decision making on proper nursing actions for evolving situations in medication administration.	Equal exchange, that is, send a disk or trade	Now	Allan Villiers, RN, MS 1603 Omar Drive Mesquite, TX 75150 (214) 270-4362
Patient Management Simulation; Pediatric Minor Illness Encounter	Patricia Woodbury, MSN	Apple II+	To be determined	Primary health care professionals	A simulation in which the student must collect subjective and objective data, make a diagnosis, and plan for care.	Upon request	Pending	Patricia Woodbury, MSN 14427 Garland Ave. Apple Valley, MN 55124 (612) 432-4698
Cardio-Respiratory Arrest, Timed Response	D. Zwarra, RN, CCRN	TRS-80 Model III Tape	BASIC	Critical care RN	Program designed for beginning-level nurses to test their knowledge of basic CPR, as well as the appropriate drug and defibrilator usage against a timed response arrest	$95	Now	Debra Case Medical Nursing Halstead 400 Johns Hopkins Hospital 600 N. Wolfe Street Baltimore, MD 21205 (301) 955-5127
Blood Gas Evaluation	D. Zwarra, RN, CCRN	TRS-80 Model III Tape	BASIC	Critical care RN	User interprets a random blood gas that is corrected and scored. User-generated graphs for pH, CO_2, HCO_3, and Aa-DO2 are included.	$95	Now	Debra Case Medical Nursing Halstead 400 Johns Hopkins Hospital 600 N. Wolfe Street Baltimore, MD 21205 (301) 955-5127
Cardiac Profile Evaluation	D. Zwarra RN, CCRN	TRS-80 Model III Tape	BASIC	Critical care RN	Nurse evaluates random ICU patient values and selects therapy; computer then prints its response.	$95	Now	Debra Case Medical Nursing Halstead 400 Johns Hopkins Hospital 600 N. Wolfe Street Baltimore, MD 21205 (301) 955-5127
Arterial Pulses	D. Zwarra RN, CCRN	TRS-80 Model III Tape	BASIC	Critical care RN	Self-learning program on physical assessment of arterial pulses and their clinical interpretation. Self-assessment is part of the program.	$95	Now	Debra Case Medical Nursing Halstead 400 Johns Hopkins Hospital 600 N. Wolfe Street Baltimore, MD 21205 (301) 955-5127

(Continued)

TABLE 15-1 *(Continued)*

TITLE	AUTHOR	COMPUTER	LANGUAGE	TARGET GROUP	SYNOPSIS	PRICE	AVAILABLE	SOURCE OF INFORMATION
Blood Gases	D. Zwarra, RN, CCRN	TRS-80 Model III Tape	BASIC	Critical care RN	Step-by-step self-learning program for the interpretation of arterial pH, CO_2, HCO_3	$95	Now	Debra Case Medical Nursing Halstead 400 Johns Hopkins Hospital 600 N. Wolfe Street Baltimore, MD 21205 (301) 955-5127
ICU Nursing Exams	D. Zwarra, RN, CCRN	TRS-80 Model III Tape	BASIC	Critical care RN	Exams designed to evaluate the new ICU nurse's knowledge of ICU skills and medications. Three exams, CCU, MICU, and ICU medications, corrected and scored	$95	Now	Debra Case Medical Nursing Halstead 400 Johns Hopkins Hospital 600 N. Wolfe Street Baltimore, MD 21205 (301) 955-5127
Computer-Animated CPR	D. Zwarra, RN, CCRN	TRS-80 Model III Tape	BASIC	RNs or nursing students	An animated computer program on basic CPR and airway management designed to supplement by graphic illustrations such programs	$65	Now	Debra Case Medical Nursing Halstead 400 Johns Hopkins Hospital 600 N. Wolfe Street Baltimore, MD 21205 (301) 955-5127
Clinical Emergencies	Nancy Reuter, RN, BSN	TRS-80 Model III Tape	BASIC	RNs or nursing students	An animated computer program consisting of seven case studies accompanied by multiple-choice questions designed to test assessment and decision-making skills in dealing with each of the following emergencies: acute CVA, seizures, acute respiratory disease, chest pain, hypotension, uncontrolled diabetes, life-threatening arrythmias. An accompanying handout illustrates various life-threatening arrhythmias.	$125 for series of 7; $30 each for each individual case study	Now	Debra Case Medical Nursing Halstead 400 Johns Hopkins Hospital 600 N. Wolfe Street Baltimore, MD 21205 (301) 955-5127
Postoperative Care Patient Simulation	Sandra Mangum, RN, MN	Apple II or Franklin	Apple Soft, BASIC	1st- and 2nd-year students	This program simulates the 3 hours of immediate postoperative care with a client who has just come back from surgery for a ruptured appendix. Students must do a baseline assessment, update that assessment every 15 to 30 minutes.Regulate the IV, decide which comfort measures are necessary, and establish a problem list and nursing diagnoses. Charting is to be done on paper using the charting form for the institution.	$200 or exchange	Now	Concepts Unlimited 692 S. 450 E. Orem, UT 84057

CPR Certification Exam	Jane Timpke, MA; Caroline Janney, MSN	Apple IIe or Apple II+	Apple Soft, BASIC	Hospital nurses, nursing students, medical personnel, general public	Two exams are on the disk; one for health professionals and one for the general public. Each exam has 90 multiple-choice questions. At the end of the exam, students are given their scores on a computer printout and an opportunity to review the questions they answered incorrectly. The computer gives feedback about the answer that was chosen and the correct answer. The test has been certified by the Long Beach California American Heart Association.	$60	Now	T.J. Designs 5905 Ironwood Ranchos Palos Verdes, CA 90274 (213) 598-1423
CPR Recertification Exam	Jane Timpke, MA; Caroline Janney, MSN	Apple IIe or Apple II+ (IBM in the near future)	Apple Soft, BASIC	Anyone who has been certified in CPR and wants to be recertified	This exam has 40 multiple-choice questions. At the end of the exam, students are given an opportunity to review the questions they answered incorrectly. The computer gives feedback on incorrect answers and gives the correct answer. The printouts can be used as permanent records for CPR certification status. The test has been certified by the Long Beach California American Heart Association.	$40	Now	T.J. Designs 5905 Ironwood Ranchos Palos Verdes, CA 90274 (213) 598-1423
Health History	Mary Sizemore, RN, EdD	Apple IIe	BASIC	Beginning-level nursing students	Taking heath history, life style patterns, and review of systems (3 disks)	Exchange	Now	M. Gail Michael, RN, MN Director, Educational Media Center University of Texas at El Paso College of Nursing/Allied Health 1101 N. Campbell El Paso, TX 79902
DDST #1 & 2	Rena Brands, RN, EdD; Betty Kinsinger, RN, PhD	Apple IIe	BASIC	Beginning-level nursing students	Procedural skills of Denver Developmental Screening Test (DDST) and testing the 4-year-old child (2 disks)	Exchange	Now	M. Gail Michael, RN, MN Director, Educational Media Center University of Texas at El Paso College of Nursing/Allied Health 1101 N. Campbell El Paso, TX 79902
DDST #3	Maria Alvarez, RN, MSN	Apple IIe with interactive video (Panasonic 8200)	BASIC plus interactive video	Beginning-level nursing students	Interactive computer video of the DDST (testing the 6-month-old child)	Exchange	Now	M. Gail Michael, RN, MN Director, Educational Media Center University of Texas at El Paso College of Nursing/Allied Health 1101 N. Campbell El Paso, TX 79902

(Continued)

TABLE 15-1 *(Continued)*

TITLE	AUTHOR	COMPUTER	LANGUAGE	TARGET GROUP	SYNOPSIS	PRICE	AVAILABLE	SOURCE OF INFORMATION
Lessons on Stress	The Oregon Department of Education	Apple II+, 48K, 1 drive	PILOT	Primarily for re-entry nurses (RNs and LPNs) but not limited to this group	Four lessons on coping with stress; part 1—stress self-assessment; part 2—anxiety stress and the general adaptation syndrome; part 3—stressors; part 4—coping with stress	$40 for the package of four disks; if purchased separately; part 1, $10; part 2, $15; part 3, $15; part 4, $10.	Now	Wanda Monthey Department of Education 700 Pringle Parkway S.E. Salem, OR 97310 (503) 378-2713
Nursing Care of Patients with Diabetes Mellitus: Part I	Patricia J. Morin, RN, PhD	TRS-80	BASIC	Nursing students, diabetics, RNs	A tutorial—questions and answers on diabetes mellitus	Upon request	Now	Patricia J. Morin, RN, PhD Department of Nursing Nebraska Wesleyan University 50th and St. Paul Lincoln, NE 68504 (402) 466-9455
Spina Bifida Case Management	MGT of America, Inc.	Apple II+, 64K, VA1 interface card, 7820 videodisk player	Super-Pilot	Pediatric chronic care nurses	Approximately 10 hours of interactive instruction, that is, computer and video that focus on the case management of spina bifida. Lessons include general information, neurology, urology, orthopedics, pressure sores, etc. Package consists of 10 diskettes, 1 videodisk and a user's guide.	Pending	Pending	Jayne Parker, RN Children's Medical Services Florida Department of Health and Rehabilitative Services 1311 Winewood Boulevard Building 5, Room 140 Tallahassee, FL 32301 (904) 487-2690
Human Genetics Training for Nurses	Center for Educational Technology, Florida State University	Apple II+, 64K, VA1 interface card, 7820 videodisk player	Super-Pilot	Nurses and other health professionals	Approximately 6 hours of instruction in basic human genetics: pedigree, index of suspicion, cell reproduction, chromosome and chromosomal problems, carrier screening, prenatal diagnosis, infant screening, autosonomal dominant/recessive/sex-linked/polygenic/teratogenic disorders. Package consists of 6 diskettes, 1 videodisk, and a user's guide (with pre- and posttesting).	Pending	Pending	Jayne Parker, RN Children's Medical Services Florida Department of Health and Rehabilitative Services 1311 Winewood Boulevard Building 5, Room 140 Tallahassee, FL 32301 (904) 487-2690
Intervention in Child Abuse and Neglect	MGT of America, Inc.	Apple II+, 64K, VA1 interface card, 7820 videodisk player	Super-Pilot	Health professionals/persons who are in contact with children	Approximately 6 hours of interactive instruction, that is, computer and videodisk, which includes lessons on physical, medical, educational, and emotional neglect; failure to thrive; physical, emotional, and sexual abuse; risk factors, identification of physical indicators; interviewing, documenting and reporting in the Florida system. Package consists of 6 diskettes, 1 videodisk, and a user's guide.	Pending	Pending	Jayne Parker, RN Children's Medical Services Florida Department of Health and Rehabilitative Services 1311 Winewood Boulevard Building 5, Room 140 Tallahassee, FL 32301 (904) 487-2690

Basic Skills Nursing Entrance Test	James Black, Sarah Wick	TICCIT	TAL, (TICCIT authoring language), APT (authoring system)	1st- or 2nd-semester nursing student	Designed to evaluate basic prerequisite nursing skills of students entering the nursing program; involves medical terminology, chemistry, and math.	Public domain	Now	James Black Phoenix College 1202 West Thomas Rd. Phoenix, AZ 85013 (602) 264-2492
Primary Nursing Assistance I (Care Management)	Prof. Theresa Rothweiler, Consulting Group on Instructional Design	Apple II+, 48K, 1 drive/IBM, 64K, 1 drive/ TERAK	Pascal	Undergraduate nurses	Tutorial: a minor illness clinical encounter; data collection of health history, physical exam, lab tests; then keyword free response diagnosis and treatment followed by recap of selected treatment	Upon request	Now	Mr. Russel Burris Consulting Group on Instructional Design University of Minnesota Minneapolis, MN 55455 (612) 373-5352
An Epidemiologic Investigation of Food-Borne Outbreak of Gastroenteritis	Prof. Dorothy Donabedian, BSN, MS, MPH	ONTEL MTS/being translated for Apple II	FOIL (File-Oriented Interpretive Language)	Mainly undergraduate nursing students	A simulation using basic epidemiologic principles for problem solving	Upon request	Apple version in September 1984	Prof. Dorothy Donabedian University of Michigan School of Nursing 400 N. Ingalls Ann Arbor, MI 48109 (313) 763-3210
Infectious Syphilis: The Gift That Keeps on Giving	Prof. Dorothy Donabedian, BSN, MS, MPH	To be translated for Apple II	BASIC	Mainly undergraduate nursing students	A simulation designed to have the nurse use and interpret data about syphilis in the application of epidemiologic principles and tools	Upon request	Apple version in September 1984	Prof. Dorothy Donabedian University of Michigan School of Nursing 400 N. Ingalls Ann Arbor, MI 48109 (313) 763-3210
Role of the Community Health Nurse in the Detection and Management of Chronic Illness: The Case of Cancer of the Female Breast	Prof. Dorothy Donabedian, BSN, MS, MPH; Prof. Avedis Donabedian, MD, MPH	Apple	BASIC	Mainly undergraduate nursing students	A case study of a chronically ill patient focusing on epidemiologic concepts and principles through illustrations presented in a clinically meaningful manner	Upon request	Apple version in September 1984	Prof. Dorothy Donabedian University of Michigan School of Nursing 400 N. Ingalls Ann Arbor, MI 48109 (313) 763-3210
Dosages and Solutions	Nursing Department Ocean County College	UNIVAC	COBOL	Beginning-level nursing students	A tutorial on mathematical concepts as they relate to medication dosages	Upon request	Now	Debbie W. Fuller, RN, MA Ocean County College College Drive Tom's River, NJ 08753 (201) 255-4000, x280
Drug Calculation	Barbara Lease, PhD; Maisie Kashka, RN, MN; Cheryl Ratliff, RN, MA	Apple II+, IIe, 1 drive, 48K	BASIC	Basic nursing students	A five-module set tutorial for junior nursing students that has a basic math review, content on oral medications, solutions, and parenteral medications	$100 per module if purchased separately, or $450 for five-module set	Now	Dr. Barbara Lease Computer Educational Resources 2705 N. Bell Ave. Denton, TX 76201 or call, Louise Chamberlain (816) 753-3730

(Continued)

TABLE 15-1 *(Continued)*

TITLE	AUTHOR	COMPUTER	LANGUAGE	TARGET GROUP	SYNOPSIS	PRICE	AVAILABLE	SOURCE OF INFORMATION
Metric I, II, III	Audree Reynolds, RN, MN	Apple IIe	BASIC	Beginning-level nursing students	A complete series of math tutorials on metric dosage calculations, apothecary to metric, and IV dosage calculations (3 disks)	Exchange	Now	M. Gail Michael, RN, MN Director, Educational Media Center University of Texas at El Paso College of Nursing/Allied Health 1101 N. Campbell El Paso, TX 79902
PROBS SET I, II	Audree Reynolds, RN, MN	Apple IIe	BASIC	Beginning-level nursing students	Practice problems on drug calculations	Exchange	Now	M. Gail Michael, RN, MN Director, Educational Media Center University of Texas at El Paso College of Nursing/Allied Health 1101 N. Campbell El Paso, TX 79902
FEABI	Audree Reynolds, RN, MN	Intecolor only (soon to be on Apple)	BASIC	Beginning-level nursing students	Clinical situations on fluid/electrolyte imbalance	Exchange	Now	M. Gail Michael, RN, MN Director, Educational Media Center University of Texas at El Paso College of Nursing/Allied Health 1101 N. Campbell El Paso, TX 79902
MISTY	Audree Reynolds, RN, MN	Apple IIe	BASIC	Beginning-level nursing students	Clinical situations on respiratory insufficiency	Exchange	Now	M. Gail Michael, RN, MN Director, Educational Media Center University of Texas at El Paso College of Nursing/Allied Health 1101 N. Campbell El Paso, TX 79902
Nasogastric Suction	Kathy Accola, MSN; Joan Stenberg	Apple II+, IIe, 48K, 1 drive	BASIC	Nursing students and nurses involved in continuing education	Two short patient care problem-solving simulations on nasogastric suction	Upon request	Pending	Kathy Accola, MSN School of Nursing University of Minnesota 308 Harvard St. 5-140, Unit F Minneapolis, MN 55455 (612) 373-7723

Chest Suction	Kathy Accola, MSN	Apple II+, IIe, 48K, 1 drive	BASIC	Nursing students and nurses involved in continuing education	Two short patient care problem-solving simulations on chest suction	Upon request	Pending	Kathy Accola, MSN School of Nursing University of Minnesota 308 Harvard St. 5-140, Unit F Minneapolis, MN 55455 (612) 373-7723
Sugar	Kathy Accola, MSN	Apple II+, IIe, 48K, 1 drive	BASIC	Nursing students and nurses involved in continuing education	Designed to help students identify symptoms of hyperglycemia and hypoglycemia	Upon request	Pending	Kathy Accola, MSN School of Nursing University of Minnesota 308 Harvard St. 5-140, Unit F Minneapolis, MN 55455 (612) 373-7723
Pre-Lab Testing	James Black, Sarah Wick	TICCIT	TAL (TICCIT authoring language), APT (authoring system)	1st- or 2nd-semester nursing students	A test of 30 pre-lab nursing tests	Public domain	Now	James Black Phoenix College 1202 West Thomas Rd. Phoenix, AZ 85013 (602) 264-2492
TESTSTAR	Lynda Joseph, RN, MSN; Allen Joseph, MBA	IBM PC, 64K, 1 disk drive or IBM compatibles/ Apple II+, Apple IIe, 48K, 1 disk drive or Apple compatibles/ TRS-80 Model III and IV, 48K, 1 disk drive	Compiled BASIC	Nursing, medical, dental, and veterinary schools, professional schools, hospitals, law schools, business schools, allied health sciences programs, colleges and universities, and high schools	A microcomputer program that assists faculty in constructing objective multiple-choice tests. It is an interactive, easy-to-use test authoring system that requires no knowledge of programming. Allows faculty to design tests based on their own criteria and objectives. Allows both drill and practice tests and assessment tests. Drill and practice examinations provide immediate stimulus response feedback to reinforce learning. Assessment tests allow the student to complete the test first and then receive computer-scored detailed analysis of performance. Rationales for correct answers and explanations for incorrect answers may also be included. Allows the use of case studies and clinical situations along with multiple-choice questions to test areas of knowledge, comprehension, application of principles skills, and analytical thinking. Will assist faculty in improving teaching strategies, revising curricula and testing. It simplifies the clerical tasks involved in preparing and revising tests. It also allows for more frequent testing.	$595 U.S.	Now	Mosby Software Division C.V. Mosby 11830 Westline Industrial Drive St. Louis, MO 63146 1-800-325-4177 MOSBYSYSTEMS provides a HOT-LINE troubleshooting service to answer all questions: 1-800-325-4177, ext. 750 (9–5 Central Time, M–F) In Missouri, call collect (314) 872-8370, ext. 452

(Continued)

TABLE 15-1 *(Continued)*

TITLE	AUTHOR	COMPUTER	LANGUAGE	TARGET GROUP	SYNOPSIS	PRICE	AVAILABLE	SOURCE OF INFORMATION
ADMINISTAR	Mosby/ENI	Apple II+, Apple IIe, 64K, printer necessary for reporting	BASIC	Educational institutions	A sorting/filing/tracking/reporting system designed for educational institutions and hospitals. It is a self-contained program that sorts, counts, and reports information from just one program. It is preformatted for nursing schools and reports in accordance with NLN requirements. Is fully editable and can be used by any school or program to report information. It allows 10 different categories and 12 different fields of information on each subject. ADMINISTAR also prints mailing labels and automatically initializes additional blank disks for unlimited storage of data.	$495 U.S.	Now	Mosby Softward Division C.V. Mosby 11830 Westline Industrial Drive St. Louis, MO 63146 1-800-325-4177 MOSBYSYSTEMS provides a HOT-LINE troubleshooting service to answer all questions: 1-800-325-4177, ext. 750 (9–5 Central Time, M–F) In Missouri, call collect (314) 872-8370, ext. 452
MONA (MOdular Nursing Administration)	Resource Group, Inc.	IBM PC, Northstar Horizon or Advantage, DEC Rainbow, plus others that use the operating systems listed to the right under Language. Minimum 5 MB (megabyte) hard disk on any of the above systems. Is network compatible.	dBase II, BASIC, and some assembly	Nursing administration	The system is designed to be purchased as individual programs or as a comprehensive package. Includes (1) management functions, such as tracking license expirations, overtime and sick time reports, and performance measurement tools and statistics; (2) quality assurance functions; (3) time management and action items, listed by due dates, priority, and person responsible. The package will soon include scheduling by preference and staffing by acuity. It offers the flexibility of user-defined databases, forms generation, policies and procedures, budgeting, electronic mail, and spreadsheets.	Upon request	Now	Resource Group, Inc. 5850 Avenida Encinas Carlsbad, CA 92008 (619) 438-3136
Computer Simulations in Clinical Nursing	Nancy Ann Corbett, RN, MEd; Phyllis Beveridge, RN, MEd	Apple II+, 48K, Apple IIe, one disk drive	Apple Pilot	Upper-level nursing students in a baccalaureate program	Provides critical decision-making practice in six simulated patient care settings, each covering different areas where students will find help in evaluating and improving their skills.	$495 for seven disks. 160-page workbook, disk folder	Now	W.B. Saunders West Washington Square Philadelphia, PA 19105 215-574-3376

Case #1: Mr. Jones: A Businessman With Indigestion	Knowledge of pathophysiology, risk factors, and symptoms of myocardial infarction; prehospital management of probable MI; factors increasing cardiac workload; how to provide emergency care; and understanding the role of the industrial nurse.
Case #2: Mr. Richardson: A Man With Newly Diagnosed Diabetes	How to evaulate patient's understanding of a treatment regimen; pathophysiology of diabetes mellitus and the general principles of its medical and nursing management; causes, symptoms, and management of hypoglycemia; developmental tasks of young adults; reaction to illness; and dietary management of diabetes
Case #3: Mrs. Shikraut: An Uncomfortable, Terminal Patient	Knowledge of hydration; urinary retention; assement and management of pain; immobility; and physical assessment (core of the program, since the patient does not speak English)
Case #4: Mrs. Gates: An Elderly Woman Experiencing Her First Hospitalization	Understanding the developmental tasks and physiologic and mental changes of aging; supporting ego integrity; recognizing responses to illness and hospitalization; utilizing communication techniques; recognizing sensory deprivation; and instituting home safety for the elderly
Case #5: Mrs. Simms: A Woman Scheduled for Hemorrhoidectomy	Knowledge of pre-operative teaching and post-operative care; individualizing pain management; providing for urinary elimination; understanding the hemorrhoidectomy procedure dealing with an uncooperative patient; mobility; and discharge planning
Case #6: Mr. Merra: A Patient With Liver Disease	Pathophysiology and medical and nursing management of hepatic encephalopathy secondary to liver disease; alcoholism; alcohol withdrawal — symptoms and management; crisis intervention; and response of the patient's family to alcoholism

(Continued)

TABLE 15-1 (Continued)

TITLE	AUTHOR	COMPUTER	LANGUAGE	TARGET GROUP	SYNOPSIS	PRICE	AVAILABLE	SOURCE OF INFORMATION
Drug Interactions	Mark Dambro, MD; H. Winter Griffith, MD	Apple II+, 48K, Apple IIe, 1 disk drive. Soon to be available for IBM PC	BASIC	Any health professional who deals with prescription drugs	Provides physicians, health care professionals, and students in health care with a quick reference to significant food and drug interactions. The database contains 350 generic drugs and 1400 brand-name drugs and their components. The program will locate all clinically significant interactions among them. All the user needs to do is to type the names or part of the names of two drugs and their interactions will appear on the screen with a statement of the level of clinical significance and a literature reference. It will also locate all interactions for a single drug.	$149 for one disk and user manual	Now	W.B. Saunders Company West Washington Square Philadelphia, PA 19105 215-574-3376
Fundamentals of Nursing Theory	Upgrade Unlimited, Inc.	Monroe EC 8800/IBM PC version available soon	Monroe Extended BASIC/MS-DOS version available soon	ADN students	A complete course for beginning students covering basic concepts, introduction to nursing process, basic interventions that are primarily nursing's responsibility, analysis of situational problems, and appropriate decision-making processes.	Upon request	Now	Upgrade Unlimited Inc. 28 Riverview Drive Tinton Falls, NJ 07724 201-741-0855
Recommended Staffing	Mary McAlindon, RN	Tektronics 4052 (being adapted for IBM PC XT)	C BASIC on Tektronics (will be in Pascal for IBM PC XT)	Nursing administrators	Units send total of their categories to be input into this program. At the beginning of each shift, a recommended staffing report is generated.	Upon request	Now	Mary McAlindon, RN McLaren General Hospital 401 South Ballenger Highway Flint, MI
Daily Report	Mary McAlindon, RN	Tektronics 4052 (being adapted for IBM PC XT)	C BASIC on Tektronics (will be in Pascal for IBM PC XT)	Nursing administrators	Generated weekly, it is the staffing that actually worked a unit. Compares all units	Upon request	Now	Mary McAlindon, RN McLaren General Hospital 401 South Ballenger Highway Flint, MI
Weekly Summary	Mary McAlindon, RN	Tektronics 4052 (being adapted for IBM PC XT)	C BASIC on Tektronics (will be in Pascal for IBM PC XT)	Nursing administrators	A summary of each day of the week generated from the weekly report (staffing report per unit by week)	Upon request	Now	Mary McAlindon, RN McLaren General Hospital 401 South Ballenger Highway Flint, MI
Payperiod Report for Each Unit	Mary McAlindon, RN	Tektronics 4052 (being adapted for IBM PC XT)	C BASIC on Tektronics (will be in Pascal for IBM PC XT)	Nursing administrators	Individual unit pay report for a 14-day period. Provides capacity and staffing by day of the week and shift	Upon request	Now	Mary McAlindon, RN McLaren General Hospital 401 South Ballenger Highway Flint, MI

Payperiod Summary	Mary McAlindon, RN	Tektronics 4052 (being adapted for IBM PC XT)	C BASIC on Tektronics (will be in Pascal for IBM PC XT)	Nursing administrators	A pay report for all units on one sheet for comparison purposes	Upon request	Now	Mary McAlindon, RN McLaren General Hospital 401 South Ballenger Highway Flint, MI
Quarterly	Mary McAlindon, RN	Tektronics 4052 (being adapted for IBM PC XT)	C BASIC on Tektronics (will be in Pascal for IBM PC XT)	Nursing administrators	Provides quarterly capacity and staffing, by unit with all units combined, by medical–surgical units combined, etc.	Upon request	In progress	Mary McAlindon, RN McLaren General Hospital 401 South Ballenger Highway Flint, MI
Shock	Virginia Nixon, RN, MN	Apple IIe, Apple II+, 48K, 1 disk drive	Apple Soft, BASIC	3rd- to 4th-year nursing students		$900 for package	Now	MEDI-SIM, INC. P.O. Box 13267 Edwardsville, KS 66113 (913) 441-2881
Module I: Pathophysiology of Shock					Provides an introduction to the major concepts of physiological alterations occurring in shock. It also provides a review of major system responses to shock.			
Module II: Types of Shock					Presents a comparison of cardiogenic, hypovolemic, neurogenic, sepatictic, and anaphylactic shock			
Module III: Assessment of Shock					Learner is presented with the major parameters for initial and ongoing patient assessment			
Module IV: Pharmacologic Aspects of Shock					Presents major pharmacologic approaches to the treatment of the patient in shock			
Module V: Complications of Shock					Provides an introduction to the potential complications of adult respiratory distress syndrome, disseminated intravascular coagulation, and acute tubular necrosis			
The Nursing Process	Virginia Nixon, RN, MN; Norma Lewis, RN, MSN	Apple IIe, Apple II+, 48K, 1 disk drive	Apple Soft, BASIC	3rd- to 4th-year nursing students		$900 for package	Now	MEDI-SIM INC. P.O. Box 13267 Edwardsville, KS 66113 (913) 441-2881
Module I: An introduction to the Nursing Process					Introduces the learner to the theory, purpose, and characteristics of the nursing process			
Module II: Components of Assessment					Learner deals with the three components of the assessment process; health history, organization of data, and nursing diagnoses are covered.			
Module III: Planning Goals and Actions					Involves continuing priority setting, writing client care goals, and planning nursing actions. The process of writing measurable goals is incorporated.			

(Continued)

TABLE 15-1 *(Continued)*

TITLE	AUTHOR	COMPUTER	LANGUAGE	TARGET GROUP	SYNOPSIS	PRICE	AVAILABLE	SOURCE OF INFORMATION
Module IV: Plan Implementation					The learner deals with validating the care plan, implementing the plan, and continuing data collection.			
Module V: Goal Evaluation					The learner is involved with a simulation to evaluate goal achievement and reassessment of the plan of care.			
Pediatric Cardiovascular	Terry Buford, RN, MSN	Apple IIe, Apple II+, 48K, 1 disk drive	Apple Soft, BASIC	3rd- to 4th-year nursing students		$900 for package	Now	MEDI-SIM INC. P.O. Box 13267 Edwardsville, KS 66113 (913) 441-2881
Module I: Assessment:					Involves admission assessment of the child with suspected tetralogy of Fallot, including evaluation, health history, risk factors, physical signs and symptoms, and laboratory results in comparison to those expected to accompany the pathophysiology			
Module II: Pre- and Postcatheterization					Involves the learner in decision making about precatheterization teaching and preparation as well as postcatheterization monitoring. Specific complications covered include arrythmias and cardiopulmonary arrest.			
Module III: The Critical Perioperative Period					The learner is exposed to nursing care in the immediate pre- and postoperative period. Included are questions about preoperative teaching and nursing care during the initial 24 to 48 hours after complete repair of tetralogy of Fallot.			
Module IV: Convalescent and Rehabilitative Care					The learner has an opportunity to apply knowledge about the care of a patient with repaired tetralogy of Fallot during the 3rd to 10th postoperative days. Included are assessment of longer term complications and discharge planning.			
Module V: Pharmacology					A comprehensive-level review of drug therapy frequently used with pediatric cardiac patients. Specific groups include digoxin, diuretics, antiarrythmics, vasopressors, and antibiotics.			

Myocardial Infarction	Evelyn Hutchinson, RN, MN	Apple IIe, Apple II+, 48K, 1 disk drive	Apple Soft, BASIC	3rd- to 4th-year nursing students		$720 for package	Now	MEDI-SIM INC. P.O. Box 13267 Edwardsville, KS 66113 (913) 441-2881
Module I: Pathophysiology of Myocardial Infarction					Deals with the pathophysiology of myocardial infarction. It includes the importance of atherosclerosis in the development of coronary artery disease and the risk factors involved.			
Module II: Diagnosis of Myocardial Infarction					Presents the common examinations used to diagnose myocardial infarction including electrocardiograms and enzyme changes			
Module III: Immediate Care					The learner deals with the acute care of the myocardial infarction patient. Included are the importance of ECG monitoring and pharmacologic agents used in the treatment of the myocardial infarction patient.			
Module IV: Long-Term Care					Presents the post-acute and rehabilitative care of the myocardial infarction patient. It includes the importance of patient education.			
Trouble Shooting The Pulmonary Artery Catheter	Anthony F. Morton, RN	Commodore 64	Not provided	Hospital nurses	The user is guided through solving four of the most common PA catheter malfunctions.	Available on cassette only. $2 to cover cost of cassette and mailing	Now	Anthony F. Morton, RN 316 Grandview Circle Muskogee, OK 74403
Rhythm ID	Anthony F. Morton, RN	Commodore 64	Not provided	Hospital nurses	A cardiac rhythm is identified by the computer after the user answers eight questions. This program is useful in ICU training or as an aid to the practitioner in decision making.	Available only on cassette. $2 to cover cost of cassette and mailing	Now	Anthony F. Morton, RN 316 Grandview Circle Muskogee, OK 74403
Nursing Pharmacology	Anthony F. Morton, RN	Commodore 64	Not provided	Hospital nurses (especially bedside nurses)	The compatibility or incompatibility of two frequently prescribed medications is found by simply entering the generic names of the drugs in question. The program also contains a listing of all names of a number of frequently prescribed medications. There is a section on drug mathematics: determining drug dosages, metric conversion, milligram/kilogram/time infusion rates and more.	Available only on cassette. $2 to cover cost of cassette and mailing	January 1984	Anthony F. Morton, RN 316 Grandview Circle Muskogee, OK 74403

(Continued)

TABLE 15-1 *(Continued)*

TITLE	AUTHOR	COMPUTER	LANGUAGE	TARGET GROUP	SYNOPSIS	PRICE	AVAILABLE	SOURCE OF INFORMATION
NURSESTAR (Institutional Version)	Lynda Joseph, RN, MSN; Allen Joseph, MBA	IBM PC, 64K, 1 disk drive or IBM PC compatibles, Apple II+, Apple IIe, 48K, 1 disk drive or Apple compatibles/TRS-80 Model III and IV, 48K, 1 disk drive	Compiled BASIC for appropriate computer	Senior nursing students and institutions	A 360-question exam formatted to test basic level of nursing knowledge. It follows the exact format of the licensure exam for nursing (NCLEX). The presentation is three 120-question tests using multiple-choice questions. Groups of questions are linked to case studies. The test taker is allowed to stop or take a break after any sequence of case studies or after every 30 questions. After 30 questions, a cumulative score is given. The test is constructed to give immediate feedback after each question or it will store the feedback until the end of the test. NURSESTAR allows multiple students to take the test and will provide individual and group scores, mean scores, and storage. Each question provides detailed rationales for the correct answers and explanations for incorrect answers. Each question is coded to the specific type of category it is intended to test (nursing behaviors, cognitive level, locus of decision making, and clinical areas).	$49 U.S. (prices in the U.S. are subject to change)	Now	Mosby Software Division C.V. Mosby 11830 Westline Industrial Drive St. Louis, MO 63146 1-800-325-4177 MOSBYSYSTEMS provides a HOT-LINE troubleshooting service to answer all questions: 1-800-325-4177, ext. 750 (9–5 Central Time, M–F) In Missouri, call collect (314) 872-8370, ext. 452
NURSESTAR (Student Version)	Lynda Joseph, RN, MSN; Allen Joseph, MBA	IBM PC, 64K, 1 disk drive or IBM PC compatibles/Apple II+, Apple IIe, 48K, 1 disk drive or Apple compatibles/TRS-80 Model III and IV, 64K, 1 disk drive	Compiled BASIC for appropriate computer	Senior nursing students and institutions	A simulated exam that reviews basic nursing knowledge, formatted to follow the NCLEX test blueprint. It is meant to be a practice/review for the actual licensure exam nurses must pass to practice. The student version will consist of four 30-question tests. The test taker chooses to receive either immediate feedback after answering a question (drill and practice), or else the program will store the student's answers until the end of each 30-question segment before giving a score (assessment). Only one student can take this exam.	$59.95 U.S.	Now	Mosby Software Division C.V. Mosby 11830 Westline Industrial Drive St. Louis, MO 63146 1-800-325-4177 MOSBYSYSTEMS provides a HOT-LINE troubleshooting service to answer all questions: 1-800-325-4177, ext. 750 (9–5 Central Time, M–F) In Missouri, call collect (314) 872-8370, ext. 452

Computerized Nursing Skills Simulation	Donna Larson, RN, PhD	Apple II+, 64K/Apple IIe/IBM PC	Apple Soft, BASIC	Beginning-level nursing students	Each of these programs allows the student to practice the skills required to accurately perform the covered procedures. The computer responds directly to the student's actions by evaluating them and providing help as needed. The student interacts with animated computer graphics, for example, IV drip chambers, to actually set the flow to the rate which the student has calculated, and sphygmomanometers to identify blood pressure sounds in mmHg.	$975 five programs, two disks each or $240 per program	Now	J.B. Lippincott Company East Washington Square Philadelphia, PA 19105 1-800-523-2945 (In PA, call collect 215-574-4443)
Calculating and Preparing Fractional Medication Dosages for Injection					A computer simulation and tutorial that assists students to calculate fractional medication dosages correctly and then to prepare these medications for injection by combining volumes in a single syringe. Throughout the program, immediate feedback is provided to the student concerning both accuracy and technique.			
Calculating and Adjusting IV Flow Rates					Presents the student with a situation in which a patient is to receive IV therapy. The student is guided through three interrelated calculations: flow rate per hour, flow rate per minute, and drops per minute. A simulated IV drip chamber appears on the screen. Drops are "infused" into the patient via animated graphics in real-time. By pressing keys on the keyboard, the student increases or slows the simulated drip rate to correspond to the calculated drip rate.			
Taking a Blood Pressure		Tape recorder for audio cassette needed			Using animated graphics and recorded Korotkoff sounds, the computer simulates taking a blood pressure. While the tape-recorded blood pressure sounds are played, the student notes the mercury level on the sphygmomanometer at which the three most significant blood pressure sounds are heard. The program verifies the accuracy of the student's readings and provides appropriate feedback.			

(Continued)

TABLE 15-1 *(Continued)*

TITLE	AUTHOR	COMPUTER	LANGUAGE	TARGET GROUP	SYNOPSIS	PRICE	AVAILABLE	SOURCE OF INFORMATION
Preparing Insulins for Injection					Presents the student with a patient who is to receive a mixture of two types of insulin. The two multi-dose insulin vials and a calibrated insulin syringe appear on the screen. The program guides the student through the steps to preparing the doses for injection. The student uses the computer keys to control the syringe plunger to draw up the required units of insulin, combining the volumes to administer in one syringe.			
Testing Urine for Sugar and Ketones					Guides the student through any one of a number of simulated urine tests for sugar and ketones. As the student conducts the test, the color of the "sample" changes. The student makes a judgment of the urine sugar and ketone concentration by comparing the color scale with the "urine sample" being tested. The program verifies the student's accuracy and prompts the student when appropriate.			
LITMAS	Eric Sohr, MD	Apple II+, 48K or Apple IIe, 2 drives	Machine language	Serious collectors of any data	This program is a rapid cross-indexing system. The user describes 512 keywords with up to 2048 synonyms to be used in indexing materials, such as journal articles or patients. More than 500 indexed items can be filed on a floppy disk. Items are searched using synonyms and the set operations, AND, OR and NOT. Changes, deletions, and additions to the data file are quick and straightforward. A text-editor is provided for entering descriptions of indexed items and for entering search requests.	$145	Now	Literature Manipulation Systems Worden, Montana 59088 (*Editor's note:* in a town as small as Worden, the above address is sufficient)
Infection Control, Including Handwashing and Gowning Techniques	Shirley Steele, RN, PhD; Helen Ptak, RN, PhD	Apple II+, 48K/Apple IIe, 1 drive	Apple Pilot, Apple, Super-Pilot	Beginning students, ADN, BSN, in-service LVNs	Basic infection control techniques. Role of infection control nurse. Handwashing principles. Gowning principles. Communicable disease and immunizations. Individualized periodic testing	$89.95	Now	Heshi Computing 17 Cedar Lawn Galveston, TX 77550
Accident Prevention	Shirley Steele, RN, PhD; Helen Ptak, RN, PhD	Apple II+, 48K/Apple IIe, 1 drive	Apple Pilot, Apple, Super-Pilot	Beginning students, ADN, BSN, client education	Accident prevention by age. Major categories of accidents by age. Accident prevention in the hospital. Individualized periodic testing	$59.95	Now	Heshi Computing 17 Cedar Lawn Galveston, TX 77550

Healthy Living	Shirley Steele, RN, PhD; Helen Ptak, RN, PhD	Apple II+, 48K/Apple IIe, 1 drive	Apple Pilot, Apple, Super-Pilot	Beginning students, ADN, BSN, client education	Risk factor determination. Ways to stay healthy. Individualized periodic testing	$59.95	Now	Heshi Computing 17 Cedar Lawn Galveston, TX 77550
Statistical Concepts	Shirley Steele, RN, PhD; Helen Ptak, RN, PhD	Apple II+, 48K/Apple IIe, 1 drive	Apple Pilot, Apple, Super-Pilot	Beginning students, BSN, remedial MSN students	Basic statistical concepts related to research design. Examples of application of statistics. Individualized periodic testing	$250	February 1984	Heshi Computing 17 Cedar Lawn Galveston, TX 77550
Test Construction	Shirley Steele, RN, PhD; Helen Ptak, RN, PhD	Apple II+, 48K/Apple IIe, 1 drive	Apple Pilot, Apple, Super-Pilot	Graduate students, in-service staff development, nursing faculty	Types of test questions. Analysis of test data. Norm-referenced against criterion-referenced testing. Individualized periodic testing	$175	April 1984	Heshi Computing 17 Cedar Lawn Galveston, TX 77550
Research Methodology	Shirley Steele, RN, PhD; Helen Ptak, RN, PhD	Apple II+, 48K/Apple IIe, 1 drive	Apple Pilot, Apple, Super-Pilot	BSN students, remedial MSN students	Basic research design and concepts. Steps of research process. Examples of application to clinical settings. Individualized periodic testing	$400	August 1984	Heshi Computing 17 Cedar Lawn Galveston, TX 77550
Injection Site Selection Drill	Linda Jelemensky, RN, PhD	TRS-80 Model I and III, 2 drives/ Apple II, 2 drives/IBM PC, 2 drives	Micro Soft, BASIC	Nursing students, nurse educators, in-service educators	Provides type of injection and requires student to enter injection site. Feedback indicates correct or incorrect response, and after the second incorrect attempt proceeds to next question.	Upon request	Now	Linda Jelemensky, RN, PhD 7312 Hartnell Drive Austin, TX 78723 (512) 928-2614
Injection Quiz	Linda Jelemensky, RN, PhD	TRS-80 Model I and II, 2 drives/ Apple II, 2 drives/IBM PC, 2 drives	Micro Soft, BASIC	Nursing students, nurse educators, in-service educators	Presents a scenario in which the student is given a client description, and order and type of injection. The student then is required to provide injection site. Calculates number of incorrect and correct responses.	Upon request	Now	Linda Jelemensky, RN, PhD 7312 Hartnell Drive Austin, TX 78723 (512) 928-2614
Equipment Selection	Linda Jelemensky, 1 N, PhD	TRS-80 Model I and II, 2 drives/ Apple II, 2 drives/IBM PC, 2 drives	Micro Soft, BASIC	Nursing students, nurse educators, in-service educators	Provides medication, dosage, amount of medicine available, and type of injection, and the student is required to give gauge and length of the needle, size of syringe, and alternate syringe. Calculates number of incorrect and correct responses. The program also provides hints if question is answered incorrectly on the first try.	Upon request	Now	Linda Jelemensky, RN, PhD 7312 Hartnell Drive Austin, TX 78723 (512) 928-2614
Dosage Calculation Exercise	Linda Jelemensky, RN, PhD	TRS-80 Model I and II, 2 drives/ Apple II, 2 drives/IBM PC, 2 drives	Micro Soft, BASIC	Nursing students, nurse educators, in-service educators	Provides medication ordered, amount ordered, frequency of administration, and amount of medication available. The student is then required to enter the correct dosage to be given. The correct solution is presented after the second incorrect response. Calculates percentage of incorrect and correct responses.	Upon request	Now	Linda Jelemensky, RN, PhD 7312 Hartnell Drive Austin, TX 78723 (512) 928-2614

(Continued)

TABLE 15-1 *(Continued)*

TITLE	AUTHOR	COMPUTER	LANGUAGE	TARGET GROUP	SYNOPSIS	PRICE	AVAILABLE	SOURCE OF INFORMATION
Calculate With Care	Helen Ferguson, EdD	Apple II+, 64K/Apple II, 1 drive/ IBM PC	Apple Soft, BASIC	Beginning-level nursing students	A comprehensive, self-study tutorial program using real life practice problems. It emphasizes instruction—"how to do it"— rather than explanations. All instructions are presented in clear, consise English. The program covers fractions, decimals, percentages, Roman numerals, ratio and proportion, systems of measurement, and problem solving. A diagnostic pretest and posttest for self-testing are included. Users learn independently at their own pace. There are six instructional programs on 12 disks.	$975 per set only	Now	J.B. Lippincott Company East Washington Square Philadelphia, PA 19105 1-800-523-2945 (In PA, call collect (215) 574-4443)
Fractions (Parts 1, 2, and 3)					Terms of a fraction and their meaning; comparing value of fractions; knowing whether a fraction is proper, improper or complex; reducing fractions to their lowest terms; converting whole or mixed number to improper fractions and vice versa; adding, subtracting, multiplying using cross cancellation, and dividing			
Decimals (Parts 1 and 2)					Reading decimals; comparing value; adding, subtracting, multiplying, dividing; converting decimals to fractions and converting fractions to decimals			
Percentages (Parts 1 and 2)					Comparing value; converting percentages to fractions and vice versa; converting percentages to decimals and decimals to percentages; finding what percentage one number is of another; and finding the given percentage of a number			
Roman Numerals					Symbols basic to the Roman system; translating Roman numerals to Arabic numerals; and writing Roman numerals			
Ratio and Proportion					Definition and use of ratio; use of ratio to express medication strength where amount is not important; comparing value; converting ratios to fractions; percents and decimals; using ratios to express amount per quantity; and using proportion to solve dosage problems when what's ordered doesn't match what's on hand			

Systems of Measurement					Recognizing each of the three systems of measurement; recognizing whether it's a solid or liquid unit of measurement; understanding the major relationships within a system; understanding the major relationships among the three systems; and using proportions to convert from one system to another			
Problem Solving (Parts 1 and 2)					Solving problems requiring both system-to-system conversions and ordered versus on-hand proportions; mixing powdered medications; calculating the amount of medication needed to last a specific amount of time and vice versa; calculating pediatric dosages involving pound/kilogram conversion; and calculating intravenous flow rate			
Care of the Pediatric Client With a Head Injury	Edith Hamilton, RN, MSN; Janet Vincent, RN, MN	Apple II+, 64K, Apple IIe	Apple, Super-Pilot	Undergraduate nurses	A simulation in which the student is presented with a series of situations that require application of the nursing process from admission to discharge. The student is required to make judgments of care based on knowledge of pathophysiology, pharmacology, development levels, communication skills, and nursing care principles.	Upon request	Spring 1984	Edith M. Hamilton, RN, MSN School of Nursing 526ET University of Kansas College of Health Sciences 39th and Rainbow Blvd. Kansas City, KS 66103 (913) 588-1660 or (913) 888-7030
Care of the Patient With Diabetes Mellitus	Edith Hamilton, RN, MSN; Ann Hess, RN, MS	Apple II+, 64K, Apple IIe	Apple, Super-Pilot	Undergraduate nurses	In this simulation, the student must apply knowledge to (1) identify patient priorities of care—both during the acute phase in the ICU and on the patient unit prior to discharge; (2) identify appropriate nursing intervention; (3) relate changes in blood glucose levels to alterations in insulin dosage, dietary intake, and patient activity levels; and (4) select the correct action of NPH and regular insulin. Finally, patient education and discharge needs are identified based on this patient's data.	$48	Now	Edith M. Hamilton, RN, MSN School of Nursing 526 ET University of Kansas College of Health Sciences 39th and Rainbow Blvd. Kansas City, KS 66103 (913) 588-1660 or (913) 888-7030
Care of Patients Requiring Isolation	Edith Hamilton, RN, MSN; Ann Hess, RN, MS	Apple II+, Apple IIe	Apple Soft, BASIC	Undergraduate nurses	In a series of four simulations, the student is required to make judgments about how the care of the simulated patients should be organized to prevent the spread of pathogenic organisms.	Upon request	Spring 1984	Edith M. Hamilton, RN, MSN School of Nursing 526 ET University of Kansas College of Health Sciences 39th and Rainbow Blvd. Kansas City, KS 66103 (913) 588-1660 or (913) 888-7030

(Continued)

TABLE 15-1 *(Continued)*

TITLE	AUTHOR	COMPUTER	LANGUAGE	TARGET GROUP	SYNOPSIS	PRICE	AVAILABLE	SOURCE OF INFORMATION
Care of the Perioperative Patient	Edith Hamilton, RN, MSN; Ann Hess, RN, MS	Apple II+, Apple IIe	Apple Soft, BASIC	Undergraduate nurses	This program (1) provides the student nurse with a review of those relevant concepts from past courses that apply directly to the care of the perioperative patient and (2) provides the student with an introduction to new concepts necessary to function in the roles of scrub and circulating nurse.	Upon request	Spring 1984	Edith M. Hamilton, RN, MSN School of Nursing 526 ET University of Kansas College of Health Sciences 39th and Rainbow Blvd. Kansas City, KS 66103 (913) 588-1660 or (913) 888-7030
Drug Proficiency Examination	Edith Hamilton, RN, MSN	Apple II+, Apple IIe	Apple Soft, BASIC	Undergraduate students	Questions can be randomly selected from a pool of 150 questions representing five content areas. Student information (name, score, questions missed) is saved on disk for the instructor.	Upon request	Spring 1984	Edith M. Hamilton, RN, MSN School of Nursing 526 ET University of Kansas College of Health Sciences 39th and Rainbow Blvd. Kansas City, KS 66103 (913) 588-1660 or (913) 888-7030
Medical Terminology	Ruth Edwards, RN; Joanne Kersten, RN	Apple II+, 48K, 1 disk drive	Apple soft, BASIC	Beginning nursing students or prenursing students	An individualized posttest producing a score.	Exchange	Now	Edith M. Hamilton, RN, MSN School of Nursing 526 ET University of Kansas College of Health Sciences 39th and Rainbow Blvd. Kansas City, KS 66103 (913) 588-1660 or (913) 888-7030
Medical Terminology Examination	Edith Hamilton, RN, MSN; Jeanne Johnson, RN, MS	Apple II+, Apple IIe	Apple Soft, BASIC	Undergraduate students	This program will generate a series of four tests, each consisting of questions randomly selected from a pool of 100 questions. The student must type in the word answer. Student information (name, score, questions missed) is saved on the disk for the instructor.	Upon request	January 1984	Edith M. Hamilton, RN, MSN School of Nursing 526 ET University of Kansas College of Health Sciences 39th and Rainbow Blvd. Kansas City, KS 66103 (913) 588-1660 or (913) 888-7030
Food and Nutrition	Shirley Steele, RN, PhD; Helen Ptak, RN, PhD	Apple II+, 48K/Apple IIe, 1 drive	Apple Pilot, Apple, Super-Pilot	Beginning students, ADN, BSN	Basic four food groups. Food requirement by age. Assessment of food requirements. Nutrients in foods. Individualized periodic testing	$69.95	Now	Heshi Computing 17 Cedar Lawn Galveston, TX 77550
Wellness–Illness Continuum	Shirley Steele, RN, PhD; Helen Ptak, RN, PhD	Apple II+, 48K/Apple IIe, 1 drive	Apple Pilot, Apple, Super-Pilot	Beginning students, ADN, BSN, Client education	Wellness–illness continuum and concepts. Risk factor identification. Individualized periodic testing.	$69.95	Now	Heshi Computing 17 Cedar Lawn Galveston, TX 77550

(Hales G [ed]: Computers in Nursing. Philadelphia, JB Lippincott, 1983)

Through the computer program, the student then receives a copy of the raw scores of the experiment and a summary of the statistical analysis of the data. The student therefore has a simulated learning experience of the research process (Newman and O'Brien, 1978).

LESS. An updated version of MESS, called LESS (Louisville Experiment Simulation Systems), is a program that allows the author to develop a model for research with more relevance to the theoretical foundations of nursing. It allows the faculty to introduce "new" research models within the design by specifying dependent variables, manipulating variables, and including unknown variables. The student then can specify the range of values, the type of data for each of the variables, and a weighting score for each variable (Newman and O'Brien, 1978).

• • •

Although the research simulation process on computers offers several advantages, no statistically significant differences appear between students who learn from computers and those who learn through the traditional research course. Table 15-3 lists five advantages of computer simulation used in teaching the research process. Most noteworthy was the positive value that students had for the research process after completing two required experimental designs and analysis on the computer during a semester (Newman and O'Brien, 1978).

Practice Examinations and Test Questions

NURSESTAR. NURSESTAR, a program compatible with a variety of microcomputers, is a practice examination for nursing licensure.

NURSESTAR has an institutional and a student version. The institutional version consists of a 360-question examination that follows the format of the nursing licensure examination and is intended to test basic nursing knowledge. The program is structured so that a student or a group of students can take the examination. Feedback on inaccurate answers can be supplied immediately, or incorrect answers can be stored for feedback at the end of the test. Scores can be compiled on an individual basis or for groups.

The institutional version has three 120-question tests using multiple choice questions linked to case studies; the student version has four 30-question tests. Like the institutional test, the student test is meant to be a practice test for nursing licensure, but only one student can take the test at a time (Mosbystar, 1983).

TESTAR. TESTAR is a test construction authoring system that allows faculty to create their own test questions, case studies, rationales, explanations, and scoring mechanisms for a test. It is a potential test bank on any subject. The tests can be administered to individuals or to groups; the results can be item analyzed, split discriminations can be done, and scores can be stored (Mosbystar, 1983).

Authoring Systems

An authoring system requires no previous programming experience of the user. NEMAS (Nursing Education Module Authoring System) is microcomputer-based instructional software that allows the user to create instructional modules on a subject. The framework for this system is nursing process. The user can create a module of any of the five steps of the nursing process: assessment, diagnosis, planning, intervention and evaluation (Grobe, 1982). This system is important because it was designed from a conceptual base and includes both nursing and instructional design components.

The program can be used on the Apple II or any microcomputer with 64K and 2 disk drives. The faculty receives an author's guide. A faculty member or student

TABLE 15-2 *Illustrative Examples of Computer-Simulated Research Process Experiments*

VARIABLES		VALUES	RESULTS				
Experiment No. 1							
Independent:	Need for achievement	High, low (2 groups)	*NEED FOR ACHIEVEMENT*	*N*	*S.D.*	$\overline{X}$	*t*
Control:	Difficulty of task	Moderate	High	50	54.18	18.02	
	Need for affiliation	Random					5.48[a]
	Fear of failure	Random	Low	50	36.72	12.39	
	Instructions to subjects	Simple	[a] $p = 0.001$				
	Number in testing group	100					
	Length of task	10 minutes					
	Sex of experimenter	Random					
	Sex of subjects	Random					
	Year in school	Random					
Experiment No. 2							
Independent:	Need for achievement	High, low	*NEED FOR ACHIEVEMENT*	*N*	*S.D.*	$\overline{X}$	*t*
Control:	Same as experiment no. 1 except for:	Female	High	50	11.57	39.16	1.38[a]
			Low	50	11.33	36.00	
	Sex of subjects		[a] $p = 0.171$				

Experiment No. 3

Independent:	Sex of subjects	Male, female	*SEX OF SUBJECTS*	*N*	*S.D.*	$\overline{X}$	*t*
Control:	Same as experiment no. 1 except for: Need for achievement	Random	Male	50	16.91	45.56	2.15[a]
			Female	50	13.63	39.00	

[a] $p = 0.034$

Experiment No. 4

Independent:	Need for achievement	High, low
	Sex of subjects	Male, female
Control:	Same as experiment no. 1	

	NEED FOR ACHIEVEMENT HIGH	LOW	ROW $\overline{X}$
Sex of Subjects			
Male	$\overline{X} = 59.18$	$\overline{X} = 34.14$	$\overline{X} = 46.66$
	S.D. = 17.74	S.D. = 13.60	
Female	$\overline{X} = 42.36$	$\overline{X} = 36.62$	$\overline{X} = 39.49$
	S.D. = 13.85	S.D. = 11.36	
Column $\overline{X}$	$\overline{X} = 50.77$	$\overline{X} = 35.38$	

SUMMARY OF ANALYSIS OF VARIANCE

SOURCE OF VARIATION	*SS*	*df*	*MS*	*F*
NACH	11842.60	1	7206.52	35.13[a]
SEXS	2570.45	1	2570.45	12.53[a]
NACH & SEXS	4656.12	1	4656.12	22.70[a]

[a] $p = 0.001$

N = number; S.D. = standard deviation; $\overline{X}$ = mean; t = Student's *t* significance; SS = sum of squares; df = degrees of freedom; [a], asterisk; p, probability significance; MS, mean squares; F, F ratio

(Newman M, O'Brien R: Experiencing the research process via computer simulation. Image 10:5–9, 1978)

TABLE 15-3 *Five Advantages of Computer Simulation for Research*

1. Computer-simulated research affords students the opportunity to gain a greater appreciation of the importance of collaboration among researchers.
2. Computer simulations allow students to connect knowledge of statistical analysis with knowledge of research design.
3. In a very short time, computer simulation teaches students how the theoretical rationale that they support determines the variables to be selected, the hypotheses to be stated, and the controls to be employed.
4. Computer simulations make research meaningful and practical to students.
5. Computer simulations require students to seek consultation from research assistants and peers as decisions are made about experiments.

(Newman M, O'Brien R: Experiencing the research process via computer simulation. Image 10:5–9, 1978)

without programming experience could write a program by following the steps outlined in the flowchart in Figure 15-1. Advantages to authoring types of CAI are listed in Table 15-4.

Inservice and Staff Education

CAI has also been developed for the nurse working in a hospital. One system used is an authoring program on drug therapy in response to a need for more staff development, especially for newly employed nurses. This program was developed on two Apple microcomputers and programmed with PASCAL. This CAI replaces a quarterly lecture series consisting of 2-hour classes twice weekly over a 6-week period. The system was designed to provide multiple choice formats for drill and practice as well as more complex strategies for creating simulations of patient management problems (Pogue, 1982).

Figure 15-2 shows a format that a staff nurse might confront. Advantages of this system in inservice education are as follows (Pogue, 1982):

1. Staff nurses are free to use the system when they have time.
2. The program reduces preparation time of nurse educators.
3. Each lesson has a means of reviewed quality control.
4. The systems are interactive with the users and provide immediate feedback for right or wrong answers.
5. The user can repeat information not learned from a single trial, which makes the system self-directing as well as self-pacing.
6. Classes need not be scheduled.
7. The dialogues are user friendly.

Computer-assisted programs have also been developed to benefit staff nurses in primary health areas. One such program is a computer simulation program using a pediatric minor illness encounter. This software uses the computer facilities at the University of Minnesota and is based on the Minnesota instructional language (MIL), which can be translated in FORTRAN. This program evaluates nurses' problem-solving skills in clinical practice.

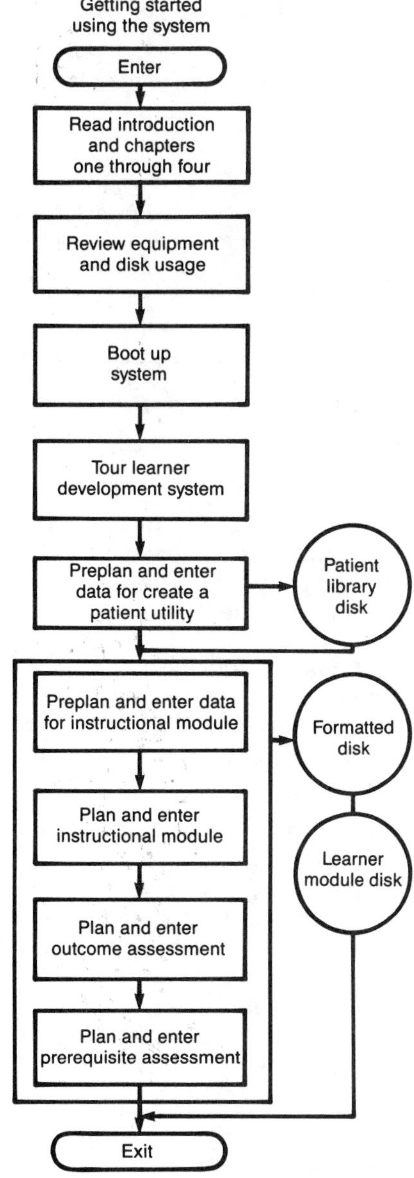

FIG. 15-1. A flowchart of the nursing education module authoring system that a faculty member or student would use. (Grobe S: NEMAS: Nursing education module authoring system: CAI software on nursing process. In Blum B [ed]: Proceedings: The Sixth Annual Symposium on Computer Applications in Medical Care. Silver Spring, MD, IEEE Computer Society Press, 1982)

The program is divided into four problem-solving areas:

Subjective or historical data about a patient
Objective data collections (*e.g.*, a physical assessment, laboratory test results)
A potential or actual diagnosis
A plan of care, with educational needs for the patient and the need for follow-up treatment.

TABLE 15-4 *Major Advantages of an Authoring System*

1. Authoring systems require no programming experience.
2. Authoring systems require less instructional design time than other systems.
3. Authoring systems prompt the user for necessary information required to write CBI media.
4. Any preprogrammed topics can be designed for instruction.
5. Content can be designed for specific types of nursing education programs (*i.e.,* diploma, associate, baccalaureate, graduate).
6. Content can be designed for varied educational levels (*i.e.,* basic, moderate, advanced concepts).

(Grobe S: NEMAS: Nursing education module authoring system: CAI software on nursing process. In Blum B [ed]: Proceedings of the Sixth Annual Symposium on Computer Applications in Medical Care. Silver Spring, MD, IEEE Computer Society Press, 1982)

Staff selections are evaluated by the supervisor. Based on a medical diagnosis model and incorporating appropriate nursing diagnosis selections based on assessment data integrated with objective test results, this program has many potentials for nursing education (Woodbury, 1982).

Patient Education

CAI for patient education has been developed on mainframes, minicomputers, and microcomputers (Table 15-5). These systems are mostly used in outpatient facilities or in areas where large numbers of persons are screened per day. The advantages include the following (Donovan and colleagues, 1983):

1. Patients feel more comfortable responding to the computer than to a nurse or physician.
2. Patients spend more time on content they do not understand by reviewing material as many times as necessary.
3. Information is printed and given to patients to review at home.
4. Patients feel that the computer reflects more time spent by the biomedical staff on their problems.

Evaluation

Because CAI has been in existence for over 20 years, significant studies have evaluated its impact (Billings, 1984). Some of its main advantages have been identified as follows (Norman, 1982):

1. CAI provides immediate feedback to the student, indicating whether answers are correct or incorrect, whether the process followed was appropriate or inappropriate, and, over time, whether the student's ability to reach correct decisions has improved.
2. The computer allows the student to respond to the program as it is received by analyzing graphics, manipulating animated forms, or answering questions. The computer responds to the student with endless patience, repeating information and offering guidance indefinitely.
3. The computer offers individualized instruction because many of the software programs allow the student to create the scenario or structure models or frameworks for study.

Question:		Isordil (isosorbide dinitrate) is often prescribed to be taken a few minutes before physical exercise or emotional situations that are known to cause angina. How would Isordil be administered in these situations? Please type your answer.
Answer 1:		sublingual+, SL, under & tongue
	Response:	
	Try 1:	You've aced this one, *student*!
	Try 2:	That's better, *student*.
	Try > 2:	Now you have it, *student*.
	Common response:	Isordil taken sublingually takes about five minutes to be effective and the effectiveness lasts about two hours.
	Branch:	19
Answer 2:		oral+, PO, mouth, swallow+
	Response:	No, *student*, oral forms of Isordil would be metabolized in the liver and then the metabolites of the drug absorbed into the systemic circulation before exerting vasodilating effects. This would take time. Please try again.
Answer 3:		ointment, topical+, cream
	Response:	An ointment would not be effective for immediate prophylaxis because ointments have to be absorbed through the skin into the circulation to be effective. This would take about 20 to 30 minutes. By the way, Isordil isn't available in an ointment. Please try again.
Answer 4:		intramuscul+, IM, I.M.
	Response:	No, Isordil is not available as an injection. Please try again.
Answer 5:		intraven+, IV, I.V.
	Response:	No, Isordil is not available as an injection. Please try again.
	Response to any other answer:	Sorry, but I don't recognize your anwer. Please check your spelling and try again. Remember, you can ask for help!
Help:		O.K., *student*, here's a hint! Nitrates can be given orally, sublingually or topically.
Give up:		Isordil is taken sublingually to keep anginal attacks from occurring. Before going to the next question, let's review why the sublingual route is faster than the oral or topical route for nitrate preparations.
	Review:	14
	Branch:	19

FIG. 15-2. An example of a computer-assisted instruction for staff nurses form. (Pogue L: Computer-assisted instruction in the continuing education process. Top Clin Nurs 4:41–50, 1982)

TABLE 15-5 *Patient Education Software Available*

CONTENT AREA	AUTHOR/VENDOR
Patient education in cancer	Cook, 1982
Hypertension information	Donovan, 1983; Ellis, 1980
Life style assessment	Hennen, 1977
Pharmacy education	Edmunds, 1982
Postmyocardial infarction	Lyons, 1982
Hypertension education	
Pacemaker instructions	
Cardiac rehabilitation	
Cardiac medications	
Postcardiac surgery instructions	
Congestive heart failure information	
Health promotion—diet, smoking, stress	Naditch, 1983
Patient instruction in an office	Somand, 1981
Prenatal education	Yates, 1982
Venereal disease	VanCura, 1975
Coping skills to alcoholics	Kadden, 1982
Nutrition plan	Dennison, 1982
Diabetes management for children	Mazzola, 1983
Diabetes patient nutrition information	Wheeler, 1983
Diet	Slack, 1976
Collecting a clean catch urine sample	Fisher, 1977
Mental health assessment	Slack, 1977
Headache survey	Dana, 1980
Nutrition and compliance with cystic fibrosis	Ellis, 1983
Allergy, cancer, cardiovascular, diabetes, neurology, nutrition, ophthalmology, orthopedic, surgery	Information Services, Primarius, 4186-C Sorrento Valley Blvd. San Diego, CA 92121
Medication information/writing prescriptions	Medical Microsystems, Inc. P.O. Box 1619 Klamath Falls, OR 97601
Home Health Guide for Children—contains information related to 155 health problems in infants, children, and adolescents and immediate actions parents should take	Clinical Reference Systems 1355 Kearney St. P.O. Box 20308 Denver, CO 80220

4. The computer terminals (provided the school has a laboratory sufficient to meet the demands for use) provides available tutorial learning when the student has the time and interest to learn. This supplements the use of the computer in the classroom.
5. CAI lays the groundwork for computer literacy as the student creates or uses the program. Students become more comfortable using computers when they are familiar with instructions.
6. Learning media can be artful and imaginative.

Other advantages of CAI have been cited (Alpert and Bitzer, 1970):

1. Computer laboratories help reduce the number of large lecture classes and provide smaller instructional groups along with a seminar atmosphere.
2. Students can proceed at a pace determined by their own capacity and motivation and not by the academic schedule.
3. Skill can be updated through simulation programs.
4. Continuing education can emanate from the academic community to the professionals in practice throughout the country.

COMPUTER-MANAGED INSTRUCTION

Many mundane functions go along with education, such as recordkeeping. Computerized reporting systems have been developed to collect, store, and process information on students, staff, and curricula. Such systems provide some type of student and program recordkeeping and thus serve to evaluate both students and educational programs. Such is the nature of a curriculum model that has been developed at Boston College in the School of Nursing. The model furnishes a framework for collecting information about nursing students, courses, clinical patient care experiences and postgraduate work experience. It also offers a method to evaluate decision-making procedures relative to program effectiveness (Sweeney and colleagues, 1980).

Types

Types of CMI include the following:

- Student records
- Student rotations
- Educational resources

Student Records

Innovative education directors have used CMI systems to record educational records that serve as documentation for outside accrediting agencies and monitor program effectiveness. One system has 14 different programs that monitor a variety of information concerning nurses educational experiences (Fig. 15-3). Evaluation summaries can be produced monthly to assess educational activities. Such a system has demonstrated more effective educational program evaluation and thus has lowered costs (Sweeney and colleagues, 1980; Moon, 1982).

Student Rotations

Just as staff assignments have been computerized (see Chap. 9), so have student rotations and schedules. An important part of student nurses' learning is balancing course preparation with clinical rotations. In some countries, certain obligatory training must be acquired at specific times. Computers have been used in Canada, North Wales, and The Netherlands for allocating student rotations, allowing for vacation leave, and tracking information on absences from sickness. The allocation and tracking of students becomes complex when more than one hospital is the site of rotations, when head nurses must be informed how many students they will have before assigning staff nurses, when variable training blocks are scheduled, and when flexibility of training must be considered. These decisions have been greatly facilitated by computers (Pritchard, 1982; Pluyter-Wenting, 1983; Ellis, 1982).

PROGRAM - NSD131

ROBINSON MEMORIAL HOSPITAL
NURSING STAFF DEVELOPMENT
SUMMARY OF TOPICS BY INSTRUCTOR
INST.#-02 NAME-MOON DAVID

PRI/ SEC	Topic ******	***Topic*** Description	Date ****	Class Hours	Clin Hours	CEU Hour	Methodology **************	Method of Evaluation	Rating Scale
P	280	MPN Orientation	3/27/79	.00	16.00	.00	Field Experience	Job Sample Test	Special
P	298	Nursing Forms/Day	5/03/79	.00	.25	.00	Clinical Practicum	O-T-J Perform Tests	Special
P	313	Concept of Cont Educa	1/03/79	1.00	.00	.00	Special Interest Grp	Inventor & Interview	Special
P	315	Tract III LPN Orient	4/30/79	23.50	89.50	.00	Short-Term Course	O-T-J Perform Tests	Standard
S	334	Near-Drowning	5/31/79	2.00	.00	.20	Symposium	Job Sample Test	Special
P	337	MPN Orientation	6/04/79	1.00	16.00	.00	Clinical Practicum	Planned Observation	Standard
P	314	Tract I RN Orientation	4/30/79	28.50	100.00	.00	Short-Term Course	O-T-J Perform Tests	Standard
P	322	Tract I Orientation	4/30/79	28.50	140.00	.00	Short-Term Course	O-T-J Perform Tests	Standard
P	335	Nurse Asst Orientation	6/11/79	18.50	13.50	.00	Short-Term Course	Planned Observation	Standard
P	271	Defibrillator CH-3	7/10/79	.00	.50	.00	Clinical Practicum	O-T-J Perform Tests	Special
P	346	NSD Overview	7/12/79	.00	2.00	.00	Special Interest Group	Inventor & Interview	Standard
P	411	Pre-CP Pat Teaching	7/23/79	.45	.00	.00	A-V Presentation	Inventor & Interview	Standard
S	414	Vital Signs/Rac Tech	8/03/79	1.50	.00	.00	Clinical Practicum	Job Sample Test	Standard
		# of Topics—13	Totals—	104.95	377.75	.20			

ROBINSON MEMORIAL HOSPITAL
NURSING STAFF DEVELOPMENT
SUMMARY OF TOPICS BY LOCATION

****** Dept.	Nurses Number	*************** Nurses Name	Topic Number	****************** Topic Description	***** Date	******Hour****** Class	Clin	CEU	PRI. Inst.	SEC. Inst.
SCU			301	Nursing Forms/Evening	5/04/79	.00	.25	.00	05	00
SCU			294	Bretylol	4/26/79	.50	.00	.00	99	00
			296	Peritoneal Dialysis	5/01/79	.50	.00	.00	99	04
			323	Feniwall Blood Filter	5/30/79	.50	.00	.00	99	00
			334	Near-Drowning	5/31/79	2.00	.0	.20	04	02
			336	New Defibrillator	6/04/79	.25	.00	.00	04	00
			341	Ventilatory Mgmt Cri	6/14/79	1.00	.00	.00	99	00
SCU			287	C.P.A.P.	4/18/79	.50	.00	.00	99	04
SCU			336	New Defibrillator	6/04/79	.25	.00	.00	04	00
SCU			294	Bretylol	4/26/79	.50	.00	.00	99	00
			306	Herpes Simplex	4/09/79	1.00	.00	.00	06	07
SCU			285	Suction Cath Kit Int	4/05/79	.25	.00	.00	05	00
SCU			287	C.P.A.P.	4/18/79	.50	.00	.00	99	04
			296	Peritoneal Dialysis	5/01/79	.50	.00	.00	99	04
SCU			336	New Defibrillator	6/04/79	.25	.00	.00	04	00
SCU			268	Adv Arrhythmia	6/28/79	16.00	.00	1.70	99	00
			285	Suction Cath Kit Int	4/05/79	.25	.00	.00	05	00
			287	C.P.A.P.	4/18/79	.50	.00	.00	99	04
			294	Bretylol	4/26/79	.50	.00	.00	99	00
			296	Peritoneal Dialysis	5/01/79	.50	.00	.00	99	04
			300	Nursing Forms/Nights	5/03/79	.00	.25	.00	01	00
			319	Airway Management	5/15/79	3.00	.00	.30	05	00
			334	Near-Drowning	5/31/79	2.00	.00	.20	04	02
			336	New Defibrillator	6/04/79	.25	.00	.00	04	00
			341	Ventilatory Mgmt Cri	6/14/79	1.00	.00	.00	99	00
			409	Pre-Op Pat Teaching	7/24/79	.45	.00	.00	03	00
			412	Pt Ed-Mi Prog 11-7	8/02/79	.45	.00	.00	03	00
SCU			413	Tract IV Orientation	8/06/79	20.00	60.00	.00	04	00
SCU			293	Electrical Hazards	4/24/79	.50	.00	.00	99	00
			294	Bretylol	4/26/79	.50	.00	.00	99	00
			306	Herpes Simplex	4/09/79	1.00	.00	.00	06	07
			336	New Defibrillator	6/04/79	.25	.00	.00	04	00
			358	Pre-Op Exercise Pat	7/17/79	.45	.00	.00	03	00
SCU			262	Cardivasc Nursing	2/01/79	30.00	.00	.00	04	05
			286	Tornados	4/18/79	.50	.00	.00	99	00
			294	Bretylol	4/26/79	.50	.00	.00	99	00

FIG. 15-3. Examples of program outputs for computer-managed instruction in in-service educational programs. (Moon D: Data processing in staff development. Nurs Manage 13:23–25, 1982)

Educational Resources

The computer has been used for storing test items, analyzing test results for individual students and groups of students, and generating test questions from test pools. Student files also provide an enormous amount of demographic data, information about career training, health records, and program flow. Through computers, student records can be profiled, trends for admission criteria to certain programs can be established, reasons for leaving school can be analyzed, and students can be compared (Davis and Williams, 1980).

The storage and retrieval capabilities of computers have been maximized by the General Nursing Council (GNC) for England and Wales. The GNC has developed a computerized system to maintain the register of nurses. The system assists nurses in the United Kingdom and the European economic community to monitor nursing training and movement of qualified persons based on skill levels (Collins, 1983).

Many systems exist in the United States to document nurse licensure and continuing education experience. Systems were developed when continuing education became mandatory by many states in order for nurses to qualify for relicensure. Currently, the presentation of continuing education credits are not monitored nationally or awarded based on successful completion of tests; however, systems that have been designed for awarding continuing education at state levels could be expanded to include such quality monitoring controls (Bolte and Denman, 1977; Dixon and colleagues, 1975; Valish and Boyd, 1975).

Evaluation

CMI has several advantages, the most important being the savings in time. Secondary gains, also important, include the following:

Enhanced communications between faculty and head nurses regarding student rotations
Planned curriculum experiences for students
Flexible schedules to incorporate holidays and vacation time
Advanced monitoring of students' health, grade, and attendance records
Training regulations matched to students' learning
Resource allocation
Minimized costs
Faculty are allowed to provide efficient programs while having time to teach

COMPUTER-ASSISTED VIDEO INSTRUCTION

The integration of computers with the color, sound, and motion of video systems has resulted in a new type of CAI—CAVI or interactive video disc (IAVD). Video instruction has its roots with television instruction; these methods have been used and evaluated for several years. Evaluating television instructions such as *Sesame Street* has demonstrated that student learning is significantly greater than with didactic classroom instruction.

Today, the integration of computers with video systems is providing students with active types of learning activities, where students interact with a motion picture or graphic video systems under computer control. The computer allows the expansion of the two technologies so that students can have individualized, user-controlled, user-paced instruction with the potential for immediate remediation and feedback during testing. After information is provided to the student through video systems, the computer controls the learning objectives, content, and test questions. If the student does not answer the question correctly, the piece of tape that provided the correct answer can be replayed (Fishman, 1984).

The computer augments the video display in several ways (Tymchyshyn, 1983):

Providing interaction between student and computer so that difficult material can be clarified
Pointing out the mechanism or exception to the current educational setting
Providing drill and practice in content areas
Using a self-assessment post test on the computer
Tracking student progress through modules

Examples of CAVI include the integration of computers with workbooks, film strips, audiotapes, videotapes, disks, movies, and television. An example of this integration is the teaching about cardiopulmonary resuscitation through the movie *The Breath of Life*. Now with interactive video, the computer provides a short lesson to illustrate new techniques in the two-person rescue procedure (Tymchyshyn, 1983).

Another example of interactive video instruction is the computer program added to the Massachusetts General Hospital videotape entitled *Cancer Chemotherapy*. This tape provided oncology nurses a continuing education workshop; computer integration was added so that objectives, content, and test questions could be included (Fishman, 1984).

Few evaluations of CAVI have been done, but it seems to be an effective method of education.

OTHER EDUCATIONAL APPLICATIONS

Specifically, the following applications will be discussed:

- Expert systems — COMMES
- Knowledge synthesizers
- Mainframe patient education systems
- Nurse extenders
- Discharge education plans
- Potentials for home computers

Expert Systems — COMMES

COMMES (Creighton On-line Multiple Medical Education Services), an artificial intelligence system that draws on knowledge prepared by experts, can interact with and learn from users, attempts to understand a user's interests, and uses heuristic search techniques to offer a variety of options that a user might request. COMMES works by being a sophisticated educational consultant that can understand a user's request for instructional assistance. For example, a nurse can request information about the standards of care for a pulmonary patient with emphysema. The COMMES system would respond with the information shown in Figure 15-4 (Evans, 1983; Ryan, 1983).

COMMES will create and print a test at a terminal for any educational goals a nurse needs. For example, it allows users to obtain continuing education credits from Creighton University on successful completion of a test. A nurse could use the computer to attend a continuing education program and then complete an examination, mail it to Creighton University, and, if the answers are correct, receive continuing education credit for the material learned (Evans, 1983; Ryan, 1983).

(COMMES prompts the user:)
ENTER ONE OR MORE KEYWORDS JOINED BY THE CONNECTORS
.AND. .OR. .IN THE CONTEXT OF.

(user identifies his interest:)
> patient care .and. emphysema .in the context of. rehabilitation

(after several interactions, the system responds with the following recommendation:)
NURSING PRACTICE PROTOCOL FOR THE FOLLOWING GOAL:

REHABILITATION: FORMULATE A PLAN OF CARE WHICH PROMOTES THE REHABILITATION OF THE PATIENT WITH PULMONARY DISTURBANCES.

NURSING PRACTICE SHOULD INCORPORATE THE FOLLOWING PATIENT CARE ISSUES:

1. THE NEED FOR BOTH PHYSICAL AND EMOTIONAL ADJUSTMENT IN COPING WITH PULMONARY DISEASES.

   RESOURCE—Luckmann & Sorensen. *Med-Surg. Nurs.,* 1980, pp. 1223–1226

   Specific aspects of physical adjustment might include environment, breathing pattern, hydration, activity, occupation, and no smoking.

   Specific aspects of emotional adjustment might include reinforcement, motivation, reward, and family response.

2. AN APPROPRIATE AND COMPREHENSIVE TEACHING PLAN TO PROMOTE REHABILITATION OF A PATIENT WITH PULMONARY DISEASE, INCLUDING ENVIRONMENTAL, PSYCHOLOGICAL AND PHYSICAL FACTORS.

   RESOURCE—Luckmann & Sorensen. *Med-Surg. Nurs.,* 1980, pp. 1223–1226

   Specific aspects of teaching plan might include self care, environmental adjustment, family cooperation, and coping mechanism.

   Specific aspects of rehabilitation might include physical rehabilitation, physical adjustment, pyschological rehabilitation, pulmonary rehabilitation, and environmental adjustment.

   Specific aspects of environmental factors might include home setting, air pollutant, humidity, temperature, and social interaction.

   Specific aspects of psychological factors might include depression, mentation, incentive, coping mechanism, family concern, emotional response, and self image.

   Specific aspects of physical factors might include physical strength and energy.

3. DEFENSE MECHANISMS AND COPING STRATEGIES EMPLOYED BY PATIENTS WITH PULMONARY PROBLEMS AND THEIR FAMILIES AND DISCUSS APPROPRIATE INTERVENTIONS.

   RESOURCE—Luckmann & Sorensen. *Med-Surg. Nurs.,* 1980, pp. 1227–1228

   Specific aspects of defense mechanisms might include denial avoidance, fantasy, and regression.

   Specific aspects of coping strategies might include reality rehearsal, personal value system, attitude, problem-solving, and resource use.

   Specific aspects of family include family anxiety and family support.

   Specific aspects of interventions might include assessment of needs, goal setting, problem solving, and resource use.

FIG. 15-4. COMMES standards of care for the pulmonary patient. (Evans S: Nursing applications of an expert information system. In Van Bemmel J et al [eds]: Medinfo 83, pp 182–85. Amsterdam, North-Holland, 1983)

Knowledge Synthesizers

Another knowledge base system was developed at the National Library of Medicine (NLM) in the Lister Hill National Center for Biomedical Communications. This program involved the design, development, demonstration, testing, and evaluation of knowledge-based computer systems in specialized areas of biomedicine. Although this application was tested for medicine, it had nursing applications (National Library of Medicine Fact Sheet, 1982).

The computer-based system includes the capability to acquire, represent, and modify knowledge structures of biomedical information from the enormous sources of literature available today. Three content areas have been developed: viral hepatitis, peptic ulcer disease, and human genetics. In the area of viral hepatitis the system addresses background information necessary to make a precise diagnosis. A pilot description of this system has been published (Mosley and Galambos, 1975; Bernstein and colleagues, 1980; Roderer and colleagues, 1981).

The peptic ulcer program focuses on this common chronic disease for which diagnosis and treatment depend on rapidly evolving technologies. The system describes the major variables in making a clinical diagnosis and determining management concepts. The content format comes from standard gastrointestinal textbook material (Sleisinger and Fordtran, 1978).

The content of the human genetics system covers basic science and clinical concepts that may be unfamiliar to a practicing rural physician. Included in this content are the anatomy, physiology, and biochemical information needed to understand human genetics. This system has already undergone an update with the assistance of a panel of experts (National Library of Medicine Fact Sheet, 1982).

• • •

Both the examples above boast of the type of technology transfer that can be expected to occur in the future. With the development of intelligent, decision-making software, computers can facilitate reasoning, provide advice, give lectures, solve problems, and test the user. In this way the knowledge of an expert faculty member can be transmitted to schools that do not have the resource, to in-service education programs, and to rural areas to develop continuing education for nurse practitioners.

Mainframe Patient Education Systems

One of the first applications developed for an IBM HIS was the patient education component of the patient care system. When computer capability to store large volumes of reference materials is capitalized on, medication information can be made available not only to staff nurses administering the medication but to the patients, who are given a printout in the emergency room or after discharge from an extended hospitalization. The computer printout can include the specific medications prescribed for the patient and describe in lay terms the purpose of the medication, the possible side-effects, appropriate dietary or activity restrictions, and symptoms that should be reported to a physician or nurse (Edmunds, 1982).

Nurse Extenders

When not enough nurses are available to structure patient education programs, computers can serve as nurse extenders in providing educational materials for patients. One creative way that computers can be used for patient education is as a consultant for patient inquiries. For example, computers have been used by nurses to provide a training program for persons with diabetes. The training program involves two parts: health facts, which includes content on the symptoms of hypoglycemia and hyperglycemia, insulin administration, foot care, and urine testing, and diet management. After preliminary information is entered this program calculates appropriate caloric intakes for a patient, who receives individualized information from the printer.

A nurse shows the patient how to use the computer; thereafter the patient answers several questions, including the type of instruction that is needed. The flow or sequence of the program is then based on the patient's response. In this way, patients control the flow of information that they receive by answering yes or no to multiple-choice questions. The system can monitor what information patients have selected and allow patients to return to the computer later to continue instructions where they left off (Cook, 1982). It runs on a microprocessor with typing keys, a black and white television screen, a printer, and a tape recorder. A comparable unit is a Hewlett-Packard 85.

A patient education program for cardiac patients has been written for a small microcomputer (Lyons and colleagues, 1982). However, limited speed and memory led to the development of a patient education system on a more robust microcomputer. The programs are written in BASIC and include such content as postmyocardial infarction instruction, hypertensive patient education, pacemaker patient instruction, cardiac rehabilitation, cardiac medication, postcardiac surgery instruction, and education of patients with congestive heart failure.

The main advantage of this system was that patients had documented improved learning. The computer was supplemental to teaching provided by staff nurses. This program will probably be expanded to include content related to basic cardiology principles, dietary instructions, precardiac catheterization instructions and informed consent, risk modification, coronary artery disease, sex and the cardiac patient, and explanations of several diagnostic studies used in cardiac patients. The goal of this program is to have patient education centers established in hospitals, consisting of 3 to 6 video terminals, one or two printers, audiovisual supplements such as visual slide graphics, and a complete reference library of educational materials (Lyons and colleagues, 1982).

Discharge Education Plans

Computers have been used in several hospitals to identify and solve problems in patient education. Some of these problems relate to the number of staff available to teach, others to patients' educational needs, and still others in the continuing change in patients' diagnoses and changing educational needs. The computer facilitates patient education by providing a database that tracks patients eligible for education, identifies patients who have received education, highlights patients who have not participated in educational programs, identifies staff educational needs, and provides data on costs of such a program. Some systems also provide the patient with an educational plan on discharge.

POTENTIALS FOR HOME COMPUTERS

Several factors will influence the growth of computer-assisted patient education. There is a great deal of emphasis on health promotion and disease prevention, especially from the Department of Health and Human Services, the Office of the Surgeon General, and United States Public Health Service, calling for proper diet, exercise, smoking cessation, stress management, and the avoidance of disease-producing risks. At the same time, home computers have become less expensive and more computer-compiled programs have become available, including those that guide the consumer in assessing disease risks and counseling about health promoting behaviors. One program called BODYCHECK uses a life style personal history questionnaire. The answers are put directly into the computer through a terminal. The program operates on a Control Data 6400 computer and on IBM equipment. From this program, the patient can receive a computer-generated letter that reinforces the physicians' office visit (Hennen, 1977). STAYWELL, another program based on the same concept, is available from Control Data (PLATO software). This program counsels the patient on reducing disease-producing risks. It is being implemented in many large industries in the United States (Naditch, 1983).

SUMMARY

Although there has been more than a decade of experience with computer applications in education, nurses are like medieval scribes painstakingly lettering books when the printing press and the photocopy machines are yet to come. A generation of "microkids" will enter academic areas of higher learning within the next 10 years. They will have no fear of computers; they will be computer literate; they will want the teacher to instruct them on extending the capabilites of computers. Nurses will be prepared for the next generation of nursing students if they continue to apply technologies in education, evaluate its impact, and extend its capabilities.

Nurses have only begun to use computers in patient and staff nursing education. Although the costs of computer implementation have been an issue, this cannot be the sole reason for their absence. Too few persons in service settings have been allowed the time to develop computer applications for patient care. With the advent of prospective reimbursement, computers may be more meaningful in hospital and ambulatory care services to provide patients with the minimum requirements of knowledge to care for themselves at home. As directors of nursing analyze how to reduce costs within their department, the prospect of more computerized in-service education programs may become a more realistic option.

This chapter reviewed computer-based education or computer-assisted learning, which includes computer-assisted instruction and computer-managed instruction. Additional computer applications were computer-assisted video instruction, expert systems, knowledge synthesizers, educational applications on HISs, and nurse extenders for patient teaching.

The four major types of CAI were described, and examples of software programs available for CAI were presented. More sophisticated education applications described included the expert systems and the knowledge synthesizers. The expert system (COMMES) and its five instructional components were described. Knowledge synthesizers were also discussed.

Finally, computers are also providing patient education information on mainframes such as the IBM patient care system. Microcomputers were described as nurse extenders in patient education, and the potential for patient education with home computers was discussed.

ISSUES

1. The evaluation of CAI has developed more slowly than has CAI software. Often content validity and reliability are not known and thus not documented.
2. With home computers, interactive video, and CAI, students could stay home and attend many classes through a terminal.

3. Many intensive courses, institutes, and workshops are provided for medical students; however, similar experiences may not be currently available for nursing students.
4. Expert systems and artificial intelligence may provide technology that could be applied to the entire nursing process.
5. Most educational applications described in other countries relate to the use of CMI and less to CAI.
6. Many computer software packages for CAI are not compatible with the central computer of a university but may be specific to one or two types of microcomputers. Therefore, CAI developed for one particular computer would need extensive programming to be compatible with other hardware.
7. Although it may be appropriate to teach basic nursing skills on the computer, how well will the student interact with the patient?
8. The use of computers in teaching patients with foreign languages has yet to be explored in nursing.
9. The development of CAI and CMI usually takes a large commitment of staff time. Therefore, much that is available has been developed by software companies rather than by nursing faculty.
10. The use of computers in educating staff nurses during orientation, updating continuing education programs, and for in-service programs has been relatively unexplored.
11. Home computers could be potential patient education tools for which nurses could develop content.

SUGGESTIONS FOR HANDS-ON EXPERIENCES

1. An educational offering has been provided to medical students who wish to enroll in an intensive 8-week elective course to study computer resources at the National Institutes of Health (NIH). The course, entitled Computers in Clinical Medicine, is intended to familiarize students with the resources at the NIH, including the Clinical Center, the Division of Computer Research and Technology, and the NLM. The course has a structured curriculum taught by about 40 members of the clinical center that has an HIS and automated clinical laboratories. The Division of Computer Research and Technology (DCRT) is the world's largest and most advanced biomedical computer center, with several dozen dedicated computers for NIH clinics and laboratories. The NLM has a national responsibility for storing, retrieving, and disseminating biomedical information through computer-based information systems and CAI. The course includes exposure to computers in clinical and research practice that a person interested in computer applications in medicine might experience. An opportunity for the student to complete an independent study project in conjunction with a senior specialist in computers is offered. No such intense course currently exists in nursing.
2. Since many schools of nursing have a computer laboratory, CAI and CAVI may already be available at your school. If not, make an appointment to visit a computer laboratory in an area near you.
3. Call a software manufacturing company and request a demonstration of new software for nursing content. Be prepared with questions concerning the hardware and software that would help you evaluate its application.
4. Contact the nurse educators or nurse administrators in your nearby hospital and ask if any patient education materials are generated by computer. If the hospital

that you work in has a computer, determine if patient education or staff education is currently available. If so, generate teaching guides for patients.

5. At many conventions, terminals are being set up in an audiovisual learning center so that participants can view available audiovisual instruction and CAI. Determine if the convention that you are attending has such an exhibit and plan to spend at least 1 day there. (The American Thoracic Society/American Lung Association annual meetings usually have such an exhibit.)
6. Most HISs have a simulation of patient care using mock patients with complete nursing documentation capabilities. Contact the hospital to determine if the school of nursing could obtain a contract to use the system from terminals and modems in the school of nursing.
7. Contact any major computer company and ask to contract educational hands-on classes using its educational experts and equipment.

STUDY QUESTIONS

1. What are the two basic categories of usage within CBE (CAL)?
2. In addition to the two categories mentioned above, are there additional educational applications of computers relevant to nursing? If so, name them.
3. Name one system that includes both CAI and CMI components and thus is a CBE system.
4. Name the four major types of CAI.
5. Does any CAI software use a video disk in addition to computer software?
6. Describe an authoring system.
7. Name an authoring system relevant for nursing.
8. List three areas where CMI benefits education.
9. Name one expert system that draws on the concepts of artificial intelligence.

REFERENCES

Alpert D, Bitzer D: Advances in computer-based education. Science 167:1582–1590, 1970

Ball M, Hannah K: Using Computers in Nursing. Reston, VA, Reston Publishing Co, 1984

Bernstein L, Siegel E, Goldstein C: The hepatitis knowledge base, a prototype information transfer system. Ann Intern Med 93:169–181, 1980

Billings D: Evaluating computer assisted instruction. Nurs Outlook 32:50–53, 1984

Bolte I, Denman L: We are ready for ANA's continuing education data bank. J Cont Ed Nursing 8:5, 1977

Brennan P: Establishment of a computer assisted instruction program to teach managerial decision making. In Heffernan H (ed): Proceedings of the Fifth Annual Symposium on Computer Applications in Medical Care, pp 769–770. Silver Spring, MD, IEEE Computer Society Press, 1981

Collins S: Computer based systems for professional education and training. In Scholes M et al (eds): The Impact of Computers on Nursing, 350–355. Amsterdam, North-Holland, 1983

Control Data Learning Center Fact Sheet. Minneapolis, MN, Control Data Corporation, 1981

Cook G: The microcomputer: Physician's aid for patient education in cancer. In Blum B (ed): Proceedings of the Sixth Annual Symposium on Computer Applications in Medical Care, p 636. Silver Spring, MD, IEEE Computer Society Press, 1982

Davis J, Williams D: Learning for mastery: Individualized testing through computer-managed evaluation. Nurse Educ 5:9, 1980

Dixon J, Gouyd N, Varricchio D: A computerized education and training record. J Cont Ed Nurs 6:20–23, 1975

Donovan M, Zielstorff R, Mauldin T, et al: Using COSTAR to assist nurses in hypertension screening and education. In Dayhoff R (ed): Proceedings of the Seventh Annual Symposium on Computer Applications in Medical Care, pp 487–490. Silver Spring, MD, IEEE Computer Society Press, 1983

Edmunds L: Computer-assisted nursing care. Am J Nurs 82:1076–1079, 1982

Ellis L: Computer based patient education: Problems and opportunities. In Heffernan H (ed): Proceedings of the Fifth Annual Symposium on Computer Applications in Medical Care, p 196. Silver Spring, MD, IEEE Computer Society Press, 1981

Evans S: Nursing applications of an expert information system. In Van Bemmel J et al (eds): Medinfo 83, pp 182–185. Amsterdam, North-Holland, 1983

Evans S: Applications of a nursing knowledge based system for nursing practice: Inservice, continuing education, and standards of care. In Dayhoff R (ed): Proceedings of the Seventh Annual Symposium on Computer Applications in Medical Care, pp 491–494. Silver Spring, MD, IEEE Computer Society Press, 1983

Fishman D: Development and evaluation of a computer assisted video module for teaching cancer chemotherapy to nurses. Comp Nursing 2:16–23, 1984

Goldberg M, Green S, Moss M, et al: Computer-based instruction and diagnosis of acid-base disorders. JAMA 223:269–275, 1973

Grobe S: NEMAS: Nursing education module authoring system: CAI software on nursing process. In Blum B (ed): Proceedings of the Sixth Annual Symposium on Computer Applications in Medical Care, p 650. Silver Spring, MD, IEEE Computer Society Press, 1982

Hassett M: Computers and nursing education in the 1980s. Nurs Outlook 32:34–36, 1984

Hennen B, Shired D, Smith G: "Bodycheck"—the assessment of lifestyle risks using computer technology. In Medinfo 77, pp 739–743. Amsterdam, North-Holland, 1977

Holzemer W, Slichter M, Slaughter R, Stotts N: Development of the University of California, San Francisco microcomputer facility for nursing research and development. In Dayhoff R (ed): Proceedings of the Seventh Annual Symposium on Computer Applications in Medical Care, pp 484–486. Silver Spring, MD, IEEE Computer Society Press, 1983

Larson D: Microcomputer tutorial-simulations to teach basic nursing skills. In Blum B (ed): Proceedings of the Sixth Annual Symposium on Computer Applications in Medical Care, pp 663–667. Silver Spring, MD, IEEE Computer Society Press, 1982

Lyons C, Krasnowski J, Greenstein A, et al: Interactive computerized patient education. Heart Lung, 11:340–341, 1982

Moon D: Data processing in staff development. Nurs Manage 13:23–25, 1982

Mosbystar: NURSESTAR, TESTAR. St. Louis, MO, CV Mosby, 1983

Mosley J, Galambos J: Viral hepatitis. In Schiff L (ed): Diseases of the Liver. Philadelphia, JB Lippincott, 1975

Murphy J, Finnegan G: Hospital harnesses computers' capabilities to spot, solve problems in patient education programs. Promot Health 1:1–3, 1980

Naditch M: PLATO STAYWELL: A behavioral medicine microcomputer program of health behavior change. In Dayhoff R (ed): Proceedings of the Seventh Annual Symposium on Computer Applications in Medical Care, pp 363–365. Silver Spring, MD, IEEE Computer Society Press, 1983

National Library of Medicine Fact Sheet: Knowledge Base Research Program: An Information Transfer System in Biomedicine. Bethesda, MD, U.S. Government Printing Office, 1982

Newman M, O'Brien R: Experiencing the research process via computer simulation. Image 10:5–9, 1978

Norman S: Computer-assisted learning—its potential in nurse education. Nurs Times 78:1467–1468, 1982

Ozbolt J: A prototype information system to aid nursing decision. In Blum B (ed): Proceedings of the Sixth Annual Symposium on Computer Applications in Medical Care, p 653. Silver Spring, MD, IEEE Computer Society Press, 1982

PLATO. Urbana-Champaign, IL, University of Illinois, 1979

Pluyter-Wenting E: Computerized student-nurse training and allocation system. In Fokkens O et al (eds): Medinfo 83, pp 322–326. Amsterdam, North-Holland, 1983

Pogue L: Computer-assisted instruction in the continuing education process. Top Clin Nurs 4:41–50, 1982
Pritchard K: Computers. III. Possible applications in nursing. Nurs Times 78:465–466, 1982
Reilly D: A computerized patient information system. Nurs Manage 13:32–36, 1982
Roderer N, King D, McDonald D, Bush C: Evaluation of the Hepatitis Knowledge Base System. DHHS report NLM 78-3. Washington, DC, U.S. Government Printing Office, 1981
Ryan S: Computers in nursing practice: COMMES—a national computer-based educational consultant. Comp Nursing 1:1, 1983
Slack W, Peckham B, Van Cura L, Carr W: A computer-based physical examination system. JAMA 200:224–228, 1967
Sleisenger M, Fordtran J (eds): Gastrointestinal Diseases, 2nd ed. Philadelphia, WB Saunders, 1978
Sweeney M, Regan P, O'Malley M, Hedstrom B: Essential skills for baccalaureate graduates: Perspectives of education and service. J Nurs Admin 10:37–44, 1980
Tymchyshyn P: An evaluation of the adoption of CAI in a nursing program. In Blum B (ed): Proceedings of the Sixth Annual Symposium on Computer Applications in Medical Care, pp 543–548. Silver Spring, MD, IEEE Computer Society Press, 1982
Tymchyshyn P: New tricks for an old game: Teaching. In Van Bemmel J et al (eds): Medinfo 83, pp 190–193. Amsterdam, North-Holland, 1983
Department of Health and Human Services: Clinical Electives for Medical Students at the National Institutes of Health, catalog, 1983. Bethesda, MD, U.S. Government Printing Office, 1983
Valish A, Boyd J: The role of computer-assisted instruction in continuing education of registered nurses: An experimental study. J Cont Ed Nurs 6:13–32, 1975
Woodbury P: Computer assisted evaluations of problem solving skills of primary health care providers using a case management simulation model. In Blum B (ed): Proceedings of the Sixth Annual Symposium on Computer Applications in Medical Care, pp 539–542. Silver Spring, MD, IEEE Computer Society Press, 1982

BIBLIOGRAPHY

Abdoo Y, Strodtman L, Truax T: Microcomputer generated nursing reports based on computerized nursing assessment. In Blum B (ed): Proceedings of the Sixth Annual Symposium on Computer Applications in Medical Care, p 651. Silver Spring, MD, IEEE Computer Society Press, 1982
Barnett G, Justice N, Somand M, et al: COSTAR—a computer-based medical information system for ambulatory care. Pro IEEE 67:1226–1237, 1979
Bitzer M, Boudreaux M: Using a computer to teach nursing. Nurs Forum 8:234–254, 1969
Butler E, Howarth M: A computer system for student nurse allocation during training. Nurs Times 76:1208–1212, 1980
Cheung P: Examination: Put test questions on a computer! Nurs Mirror 149:26–28, 1979
Cobin J: Computer applications for users in schools of nursing for staff-budget control and as a teaching aid. In Fokkens O et al (eds): Medinfo 83 Seminars, pp 327–331. Amsterdam, North-Holland, 1983
Collart M: Computer-assisted instruction and the teaching-learning process. Nurs Outlook 21:527–532, 1973
CONDUIT. Iowa City, IA, University of Iowa, (Oakdale Campus)
Conklin D: A study of computer assisted instruction in nursing education. J Comp Instr 9:3, 1983
Dana D, Leviton A, Swidler C, et al: A computer-based headache interview: Acceptance by patients and physicians. Headache 29:85–89, 1980
Dennison D: The DINE System: The Nutritional Plan For Better Health. New York, Amherst, 1982
Dennison D, Isu L, Phelps J, Frauenheim K: The DINE system: A nutritional microcomputer program for patient service. In Dayhoff R (ed.): Proceedings of the Seventh Annual

Symposium on Computer Applications in Medical Care, pp 374–376. Silver Spring, MD, IEEE Computer Society Press, 1983
Dexter P, Laidig J: Breaking the education/service barrier. Nurs Outlook 28:179–182, 1980
Donabedian D: Computer-taught epidemiology. Nurs Outlook 24:12, 1976
Droste-Bielak E: The use of computer simulation in teaching interviewing techniques to beginning nursing students in a baccalaureate program. Doctoral dissertation, University of Michigan, 1980
Edmunds L: Making the most of a message function for nurse services. In Dayhoff R (ed): Proceedings of the Seventh Annual Symposium on Computer Applications in Medical Care, p 510. Silver Spring, MD, IEEE Computer Society Press, 1983
Ellis L, Petzel S, Asp E: Computer-assisted instruction for the chronically ill child. In Dayhoff R (ed): Proceedings of the Seventh Annual Symposium on Computer Applications in Medical Care, pp 366–369. Silver Spring, MD, IEEE Computer Society Press, 1983
Ellis P: Matching student with clinical experiences by computer. Nurs Outlook 30:29–30, 1982
Erikson E, Borgmeyer V Sr: Simulated decision making experiences via case analysis. J Nurs Admin 9:10–15, 1979
Evans S: Overview of the COMMES System. Omaha, NE, Creighton University Press, 1983
Evans S: The structure of instructional knowledge: An operational model. Instr Sci 2:421–450, 1974
Farrand L, Holzemer W, Schleutermann J: A study of the construct validity: Simulations as a measure of nurse practitioners; problem solving skills. Nurs Res 31:37–42, 1982
Fildes C: A step towards computerized learner nurse allocation. In Scholes M et al (eds): The Impact of Computers on Nursing, pp 356–363. Amsterdam, North-Holland, 1983
Fisher L, Johnson T: Collection of a clean voided urine specimen: A comparison among spoken, written, and computer-based instructions. Am J Publ Health 67:640–644, 1977
Goodwin J, Edwards B: Developing a computer program to assist the nursing process. Phase I—From system analysis to an expandable program. Nurs Res 24:229–305, 1975
Grobe S: Nursing process algorithm used for a nursing CAI authoring system. In Van Bemmel J et al (eds): Medinfo 83, pp 194–197. Amsterdam, North-Holland, 1983
Grobe S: Protocols for software selection, development and evaluation. In Scholes M et al (eds): The Impact of Computers on Nursing, pp 307–326. Amsterdam, North-Holland, 1983
Hales G (ed): Computers in Nursing. Philadelphia, JB Lippincott, 1983
Hannah K: Computer managed instruction in nursing education. In Van Bemmel J et al (eds): Medinfo 83, pp 1983–202. Amsterdam, North-Holland, 1983
Hannah K: Computer assisted learning in nursing education: A macroscopic analysis. In Scholes M et al (eds): The Impact of Computers on Nursing, pp 280–287. Amsterdam, North-Holland, 1983
Hartmann B: Student nurse allocation. Nurs Times 64:5–7, 1968
Holzemer W, Schleutermann J, Farrand L, Miller A: A validation study: Simulations as a measure of nurse practitioner problem solving skills. Nurs Res 39:139–144, 1981
Huckabay L, Anderson N, Holm D, & Lee J: Cognitive, affective, and transfer of learning consequences of computer-assisted instruction. Nurs Res 28:228–233, 1979
Kadden R, Wetstone S: Teaching coping skills to alcoholics using computer based education. In Blum B (ed): Proceedings of the Sixth Annual Symposium on Computer Applications in Medical Care, p 635. Silver Spring, MD, IEEE Computer Society Press, 1982
Kamp M: Index to Computerized Teaching in the Health Sciences. San Francisco, University of California Press, 1975
Kirchoff K, Holzemer W: Student learning and a computer-assisted instructional program. J Nurs Ed 13:4, 1974
Krull S: Computer assisted instruction for nursing education. In Blum B (ed): Proceedings of the Sixth Annual Symposium on Computer Applications in Medical Care, p 652. Silver Spring, MD, IEEE Computer Society Press, 1982
Larson D: The use of computer-assisted instruction to teach calculation and regulation of

intravenous flow rates to baccalaureate nursing students. Doctoral dissertation, Michigan State University, 1981

Mazzola F, Rowe B, Rowe D: Video diabetes: A teaching tool for children with insulin-dependent diabetes. In Dayhoff R (ed): Proceedings of the Seventh Annual Symposium on Computer Applications in Medical Care, p 822. Silver Spring, MD, IEEE Computer Society Press, 1983

Meadows L: Nursing education in crisis: A computer alternative. J Nurs Ed 16:13–21, 1977

Mirin S: The computer's place in nursing education. Nurs Health Care 2:500–506, 1981

Nabor S: Creative approaches to nurse-midwife education. V. Computerized nurse-midwifery management: Its usefulness as a learning-teaching tool. J Nurse Midwifery 20:26–28, 1975

Olivieri P, Sweeney M: Evaluation of clinical learning: By computer. Nurse Ed 5:26–31, 1980

Pogue R: Medical College of Georgia CAI Systems: Author Manual. Augusta, GA, Systems and Computer Services, 1981

Pogue R: The authoring system: Interface between author and computer. J Res Devel Ed 14:57–68, 1980

Porter S: Application of computer-assisted instruction to continuing education in nursing: Review of the literature. J Cont Ed Nurs 9:5–9, 1978

Ronald J: Computer and undergraduate nursing education: A report on an experimental introductory course. J Nurs Ed 18:4–9, 1979

Rubinson L, Robinson J: Computer-assisted instruction in health education: A pilot study. Intl J Instr Media 5:251–259, 1977–1978

Scholes M, Bryant Y, Barber B: The Impact of Computers on Nursing. Amsterdam, North-Holland, 1983

Schultz S: A model computing laboratory for university schools of nursing: The Michigan experience. In Blum B (ed): Proceedings of the Sixth Annual Symposium on Computer Applications in Medical Care, pp 549–550. Silver Spring, MD, IEEE Computer Society Press, 1982

Sherman J, Miller A, Farrand L, Holzemer W: A simulated patient encounter for the family nurse practitioner. J Nurs Ed 18:22–30, 1979

Simonsen R, Renshaw R: CAI—boon or boondoggle? Datamation 20:90–102, 1974

Slack W, Porter O, Witschi J, et al: Dietary interviewing by computer. J Am Dietet Assoc 69:414–417, 1976

Slack W, Clack C: Talking to a computer about emotional problems: A comparative study. Psychotherapy: Theory Res Pract 14:156–164, 1977

Steinberg E: The Evolutionary Development of CAI Courseware. Illinois, Computer Educational Research Laboratory, 1976

Sweeney M: Development of a Nursing Curriculum Evaluation Model. Final Report of a Nursing Project Grant, Division of Nursing, Department of Health, Education and Welfare. Washington, DC, U.S. Government Printing Office, 1980

VanCura L, Jenson N, Griest J, et al: Venereal disease: Interviewing and teaching by computer. Am J Publ Health 65:1159–1164, 1975

Werley H, Grier M: Nursing Information Systems. New York, Springer, 1981

Wheeler L, Wheeler M, Ours P, Swider C: Use of CAI/video in diabetes patient nutritional education. In Dayhoff R (ed): Proceedings of the Seventh Annual Symposium on Computer Applications in Medical Care, pp 961–964. Silver Spring, MD, IEEE Computer Society Press, 1983

Yates W: Computer-assisted patient prenatal education. In Blum B (ed): Proceedings of the Sixth Annual Symposium on Computer Applications in Medical Care, p 633. Silver Spring, MD, IEEE Computer Society Press, 1982

Zielstorff R: Computers in Nursing. Wakefield, MA, Nursing Resources, 1980

Glossary

Abacus The first computing device

ADA A high-level programming language (named for ADA, Countess of Lovelace)

ALGOL (*ALGO*rithmic *L*anguage)
A high-level international algebraic programming language

Algorithm A series of steps that outline the solution to a problem in a program

Analog computer A computer that operates on continuous data and measures analogous quantities (*e.g.*, voltages, currents, temperatures, pressures)

Analytical machine The first design of the modern computer developed by Charles Babbage

Application program A program written in a programming language by or for a user; stored in random access memory (RAM)

Arithmetic and logic unit (ALU) The part of the central processing unit (CPU) that performs the computer's mathematical and logical operations

Artificial intelligence A term used to describe the fifth-generation computers, which will solve complex problems similar to human reasoning

ASCII (*A*merican *S*tandard *C*ode for *I*nformation *I*nterchange)
A coding scheme in which seven bits are used to represent one character (byte of data)

Assembler A program that translates assembly languages into machine language

Assembly language A low-level language that uses abbreviations and mnemonic codes instead of binary digits

BASIC (*B*eginners *A*ll-purpose *S*ymbolic *I*nstruction *C*ode)
A high-level programming language used interactively

Batch processing The processing of like groups of data, at one time, as needed

Binary numbering system System that uses the digits 0 and 1 and has a base of 2

Bit (*BI*nary digi*T*)
The components of the binary numbering system that use 0 or 1

Bug An error in a computer system

Byte A string of seven or eight bits. The smallest logical entity stored in the computer; also called a character

Cathode ray tube (CRT) terminal An input/output device used to communicate with the computer, consisting of a keyboard and a video display screen; also called a video display tube (VDT)

Central processing unit (CPU) The "brain" of the computer; controls and supervises the entire computer system

Character A number, letter, or symbol; called a byte

Character printer An impact printer that prints one character at a time

Chip A thin square piece of silicon on which electronic circuits are etched

COBOL (*C*ommon *B*usiness *O*riented *L*anguage)
A high-level programming language for business applications

Code A set of numbers, letters, or symbols used to represent data

Compiler A program that translates high-level languages into machine language

Computer An electronic machine that automatically processes data as directed by a stored program (a sequence of instructions)

Computer generations The major milestones in computer development marked by the electronic components

Computer output microfilm (COM) Computer output represented by miniaturized images on a reel of film (microfilm) or a sheet (microfiche)

Control unit That part of the CPU that supervises and controls the whole computer system

Daisy wheel A "special ball" used by a character printer to print single characters one at a time

Data A collection of raw facts communicated, stored and processed by a computer

Database A collection of interrelated files of data organized and stored together

Database management system (DBMS) A software package (set of programs) with its own query language designed to create, access, manage, and monitor a database

Data processing The interaction between hardware and software to transform data into information

Debugging The process of checking a computer program to ensure it is errorfree

Digital computer A computer system that uses binary digits (0 and 1) to represent data

Disk (disc) drive A device by which data are written on and read from magnetic disks

Dot matrix printer A character printer that prints characters constructed of a series of dots

Dumb terminal A terminal that only transmits keyed data to and from the computer without processing data in any way

EBCDIC (*E*xtended *B*inary *C*oded *D*ecimal *I*nterchange *C*ode)
A coding scheme in which eight bits are used to represent one byte (character)

EDSAC (*E*lectronic *D*elay *S*torage *A*utomatic *C*alculator)
An early experimental computer

EDVAC (*E*lectronic *D*iscrete *V*ariable *A*utomatic *C*omputer)
An early experimental computer

ENIAC (*E*lectronic *N*umerical *I*ntegrator *A*nd *C*alculator)
The first electronic digital computer, developed by Presper Echert Jr. and Dr. John Mauchley

Floppy disk (disc) A flexible plastic-coated magnetic disk (about the size of a 45 rpm record) that can function as both an input/output and auxillary storage device; also called a diskette

FORTRAN (*FOR*mula *TRAN*slator)
A high-level programming language used primarily for scientific and mathematical applications

Flowchart A series of symbols used to illustrate the logical solution to a problem graphically

Field A collection of characters stored together to represent a single item of data

File A collection of related records of data organized and stored together

Graphic display terminal A display device used for input/output of both alphanumeric and graphic data

Hard copy Copy (output) printed primarily on paper

Hard disk (disc) A rigid metal disk that can function as an input/output and auxillary storage device; also called a Winchester

Hardware The physical components of the computer

High-level language A programming language that approximates normal English language and does not reflect a specific computer

Hollerith tabulator The first electric tabulator and sorter, developed by Herman Hollerith

Hybrid computer A computer that contains features of both analog and digital computers

Information The results of data processed by a computer system

Integrated circuits (IC) The electronic circuits etched on small silicon wafers used in third-generation computers

Intelligent Terminal See Smart terminal

Input unit A unit by which data are entered into a computer system

Interactive processing The processing of data in which a user interacts with the computer

Jacquard loom The first automatic weaving machine, developed by Joseph Jacquard

K The abbreviation for kilo (1024 bytes), used to describe the number of bytes a computer can store (*e.g.*, a computer with a storage capacity of 128K can store approximately 128 thousand bytes)

Keyboard An input device that resembles a typewriter and is an integral part of a terminal

Large scale integration (LSI) The microminiaturized electronic circuits etched on a single silicon chip used in fourth-generation computers

Loop A flowchart symbol that graphically illustrates a repititious instruction in a computer program

Leibniz calculator The first mechanical calculator, developed by Goffried von Leibniz

Line printer An impact printer that prints one line at a time

Machine language The low-level language (consisting of binary digits 0 and 1) that only the computer understands and uses

Magnetic disk (disc) Input/output and storage medium; a metal plate that resembles a phonograph record, on which data are stored as magnetized spots

Magnetic ink character recognition (MICR) Input medium that uses a device to read characters imprinted with special magnetic ink

Magnetic tape Input/output and storage medium; a tape that resembles a ½-inch reel of film strip, on which data are stored as magnetized spots

Mainframe The largest, fastest computer that can collect, store, and process extensive amounts of data

MARK I The first large-scale digital calculator, developed by Howard Aiken

Megabyte One million characters (bytes)

Memory, auxillary Storage (*e.g.*, on magnetic disk) used to expand the memory capacity of the computer; also called secondary storage

Memory, main The unit within the CPU that stores all data for immediate access; also called primary storage

Memory unit The computer unit that stores the data and instructions that the computer will process

Menu Lists of options, displayed on a terminal video screen, offered for selection by a computer program

Microcomputer The smallest type of computer, in which all the hardware is built into one unit; also called personal computer, desktop computer, or home computer

Microprocessor on a chip The electronic circuits of the CPU etched on a silicon chip; a computer on a chip

Minicomputer A computer that is smaller but similar to a mainframe. It generally has a smaller storage capacity and a slower processing time

Model A representation of a real situation

Modem A device that translates (encodes and decodes) digital data into waves (analog signals) so that they can be transmitted over communication lines (*e.g.*, telephone lines) to or from a computer system

Multiprocessing The integrated processing of data by two or more computer systems

Multiprogramming The concurrent processing of two or more programs by one computer system

MUMPS (*M*assachusetts General Hospital *U*tility *M*ulti *P*rogramming *S*ystem) A high-level programming language developed for clinical health care applications

Napier bones An early computing device for multiplication and division, developed by John Napier

On-line (processing) Processing in which data are communicated through an on-line terminal, to the computer

Operating system The system programs that supervise and control the computer resources, manage the data, and execute computer programs

Optical character recognition (OCR) Input medium that uses a scanning device to read (sense) specially printed marks or characters

Output unit The unit that conveys the information generated by the computer

PASCAL A high-level programming language with many applications used in interactive processing, named for Blaise Pascal

Pascal calculator The first mechanical calculator to add and subtract, developed by Blaise Pascal

Peripheral All devices external to the CPU

PLI (*P*rogramming *L*anguage *I*) A general all-purpose high-level programming language

Plotter An output device that produces hard copy in graphic form

Printer An output device that converts information generated by the computer into hard copy in printed form

Program A set of instructions, organized in sequence, stored in the computer, and used to solve a problem

Programming The process of writing a computer program

Programming language A language that uses a precise set of rules to communicate with the computer

Punched card A paper card with 12 rows and 80 columns in which combinations of holes are punched to represent data

RAM (*R*andom *A*ccess *M*emory) Memory in which data and instructions may be added or altered by the user

Random access Method of processing data that has been organized randomly; data are accessed directly as they occur

Real-time processing Processing of on-line interactive data as they occur (to affect decision making)

Record A collection of related fields of data organized and stored together

ROM (*R*ead *O*nly *M*emory) Memory that contains programs and data that cannot be altered by the user

RPG (*R*eport *P*rogram *G*enerator)
A high-level programming language used to allow easy generation of business reports

Security Safeguards designed to protect a computer system and data from deliberate destruction, accidental access, or loss by unauthorized persons

Sequential access Method of processing data that have been organized in sequence; data are accessed one after another

Smart terminal A terminal able to store, edit, and minimally process data before transmitting them to the computer

Soft copy Information conveyed as a video display

Software Computer programs that run the computer; all nonhardware computer components

Software package A set of computer programs developed for a specific function and sold to many computer users in ready-to-use form

Storage, primary See memory, main

Storage, secondary See memory, auxillary

Stored program Concept of the stored computer program, developed by John von Neumann

System A whole unit composed of interrelated parts or elements

System programs Programs stored in ROM that carry out, maintain, supervise, and control the automatic functions of the computer

Teleprocessing The use of telecommunication equipment to communicate from terminals in remote locations with a computer

Teletypewriter See hard copy terminal

Template A display menu of headings that formats the input of data into the computer; a tool used to draw the symbols of a flowchart

Terminal An input/output device used to communicate (send or receive data to or from) with the computer

TimeSharing A computer system that allows many users to access it at the same time to run different programs

Transistor A small semiconductor electronic device used in second-generation computers

Translation program The systems programs that translate the programming language into machine language; also called compiler, interpreter, or assembler

Vacuum tube A light bulblike two-state device used for the electronic component of first-generation computers

Video display tube (VDT) See cathode ray tube (CRT) terminal

UNIVAC I (*UNIV*ersal *A*utomatic *C*omputer *I*)
The first commercial computer

User friendly A program, written in English-like words, that is easy to use

Voice input A special audio device that converts voice input into digital form that the computer can understand

Voice output A special device that converts computer output into vocalized sounds

Whirlwind I An early experimental computer

Answers to Study Questions

CHAPTER 1

1. List the needs of the nursing profession that influenced the introduction of the computer into nursing.
   1. Nursing practice
   2. Nursing standards
   3. Nurse supply
   4. Nursing services
   5. Nursing education
   6. Nursing research

2. Name the nurse who greatly influenced nursing practice, education, and research

   Florence Nightingale

3. Who sets the standards for nursing practice in hospitals?

   Joint Commission of Accreditation for Hospitals

4. Who conducted the first inventory of all registered nurses and when was it conducted?

   1. American Nurses' Association 2. 1949

5. List the four key people who conducted studies in nursing education.
   1. Goldmark
   2. Brown
   3. Bridgmen
   4. Lysaught

6. In what year did nursing research begin to receive federal support?

   1955

7. Name at least three legislative acts that influenced the introduction of the computer into nursing.
   - Nurse Training Act of 1964
   - Omnibus Budget Reconciliation Act of 1981
   - Social Security Amendment of 1965 (Medicare and Medicaid)
   - Quality Assurance Program of 1972
   - National Health Planning and Resources Development Act of 1974
   - Health Services Research, Health Statistics, and Medical Libraries Act of 1974
   - Social Security Amendments of 1984 (DRGs)

8. Name three of the five early hospital computer applications.
   1. Burroughs/Medi Data HIS
   2. Texas Institute for Rehabilitation and Research system
   3. Institute of Living system
   4. PROMIS
   5. Technicon MIS

9. What is COSTAR and what does the acronym stand for?
   1. An ambulatory care system
   2. *CO*mputer *ST*ored *A*mbulatory *R*ecord system

10. Name the first computer-based education system.
PLATO

11. What is MEDLINE and what does the acronym stand for?
   1. The world's largest document retrieval system
   2. *MED*ical *L*iterature *A*nalysis and *R*etrieval *S*ystem on *L*ine

12. Who sponsored the first national conference on management information system for public and community health agencies in 1973?
Division of Nursing, U.S. PHS, in cooperation with the National League for Nursing

13. When and where was the first international computer meeting involving nurses held?
1. 1982   2. London

14. Name an organization that annually sponsors a symposium on computer application in medical care that offers nursing sessions.
The Annual Symposium on Computer Application in Medical Care (SCAMC), sponsored by George Washington Medical Center, Office of Continuing Medical Education

15. What is the name of the first nursing journal on computers and when was it first published?
1. Computers in Nursing (CIN)   2. 1984

CHAPTER 2

1. What five inventions or people influenced the early development of the computer?

INVENTIONS	*NAMES*
Abacus	
Napier bones	Jones Napier
Calculator	Blaise Pascal
Calculator	Gottfied von Leibniz
Analystical engine	Charles Babbage
Tabulator	Herman Hollerith

2. Who is considered the father of the computer?
Charles Babbage

3. Who built Mark I, the first large-scale computer, and where was it built?
1. Professor Howard Aiken   2. Harvard University

4. What is the name of the first electronic computer?
ENIAC (*E*lectronic *N*umerical *I*ntegrator *A*nd *C*alculator).

5. Who was responsible for the stored-program concept?
Dr. John von Newmann

6. Name the three experimental computers used to develop the modern computer.

1. EDSAC (*E*lectronic *D*elay *S*torage *A*utomatic *C*alculator)
2. EDVAC (*E*lectronic *D*iscrete *V*ariable *A*utomatic *C*omputer)
3. WHIRLWIND I

7. What is the name of the first commercially available computer?
UNIVAC I

8. How many generations of computers are there to date?
Four

9. List the type of electronic component for each of the computer generations.
First generation—vacuum tube
Second generation—transistor
Third generation—integrated circuit (IC)
Fourth generation—large-scale integrated (LSI) circuit

10. In what form was the first microcomputer introduced in 1975?
As a hobbyist kit

CHAPTER 3

1. What are the three broad classes of computers?
1. Analog
2. Digital
3. Hybrid

2. Name four major characteristics of a computer.
1. Automatic
2. Electronic
3. General purpose
4. Digital

3. Name the three types of computers.
1. Mainframe
2. Minicomputer
3. Microcomputer

4. Name the five functional components of a computer.
1. Input
2. Output
3. Control unit
4. Memory unit
5. Arithmetic and logic unit (ALU)

5. Name the most common input device.
Cathode Ray Tube (CRT) Terminal—contains keyboard and CRT video display

6. Name the two types of terminals.
1. Dumb terminal
2. Smart terminal

7. Name the input media for the early computers.
Punched card

8. Name the three units in the CPU.
1. Control unit
2. Arithmetic and logic unit
3. Main memory

9. What are the two operations that the arithmetic and logic unit performs?
1. Arithmetic calculation
2. Logical operations

10. What are the three basic comparisons the arithmetic logic unit performs?
1. Equal to
2. Less than
3. Greater than

11. Name the two types of memory units.
1. Main memory (primary storage)
2. Auxiliary memory (secondary storage)

12. Name the two types of memory storage.
1. Read Only Memory (ROM) 2. Read Access Memory (RAM)

13. Name the four types of auxiliary memory (secondary storage) media.
1. Magnetic tape 3. Floppy disk (diskette)
2. Magnetic disk 4. Hard disk

14. Name two auxiliary storage media used by the microcomputer.
1. Floppy disk (diskette) 2. Hard disk

15. Name six major output devices.
1. Printer 4. Voice output
2. Microfilm/microfiche 5. CRT terminal
3. Graphic display 6. Terminals

CHAPTER 4

1. What does computer software do?
Makes the computer run

2. A computer program is a set of organized instructions written in sequence and stored in computer memory. True or false?
True

3. Who first described the stored computer program?
Ada, Countess of Lovelace, Lord Byron's daughter

4. Who proposed the stored program concept for the modern computer?
Dr. John von Neumann

5. Name the two major categories of programs.
1. System programs 2. Applications programs

6. Name two functions performed by system programs.
Any two of the following are correct:
1. Operating systems 3. Utility programs
2. Translation programs

7. Name the three translation programs.
1. Compiler 3. Assembler
2. Interpreter

8. Application programs are stored in what type of memory?
Random access memory (RAM)

9. Name three types of softwares packages.
Any one is correct:
1. Database management systems 3. Statistical software packages
2. Authoring systems 4. Work processing systems

10. Name the two types of displays on a CRT screen.
1. Menu 2. Template

11. Name the three levels of computer programming languages.

1. Machine language
2. Assembly language
3. High-level language

12. Which language consists of the binary digits 0 and 1?
Machine language

13. What language requires on assembler?
Assembly language

14. Which language uses English-like words?
High-level languages

15. Name the most common business high-level language.
COBOL (*co*mmon *b*usiness *o*riented *l*anguage)

16. Name the language used primarily for scientific and mathematical applications.
FORTRAN (*for*mula *tran*slator)

17. Name the language developed for clinical health care applications.
MUMPS (*M*assachusetts General Hospital *u*tility *m*ulti *p*rogramming *s*ystem)

18. Name the five steps in preparing a computer program (programming).
1. Problem definition
2. Program design
3. Program preparation
4. Program testing
5. Program implementation/documentation

19. What is used to illustrate graphically the logical solution to a program?
Flowchart

20. What is used to represent graphically the repetitive operation in a computer program?
Loop

CHAPTER 5

1. What does data processed by the computer produce?
Information

2. Name five common operations the computer performs.
Any five listed below are correct:
1. Input
2. Storage
3. Update
4. Sort
5. Classify
6. Compare
7. Compute
8. Summarize
9. Query
10. Retrieve
11. Output

3. Name the six logical entities in which data are organized and stored in the computer.
1. Bit
2. Character
3. Field
4. Record
5. File
6. Database

4. How many numbers are used in the binary numbering system?
Two

5. A bit can have what two values?
1. Zero (0) 2. One (1)

6. What is another name for a character?
Byte

7. Code the number 2 using the binary numbering system with 8 bits.
0000 0010

8. What are the two standards the computer uses to code bytes?
1. EBCDIC (*e*xtended *b*inary *c*oded *d*ecimal *i*nterchange *c*ode)
2. ASCII (*a*merican *s*tandard *c*ode for *i*nformation *i*nterchange)

9. How many bytes are described by the letter K (kilobyte)?
1024 bytes or 1000 bytes

10. Name the two types of record lengths.
1. Fixed length 2. Variable length

11. A field represents a single piece of information. True or false?
True

12. Name three types of files.
1. Master files
2. Transaction/update files
3. Report/sort files

13. Name three different file structures.
1. Sequential file
2. Direct/random file
3. Indexed file

14. Name the three different database structures.
1. Hierarchical structure
2. Network structure
3. Relational structure

15. Name two major characteristics of a DBMS.
1. Software package 2. Query language

16. What are the two methods of data processing?
1. Sequential access 2. Random access

17. Name three types of data processing.
1. On-line processing
2. Interactive/real-time processing
3. Batch processing

18. How are data entered into the computer in interactive/real-time processing?
CRT terminals

19. Card-key methods to access the computer are installed for what purpose?
To promote physical security of the computer

20. Can the Social Security number of citizens be used in any nongovernmental computer system?
No

CHAPTER 6

1. Who first introduced general systems theory?
Ludwig von Bertalanffy

2. What event caused systems theory to emerge?
   World War II

3. What is a system?
   1. A whole unit composed of interrelated subunits
   or
   2. A set of interrelated elements

4. Name four types of systems.
   1. Mechanical 3. Human
   2. Organizational 4. Combination of above

5. What are the five major elements of a system?
   1. Input 4. Feedback
   2. Process 5. Control
   3. Output

6. Name two characteristics of systems.
   1. Open 2. Closed

7. Define a computer system.
   The application of systems theory to a computer

8. Name the five common types of information systems.
   1. Dedicated 4. Monitoring
   2. Transaction 5. Word processing
   3. Retrieval

9. What is the purpose of a menu in a word processing system?
   To display options

10. What is the purpose of a template in a word processing system?
    To enter data

11. What are the three functional levels addressed in a MIS?
    1. Strategic planning 3. Staff operations
    2. Management control

12. Name the three personnel levels in an organization.
    1. Top level 3. Lower level
    2. Middle level

13. What is the purpose of a HIS?
    To facilitate communication and integration of data needed to deliver patient care

14. Name the three types of HIS applications.
    1. Administrative 3. Special purpose
    2. Clinical

15. Several minicomputers connected together form what system configuration?
    Network system

CHAPTER 7

1. Define a NIS.
   A NIS uses a computer to process data into information to support all types of nursing activities or functions

2. What organization defined nursing in its social policy statement?
American Nurses' Association

3. Name three nurse theorists or authors who have described different ways patient care is provided.
Any three listed below are correct:
1. Rogers
2. Orem
3. Yura and Walsh
4. Putt
5. Donnelly, Mangel, and Sutterley
6. McFarland, Leonard, and Morris

4. In what organizational structures does nursing information exist?
Facilities that employ nurses

5. List three major types of facilities where NISs exist.
Any three listed below are correct:
1. Hospital/institution
2. Public/community health
3. Occupational/industry
4. Schools/boards of education
5. Educational institution
6. Research setting

6. Name the various groups that have defined a NIS.
1. Study group on NISs
2. Flynn, Forest, and Heffron
3. Saba and McCormick

7. Name the four major nursing areas where NISs are found.
1. Nursing administration
2. Nursing practice
3. Nursing research
4. Nursing education

8. In which two major in-hospital nursing areas are NISs generally found?
1. Nursing service 2. Nursing unit management

9. Name a system specific for nursing practice.
Physiologic monitoring system

10. Name two areas in research where computers are used.
1. Document retrieval systems 2. Data management systems

11. What is included in computer-based education?
1. Computer-assisted instruction (CIA)
2. Computer-managed instruction (CMI)

12. An expert system is a form of artificial intelligence. True or False?
True

CHAPTER 8

1. Name the three ways a NIS is designed.
1. Separate stand-alone system
2. Subsystem of a larger system
3. Component of another system

2. Name the five phases in developing a NIS.
1. Planning phase
2. Analysis phase
3. Design phase
4. Development phase
5. Implementation/evaluation phase

3. Name the two groups of people needed to begin developing a NIS.
1. Project staff 2. NIS committee

4. What is another name for the planning phase?
Initial phase or preliminary phase

5. List one critical step in the planning phase.
Any of those listed below is correct:
1. Define problem
2. Conduct feasibility study
3. State objectives
4. Determine scope
5. Determine information needs
6. Allocate resources

6. What factors are considered in allocating resources?
1. Personnel
2. Time frame
3. Cost/budget
4. Facilities and equipment

7. Name the three major steps in the system analysis phase.
1. Collect data
2. Analyze data
3. Review data

8. What are the four major sources of data for the fact-finding activity?
1. Written documents
2. Questionnaires
3. Interviews
4. Observations

9. What five tools of the trade are used to analyze data?
1. Flow chart
2. Grid chart
3. Decision table
4. Organizational chart
5. Model

10. What four major steps are carried out in the design phase?
1. Design outputs
2. Design inputs
3. Design files and databases
4. Design system controls

11. Name three factors that must be considered in designing outputs.
Any of those listed below is correct:
1. Content
2. Format
3. Medium
4. Estimated volume
5. Frequency
6. Distribution

12. Name the scope of data inputs.
Smallest definable data element

13. What two approaches are used in developing data files?
1. Bottom up
2. Top down

14. What are the three major steps in selecting a system contract service?
1. Request for proposal (RFP)
2. Evaluate responses
3. Negotiate contract

15. Name the four steps in the system development phase.
1. Select hardware
2. Develop software
3. Test system
4. Document system

16. What dictates the type of hardware selected?
1. System design
2. System application
3. Software required

17. Who writes the computer software programs?
Programmer

18. What type of data are used to test the system?
Live data (real facts)

19. Name the three manuals that should be prepared to document the system.
1. User's manual
2. Operator's manual
3. Maintenance manual

20. Name the four steps in the implemenation and evaluation phase.
1. Implement system
2. Train users
3. Manage and maintain system
4. Evaluate system

21. What are the four possible approaches to implement the system?
1. Parallel
2. Pilot
3. Phased
4. Crash

22. Name two levels of training.
1. General overview
2. In-depth level

23. Who manages and maintains the system?
Computer unit staff

24. Name three tools that can be used to evaluate a system.
1. Record review
2. Time study
3. Satisfaction questionnaire

25. Name four approaches that can be used to evaluate a system.
1. Patient care benefits
2. Morale of nursing personnel
3. Nursing department operations benefits
4. Technical and functional performance

CHAPTER 9

1. What are the two main categories of administrative applications?
1. Nursing services administration information
2. Nursing unit management information

2. What are the essential components of a nursing services administration information system?
1. Quality assurance
2. Personnel files
3. Communications
4. Budgeting
5. Census reports
6. Summary reports
7. Forecasting and planning

3. What are the essential components of nursing unit management systems?
1. Classifications
2. Staffing based on acuity
3. Schedules
4. Inventory
5. Patient bills/charge compilations
6. Incident and other reports
7. Shift reports

4. Describe a quality assurance system in which the computer is the central processor.
1. See Figure 9-1 or any mainframe or microcomputer versions of systems that provide quality assurance (*e.g.*, Technicon, IBM, Shared Medical Systems,

Medical Information Technology, MEDICUS, or Hospital Data Center of Virginia)

5. List important information that can be provided on payroll systems.
   1. Mailing lists
   2. Educational programs
   3. Promotion eligibility
   4. Census
   5. Float pools
   6. Personnel budget expenditures
   7. Location of personnel
   8. License validation
   9. Certification updates
   10. Profile analysis of nursing personnel

6. Define a patient classification system
   A scheme by which patient needs or nursing services are assessed

7. How is patient classification converted by computers to workload measures?
   The translation of classification to a workload measure is the acuity.

8. List the components of a budget system.
   1. Accounts receivable
   2. Patient account
   3. Accounts payable
   4. General ledger
   5. Property ledger accounting
   6. Debts
   7. Collections
   8. Preventive maintenance costs
   9. Medicare/Medicaid patient profiles
   10. Cost allocation
   11. Cash control

9. What types of unit reports can be generated with computers?
   1. Incident
   2. Poison control
   3. Allergy and drug reactions
   4. Identification of patients at risk
   5. Infection control

10. How many mainframe and minicomputer systems have all the administrative and management applications?
    None

11. How many microcomputer systems have all the administrative and unit management applications?
    None

12. Discuss one issue confronting the administrative applications of computers.
    Careful consideration of what nursing includes in its budgeting rosters.

CHAPTER 10

1. Which public law placed Medicare beneficiaries on a prospective payment system? In what year did this occur?
   PL 98-21; 1983

2. What unit of payment and method or mechanism for price setting was established by HCFA?
   Per case, with a formula approach

3. What advantages do computers have with nursing information under cost containment efforts?
   To link patient care, financial, and management information

4. Useful nursing management information can be obtained from what 15 areas?

1. Skill and patient mix by unit (patient classification acuity)
2. Staffing patterns (workload)
3. Absenteeism
4. Patient occupancy patterns (census)
5. Nursing costs by unit
6. Cost of other services by unit
7. Quality assurance information (documentation against standards)
8. Discharge planning
9. Staff recruitment
10. Performance and productivity evaluation
11. Risk management and incident reports
12. Payment mechanisms
13. Nursing orders
14. Transfer notes
15. Patient's DRG status

5. What is the major benefit of computerized information for prospective payment?
Timely information

6. How could existing software packages be classified?

1. Product-line costing
2. Case cost accounting
3. Profile physician admissions, costs, and results consumption
4. Manage the total cost per case

7. Identify 20 essential components of an integrated hospital system for prospective payment

1. Planning
2. Budgeting
3. Medical and nursing performance evaluation
4. Marketing
5. Staff recruitment
6. Quality assurance
7. Utilization review
8. Discharge planning
9. Payment mechanism
10. Other management reports (*e.g.*, risk management and incident reports)
11. Census
12. Patient bills
13. Accounts receivable
14. Order entry
15. Case mix
16. Patients' conditions
17. DRG assignment
18. Communications
19. Results reports
20. Litigations (malpractice suits)

8. Name a case-mix information system that integrates clinical and financial data,

incorporates case-mix classification systems, and produces planning, budgeting, and clinical management reports.
PBCS

9. What is the name of the Dynamic Control Corporation system?
Hospital patient management system

10. Which system provides rate setting, financial modeling, budgeting, and DRG grouping?
MediFlex

11. Which system combines mainframes with microcomputer terminals?
Hospital Workstations

12. Which system integrates nursing-based patient acuity ratings with costs?
Medicus NPAQ

13. Which system offers nursing care hours accounting within a microcomputer?
Janna+

14. What, if any, system examines nursing procedures?
GRASP

15. What New Jersey system supplements DRGs with nursing costs?
Relative intensity measures (RIMS)

16. Has nursing diagnosis been computerized?
Yes

17. Name one medical diagnosis or procedure-based system.
1. CRVS 4. ICD-9-CM
2. CPT-4 5. MDC
3. GPMP 6. Severity of illness

18. Discuss one nursing management change that computerized prospective payment will have on future nurse administrators.
Provision of timely information

CHAPTER 11

1. What major piece of legislation influenced the expansion of community health nursing services in this county?
Medicare and Medicaid (Social Security Amendments of 1965)

2. Computer application in community health centers around what three major areas?
1. Community health management information systems.
2. Ambulatory care systems
3. Special-purpose applications

3. Name the three types of community health management information systems.
1. Financial and billing 3. Patient care
2. Statistical reporting

4. Name at least three applications provided by financial and billing systems.
Any three are acceptable:
1. General ledger 2. Accounts receivable

3. Accounts payable
4. Payroll
5. Billing

5. Name at least three applications provided by statistical reporting systems.
Any three are acceptable:
   1. Visit reports
   2. Service statistics
   3. Patient registration
   4. Patient case load
   5. Census
   6. Patient scheduling

6. List the three system options that community and home health agencies can select from service bureau or vendors.
   1. Batch processing
   2. Remote entry
   3. Complete package

7. In what state is the only on-line statewise client information system found?
Florida

8. Name three local community health agencies that offer a management information system.
   1. Visiting Nurse Association of Omaha, NE
   2. Visiting Nurse Association of Houston, TX
   3. Ramsey County Public Health Nursing Service

9. Name the three instruments that can be used to assess community health patients.
   1. Psychosocial assessment
   2. Activities of daily living
   3. Family coping scale

10. Name the most widely used ambulatory care system.
COSTAR (*co*mputer-*st*ored *a*mbulatory *r*ecord system)

11. In what two states is the Indian health service system (patient care information system) found?
   1. Arizona
   2. Alaska

12. List the four types of community health special applications.
   1. Special statistical studies
   2. Screening programs
   3. Epidemiologic projects
   4. Prevention projects

CHAPTER 12

1. What major standards govern nursing documentation?
   1. Practice acts
   2. JCAH standards
   3. ANA standards
   4. Hospital policies,
   5. Current legal thinking

2. Define the two basic categories of documentation of patient care.
   1. Direct patient care
   2. Nursing unit management reports

3. How are the potential components of documenting direct patient care universally organized in mainframe systems?
Nursing process: assessing, planning, implementing, evaluating

4. Name five records that could be produced from a direct patient care system.
   1. Admission assessment
   2. Nursing care plan/Kardex
   3. Nursing progress note
   4. Medication administration sheets
   5. Vital signs and other flowsheets
   6. Nursing order summary
   7. Automatic schedule summaries
   8. Discharge care plan
   9. Summary

5. Name five major vendors of mainframe computers with nursing documentation capabilities.
   1. Burroughs
   2. Datacare
   3. IBM
   4. SMS
   5. Technicon
   6. Martin Marietta
   7. NCR/MEDNET
   8. HBO MEDPRO

6. Nursing content can be integrated with risk management information. True or False?
   True

7. If so, where has this been done and on what system?
   New York University Hospital; IBM Hardware/Technicon MATRIX MIS

8. What three areas of documentation are found within the Technicon System?
   1. Interdependent nursing
   2. Independent nursing
   3. Interrelationship between the two

9. The Technicon system uses pattern, impairment, and aid as one example of content flow. From the other examples provided, what is another content flow?
   Improvement, stabilization, and deterioration

10. What are the five components of a discharge care plan?
    1. Admission summary assessment
    2. Summary of learning needs
    3. Multi-disciplinary plan
    4. Medications and procedures
    5. Summary of patient outcomes that the patient should have achieved during hospitalization

11. Describe the seven essential elements to consider in a microcomputer for documenting nursing practice
    1. Amount of memory
    2. Input mode
    3. Output features
    4. Language
    5. Communication
    6. Software availability
    7. Flexibility

12. Are any documentation systems available on microcomputers?
    RNact or DIALAZA

CHAPTER 13

1. What are the seven major capabilities of computers in the ICU, ER, and OR?
   1. Microprocess physiologic data
   2. File documentation of patient care
   3. Graph trend data
   4. Regulate physiologic equipment through microprocessors

5. Microprocess diagnostic equipment
6. Recognize by an alarm deviations from normal preset ranges
7. Compare and evaluate patients with similar diagnoses

2. What are the three types of computer applications in the ICU?
1. Arrhythmia monitors
2. Physiologic monitors
3. Special-purpose systems

3. Name the basic elements of an arrhythmia monitor.
1. Sensor
2. Signal conditioner
3. Cardiograph
4. Pattern recognition
5. Rhythm analysis
6. Diagnosis
7. Written report

4. Identify the types of arrhythmia systems
Detection surveillance and diagnostic/interpretive

5. Name a vendor of an arrhythmia monitoring system.
1. IBM Bonner
2. Telemed
3. CAPOC
4. Hewlett-Packard
5. Phone-a-Gram System

6. List the five basic parts of physiologic monitoring systems.
1. Sensor
2. Signal conditioner
3. File
4. Computer processor
5. Evaluator

7. What are the three basic types of physiologic monitoring systems?
1. Detection/surveillance
2. Diagnostic/interpretive
3. Treatment intervention

8. Name a distributed physiologic monitoring system.
Hewlett-Packard to IBM or IBM TO IBM PDMS (must be two systems linked)

9. Describe two modular systems that extend the concept of distributed systems.
Burdick and Trinity

10. Define an integrated physiologic monitoring system.
An integrated system is one that combines physiologic monitoring systems and patient data management systems

11. Name the seven special-purpose systems that nurses may use in hospital practice today.
1. Ventilators
2. Blood gas analyzers
3. Pulmonary functions systems
4. Intracranial pressure monitors
5. Cardiac and other diagnostic systems
6. Drug administration systems
7. Newborn nursery systems

12. What are the basic elements of an emergency medical system?
1. Continuous patient monitorings
2. Communication with interpretive and diagnostic centers
3. Consultation using immediate access to large databases

13. What are the basic elements of an OR management system?

1. OR schedules and nursing personnel schedules
2. Budgeting supplies
3. Infection control
4. Documenting medications given
5. Intake and output
6. Retrospective chart audit

14. What surgical procedure may be facilitated by computers?
    1. Arteriography
    2. Angiography
    3. Autotransfusion
    4. Reconstructive surgery

CHAPTER 14

1. What are two main applications of computers for nursing research?
   1. Nursing research process 2. Clinical nursing research
2. What are the six uses of computers in the research process?
   1. Information retrieval
   2. Data processing
   3. Statistical analysis
   4. Graphics
   5. Database management
   6. Text editing
3. Name the MEDLARS on-line database that is the largest information retrieval system in the world.
   MEDLINE
4. Name two databases relevant to nursing.
   ERIC and SOCIAL SCISEARCH
5. Identify the four main steps in transforming raw data into a computer file.
   1. Edit the raw data
   2. Code, score, and scale the data
   3. Communicate the data through acoustic couplers, satellite, or microwave
   4. Input the data
6. What are the ten main components of a file?
   1. Problem, title, or label
   2. Input paragraph
   3. Variable paragraph
   4. Group, box, head category
   5. Lines or blocking factors
   6. Columns
   7. Cells
   8. Body
   9. Footnotes
   10. Source
7. What are the seven major categories of statistics software packages?
   1. General purpose
   2. Restricted applications
   3. Database management packages
   4. Editing packages
   5. Tabulations packages
   6. Survey analysis
   7. Subroutine libraries
8. Discuss the five essential characteristics of a statistical software package.
   1. Capabilities
   2. Portability
   3. Ease of learning
   4. Reliability
   5. Cost
9. What are three major capabilities of a statistical software package?

1. Statistical analysis 3. Mathematical
2. Sample survey

10. Name the three major statistical software packages on mainframes and minicomputers.
1. SPSS 3. BMDP
2. SAS

11. List ten major statistical programs on microcomputers

1. ABSTAT	13. SpeedSTAT
2. AIDA	14. SPS
3. Dynacomp	15. STAN
4. A-STAT	16. Statpro
5. EDA	17. SYSTAT
6. HSD	18. TWG ELF
7. INTROSTAT 2.1	19. TWG ARIMA
8. MICROSTAT	20. Wallonick Statpac
9. Micro-TSP	21. PFS
10. Number Cruncher	22. UISACALC
11. NWA STATPAK	23. MUHPLAN
12. SAM	

12. Name a software package for graphically displaying data
Prime Plotter

13. Name a program for text editing.
1. Wylbur 3. TEK
2. Scribe 4. ATMS

14. Describe two essential preconditions for a nursing database
1. Structure is valid 2. Content is reliable

15. Identify three categories of data available for clinical nursing information.
1. Nursing science
2. Efficacy of strategies
3. Nursing care organization and delivery

16. Discuss one issue confronting the nursing profession resulting from the impact of computers on nursing research.
Take any one listed in chapter.

CHAPTER 15

1. What are the two basic categories of usage within CBE (CAL)?
1. CAI 2. CMI

2. In addition to the two categories mentioned above, are there additional educational applications of computers relevant to nursing? If so, name them.
Yes.
1. CAVI
2. Expert systems
3. Knowledge synthesizers
4. Educational applications with mainframes
5. Nurse extenders

6. Discharge education plans
7. Potentials for home computers

3. Name one system that includes both CAI and CMI components and thus is a CBE System.
PLATO

4. Name the four major types of CAI.
1. Problem solving
2. Drill and practice
3. Tutorials
4. Simulations

5. Do any CAI software use a video disk in addition to computer software?
Yes

6. Describe an authoring system.
One that requires no previous programming experience

7. Name an authoring system relevant for nursing.
NEMAS (*n*ursing *e*ducation *m*odule *a*uthoring *s*ystem)

8. List three areas where CMI benefits education.
1. Student records
2. Student rotations
3. Educational resources

9. Name one expert system that draws on the concepts of artificial intelligence.
COMMES

Index

Figures followed by *f* indicate illustrations; *t* following a page number indicates tabular material.

Abacus, 409
  as early computer, 27, 28f
Acuity systems, 188–189, 190t–191t, 192, 194–195
  staffing based on, 177
ADA, 78, 409
ADMINISTAR, 196
ALGOL, 78, 409
Algorithm, 409
Algorithmic language. *See* ALGOL
Allergy, lists of, 179
Ambulatory care. *See also* COSTAR
  military study, 251
  nursing model, 229, 230f
  nursing responsibility, areas of, 229, 230f
Ambulatory care systems, 217–218, 245–249, 250f
  COSTAR, 246–247, 247f, 248, 249t. *See also* COSTAR
American Association for Medical Systems and Informatics (AAMSI), 19
American Standard Code for Information Interchange. *See* ASCII
Analog computer, 409
Analytical machine, 409
ANSOS, nursing administration applications, 196, 197f
Application programs, 75, 409
Arithmetic/logic unit, 58–59, 409
Arrhythmia monitors, 302–304
  components, 302, 302t
  examples of systems, 303–304
  types, 302–303
Artificial intelligence, 398, 409
ASCII, 89, 409
Assembler, 409
Assembly language, 77, 409
Assessment criteria, changes in, 4, 4t
Authoring system, computer-assisted, 387, 390, 391f

Babbage, C.
  analytical engine, 28
  difference engine, 28, 30, 30f
  difference machine, 29, 31f
BASIC, 78, 409
Batch processing, 94, 239, 409
Bertalanffy, L. von, 100
Billing, 178, 231
Binary coding. *See* EBCDIC coding system
Binary digit. *See* Bit
Binary numbering system, 409
Bit, 60, 88, 409
Blood gas analysis, microprocessor regulation, 317
Blue Cross, cost management system, 218
BMDP, 342
Boole, G., 59
Boolean true–false propositions, 59, 59f
Budgeting, 172–173
Buffalo Project, 11
Bug, 409
Burdick physiologic monitoring system, 305–306, 307f
Burroughs
  Medi-Data system, 9
  nursing documentation capabilities, 271
Byte, 88–89, 409

CAI. *See* Computer-assisted instruction
Calculators, as early computers, 27, 28f, 29f
CAPOC arrhythmia monitors, 204
CARDIONET system, 321
Casalud, 242
Caseload/Workload planner project, 253
Case-mix information system, 208, 209
CASS, 252

Cathode ray tube (CRT), 409
as output device, 65
terminal, 53, 54f
Census
Hospital Data Center of Virginia and, 187
Shared Medical Systems and, 188
system, 173, 175f
Central processing unit, 409
components of, 58–64
arithmetic/logic unit, 58–59
control unit, 58
memory, 58–64
Character, 88–89, 410
Character printer, 410
Charts
grid, 132, 134f
organizational, 132, 135f
Client management information system, 226, 228, 228f. *See also* Management information system
Chips, 38, 39f, 40f, 410
configuration, 39f
earliest, 40f
COBOL, 78, 410
Code, 410
Coding systems, 89. *See also* EBCDIC coding system; ASCII
COMMAND, in Shared Medical Systems, 188
COMMES, 398, 399f
Communication networks, features and functions, 169, 171, 171f
Community health
agencies, development of computer use in, 224–225
computer applications, 10–12, 229
information systems
nursing models used in, 225–229
special applications, 249, 251
nursing process model, 118f
nursing role in, 224
nursing survey 1979, 251–252
nursing workload assessment, 253
programs, nursing information system and, 119, 122
Compiler, 410
Computer applications
in community health, 10–12
educational, 12
in hospitals, 9–10
in nursing, 8–13
in research, 12
Computer-assisted instruction
advantages of, 392, 394–395
evaluating studies, 392, 394–395
in hospital information systems, 112
software available, 364–365, 366t–386t, 387–395
types of, 363–364
Computer Resources, Inc., 240–241
Computer systems, 105. *See also specific types of systems*
components, 207–208, 208t
Computers, 410
characteristics, 47–48
classes, 47
defined, 46
fifth generation, 39, 41
first generation, 35–37
fourth generation, 38–39
functional components, 50–70
central processing unit, 58–64
input unit, 52–58
output unit, 65–70
generations of, 34–41
hardware. *See* Hardware
historical development, 26–30
industry growth, 41
integrated circuits, 37
large scale, 38
nursing and, landmark events, 13–21
output, microfilm, 410
recent developments, 27t, 31, 33–35, 37
second generation, 36
third generation, 37–38
transistors, 37
types, 48–50. *See also specific types*
uses, in nursing, 3–8
vacuum tubes, 35, 36t
World War II development, 31
Computers in Nursing, establishment, 19
COMSHARE, intake/output system, 322, 324
Control unit, 410
Cost management
alternate payer system, 218
module, Medicus system, 214f, 215f
COSTAR, 11, 246–247, 247f, 248f, 249f
adaptations, 246–247
language used, 246
modules contained, 246
CPU. *See* Central processing unit
Crash implementation, 150, 151
CRT. *See* Cathode ray tube
Cumulative Index to Nursing and Allied Health Literature (CINAHL), 334

Daisy wheel, 410
Data, 10
  field, 90
  file, 91
  hierarchy, 88
  vs information, 105
  record, 90–91
  security, 94–95
  storage organization, 88–89, 90f
Database, 91–93, 410
  hierarchical, 92
  network, 92
  relational, 92
  structure, 92–93
Database management systems, 92–93, 410
  nursing research applications, 344, 347–348
  vendors, 352t
Data bus, 87
Data entry forms, 231, 232f, 233f, 234f, 235f
Data models, 133
Data processing, 410
  batch, 94
  defined, 87
  interactive, 94
  methods, 93
  nursing research applications, 339–344
  on-line, 93–94
  operations, 88
  real-time, 94
  types, 93–94
Data trees, 274f, 275f
DBMS. *See* Database management systems
Debugging, 83, 410
Decision table, 132, 135f
Dedicated systems, 106
Delta Computer Systems, Inc., 241
Diagnosis, medical, systems for, 214
Diagnosis related groups, 7–8, 204–205. *See also* Prospective payments
  in Dynamic Control Corporation's hospital management system, 209
  international system and, 218
  military, 218
DIALAZA, 291
Digital computer, 410
Digital Equipment Corporation, 37, 193
Discharge care planning, 278–279, 282f
Discharge education, 401
Discharge plan summary, example, 290f
Disease prevention projects, 253
Disease surveillance system, 252
Disk
  floppy, 64
  hard, 64, 411
Disk drive, 410
Diskette, 64
Diversified Computer Applications. *See* IMI Health Systems, Inc.
Document retrieval, vendors, 337, 339t
Document retrieval systems, nursing research applications, 331–338
Document systems, for information systems, 149–150
Dot matrix printer, 410
DRGs. *See* Diagnosis related groups
Drug administration, microprocessor regulated, 321–324
Drug reactions, lists of, 179
Dumb terminal, 410
Dynamic Control Corporation, hospital patient management system, 209–210, 210t

EBCDIC coding system, 89, 89f, 410
EDSAC, 34, 410
Education, *See also* Instruction, computer-assisted; Nursing education; Patient education
  computer applications, 12
  computer-based, PLATO, 363
  expert systems, 398
  inservice, computer-assisted, 390–392
  knowledge synthesizers and, 400
  of nursing staff, computer-assisted, 390–392, 393f
  of patients, computer-assisted, 392, 394t
EDVAC, 34, 410
Emergency medicine
  computer applications, 324–325
  poison indexes, 325
ENIAC, 33, 35f, 411
Epidemiology projects, computer applications, 252
ERIC database, 335, 338t
Excerpta Medica database, 334
  abstract journals, 336t–337t
Extended Binary Coded Decimal Interchange Code. *See* EBCDIC coding system

Fair Credit Act, 95
Feasibility studies, for nursing information system, 128–129
Feedback, 102–103
Field, 90, 411
File, 411
  components, 339–340
  direct/random, 91
  indexed, 91
  master, 91
  report/sort, 91
  sequential, 91
  structure, 91
  transaction/update, 91
  types, 91
Financial systems, 172–173
Fleet Information Systems, Inc., 241
Floppy disk, 64, 411
Florida Client Information System, 243, 244, 244f, 245f
Flowchart, 80–81, 80f, 81f, 411
  in data analysis, 132, 133f
  with loop, 83f
  template, 82f
Forecasting, information system application, 173, 175–176
FORTRAN, 78, 411

Graphics, chart, 68f, 69f
Graphics display, 344, 347f, 348f, 349f, 350f
  output, 66, 68f, 69f
  terminal, 411
GRASP system, 212
  nursing administration applications, 188–189, 190t–191t, 192
Grid chart, 132, 134f

Hard copy, 411
Hardware, 411. *See also* Computers; *specific hardware*
  defined, 46
Health assessment, preschool, 252
HELP
  intensive care patient care data system, 306, 310f, 310t, 312f
  nursing administration applications, 192
Hewlett-Packard
  arrhythmia monitoring system, 303
  IBM link, 311
  patient data management system, 306, 309–311
High-level language, 411
HIS. *See* Hospital information system
HMO Act of 1973, 245
Hollerith tabulator, 30, 32f, 411
Home computers, patient education and, 401–402
Home health, information systems applications, 240–242. *See also* Ambulatory care; Community health
Hospice system, 217
Hospital Data Center of Virginia, nursing administration applications, 187–188
Hospital information system (HIS), 110–112
  administrative applications, 110
  Burroughs/Medi-Data, 9
  clinical applications, 110
  combination systems, 112
  configurations, 111–112
  CRT use in, 111
  defined, 110
  functions, 166t
  Institute of Living, 9
  microcomputer use in, 112
  network system, 112
  on-line, interactive, 111, 111f
  patient education and, 112
  PROMIS, 9–10
  stand-alone system, 111
  Technicon MIS, 10
  Texas Institute for Rehabilitation and Research, 9
  types, 110
Hospital Workstation system, 211–212
  principal components, 211
Hybrid computer, 411

IBM
  HIS, administrative applications, 181, 184f
  minicomputer review system, 217
  patient care system, 267, 270, 270f
Illness severity index, 216–217

IMI Health Systems, Inc., 241
Implementation of information systems, 150–151
Index to Dental Literature, 333
Index Medicus, 13, 333
Indian Health Service system, 12
  ambulatory care system, 247–249
Infant monitors, microprocessor regulated, 324
InfoMed, 241
Information, 411
  vs data, 105
Information Sciences, Inc. *See* Fleet Information Systems, Inc.
Information systems. *See also* Hospital information system; Management information system; Nursing information system
  applications
    billing, 178
    budgeting, 172–173, 174f
    census, 173, 175f
    disease prevention, 253
    epidemiology, 252
    forecasting, 173, 175–176
    infection control, 179
    inventory, 177–178
    patient classification, 176–177
    payroll, 172–173
    personnel files, 168–169
    poison control, 178
    quality assurance, 165, 166f–167f, 167–168
    reports, 173, 174f, 175f, 178–179
    scheduling, 177
    screening, 252
    staffing, 177
    unit reports, 179
    utilization review, 179
  dedicated, 106
  defined, 105
  financial functions, 172–173
  monitoring, 107
  retrieval, 106–107
  transaction, 106
  types, 105–108
  word processing, 107–108
Input, 102
  devices and media, 52–58
  unit, 411
Institute of Living, information system of, 9
Instruction
  computer-assisted, 363–365, 366t, 386t, 387–395
    video, 397–398
  computer-managed, 395–397
    education resources, 396–397
    evaluation of, 397
    student records, 395
    student rotations, 395–396
Integrated circuits, 37, 411
  large-scale, 38
Intelligent terminal, 411
Intensive care
  computer applications, 301–324
    arrhythmia monitors, 302–304
    physiologic monitors, 304–313
    special purpose, 314–324
  minicomputer function in, 315t
Interactive processing, 411
International Classification of Diseases, computerized, 214
International Medical Information Association, 9
International Nursing Index, 13, 333, 334, 338t
Intracranial pressure monitoring, microprocessor regulation, 319
Inventory, information system applications, 177–178

Jacquard loom, 411
  as early computer, 27, 29f
Janna+, 212, 216f
  nursing administration applications, 194–195
Janna Medical Systems, program applications, 194f
Joint Commission on Accreditation of Hospitals, 4
Joint Committee on Accreditation of Hospitals (JCAH), quality assurance by information system, 165, 167–168, 169t
Journal, on computers in nursing, 19, 20f

K, 411
Keyboard, 53, 411
Knowledge synthesizers, 400

Languages. *See* Programming languages
Large-scale integration, 412
Legislation, requiring computer assistance, 6–8
Leibniz calculator, 27, 412
Line printer, 67f, 412
Logic operations, 58–59
Loops, 73, 81, 83f, 412

Machine language, 76, 412
Magnetic disks
  floppy, 64
  hard, 64
  memory, 61f, 62–64
Magnetic ink character recognition (MICR), 412
  as input medium, 56–57, 58f
Magnetic media, as input media, 57, 60f, 61f
Magnetic tape, 412
Magnetic tape drive, 63f
Mainframe, 48, 49f, 412
  nursing administration applications, 180t
Maintenance manual, for information systems, 149–150
Management information system (MIS), 108–110
  benefits, 229, 231
  community health applications, 231–237
    local systems, 242–243
    state systems, 243–244, 244f, 245f
    system options, 237, 239–242
  defined, 229
  financial and billing systems, 231
  functional levels in, 108–109, 108f
  information flow in, 109f
  modules in, 228
  patient care, 233, 235
  processing configuration, 226f
  statistical reporting, 231
MARK I, 32f, 33, 412
"Mark sense," 183, 185f
Martin Marietta, nursing documentation system, 270
Medical query language (MQL), 246
Medicare, prospective payment system, 205
Medication information, on computer screen, 286f, 287f
Medicus system
  cost management module, example of, 214f, 215f
  nursing administration applications, 181, 183–184, 185f, 186
  nursing productivity and quality, 212
Mediflex system, 210–211, 211t
  modules of, 210
MEDINFO 1983, 18f, 19
MEDI-VISIT information system, 241
MEDLARS database, 7, 12–13, 331–332, 333t
MEDLINE, 13, 332–334, 338t
Mednet system, nursing documentation capabilities, 271
Megabyte, 412
Memory access
  random, 93
  sequential, 93
Memory
  auxiliary, 61–64, 412
  magnetic disk, 61f, 62–64
  magnetic tape, 63–64
  main unit, 59–70, 412
  media, 59–60
  random access, 60
  read only, 60
  secondary storage, types, 61–64
  storage types, 60
Menu, 76, 412
Michigan State system, 243–244
Micro-Budget, nursing administration applications, 195
Microcomputer, 38–39, 49–50, 51f, 412
  clinical research applications, 354
  integrated patient data management systems, 312–313
  nursing administration applications, 192–197
  nursing documentation capabilities, 283–284, 289, 291
  statistical analysis on, 342–344, 343t, 345t
    program characteristics, 343–344
Microfiche, 66, 68f
Microfilm, 66, 67f
Micro Personnel, 196
Micro-Planning, 195–196
Microprocessor, 38
  on chip, 412
  regulation of equipment with, 314–326
Military ambulatory care study, 251
Military system, diagnosis related groups and, 218
Minicomputer, 37–38, 48–49, 50f, 412. *See also specific minicomputers*

intensive care applications, 315t
nursing administration applications, 180t, 188–192
MIS. *See* Management information system
Model, 412
Modem, 52, 53f, 412
Monitoring, 107
Multiprocessing, 412
Multiprogramming, 413
MUMPS, 79, 246, 413

Napier bones, 413
as early computer, 27, 28f
National Cash Register
nursing administration applications, 188
nursing documentation capabilities, 271
National Center for Health Services Research, 7
National Health Planning and Resources Development Act, 7
National Institutes of Health
conference on computer applications, 17, 19
nursing documentation system, 272–273
National League for Nursing
conference on management information systems, 13, 16f
statistical reporting model, 225, 227f
National Library of Medicine, 12, 331
Network planning models, 135–136
New Jersey Project, 11
New York University Medical Center, nursing documentation system, 276–277
NIS. *See* Nursing information system
Notation, computerized system of, 312
Nurse Training Act of 1964, 6
Nurses, supply of, 4–5
Nursing
computers and, landmark events, 13–21
definitions, 117
intensity index, 216–217
productivity, Medicus system for, 212
Nursing administration
hospital information system applications, 164–176
prospective payment impact on, 219–220
Nursing assessment
IBM Technicon system, 276f
menu, 184f
Nursing care plan, example, 285f
Nursing diagnosis, computerized, 214
Nursing documentation
categories, 263
changes in methods, 260–261
computerized
examples, 282–283, 283f–290f
standards governing, 261, 262t
direct patient care system, 263–265
discharge planning, 278–279
international systems, 277–278
microcomputer use for, 283–284, 289, 291
system capabilities, 266–267, 268t–269t
vendors, 265–279. *See also specific vendors*
Nursing education
history of computer use in, 5–6
information system applications, 122–123
Nursing information systems
administration applications, 122, 180–197
analysis phase, 131–136
applications, 120–123, 121f
background, 116–120
committee and project staff, 125–126
controls design for, 146
cost/budget for developing, 10
cost containment and, 206–207
data collection for, 131–136
database design, 146
dedicated, 119
definitions, 120
design phase, 136–146
development phase, 147–150
document system for, 149–150
in educational institutions, 119
facilities and equipment needed, 130
feasibility study, 128–129
file design, 146
hardware selection, 147
implementation and evaluation phase, 150–151, 153, 157–159
information needs and, 128–129
input design, 140, 142f, 143f, 144f, 144–145
mainframes in, 119
maintenance manual, 149–150
microcomputer in, 119
NLN conference on, 13
nursing definitions and, 117
nursing education and, 122–123
nursing practice and, 122
nursing research and, 122
nursing theory and, 117–119

nursing unit management and, 176–180
operator's manual, 149
organizations implementing, 119
output design, 137, 138f, 139f, 140, 141f
patient data management and, 122
planning phase, 127–131
request for proposal, 147
Research Conference on, 13, 16
research retrieval, 353, 353t
resource allocation for, 129–131
scope, 128
software development, 148–149
as subsystem, 119
Tri-Service Medical Information Systems (TRIMIS), 16
user's manual, 149
user training, 150
uses, 2
Nursing notes, automated, 261
Nursing practice
documenting, 260–261
history of computer use in, 3–4
information system applications, 122
standards of, 4
Nursing process, general model, 118f
Nursing research
clinical
mainframe and minicomputer use, 351–354
microcomputer use, 354
database management systems, 344, 347–348
data processing, 339–344
document retrieval, 331–338
graphics display, 344
history of computer use, 6
information system applications, 122
state of the art of computer use, 350
text editing, 348–350
Nursing services, studies, 5
Nursing skills, computer-assisted, 364–365
Nursing systems, 117–119
Nursing theory, information system applications, 117–119
NURSTAR, 387
NURSystem
nursing administration applications, 193
reports generated by, 193

On-line processing, 93–94, 413
hospital applications, 111
Operating room management, computer applications, 325–326
Operating systems, 74, 413
Operator's manual, for information systems, 149
Optical character recognition, 413
as input medium, 56, 57f
Organizational charts, 132, 135f
Outpatient care system, 217–218
scheduling, 290, 291f
Output, 102
devices and media, 65–70
voice, 66
unit, 413

Parallel implementation, 150
PASCAL, 79, 413
Pascal calculator, 27, 28f, 413
Patient hour chart, 189, 190t–191t
Patient care information system (PCIS), 233, 235–236, 236f, 237f, 238f, 247, 249, 250f, 263
components, 263–264
examples, 264–265
Patient classification systems, 176–177
Medicus system, 186
Patient data management system, 122, 209–210, 210t
Hospital Data of Virginia, 187–188
integrated with physiologic system, 306, 309, 311–313
Patient discharge summary, 213f
Patient education
computer as nurse extender, 400–401
home computer use, 401–402
on mainframe, 400
Payrolls, processing with information systems, 172–173
PDP series, of computers, 37–38
Performance monitors, Medicus system for, 184, 186
Peripheral, 413
Personnel
files, information system use in, 168–169, 170t
productivity, ANSOS and, 196
PERT, 135, 136f
PETO system, 189
Pharmacy systems, 321–322
Phased implementation, 150–151
Philadelphia Project, 11
Phone-a-Gram system, arrhythmia monitor, 303–304

Physical examination, computer-assisted instruction in, 365
Physiologic monitors, 304–313
  bedside systems, 305–306
  integrated systems, 306, 309, 311–313
  types, 305
Pilot implementation, 150
PLATO system, 12, 363
PLI, 79, 413
Plotter, 413
Poison indexes, computerized, 325
POMR (problem-oriented medical record), nursing documentation capabilities, 277
Practice exams and test questions, computer-assisted, 387
Prime Plotter, graphics examples, 247f–250f
Printer, 413
  line printer, 67f
  as output device, 66, 67f. *See also specific types of printers*
Privacy
  legislation, 95–96
    Fair Credit Act, 95
    Privacy Act of 1974, 95–96
  for personal data, 95–96
Privacy Act of 1974, 95–96
Problem-oriented information system. *See* PROMIS
Problem-oriented medical record. *See* POMR
Process, 102
Processing
  interactive, 411
  on-line, 413
  real-time, 413
  tele-, 414
Program, 413
  application, 75
  history, 73–74
  storage concept, 34
  system. *See* Systems programs
  translation, 74–75
  utility, 75
Programming, 413
  definition, 79
  design, 79–81
  documentation, 83–84
  implementation, 83–84
  steps in, 79
  testing, 82–83
  preparation, 82
Programming language, 76–79, 413. *See also specific languages*
  assembly, 77
  high-level, 77–79
  levels of, 76, 77f
  machine, 76
  selection, 78–79
PROMIS system, 9–10, 277
Prospective payment
  defined, 203–204
  diagnosis related groups (DRGs) and, 204–205
  implementation, 205
  Medicare system of, 205
  nursing administration impact, 219–220
  pricing mechanisms, 204
  vs retrospective payment, 204
  trends in, 206
  units, 204
Public health, computer applications, 10–12
Pulmonary function, microprocessor regulation of, 317–319, 320f
Punched cards, 413
  as input, 54–55, 55f, 56f

Q.S., Inc., 241–242
Quality assurance
  information system applications, 165, 167–168, 168f, 169t
  Medicus system for, 181, 183–184, 185f, 186
  program of 1972, 7
Quantitative Sentinel patient data management system, 311–312, 316f
Query language, 75

RAM. *See* Random access memory
Ramsey County Public Health Nursing Service of St. Paul, 243
Random access, 93, 413
Random access memory, 60, 413
Read only memory, 60
Real-time processing, 94, 413
Record, 90–91, 413
Record review, 152f, 153, 154f–155f
Record systems, computerized, 243
Relative intensity measures, 212, 214
Remote entry, 239
Reports
  incident, 178–179
  information system applications, 173, 174f

Research. *See* Nursing research
Research Conference on Nursing Information Systems, 13, 16
Respitrace, ventilation monitoring, 317, 319t
Request for proposal, for information system development, 147
Retrieval system, 106–107
Retrospective payment, vs prospective payment, 204
RNact, 289
Rockland County Project, 10–11
ROM, 413. *See* Read only memory
RPG (Report Program Generator), 79, 414

SAS, 342
Scheduling
  ANSOS and, 196–197
  Janna+ and, 194–195
  Medicus system for, 186
  systems, 177
Schwirian's cube, 352f, 353
Screening programs, computer applications, 252
Security, of data, 94–95, 414
SensorMedics, MMC Horizon System, 317, 318f, 319f
Sequential access, 93, 414
Service bureaus, 239–242, 240t. *See also specific bureaus or vendors*
Shared Medical Systems
  nursing administration applications, 188
  nursing documentation capabilities, 270–271
Smart terminal, 414
SOCIAL SCISEARCH database, 335, 337, 338t
Soft copy, 414
Software, 414
  ADMINISTAR, 196
  capabilities of, 207
  defined, 73
  packages, 73, 75–76, 414
    variations in, 75–76
  sys/PLANR, 195
SPSS, 342
Staffing
  ANSOS and, 196–197
  projections for, 184, 186, 186t
STAT information system, 240–241
Statistical analysis, 340–344
  capabilities, 340–342
  categories, 340–342
  characteristics, 241, 241t
  evaluations, 344
  forecasting, 241–242
  on microcomputers, 342–344, 343t, 345t, 346t
  software packages, 342, 346t
Statistical reporting, information system use in, 231
Statistical studies, computer applications, 251–252
Storage
  primary, 414
  secondary, 414
Stored program, 414
Surgery, computer-assisted, 325–326
Survey of Community Health Nursing 1979, 251–252
Symposium on Computer Applications in Medical Care, 17, 18f, 19
sys/PLANR software, 195
SysteMetrics Inc., Hospital Workstation system, 211–212
System programs, 414
  functions of, 74–75
Systems, 414. *See also* Computer system; Hospital system; Management system; *specific types of systems*
  characteristics, 104
  closed, 104
  control, 102–103
  dedicated, 106
  defined, 101
  elements, 102–104, 103f, 104f
  feedback, 102–103
  human, 102, 103f
  mechanical, 101
  monitoring, 107
  open, 104
  organizational, 102, 102f
  retrieval, 106–107
  transaction, 106
  types, 101–102
  word processing, 107–108
Systems analysis. *See* Systems theory
Systems architecture, nursing administration applications, 189, 192
Systems theory, 100–101

Technicon Matrix Medical Information System, 10, 272–277
  administration applications, 180–181, 182t–183t

- data trees, 274f, 275f
- documentation areas, 273–274
- file structure matrix, 274–276, 274f, 275f
- at National Institutes of Health, 272–273
- at New York University Medical Center, 276–277, 276f, 277f
- nursing formats, 273f

Teleprocessing, 414
Teletypewriter, 414
Template, 76, 414
- screens, 231f, 233f, 234f, 235f

Terminals, 52–53, 54, 414
- cathode ray tube (CRT), 53
- dumb, 410
- hand-held, 54
- hard copy, 54
- intelligent, 53, 411
- portable, 54, 55f
- teletypewriter, 54

TESTAR, 387
Texas Institute for Rehabilitation and Research, information system of, 9
Timesharing, 53, 414
Time study, 153, 156f, 157f
Total child health data system, 253
Transaction systems, 106
Transistors, 37, 414
Translation programs, 74–75, 414
Treatment plans, computer-generated, 236f, 237f, 238f
TRIMIS conference, 16
Trinity physiologic monitor, 306–308, 309f
Tri-Service Medical Information Systems. *See* TRIMIS
Turnkey system, 239

UNIVAC I, 34, 35f, 414
User friendly software, 75, 415
User satisfaction, evaluation of, 153, 157–159, 158f, 159f
User's manual, for information system, 149
Utility programs, 75
Utilization review, in Shared Medical Systems, 188, 194f

Vacuum tubes, 34, 35f, 414
VDT. *See* Video display terminal
Vendor systems, 239–242, 240t. *See also specific services or vendors*
Ventilators, microprocessor regulated, 314–315, 317
Video display terminal (VDT), 414
Visiting Nurse Association of Houston, management information system developed by, 242
Visiting Nurse Association of Omaha, management information system developed by, 242
Voice/image input, 58
Voice input, 415
Voice output, 66, 415

WHIRLWIND I, 34, 415
Word processing
- defined, 107
- menu for, 107
- processing system, 107–108

Workload management, GRASP system and, 188–189